Obstructive
Sleep Apnoea

Edited by
Ferran Barbé and Jean-Louis Pépin

Editor in Chief
Tobias Welte

This book is one in a series of *ERS Monographs*. Each individual issue provides a comprehensive overview of one specific clinical area of respiratory health, communicating information about the most advanced techniques and systems required for its investigation. It provides factual and useful scientific detail, drawing on specific case studies and looking into the diagnosis and management of individual patients. Previously published titles in this series are listed at the back of this *Monograph*.

ERS Monographs are available online at www.erspublications.com and print copies are available from www.ersbookshop.com

Continuing medical education (CME) credits are available through many issues of the *ERS Monograph*. Following evaluation, successful *Monographs* are accredited by the European Board for Accreditation in Pneumology (EBAP) for 5 CME credits. To earn CME credits, read the book of your choice (it is clearly indicated on the online table of contents whether CME credits are available) then complete the CME question form that is available at www.ers-education.org/e-learning/cme-tests.aspx

Editorial Board: Antonio Anzueto (San Antonio, TX, USA), Leif Bjermer (Lund, Sweden), John Hurst (London, UK) and Carlos Robalo Cordeiro (Coimbra, Portugal).

Managing Editor: Rachel White
European Respiratory Society, 442 Glossop Road, Sheffield, S10 2PX, UK
Tel: 44 114 2672860 | E-mail: Monograph@ersj.org.uk

Published by European Respiratory Society ©2015
March 2015
Print ISBN: 978-1-84984-059-0
Online ISBN: 978-1-84984-060-6
Print ISSN: 2312-508X
Online ISSN: 2312-5098
Printed by Charlesworth Press, Wakefield, UK

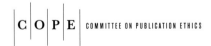

This journal is a member of and subscribes to the principles of the Committee on Publication Ethics.

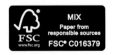

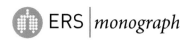

Contents

Obstructive Sleep Apnoea

Number 67
March 2015

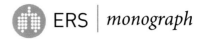

ERS | *monograph*

Preface

Tobias Welte, Editor in Chief

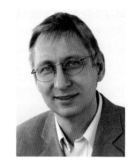

When the first prevalence studies on OSA were published 50 years ago, it was considered a rare disease. In 1981, a letter to the *Lancet* even questioned whether OSA existed in the UK [1]. With the improvement of diagnostics, however, it become clear that OSA is a common disorder with serious consequences for the morbidity and mortality of patients, and with a tremendous influence on quality of life. Today, the prevalence of moderate-to-severe OSA (defined by an AHI of $\geqslant 15$ events·h^{-1}) is >10%. The prevalence increases with age and the disease is more common in women than in men. Both the costs of the disease itself (*i.e.* limited working capacity, rate of traffic accidents due to sleeping while driving) and the costs of the resulting comorbidities (particularly cardiovascular and metabolic diseases) are significant.

With the introduction of nocturnal CPAP therapy, the prognosis and quality of life of OSA patients significantly improved. Ventilators have now become more powerful, less noisy and better to use, thanks to rapid technological development. New ventilation modes have also been developed that allow a more individualised therapy, better adapted to the patient's needs. A number of other treatment options besides CPAP have also been introduced into the therapeutic portfolio of OSA.

In the beginning, the management of OSA patients was more art than science. Evidence increased rapidly and sleep medicine became an evidence-based specialty of pulmonary medicine. The requirements for training specialists, however, have been constantly growing over time. This issue of the *Monograph* summarises the current knowledge about sleep apnoea, from basic research to clinical practice; future developments are also presented. I want to congratulate Ferran Barbé and Jean-Louis Pépin for compiling such an extensive book. We hope this *Monograph* will be helpful to clinicians and scientists involved in the management of this disease, as well as public health bodies and industry connected with this condition.

Reference

1. Shapiro CM, Catterall JR, Oswald I, *et al.* Where are the British sleep apnoea patients? *Lancet* 1981; 2: 523.

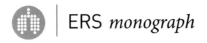

ERS *monograph*

Guest Editors

Ferran Barbé

Ferran Barbé received his degree in medicine in 1985 and his PhD in 1999 from the University of Barcelona (Barcelona, Spain). He followed a training programme in respiratory medicine at the Hospital de Bellvitge (Barcelona, Spain). In 1992, he received the Diplome D'Universite in Sleep Physiology from the University René Descartes (Paris, France). He was the Director of the Sleep Unit at the Son Dureta University Hospital (Palma de Mallorca, Spain) for 14 years. In 2005, he moved to Lleida (Spain) as Head of the Respiratory Department at the Arnau de Vilanova University Hospital and Professor of Respiratory Medicine at the University of Lleida. He achieved his European certification in sleep medicine in 2013. Since May 2014 he has been the Director of the Biomedical Research Networking Center Consortium for Respiratory Diseases (CIBERES, Madrid, Spain).

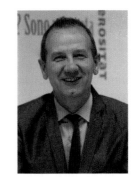

Ferran Barbé's work focusses on sleep apnoea and CVDs. His research aims to achieve a better understanding of the pathogenesis of the cardiovascular consequences for sleep apnoea patients, and to evaluate new diagnostic and therapeutic options in such patients.

Ferran Barbé has had 150 papers published in peer-reviewed journals; these papers have received over 3300 citations. His H-index is 31. He is a member of the Editorial Advisory Board for *Lancet Respiratory Medicine*.

Jean-Louis Pépin

Jean-Louis Pépin received his medical doctorate from Montpellier University (Montpellier, France) in 1987. He was a resident in respiratory medicine at Montpellier University and obtained his certificate as a specialist in sleep medicine during 1987–1989. In 1990, he obtained a Master's Degree in animal biophysiology (neuroscience) from Claude Bernard University of Lyon (Villeurbanne, France). He gained his PhD in biology (cardiovascular adaptations induced by chronic hypoxia) from Joseph Fourier University (Grenoble, France) and was a visiting professor at the Laboratory of Pulmonary Physiology of Harvard University in 1999 (Boston, MA, USA). He achieved his European certification in sleep medicine in 2013.

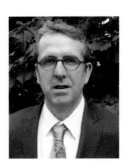

Jean-Louis Pépin's education, training and research has focussed on clinical and translational research into the cardiovascular consequences associated with chronic and IH, sleep apnoea, COPD, chronic respiratory failure and noninvasive ventilation.

Jean-Louis Pépin is currently: Professor of Clinical Physiology and Medical Director of the Regional Homecare System for Chronic Respiratory Failure at Joseph Fourier University; Head of the HP2 Laboratory Clinical Research Team (INSERM U1042, Grenoble, France) (hypoxia pathophysiology: cardiovascular consequences of IH); and a member of the Faculty of Medicine at the Joseph Fourier University, where he holds a 5-year INSERM Interface full-time research contract. He is Head of the Clinic of Physiology, Sleep and Exercise Department, Scientific Director of Clinical Research Administration and presides over the Research Division at Grenoble University Hospital (Grenoble, France). He runs the French registry of sleep apnoea (which includes more than 90 000 individuals) and is involved in the European Sleep Apnoea Database (ESADA). He is involved in several European Respiratory Society (ERS) and American Thoracic Society (ATS) Task Forces.

Jean-Louis Pépin is the co-author of over 250 published scientific papers (H-index 38). He is the former President of the French Sleep Research and Medicine Society, a member of the ERS and ATS, and an associate editor of *Thorax* for the sleep medicine field.

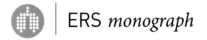

Introduction

Ferran Barbé[1,2] and Jean-Louis Pépin[3,4,5]

OSA is a syndrome caused by recurrent episodes of partial or complete pharyngeal collapse during sleep. It is a common and progressive chronic disease that is responsible for a high number of comorbidities and it is related to an increase in mortality, including a rise in the rate of sudden cardiac death. OSA affects millions of people worldwide; it is a heterogeneous condition with distinct phenotypes, varying from lean young adults with maxillofacial abnormalities and limited IH, to obese middle aged OSA patients with metabolic syndrome, obesity hypoventilation syndrome or overlap syndrome (*i.e.* a combination of OSA and COPD). Two-thirds of HF patients exhibit CSA or OSA. OSA is highly prevalent in specific populations, such as those with hypertension, stroke, coronary heart disease and patients exhibiting arrhythmias. Sleep fragmentation and chronic IH, the markers of OSA, induce intermediate mechanisms, such as oxidative stress, sympathetic nervous system activation and systemic inflammation, responsible for symptoms and cardio-metabolic consequences.

This issue of the *ERS Monograph* begins by addressing the pathogenesis of OSA, with new insights from animal models and integrated physiology. These chapters provide new clues to understanding OSA-related cardiovascular morbidity, as well as ways of phenotyping patients for better prediction of their response to different therapeutic modalities. Leg fluid volume shift from the legs to the neck during the night, a recently demonstrated mechanism that may precipitate UA collapse, is also put into clinical perspective. Another recent hot topic is the link between OSA and cancer; the excess mortality associated with OSA has not only been attributed to cardio-metabolic consequences but also to cancer. This was first suggested in animal studies that demonstrated an association between IH, carcinogenesis and the acceleration of tumour growth; this has recently been confirmed in clinical and epidemiological studies.

The individual populations in which OSA is highly prevalent are considered in subsequent chapters. Specific diagnostic strategies are necessary because OSA recognition modifies risk stratification and requires therapeutic intervention. The authors provide state-of-the art updates on various clinical scenarios, including OSA in children, during pregnancy, in overlap and obesity hypoventilation syndromes and in patients undergoing bariatric surgery.

[1]Respiratory Dept, Hospital Universitari Arnau de Vilanova and Santa Maria, IRB Lleida, Lleida, Spain. [2]Centro de Investigación Biomédica en Red de Enfermedades Respiratorias (CIBERES), Madrid, Spain. [3]Grenoble Alpes University, HP2 Laboratory, Grenoble, France. [4]INSERM U1042, Grenoble, France. [5]Clinique Universitaire de Physiologie et Sommeil, Pôle Thorax et Vaisseaux, Hôpital A. Michallon, Grenoble, France.

Correspondence: Jean-Louis Pépin, Laboratoire EFCR, CHU de Grenoble, BP217X, 38043 Grenoble cedex 09, France. E-mail: jpepin@chu-grenoble.fr

Comorbidities are of major importance in OSA because they have a significant impact on healthcare use and mortality. Effective OSA treatment may represent an important target for improving cardio-metabolic risk. However, CPAP, the first-line therapy for OSA, fails to alter metabolic or inflammatory markers in obese OSA patients. This emphasises the need to offer a combination of multiple treatment modalities, including weight loss through lifestyle intervention, bariatric surgery or physical activity, and new medications for the reduction of cardiovascular risk that are specifically dedicated to OSA patients. As OSA-related comorbidities lie in different medical specialties, patients may not receive a totally integrated treatment regime due to poor collaboration across different medical services. It is necessary to establish whether an integrated, remote monitoring approach actually improves patient medical outcomes in a cost-effective manner. Telemedicine could be used not only to monitor CPAP compliance, leaks and residual events but also to record physical activity and self-measurements of BP and oximetry at home. This would allow the implementation of individually tailored therapeutic strategies. A panorama of the different therapeutic modalities and strategies together with OSA e-health are presented in the final chapters of this *Monograph.*

As editors, we hope that you will find this issue of the *Monograph* a useful overview of OSA that aids understanding of the condition and may influence your management of the disease. The chapters are well referenced and should stimulate research initiatives and new management pathways. We are very grateful to all the authors who have contributed excellent chapters to this *Monograph.*

List of abbreviations

AHI	Apnoea–hypopnoea index
BMI	Body mass index
BP	Blood pressure
BPAP	Bilevel positive airway pressure
COPD	Chronic obstructive pulmonary disease
CPAP	Continuous positive airway pressure
CSA	Central sleep apnoea
CVD	Cardiovascular disease
DBP	Diastolic blood pressure
EDS	Excessive daytime sleepiness
EPAP	Expiratory positive airway pressure
ESS	Epworth Sleepiness Scale
FEV$_1$	Forced expiratory volume in 1 s
FRC	Functional residual capacity
FVC	Forced vital capacity
HF	Heart failure
IH	Intermittent hypoxia
IL	Interleukin
IPAP	Inspiratory positive airway pressure
MAD	Mandibular advancement device
ODI	Oxygen desaturation index
OSA	Obstructive sleep apnoea
PAP	Positive airway pressure
PSG	Polysomnography
RCT	Randomised controlled trial
RDI	Respiratory disturbance index
REM	Rapid eye movement
SBP	Systolic blood pressure
TNF	Tumour necrosis factor
UA	Upper airways

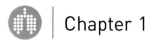

Chapter 1

Animal and physiological settings of IH exposure

Renaud Tamisier[1,2,3], Anne Briançon[1,2], Patrick Lévy[1,2,3] and Jean-Louis Pépin[1,2,3]

OSA syndrome causes nocturnal chronic IH, sleep fragmentation, intrathoracic pressure swings and carbon dioxide surges. Clinical studies demonstrate a close relationship between IH and excess cardiovascular morbidity. To explore the consequences of IH *per se*, we and others have used different settings of IH in animals, cells and healthy humans to characterise the different pathways driven by IH that alter cardiovascular physiology, from vascular inflammation to atherosclerosis and excessive sympathetic tone to high BP. These different settings are clearly bringing different and complementary insights, independently of cofactors such as age, obesity and associated metabolic disease and CVD. Moreover, they allow us to trigger exposure in specific target cells or organs using different exposure durations, or using transgenic animals or a specific diet. In this chapter, we briefly review the different settings allowing IH exposure and summarise the mechanisms that have been proposed to reflect those underlying the cardiovascular morbidity associated with OSA syndrome.

OSA is the most frequent sleep breathing disorder and is responsible for severe cardio-metabolic complications. OSA includes different respiratory events occurring during sleep, which depend on the severity of UA narrowing, starting with snoring and including UA resistance episodes, hypopnoea and apnoea following a complete collapse. Apart from snoring, all of these end due to an arousal from sleep, the brain response to an unsustainable respiratory effort. Apnoea and hypopnoea causing transitory changes in carbon dioxide and oxygen levels that repeat over time is named IH. Thus, OSA is characterised by three stimuli: IH, sleep fragmentation and change in respiratory efforts. Although these stimuli are well defined and characterised, OSA should be considered as a heterogeneous condition due to the large variations in severity, patient history, duration of disease and association with other components (risk factors and diseases). OSA is a multicomponent disease almost always associated with obesity, hypertension or other cardiovascular and metabolic diseases, and is a heterogeneous clinical entity in terms of severity (*i.e.* the number and type of respiratory events, and hypoxia length and depth) and duration of exposure to the disease, with different consequences according to individual susceptibility. Due to all these factors, understanding the physiopathology that binds OSA *per se* and CVD is a difficult task in a clinical population.

[1]Grenoble Alpes University, HP2 Laboratory, Grenoble, France. [2]INSERM U1042, Grenoble, France. [3]Clinique Universitaire de Physiologie et Sommeil, Pôle Thorax et Vaisseaux, Hôpital A. Michallon, Grenoble, France.

Correspondence: Renaud Tamisier, Laboratoire EFCR, CHU de Grenoble, CS 10217, 38043 Grenoble Cedex 09, France. E-mail: rtamisier@chu-grenoble.fr

Copyright ©ERS 2015. Print ISBN: 978-1-84984-059-0. Online ISBN: 978-1-84984-060-6. Print ISSN: 2312-508X. Online ISSN: 2312-5098.

The mechanisms by which OSA and nocturnal hypoxia contribute to CVD and metabolic (glucose and lipid) disease are thus a major topic of interest. To study these mechanisms, a natural approach was to build models that could mimic sleep apnoea in a setting allowing control of the different parameters (sleep, respiratory effort, carbon dioxide) and associated factors (obesity, CVD and risk).

Chronic IH has been applied to intact animals [1]. FLETCHER et al. [2] were the first to build a device that allowed small animal exposure to chronic IH. BROOKS et al. [3] later conceived an interesting unique model in dogs that combined the three stimuli characterising OSA (i.e. augmented respiratory effort, asphyxia and arousal from sleep). Both models have been shown, in elegant studies, to produce elevations of arterial BP that persist after termination of the hypoxic exposure. Different pathways inducing BP elevation have been studied. Fletcher's model is now used extensively with rodents to explore the mechanisms that link OSA to cardiovascular and other morbidity. IH is also now applied to cell cultures in order to provide insight into how IH modulates cell signalling pathways. This particular technique has the advantage of exposing specific cells (e.g. endothelial or adipocyte) and allowing study of the specific response of these cells to IH [4]. Finally, we and others have investigated how healthy subjects might adapt their physiology to IH during the daytime [5, 6] and during sleep [7].

Several review articles have been published about the possible different settings of IH exposure in animals, cells and humans, including a complete discussion of the methodological strengths and pitfalls of these settings [8]. The purpose of the current chapter is to present a summary description of each model and describe what these have added to the field.

Experimental models

All models that have been proposed, apart from the dog model, are models of IH with or without sleep disturbance. The goal is to mimic the IH that occurs in sleep apnoea patients (fig. 1 and table 1). Apart from the dog model, no other paradigms can be literally qualified as models of sleep apnoea. Indeed, only the dog model was able to reproduce repetitive asphyxia induced by the onset of sleep and relieved by the occurrence of microarousal from sleep, which characterises OSA [3]. OSA is a specific composite stimulus associated with asphyxia (hypoxia plus hypercapnia with respiratory effort) lasting 3–10 breaths, occurring during sleep and fragmenting sleep. However, models of this complexity have not been reproduced except by the initial studies with samples of only a few animals.

Experimental models of IH in animals

Animal settings with IH have considerably improved over the years in order to obtain, as far as possible, a pure IH exposure. Handling is minimised, with settings allowing exposure of animals in their usual chambers and not in small specific exposure chambers as was done initially. This may be a major confounding factor, although it is not clear how much this would interfere with the effect of IH per se [9]. Noise induced by IH systems has also been improved, which may reduce the impact on sleep fragmentation induced by these systems.

Apart from in the model proposed by TAGAITO et al. [10], which by design was inducing sleep fragmentation in line with hypoxic events, it is not clear to what extent sleep is fragmented using these models. Indeed, most models of IH in rodents do not assess sleep during exposure. Even though the exposure occurs during daylight hours, which is supposed to be

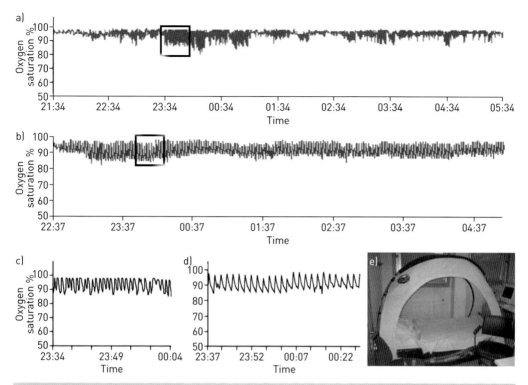

Figure 1. Examples of oxymetric traces from a) a patient with OSA and b) a healthy subject exposed to IH. c and d) Magnification of regions in boxes from parts a and b, respectively. The exposure to IH of about 30 cycles per hour induced associated sleep fragmentation (table 1). e) Equipment used for these measurements. Parts a and b reproduced and modified from [23] with permission from the publisher.

sleeping time in rodents, the total amount of sleep and its quality is poorly monitored. When it is monitored, it is clear that IH induces both sleep fragmentation and reduction of sleep duration, which seem to occur during the IH exposure time [11]. This is a concern, as many studies have demonstrated the impact and possibly the synergistic effect of IH and sleep fragmentation on cardio-metabolic changes [12]. Thermoneutrality may also be of importance since, depending on the temperature of the housing, the effects of IH on metabolism may vary [13]. In this study by Jun et al. [13], the temperature changed the level of lipolysis.

IH exposure is mainly chronic in animal models. However, the duration of exposure can vary from weeks to months. This has some importance in showing the different types of

Table 1. Measurements of ODI and microarousals from sleep in healthy subjects before and after exposure to IH

	Pre-exposure	Night 1	Night 14
ODI events·h^{-1}	0.4±0.7	37.8±7.7***	33.9±9.4***
Microarousals events·h^{-1}	19.6±9.5	36.6±10.9**	33.9±9.4*

Data are presented as mean±SD. *: p<0.05; **: p<0.01; ***: p<0.001. Data from [7].

adaptation to acute or chronic exposure. As an example, the effect of IH may be different depending on the intensity and the duration of exposure. A short exposure (8 h) has been shown to enhance cardiac muscle protective mechanisms against ischaemia [14], while longer exposures have the opposite effect, worsening the infarct size in the heart after transient ischaemia [15]. This also applies to nitric oxide synthase expression in the brain, with no change or upregulation upon acute exposure and downregulation when exposure is prolonged [16]. Cycling should also be discussed as an important parameter. The time duration of hypoxia *versus* normoxia in these animal models of IH exposure is mostly driven by technical considerations, as the oxygen fraction in the chamber has to be decreased sufficiently to induce oxygen desaturation in the animals. It should also be borne in mind that the ratio of hypoxia time duration to number of breaths during the episode is totally different in animals compared with sleep apnoea patients. Finally, although adding carbon dioxide during the hypoxic phase has been shown to account for a minimal effect in animal exposure models, it is likely that carbon dioxide may enhance the hypoxic response and alter the results that are commonly accepted in the field.

A concern when using animal models of IH is what conclusions can be drawn for animals that are applicable to humans, as OSA is a human disease. Indeed, human physiology may be quite different when compared with rodent physiology. Despite the considerable amount of data derived from studies conducted in animals, because of all the aforementioned limitations, caution should be taken when interpreting animal data before translating these to humans. However, there are enough data that have been demonstrated both in human patients and animals regarding the different pathways triggered by IH, to continue to use and improve IH models. This will undoubtedly enhance our knowledge of IH-triggered mechanisms, which will help us to understand those that are involved in patients.

IH in cells

In recent years, several models of cellular IH have been developed. Such models have to address a technical challenge, namely achieving rapid and precise oxygen saturation oscillations in the cell culture media. Indeed, while rapid oxygen cycles in ambient air are easily obtained, equilibration of oxygen in a liquid phase by diffusion is very slow in the absence of any mixing [17]. Moreover, convective mixing in the culture media exists but can be variable; thus, the precision of oxygen saturation achieved at the cellular level is poor. In view of these limitations, different strategies have been adopted by several teams to develop systems for cell exposure to IH.

In 2003, the first system was published [18]. A humidified Lucite chamber was used, which had a flow of gas containing 1% oxygen (15 s) then 21% oxygen (3 min), thus achieving very rapid cycles. The partial pressure of oxygen (P_{O_2}) in ambient air cycled between 110 mmHg in the normoxic phase and 20 mmHg in the hypoxic phase. However, the P_{O_2} in the culture medium only cycled between 70 mmHg in the normoxic and 50 mmHg in the hypoxic phase (approximately corresponding to 9.5% and 6.8% oxygen, respectively). Thus, this system shows that the amplitude of oxygen variations in culture medium is greatly attenuated compared with the amplitude in air; however, using this system, the authors demonstrated that IH profoundly affected cell activity [18].

To increase the amplitude of oxygen variations, another team decided to increase the duration of the cycles [19]. In this system, the oxygen in the air was set at 21% for 25 min followed by 0.1% for 35 min. The actual oxygen in the culture medium was measured and reached $\leqslant 2\%$ for $\geqslant 6$ min in each 1-h cycle and $\geqslant 15\%$ for $\geqslant 14$ min in each cycle. The same type of IH was performed by another team [20]. Cells were exposed to 1 h of hypoxia (1% oxygen) and 30 min of normoxia (21% oxygen), and it was observed that during hypoxia a level of 10 mmHg (approximately 1.3% oxygen) is achieved in about 10 min while under normoxia a level of 120 mmHg (approximately 16% oxygen) is reached within 2 min. In these experiments, the authors thus achieved a high amplitude of actual oxygen variation between 15% and 1–2%, but the cycles lasted for 1 h or more. This probably limits the extrapolation of results obtained with this system to actual variation in the blood of sleep apnoea patients, in which cycles of hypoxia/reoxygenation are much faster.

Another strategy was to use pre-equilibrated culture medium [17, 21]. In the work of RYAN *et al.* [21], a hypoxic chamber was used in combination with media pre-equilibrated at 1% oxygen (5 min) or at 21% oxygen (10 min), to achieve cycles of 15 min. BAUMGARDNER and OTTO [17] developed a system for forced convection cell culture using capillary tubes, achieving a response time for cycling of P_{O_2} of 1.6 s. This system thus allows very rapid cycles without limitation of the amplitude of oxygen saturation variations. In these two systems, the use of pre-conditioned medium ensured an instantaneous perception of oxygen changes at the cellular level. However, medium is changed very frequently and it is thus more complicated to measure variation of soluble factors such as cytokines in the culture medium, unless the flushed medium is re-used. Moreover, the cells are probably submitted to significant shear stress during the medium changes, which can have an impact on cell activity and metabolism.

Finally, more recently, a team proposed a system in which gas was directly bubbled into the culture medium [22]. They alternated 5 min of 16% oxygen and 5 min of 0% oxygen, leading to six cycles per hour, which was the highest frequency leading to the desired oxygen variation amplitude.

In conclusion, the various systems that have been developed show various advantages and disadvantages in terms of cycle duration, oxygen variation amplitude and cell growth. New systems are currently being developed by several teams to avoid these limitations using new technical strategies, such as the use of gas-permeable dishes, and these will soon allow cellular IH that closely resembles that really observed in sleep apnoea patients.

IH in humans

The principal message that can be drawn from IH exposure in human healthy subjects is their high physiological adaptation capacity. Although healthy subjects have been exposed to IH for a period of weeks, the overall change in BP is a minimal 6% increase [23], compared with a 28% increase after a long period of time at high altitude [24]. This may be related to activation of mechanisms that both promote and mitigate the increase in BP. Three settings have been proposed to expose young healthy subjects to acute and sub-acute IH. It is worth noting that, despite being able to expose subjects for 1 month, we should consider our exposure to be relatively short, owing to the adaptation of human physiology. Sleep apnoea patients are usually exposed to IH for years.

Several groups, including our own, have exposed healthy subjects to IH for a period of between 20 min and 2 h during the daytime when the subjects were awake [25, 26].

The time duration of hypoxic events was quite heterogeneous and not all designs controlled for carbon dioxide. However, this setting was able to demonstrate a significant increase in sympathetic activity with or without an increase in vascular resistance. This was similar to what occurs with sustained short hypoxic exposure, when there is both an increase in sympathetic activity and an increase in circulating factors causing vascular relaxation, which results in a lack of increase in vascular resistance [27]. Adding carbon dioxide during hypoxic exposure to a level above baseline enhances sympathetic activation [28]. However, these settings did not account for the human physiology adaptation that may occur with longer exposure. Indeed, respiratory control plasticity has been demonstrated to change across time duration of hypoxic exposure [29]. With this in mind, two approaches have been proposed, one using a mask interface allowing the control of both hypoxia and carbon dioxide content [6, 30], and the other having the subject free in a hypoxic chamber with the ability to sleep [7]. Using these settings, several pathways of IH have been highlighted.

First, IH-driven sympathetic hyperactivity has been well demonstrated, with a magnitude that increases with exposure duration, which reinforces the importance of sympathetic activation in the pathophysiology of CVD in OSA [23]. Secondly, there is a clear change in peripheral hypoxic chemosensitivity [7, 30], which reinforces the hypothesis that IH-driven sympathetic activity is related to an increase in peripheral chemosensitivity, as it was demonstrated in OSA patient [31]. Moreover, it was initially demonstrated that a denervated carotid body could prevent the increase in BP induced by IH in rats [32]. Additionally, using the carbon dioxide rebreathing technique, central chemosensitivity was amplified with IH exposure [7], which may also be linked to an increase in oxidative stress [33], although this has been not demonstrated in the brain.

The human autonomic nervous system is continuously adapting its control in order to prevent vascular resistance increase (*i.e.* vascular sympathetic gain) and increase in heart rate (*i.e.* baroreflex gain). Thus, physiological adaptation to an increase in sympathetic activity would suggest a decrease in vascular sympathetic gain and an increase in baroreflex gain in order to protect against hypertension. However, in OSA patients there is a sustained vascular gain (personal unpublished data) and a decrease in baroreflex gain [34]. Interestingly, IH exposure decreases baroreflex gain, which may promote the rise in BP in conditions of stress [23].

Using acute 6-h IH exposures during the daytime, FOSTER *et al.* [35] demonstrated that the renin–angiotensin system was involved through the type I angiotensin II receptor. Losartan was able to prevent the increase in BP induced by IH exposure. Despite the fact that neither plasma renin activity nor aldosterone was increased with IH exposure, the fact that type I angiotensin II could prevent the increase in BP is likely to demonstrate that the renin–angiotensin–aldosterone system is involved in BP rise.

BP does indeed increase after IH exposure. Although 2 h are not enough to produce an increase [26], 8 h, 6 days, 15 days or 4 weeks have demonstrated a significant increase in BP [5, 7, 23, 30, 35]. However, the magnitude of increase seems to decrease with longer exposure, with an increase in DBP of more than 8 and 4 mmHg after 6 h and 4 days of IH, respectively, but of only 5 and 2 mmHg after 2 and 4 weeks of IH exposure, respectively. Interestingly, the increase in BP was mainly due to an increase during the awake state, with major increases during the afternoon and not during the exposure time [23]. This may be related to the inability to prevent BP rises due to increased sympathetic tone and decrease in baroreflex gain [23].

Vascular inflammation is one of the major pathways that have been proposed to cause atherosclerosis in OSA patients. Despite an increase in oxidative stress after a short time of exposure [30], we were not able to find any change in many circulating cytokines (IL-1, IL-8, MCP-1, RANTES and TNF-α) and vascular mediators of vascular inflammation (hsCRP, adiponectin, leptin and sICAM-1) [23].

Compared with the daytime setting of IH exposure, our model of exposure during sleep had a significant impact on sleep fragmentation and thus may act through both IH stimulus and sleep fragmentation, since sleep disruption *per se* has been demonstrated to impair cardiovascular regulation [7].

Conclusion

Using different settings of IH in animals, cells and human healthy subjects, we are now able to target different tissues, organs and physiological mechanisms that may be altered by IH. The relatively broad variety of models that are available should allow us to conduct comprehensive research, from cultured cells to human physiology. The particularly favourable aspect of the rodent model is its capacity for running experiments in animal subjects with specific diets or lifestyles and for exposing animals with specific knockout or expressed genes. IH is, however, a quite unique risk factor that it is now possible to introduce for a short duration to human healthy subjects with sufficient confidence of no adverse effects, thus allowing study of the effect of exposure on human physiology in order to better understand how to prevent the deleterious effects that this exposure may have after many years.

References

1. Fletcher EC. Invited review. Physiological consequences of intermittent hypoxia: systemic blood pressure. *J Appl Physiol* 2001; 90: 1600–1605.
2. Fletcher EC, Lesske J, Qian W, *et al.* Repetitive, episodic hypoxia causes diurnal elevation of blood pressure in rats. *Hypertension* 1992; 19: 555–561.
3. Brooks D, Horner RL, Kozar LF, *et al.* Obstructive sleep apnea as a cause of systemic hypertension. Evidence from a canine model. *J Clin Invest* 1997; 99: 106–109.
4. Taylor CT, Kent BD, Crinion SJ, *et al.* Human adipocytes are highly sensitive to intermittent hypoxia induced NF-κB activity and subsequent inflammatory gene expression. *Biochem Biophys Res Commun* 2014; 447: 660–665.
5. Foster GE, Brugniaux JV, Pialoux V, *et al.* Cardiovascular and cerebrovascular responses to acute hypoxia following exposure to intermittent hypoxia in healthy humans. *J Physiol* 2009; 587: 3287–3299.
6. Louis M, Punjabi NM. Effects of acute intermittent hypoxia on glucose metabolism in awake healthy volunteers. *J Appl Physiol* 2009; 106: 1538–1544.
7. Tamisier R, Gilmartin GS, Launois SH, *et al.* A new model of chronic intermittent hypoxia in humans: effect on ventilation, sleep, and blood pressure. *J Appl Physiol* 2009; 107: 17–24.
8. Foster GE, Poulin MJ, Hanly PJ. Intermittent hypoxia and vascular function: implications for obstructive sleep apnoea. *Exp Physiol* 2007; 92: 51–65.
9. Whittaker AL, Howarth GS, Hickman DL. Effects of space allocation and housing density on measures of wellbeing in laboratory mice: a review. *Lab Anim* 2012; 46: 3–13.
10. Tagaito Y, Polotsky VY, Campen MJ, *et al.* A model of sleep-disordered breathing in the C57BL/6 J mouse. *J Appl Physiol* 2001; 91: 2758–2766.
11. Kaushal N, Ramesh V, Gozal D. Human apolipoprotein E4 targeted replacement in mice reveals increased susceptibility to sleep disruption and intermittent hypoxia. *Am J Physiol Regul Integr Comp Physiol* 2012; 303: R19–R29.
12. Lévy P, Pépin JL, Arnaud C, *et al.* Intermittent hypoxia and sleep-disordered breathing: current concepts and perspectives. *Eur Respir J* 2008; 32: 1082–1095.

13. Jun JC, Shin MK, Yao Q, *et al.* Thermoneutrality modifies the impact of hypoxia on lipid metabolism. *Am J Physiol Endocrinol Metab* 2013; 304: E424–E435.

14. Béguin PC, Joyeux-Faure M, Godin-Ribuot D, *et al.* Acute intermittent hypoxia improves rat myocardium tolerance to ischemia. *J Appl Physiol* 2005; 99: 1064–1069.

15. Joyeux-Faure M, Stanke-Labesque F, Lefebvre B, *et al.* Chronic intermittent hypoxia increases infarction in the isolated rat heart. *J Appl Physiol* 2005; 98: 1691–1696.

16. Huang J, Tamisier R, Ji E, *et al.* Chronic intermittent hypoxia modulates nNOS mRNA and protein expression in the rat hypothalamus. *Respir Physiol Neurobiol* 2007; 158: 30–38.

17. Baumgardner JE, Otto CM. *In vitro* intermittent hypoxia: challenges for creating hypoxia in cell culture. *Respir Physiol Neurobiol* 2003; 136: 131–139.

18. Kumar GK, Kim DK, Lee MS, *et al.* Activation of tyrosine hydroxylase by intermittent hypoxia: involvement of serine phosphorylation. *J Appl Physiol* 2003; 95: 536–544.

19. Dyugovskaya L, Polyakov A, Lavie P, *et al.* Delayed neutrophil apoptosis in patients with sleep apnea. *Am J Respir Crit Care Med* 2008; 177: 544–554.

20. Toffoli S, Delaive E, Dieu M, *et al.* NDRG1 and CRK-I/II are regulators of endothelial cell migration under intermittent hypoxia. *Angiogenesis* 2009; 12: 339–354.

21. Ryan S, Taylor CT, McNicholas WT. Selective activation of inflammatory pathways by intermittent hypoxia in obstructive sleep apnea syndrome. *Circulation* 2005; 112: 2660–2667.

22. Polotsky VY, Savransky V, Bevans-Fonti S, *et al.* Intermittent and sustained hypoxia induce a similar gene expression profile in human aortic endothelial cells. *Physiol Genomics* 2010; 41: 306–314.

23. Tamisier R, Pépin JL, Rémy J, *et al.* 14 nights of intermittent hypoxia elevate daytime blood pressure and sympathetic activity in healthy humans. *Eur Respir J* 2011; 37: 119–128.

24. Calbet JA. Chronic hypoxia increases blood pressure and noradrenaline spillover in healthy humans. *J Physiol* 2003; 551: 379–386.

25. Cutler MJ, Swift NM, Keller DM, *et al.* Periods of intermittent hypoxic apnea can alter chemoreflex control of sympathetic nerve activity in humans. *Am J Physiol Heart Circ Physiol* 2004; 287: H2054–H2060.

26. Tamisier R, Anand A, Nieto LM, *et al.* Arterial pressure and muscle sympathetic nerve activity are increased after two hours of sustained but not cyclic hypoxia in healthy humans. *J Appl Physiol* 2005; 98: 343–349.

27. Tamisier R, Norman D, Anand A, *et al.* Evidence of sustained forearm vasodilatation after brief isocapnic hypoxia. *J Appl Physiol* 2004; 96: 1782–1787.

28. Tamisier R, Nieto L, Anand A, *et al.* Sustained muscle sympathetic activity after hypercapnic but not hypocapnic hypoxia in normal humans. *Respir Physiol Neurobiol* 2004; 141: 145–155.

29. Powell FL, Milsom WK, Mitchell GS. Time domains of the hypoxic ventilatory response. *Respir Physiol* 1998; 112: 123–134.

30. Pialoux V, Hanly PJ, Foster GE, *et al.* Effects of exposure to intermittent hypoxia on oxidative stress and acute hypoxic ventilatory response in humans. *Am J Respir Crit Care Med* 2009; 180: 1002–1009.

31. Somers VK, Dyken ME, Clary MP, *et al.* Sympathetic neural mechanisms in obstructive sleep apnea. *J Clin Invest* 1995; 96: 1897–1904.

32. Fletcher EC, Lesske J, Culman J, *et al.* Sympathetic denervation blocks blood pressure elevation in episodic hypoxia. *Hypertension* 1992; 20: 612–619.

33. Brugniaux JV, Pialoux V, Foster GE, *et al.* Effects of intermittent hypoxia on erythropoietin, soluble erythropoietin receptor and ventilation in humans. *Eur Respir J* 2011; 37: 880–887.

34. Carlson JT, Hedner JA, Sellgren J, *et al.* Depressed baroreflex sensitivity in patients with obstructive sleep apnea. *Am J Respir Crit Care Med* 1996; 154: 1490–1496.

35. Foster GE, Hanly PJ, Ahmed SB, *et al.* Intermittent hypoxia increases arterial blood pressure in humans through a renin-angiotensin system-dependent mechanism. *Hypertension* 2010; 56: 369–377.

Disclosures: **None declared.**

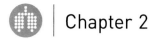
Physiological phenotypes

Danny Joel Eckert[1] and Andrew Wellman[2]

OSA is a multifactorial disorder with several physiological phenotypes. Pharyngeal anatomy/collapsibility is the primary abnormality in most OSA patients. However, the extent of UA anatomical compromise varies widely between OSA patients. Many have only a modest degree of anatomical impairment. Accordingly, a number of other non-anatomical contributors also play a role. These include an oversensitive ventilatory control system, a low respiratory arousal threshold, and poor pharyngeal muscle responsiveness or effectiveness during sleep. The contribution of these non-anatomical factors has only recently been recognised. This chapter reviews the data establishing the importance of these variables and describes a graphic, physiological model integrating them to illustrate their relative contribution. Ultimately, such a model could be useful for guiding therapy and advancing the field of OSA management beyond the "one size fits all" approach of CPAP.

OSA is a common disorder characterised by repetitive pharyngeal collapse during sleep [1]. It has a number of adverse cardiovascular [2–9], neurocognitive [10] and quality of life [11] consequences. Therefore, understanding the pathophysiology and developing novel treatments is important. This chapter describes the physiological variables, or phenotypic traits, that cause OSA and how understanding their pathogenic role in each patient could lead to new therapies. This is particularly important, since existing therapies for OSA are either poorly tolerated (*e.g.* CPAP) or have variable efficacy (*e.g.* oral devices or pharyngeal surgery).

Recent evidence suggests that OSA is a multifactorial disorder [12, 13]. Contributing factors include a small or collapsible pharyngeal airway [14–16], a high loop gain (large ventilatory response to a ventilatory disturbance) [17–22], a low respiratory arousal threshold [23–28], and poor pharyngeal muscle responsiveness or effectiveness during sleep [29–36]. The relative contribution of these traits varies substantially between individuals [12, 13, 37], and will be discussed in detail later.

Role of pharyngeal anatomy in OSA

The size, or collapsibility, of the UA is probably the most important variable in the pathogenesis of OSA. Since the disorder is characterised by UA obstruction, all individuals must have at least some underlying predisposition to pharyngeal collapse.

[1]Neuroscience Research Australia (NeuRA) and the School of Medical Sciences, University of New South Wales, Randwick, Australia. [2]Division of Sleep Medicine, Brigham and Women's Hospital, Harvard Medical School, Boston, MA, USA.

Correspondence: Danny J. Eckert, Neuroscience Research Australia (NeuRA), PO Box 1165, Randwick, Sydney, New South Wales 2031, Australia. E-mail: d.eckert@neura.edu.au

The "collapsibility" of the pharynx can be measured by lowering CPAP, sometimes to negative pressures (suctioning the airway), until the airway collapses. The airway lumen pressure at which collapse occurs is called the critical pressure (Pcrit) and is a measure of collapsibility [38]. For an example of a single trial used to obtain a Pcrit measurement see figure 1. Poor anatomy (*e.g.* a narrow or crowded UA) leads to collapse at a high airway luminal pressure, typically above atmospheric pressure. Normal or "good" pharyngeal anatomy prevents collapse until the airway pressure decreases below -5 cmH$_2$O, *i.e.* vacuuming (or suction) pressure must be applied to close the airway.

Individuals with OSA have, on average, a higher Pcrit than people without OSA [14, 39], although there is considerable overlap between patients with OSA and normal controls. Indeed, Pcrit can vary from -5 to $+5$ cmH$_2$O or more in patients with OSA [12, 39]. 20% of OSA patients also have identical Pcrit values to many normal controls [12]. Thus, a number of other non-anatomical variables must come into play and ultimately dictate whether the airway closes or remains patent during sleep. The role of these other non-anatomical variables, or traits, and how they interact with the anatomy to produce OSA is the focus of this chapter.

Another feature that could contribute to the development of OSA and is likely to be related to UA anatomical characteristics is the amount of inspiratory negative effort dependence (NED) present. Some individuals exhibit substantial reductions in flow rate with increasing inspiratory effort (fig. 2) [40]. NED can occur not only within breaths, as shown in figure 1, but also across breaths, for example, the peak flow decreases from one breath to the next as respiratory effort progressively increases. In individuals with significant NED, the force of inspiration can play a substantial contributing role in collapse. The anatomical features in the airway responsible for producing more or less NED in an individual are currently incompletely understood [41]. However, given the variable sites and mechanisms of collapse (*e.g.* palate, tongue, lateral walls and epiglottis), it is not surprising that there is variability in NED between patients [41, 42].

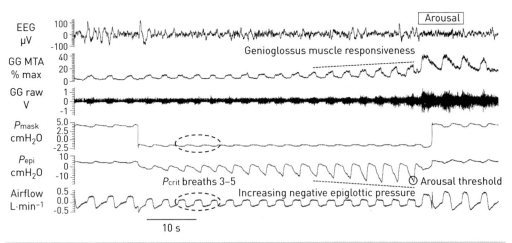

Figure 1. Example of a CPAP drop technique used to calculate the critical closing pressure of the UA (Pcrit), genioglossus (GG) muscle responsiveness and the respiratory arousal threshold. EEG: electroencephalography; MTA: 100 ms moving-time average of the rectified raw electromyographic activity; Pepi: epiglottic pressure; Pmask: mask pressure. Reproduced from [12] with permission from the publisher.

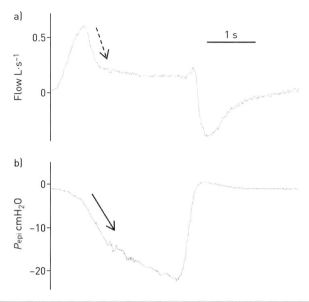

Figure 2. Negative effort dependence (NED) can substantially limit ventilation. In this individual with NED, there is a high peak flow initially (a), indicating an open airway on expiration and early inspiration. However, with further inspiratory suction force (arrow in b), the airflow drops dramatically (dashed arrow in a). P_{epi}: epiglottic pressure.

Role of loop gain in OSA

There is increasing evidence that an oversensitive ventilatory control system, or high loop gain, plays a contributing role in the pathogenesis of OSA [12, 43, 44]. We emphasise here that it plays a contributing role, and that patients must have an underlying predisposition to UA collapse to develop OSA. A high loop gain alone can produce central, but not obstructive, sleep apnoea. Consequently, loop gain (and the other non-anatomical traits described later) has a lower effect size than anatomical metrics but, as will be pointed out, such traits are nevertheless important to consider as therapeutic targets.

Ventilatory control sensitivity is quantified as the gain of the ventilatory control feedback loop, i.e. loop gain. Figure 3 illustrates this concept by showing how a disturbance in ventilation leads to a response that can be used to quantify loop gain. A large loop gain ratio indicates an unstable system prone to oscillations. A low loop gain signifies a stable system. YOUNES et al. [18] measured loop gain in patients with OSA using a proportional assist ventilator and found that severe OSA patients had a higher loop gain than mild/ moderate patients. These results are supported by several additional studies showing that certain patients with OSA have a more sensitive ventilatory control system [12, 17, 19, 20]. However, patients with OSA (as opposed to CSA) generally do not have a loop gain high enough to produce self-sustaining oscillations. Nonetheless, measured using a CPAP drop technique (fig. 4) [13], more than one third of OSA patients have high loop gain such that a 1 $L \cdot min^{-1}$ reduction in minute ventilation results in a more than 5 $L \cdot min^{-1}$ increase in minute ventilation [12]. High loop gain is likely to make an important contribution to OSA pathogenesis in these patients [12]. Consistent with the importance of the interaction between anatomical and non-anatomical features, loop gain is almost twice as high in OSA

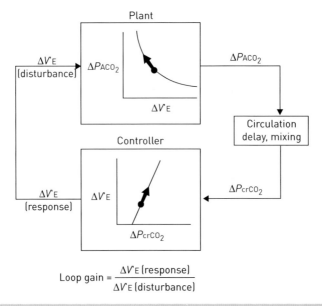

Loop gain $= \dfrac{\Delta V'\text{E (response)}}{\Delta V'\text{E (disturbance)}}$

Figure 3. The sensitivity of the ventilatory control system is quantified as the loop gain, which is the ratio of ventilatory response to a ventilatory disturbance. Starting in the upper left corner, a ventilatory disturbance (change in minute ventilation ($\Delta V'$E), such as a hypopnoea) produces a change in alveolar CO_2 tension ($\Delta P\text{ACO}_2$). The amount of change in CO_2 tension depends on the properties of the plant. The plant is the lungs, blood and body tissues where CO_2 is stored (thus, factors such as lung volume, metabolic rate and dead space affect the relationship between $P\text{ACO}_2$ and ventilation in the plant). The altered $P\text{ACO}_2$ then mixes with the existing blood in the heart and arteries and undergoes a circulatory delay before changing CO_2 tension at the chemoreceptors ($\Delta P\text{crCO}_2$). A change in $P\text{crCO}_2$ produces a change in ventilation ($\Delta V'$E response) that acts to correct the initial disturbance. This last step (the $\Delta V'$E for a given $\Delta P\text{crCO}_2$) is known as the controller gain and is influenced by the inherent sensitivity of the chemoreceptors (carotid body and central chemoreceptor) as well as respiratory muscle strength and mechanics. Loop gain, which takes into account the plant, circulation delay and mixing, and the controller gain, is defined as the magnitude of the ventilatory response divided by the magnitude of the original ventilatory disturbance (Loop gain=$\Delta V'$E response/$\Delta V'$E disturbance).

patients who only have a modestly collapsible UA (<-2 cmH$_2$O) when compared with non-OSA individuals with the same degree of anatomical compromise as measured by Pcrit [12].

The mechanisms as to how high loop gain contributes to OSA are two-fold. First, in patients with NED (who suck the airway (partially) closed on inspiration) increasing respiratory effort can cause clinically important obstruction. As individuals with a high loop gain generate a large inspiratory force in response to an increase in CO_2 tension, this could be a potential mechanism of collapse in these individuals. The second way in which a high loop gain can contribute to OSA is based on the neuro–anatomical linkage between the UA muscles and the central respiratory centre in the brainstem (fig. 5). The UA muscles, like the diaphragm, receive neural input from the central respiratory centre. Thus, oscillations in ventilatory drive, due to a high loop gain, can produce periods of low ventilatory drive which will not only diminish diaphragm activity but also pharyngeal dilator muscle activity. If the drive to the UA falls to critically low levels, or if there is a mismatch in drive to the pump and UA dilators, UA obstruction can occur. Thus, in individuals with an anatomically susceptible airway, reductions in ventilatory drive may cause clinically significant UA obstruction [12, 45–47].

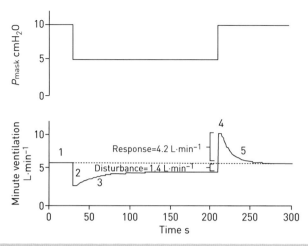

Figure 4. Determination of loop gain from a CPAP drop. 1) Prior to the drop, the patient's airway is open and ventilation is at eupnoea. 2) When CPAP is dropped, the UA narrows and limits ventilation. 3) As a result, CO_2 increases and, in many individuals, activates/stiffens the pharyngeal muscles and increases ventilation slightly (although it typically remains below eupnoea). In this example, the disturbance is a change in ventilation of -1.4 L·min^{-1}. 4) The response to this disturbance is a determined by reopening the airway with CPAP and measuring the ventilatory overshoot, which is 4.2 L·min^{-1}. Therefore, the loop gain is $4.2/-1.4=-3$, i.e. for every L·min^{-1} reduction in ventilation, there is a three-fold increase in ventilatory drive. 5) After the airway is reopened and the excess CO_2 is blown off, ventilation returns back to eupnoea. P_{mask}: mask pressure. Refer to the text and [13] for further detail. Reproduced from [12] with permission from the publisher.

Further evidence for the role of loop gain in OSA comes from studies in which loop gain was pharmacologically reduced. WELLMAN *et al.* [22] administered oxygen to OSA patients with a high loop gain and found that it significantly lowered the loop gain as well as the AHI, indicating the important role that loop gain played in these individuals. However, there was incomplete resolution of OSA (a 53% reduction in AHI), indicating the importance of the other traits. Similarly, EDWARDS *et al.* [48] halved loop gain using acetazolamide and found a similar improvement in AHI. These studies provide compelling evidence that loop gain plays a major role in OSA pathogenesis in certain patients.

Role of arousals in OSA

Frequent arousals from sleep due to a low respiratory arousal threshold can contribute to the development of OSA in several ways: 1) by preventing deeper sleep which is associated with more stable breathing, 2) by perpetuating respiratory control instability, and 3) by limiting build-up of essential respiratory stimuli required to increase neural drive to the UA dilator muscles [24, 28, 49]. These mechanisms and the potential to manipulate the arousal threshold as a novel therapeutic target have been the subject of a comprehensive review article and commentary articles [27, 28, 49, 50]. Thus, this topic is only covered briefly in the current chapter.

When the UA narrows or closes, as occurs repetitively in OSA, respiratory drive increases. This causes an increase in negative intrathoracic pressure which is believed to be the trigger for respiratory-induced arousal [51]. The arousal threshold can be quantified using an oesophageal or an epiglottic pressure catheter (fig. 1).

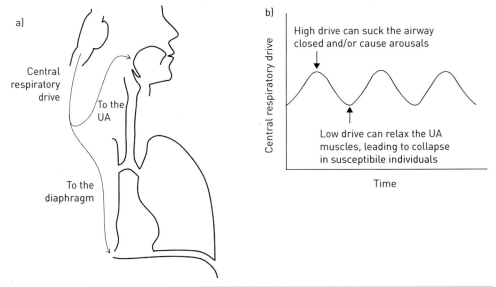

Figure 5. Due to the linkage between central respiratory drive and the UA and diaphragm (a), fluctuations in ventilatory drive due to a high loop gain can contribute to UA collapse (b).

Deeper stages of sleep, in particular slow wave sleep, are associated with an increase in the arousal threshold, increased UA muscle activity and an accompanying reduction in the AHI in patients with OSA compared with lighter stages of sleep [31, 52, 53]. Frequent arousals destabilise sleep and can prevent the progression into deeper sleep and, thus, breathing stability. Arousals are also associated with transient hyperventilation (a few breaths) [54], especially following an obstructive event. This hyperventilation can lead to a reduced CO_2 tension level yielding transient hypoventilation (reduced ventilatory drive), which could contribute to the next obstruction for the reasons described above for loop gain. Arousals can also interrupt the "compensatory upper airway response" [37]. If UA obstruction occurs during sleep, then ventilatory drive will increase and in many individuals this also stimulates the UA musculature. In some patients, this may partially or completely reopen the airway without arousal (*i.e.* effective compensation). In others, arousal may occur at a lower level of ventilatory drive than is needed to reopen the airway (*i.e.* ineffective or incomplete compensation) and, thus, stable sleep cannot be established. As a result, a low arousal threshold is probably important in OSA pathogenesis in at least one third of OSA patients [12, 26, 28]. Certain sedatives can increase the arousal threshold and reduce OSA severity in patients who have a low respiratory arousal threshold [25, 26].

Role of the UA muscles in OSA

Because the human UA lacks rigid bony support, pharyngeal patency relies heavily on the activity of dilating muscles. Although the loss of dilator muscle activity at sleep onset is an important mechanism in apnoea pathogenesis [55–57], these muscles nevertheless retain some ability to respond to mechanical and chemical stimuli during sleep in most individuals (fig. 1) [12, 58, 59]. However, one third of OSA patients generate very little or no electrical activation of the largest UA dilator muscle, genioglossus, during experimentally induced hypopnoeas and apnoeas [12]. Thus, there are differences between individuals in the ability of these muscles to respond [12, 30], which impacts the development of sleep apnoea and its severity. In addition to our sleep apnoea phenotyping study [12], other studies support this concept. YOUNES [33] found that only 34% of the variability in apnoea severity could be accounted for by "mechanical load" (*i.e.* anatomical deficiency) while "compensatory effectiveness" (UA dilator muscle response) accounted for a considerably greater proportion of this variability. PATIL *et al.* [60] also reported that some individuals with deficient UA anatomy, in whom OSA would otherwise be expected, may be protected by pharyngeal dilator muscles that remain responsive during sleep.

The UA response also consists of the translation of neural activation into a mechanical effect (neuro–mechanical coupling). Activation of the UA muscles must be converted into airway stiffening/dilation to have the desired effect. Recent studies using novel magnetic resonance imaging tagging to track the motion of genioglossus muscle activity throughout the respiratory cycle show clear differences in movement patterns between individuals [61]. Specifically, some OSA patients show very little movement (typically very severe patients), while others show quite pronounced movement which is counterproductive in terms of airway dilation (typically moderately severe patients) [61]. By contrast, many overweight and obese individuals without OSA have major genioglossus movement and very high levels of genioglossus activation during sleep, both of which are likely to be protective in these individuals [62, 63]. Recently, DOTAN *et al.* [36] also reported a dissociation between electromyographic (EMG) activity of the UA dilators and the mechanical response in many OSA patients during propofol anaesthesia. Anecdotally, we have seen several instances of OSA patients with good muscle responsiveness as measured *via* EMG but no improvement in airway mechanics. The UA response is, therefore, composed of two key components: 1) the ability to sense and develop neural activation of the UA muscles in response to a respiratory load, and 2) translation of neural activation into airway reopening (effectiveness). A breakdown in either component could lead to a poor UA response. The extent to which these components are impaired probably varies considerably between OSA patients [12, 32, 61, 64].

Interaction between the traits to cause OSA

All of these factors (a narrow/collapsible UA, ventilatory control instability, a low respiratory arousal threshold and a poor UA response) and other modifiers of these traits (*e.g.* rostral fluid shifts which may increase UA collapsibility) [65] interact with one another to produce OSA. Regardless of the underlying cause, CPAP almost always works because it mechanically splints the airway open with positive pressure. However, many patients find it unacceptable or intolerable [66, 67]. Nevertheless, there is little else available and, thus, the majority of patients are prescribed CPAP.

If, however, the relative contribution of each physiological trait could be determined in a particular individual, then there is the potential to target one or more of the traits with specific therapies (fig. 6). Such an individualised approach to treating OSA is not possible with the current diagnostic method used for OSA (PSG), which only provides information about the frequency of events·h^{-1}. Newer procedures with potential clinical applications are being developed to measure and model each of these traits [13, 44]. These include new approaches to estimating the phenotypic traits using standard overnight PSG and clinical measures [68, 69]. Such techniques could be used by clinicians to choose potentially effective treatments. These approaches may be useful in optimising success rates for existing

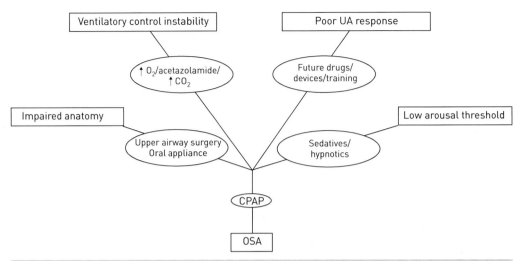

Figure 6. Targeting the "upstream" mechanisms of OSA may allow some people to be treated without CPAP.

therapies, including CPAP, oral devices and pharyngeal surgery, for newly diagnosed patients rather than the current costly and time consuming trial and error approach. Alternatively, these techniques could be used to test the utility of new therapeutic approaches including combined targeted strategies that may be particularly useful in those who fail with existing therapies. For example, pharyngeal surgery and a sedative might be effective in a patient with a small airway and a low arousal threshold [12, 26]. If the ventilatory control system is also unstable, then adding oxygen or acetazolamide (which stabilise the ventilatory control system [70–75]) might be useful. If recent advances in implantable devices are realised [76, 77] or if in the future drugs [78–81] that stimulate the UA muscles are developed, they will probably need to be combined with one of these other treatments to completely treat the OSA in many patients. Strategies to improve UA muscle function, such as training, may also be beneficial in certain OSA patients [82, 83]. Other interventions may improve multiple traits. For example, CO_2 may increase UA muscle tone and prevent respiratory control instability [35, 84].

Wellman and colleagues [13, 44] have developed a physiological model to illustrate the relative contribution of each trait in the pathogenesis of OSA. The importance of such a model becomes clear later when alternative treatments for OSA are discussed. The methods for measuring the traits are not described here except where needed to clarify the model. Rather, the focus is on the physiological meaning and interrelationship of each trait. The traits are plotted on a two-dimensional graph, with ventilatory drive on the x-axis and ventilation on the y-axis. The following paragraphs describe the model in detail and outline how each physiological trait is represented on the graph.

Eupnoeic ventilatory demand

Since most individuals with OSA do not have gas exchange or pulmonary mechanical abnormalities, the eupnoeic ventilation when the airway is fully patent during sleep is a reasonable measure of basal ventilatory demand. This value is represented by a dot along the line of identity in the model, *i.e.* ventilation matches ventilatory demand when the airway is patent, for example, on CPAP (fig. 7a).

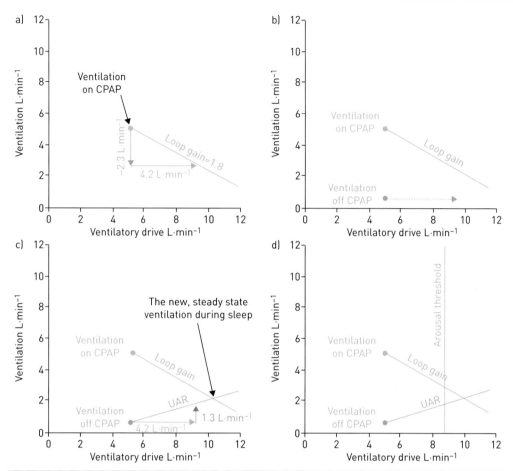

Figure 7. a) The ventilation on CPAP is a measure of ventilatory demand. Loop gain is plotted using a vector diagram of the disturbance (downward arrow) and the response (rightward arrow). b) The anatomy trait is represented as the ventilation off CPAP at the eupnoeic level of ventilatory drive. c) The UA response (UAR) is depicted as a slope. A flat slope indicates no compensatory responsiveness, whereas a positive slope (as shown here) indicates improving pharyngeal muscle responsiveness/effectiveness. d) The arousal threshold is represented as a vertical line. In this example, arousals occur when the ventilatory drive exceeds 9 L·min^{-1}.

Loop gain

Recall from figure 3 that loop gain is the ratio of the ventilatory response to a ventilatory disturbance. This ratio can be represented on the graph as a slope. For example, conceptually, if the loop gain is 1.8, then a reduction in ventilation of 2.3 L·min^{-1} will produce an increase in ventilatory drive to 4.2 L·min^{-1} (figs 4 and 7a). Note that an oversensitive ventilatory control system (high loop gain) would have a large ventilatory response for the same disturbance and, thus, a flatter loop gain slope on this graph. A low loop gain, on the other hand, would produce a steeper slope. The physiological meaning of the steepness/flatness of the loop gain slope will become clear as the other phenotypic traits are added to the graph.

UA anatomy/collapsibility

The anatomy/collapsibility trait is quantified as the level of ventilation that would occur on no CPAP (0 cmH$_2$O) at the eupnoeic level of ventilatory drive. This value is similar to the pharyngeal critical pressure measurement [85], except that the ventilation at zero pressure, rather than the pressure at zero flow, is used to quantify pharyngeal collapsibility. This allows the anatomy parameter to be incorporated directly into the OSA model with the correct units of $L \cdot min^{-1}$. Figure 7b shows the OSA model with the loop gain and anatomy parameters plotted. The model indicates that on CPAP, ventilation is 5.1 $L \cdot min^{-1}$. However, off CPAP, at eupnoeic ventilatory drive, ventilation is only 0.7 $L \cdot min^{-1}$. A reduction in ventilation of this magnitude would, according to the loop gain, lead to an increase in ventilatory drive to above 12 $L \cdot min^{-1}$ (dashed arrow in fig. 7b), which is not sustainable and, in the absence of compensatory reopening of the airway, would cause arousal.

UA response

During sleep, particularly in patients with OSA, the UA may partially or completely obstruct, thereby reducing ventilation and yielding increasing CO_2 tension. As a result, ventilatory drive increases. The increase in ventilatory drive will stimulate the diaphragm and UA muscles. Thus, ventilation may recover slightly. The amount of recovery depends, in part, on the amount that the UA stiffens/dilates in response to the increase in drive as well as the negative pressure reflex in the pharyngeal airway. This characteristic or trait, which has been labelled the "upper airway response", can be represented in the model as a slope. The representative subject in figure 7c has a positively sloped UA response of 0.3, which means that an increase in ventilatory drive of (for example) 4.2 $L \cdot min^{-1}$ will stiffen the UA muscles, yielding an increase in ventilation of 1.3 $L \cdot min^{-1}$. Consistent with EMG recordings of the genioglossus [12], Wellman and colleagues found that some patients have a flat or even a negatively sloped UA response, indicating a complete inability to compensate [13, 44].

The intersection of the UA response line and the 1/loop gain line is the new, steady state ventilation that would occur during sleep in the absence of CPAP. That is, if this individual were initially breathing at 5.1 $L \cdot min^{-1}$ on optimum CPAP, and then CPAP was turned off, ventilation would decrease to 0.7 $L \cdot min^{-1}$. Then, as ventilatory drive increases, ventilation would also increase along the slope of the UA response line until it reaches the loop gain line, at which point it stops, *i.e.* the new steady state level of ventilation. The reason that ventilation (and ventilatory drive) eventually settle at the intersection of the UA response and loop gain lines is because this is the simultaneous solution to the equations for each line. Thus, any movement away from the intersection would be transient, and ventilation and ventilatory drive would eventually be drawn back to this point.

Arousal threshold

The last trait to be added to the model is the arousal threshold. As stated earlier, the arousal threshold is the level of ventilatory drive that causes arousal from sleep. This is depicted in the model as a vertical line at the threshold level of ventilatory drive (fig. 7d). The model is now complete and says that the individual will have OSA for the following reasons: during sleep in the absence of CPAP, ventilation is initially 0.7 $L \cdot min^{-1}$ (see dot labelled ventilation off CPAP). As ventilatory drive increases, ventilation increases along the UA response line. However, before the steady state point (intersection of the loop gain line and UA response line) can be reached, arousal occurs. Therefore, according to the model, if the arousal threshold is lower than (to the left of) the steady state ventilation point, then

OSA will occur. If the arousal threshold is above (to the right of) the steady state ventilation point, then OSA should not occur.

Implications of the different phenotypes

Despite the considerable resources devoted to developing alternative treatments for OSA, CPAP remains the most consistently effective option for many patients although oral appliances are also quite effective in many instances [86]. Non-PAP therapies, such as uvulopalatopharyngoplasty [87], oxygen [88–91], acetazolamide [92–96] and sedatives [97–101] have been studied in unselected populations. In most cases, the interventions had a modest effect on apnoea severity, although in almost every study a proportion of patients exhibited more complete responses. Better matching of the agent (or combinations of agents) to the abnormal trait(s) may improve treatment effectiveness and patient outcomes.

Using the model to choose appropriate therapy

Modelling the parameters in individual patients has limitations and relies on several underlying assumptions. For example, while some of the traits can vary with sleep state [28], current approaches are limited to non-REM sleep (predominately S2) as this is the sleep state in which most of the physiological and intervention data have been obtained [28]. Nonetheless, using either the technique presented or a similar procedure could be useful for choosing therapies. For instance, in the current example, manipulation of pharyngeal anatomy would be helpful. The effect of such a manipulation could be modelled by shifting the "anatomy" dot upwards slightly (fig. 8). The amount it is shifted upwards depends on the effect size of the intervention chosen to change the anatomy (*e.g.* UA surgery, weight loss, oral appliance or positional therapy). Figure 8 shows how a small improvement in pharyngeal anatomy (*e.g.* following UA surgery) might affect the development of OSA. In this example, if this were the only intervention used, OSA may persist to some extent because the steady state point still lies to the right of the arousal threshold line. In this situation, the addition of a sedative (to shift the arousal threshold to

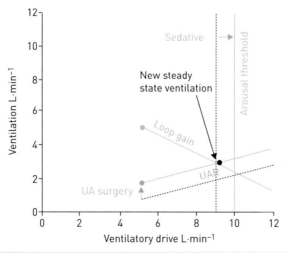

Figure 8. Small improvements in UA anatomy and arousal threshold could, in some individuals, bring the steady state point into the stable region (to the left of the arousal threshold line). UAR: UA response.

the right) might be needed to move the steady state point into the stable region (to the left of the arousal threshold line) to fully treat OSA. These types of predictions need to be studied carefully by testing the effect of various drugs/agents on the phenotypic traits. This is a future direction for OSA research that shows great potential.

Conclusion

In summary, the multifactorial nature of OSA pathogenesis is largely underappreciated. While anatomy is clearly the most important variable, a handful of other traits play a contributory role and present themselves as potential therapeutic targets in selected patients, particularly if combination therapy is applied. Nevertheless, OSA continues to be treated largely with monotherapy. To advance the field of OSA management, procedures for phenotyping in the clinical arena, such as the one described here, are needed. Moreover, the effect size of various non-PAP agents on the traits needs to be carefully determined and how responses may vary according to different phenotypes. If these goals can be accomplished, the future of OSA management could involve a more individualised approach that some patients might find more tolerable.

References

1. Young T, Peppard PE, Gottlieb DJ. Epidemiology of obstructive sleep apnea: a population health perspective. *Am J Respir Crit Care Med* 2002; 165: 1217–1239.
2. Somers VK, Dyken ME, Clary MP, *et al.* Sympathetic neural mechanisms in obstructive sleep apnea. *J Clin Invest* 1995; 96: 1897–1904.
3. Nieto FJ, Young TB, Lind BK, *et al.* Association of sleep-disordered breathing, sleep apnea, and hypertension in a large community-based study. Sleep Heart Health Study. *JAMA* 2000; 283: 1829–1836.
4. Peppard PE, Young T, Palta M, *et al.* Prospective study of the association between sleep-disordered breathing and hypertension. *N Engl J Med* 2000; 342: 1378–1384.
5. Wessendorf TE, Thilmann AF, Wang YM, *et al.* Fibrinogen levels and obstructive sleep apnea in ischemic stroke. *Am J Respir Crit Care Med* 2000; 162: 2039–2042.
6. Hoffstein V, Mateika S. Cardiac arrhythmias, snoring, and sleep apnea. *Chest* 1994; 106: 466–471.
7. Shahar E, Whitney CW, Redline S, *et al.* Sleep-disordered breathing and cardiovascular disease: cross-sectional results of the Sleep Heart Health Study. *Am J Respir Crit Care Med* 2001; 163: 19–25.
8. Brooks D, Horner RL, Kozar LF, *et al.* Obstructive sleep apnea as a cause of systemic hypertension. Evidence from a canine model. *J Clin Invest* 1997; 99: 106–109.
9. Hung J, Whitford EG, Parsons RW, *et al.* Association of sleep apnoea with myocardial infarction in men. *Lancet* 1990; 336: 261–264.
10. Redline S, Strauss ME, Adams N, *et al.* Neuropsychological function in mild sleep-disordered breathing. *Sleep* 1997; 20: 160–167.
11. Findley LJ, Unverzagt ME, Suratt PM. Automobile accidents involving patients with obstructive sleep apnea. *Am Rev Respir Dis* 1988; 138: 337–340.
12. Eckert DJ, White DP, Jordan AS, *et al.* Defining phenotypic causes of obstructive sleep apnea. Identification of novel therapeutic targets. *Am J Respir Crit Care Med* 2013; 188: 996–1004.
13. Wellman A, Eckert DJ, Jordan AS, *et al.* A method for measuring and modeling the physiological traits causing obstructive sleep apnea. *J Appl Physiol* 2011; 110: 1627–1637.
14. Gleadhill IC, Schwartz AR, Schubert N, *et al.* Upper airway collapsibility in snorers and in patients with obstructive hypopnea and apnea. *Am Rev Respir Dis* 1991; 143: 1300–1303.
15. Isono S, Remmers JE, Tanaka A, *et al.* Anatomy of pharynx in patients with obstructive sleep apnea and in normal subjects. *J Appl Physiol* 1997; 82: 1319–1326.
16. Schwab RJ. Upper airway imaging. *Clin Chest Med* 1998; 19: 33–54.
17. Hudgel DW, Gordon EA, Thanakitcharu S, *et al.* Instability of ventilatory control in patients with obstructive sleep apnea. *Am J Respir Crit Care Med* 1998; 158: 1142–1149.
18. Younes M, Ostrowski M, Thompson W, *et al.* Chemical control stability in patients with obstructive sleep apnea. *Am J Respir Crit Care Med* 2001; 163: 1181–1190.

19. Asyali M, Berry RB, Khoo MC. Assessment of closed-loop ventilatory stability in obstructive sleep apnea. *IEEE Trans Biomed Eng* 2002; 49: 206–216.

20. Wellman A, Jordan AS, Malhotra A, *et al.* Ventilatory control and airway anatomy in obstructive sleep apnea. *Am J Respir Crit Care Med* 2004; 170: 1225–1232.

21. Salloum A, Rowley JA, Mateika JH, *et al.* Increased propensity for central apnea in patients with obstructive sleep apnea: effect of nasal continuous positive airway pressure. *Am J Respir Crit Care Med* 2010; 181: 189–193.

22. Wellman A, Malhotra A, Jordan AS, *et al.* Effect of oxygen in obstructive sleep apnea: role of loop gain. *Respir Physiol Neurobiol* 2008; 162: 144–151.

23. Jordan AS, Eckert DJ, Wellman A, *et al.* Termination of respiratory events with and without cortical arousal in obstructive sleep apnea. *Am J Respir Crit Care Med* 2011; 184: 1183–1191.

24. Younes M. Role of arousals in the pathogenesis of obstructive sleep apnea. *Am J Respir Crit Care Med* 2004; 169: 623–633.

25. Eckert DJ, Malhotra A, Wellman A, *et al.* Trazodone increases the respiratory arousal threshold in patients with obstructive sleep apnea and a low arousal threshold. *Sleep* 2014; 37: 811–819.

26. Eckert DJ, Owens RL, Kehlmann GB, *et al.* Eszopiclone increases the respiratory arousal threshold and lowers the apnoea/hypopnoea index in obstructive sleep apnoea patients with a low arousal threshold. *Clin Sci (Lond)* 2011; 120: 505–514.

27. Eckert DJ, White DP, Jordan AS, *et al.* Reply: arousal threshold in obstructive sleep apnea. *Am J Respir Crit Care Med* 2014; 189: 373–374.

28. Eckert DJ, Younes MK. Arousal from sleep: implications for obstructive sleep apnea pathogenesis and treatment. *J Appl Physiol* 2014; 116: 302–313.

29. Patil SP, Schneider H, Marx JJ, *et al.* Neuromechanical control of upper airway patency during sleep. *J Appl Physiol* 2007; 102: 547–556.

30. Jordan AS, Wellman A, Heinzer RC, *et al.* Mechanisms used to restore ventilation after partial upper airway collapse during sleep in humans. *Thorax* 2007; 62: 861–867.

31. Jordan AS, White DP, Lo YL, *et al.* Airway dilator muscle activity and lung volume during stable breathing in obstructive sleep apnea. *Sleep* 2009; 32: 361–368.

32. Younes M, Loewen AH, Ostrowski M, *et al.* Genioglossus activity available *via* non-arousal mechanisms *vs.* that required for opening the airway in obstructive apnea patients. *J Appl Physiol* 2012; 112: 249–258.

33. Younes M. Contributions of upper airway mechanics and control mechanisms to severity of obstructive apnea. *Am J Respir Crit Care Med* 2003; 168: 645–658.

34. Eckert DJ, Lo YL, Saboisky JP, *et al.* Sensorimotor function of the upper-airway muscles and respiratory sensory processing in untreated obstructive sleep apnea. *J Appl Physiol* 2011; 111: 1644–1653.

35. Jordan AS, White DP, Owens RL, *et al.* The effect of increased genioglossus activity and end-expiratory lung volume on pharyngeal collapse. *J Appl Physiol* 2010; 109: 469–475.

36. Dotan Y, Pillar G, Tov N, *et al.* Dissociation of electromyogram and mechanical response in sleep apnoea during propofol anaesthesia. *Eur Respir J* 2013; 41: 74–84.

37. Younes M, Ostrowski M, Atkar R, *et al.* Mechanisms of breathing instability in patients with obstructive sleep apnea. *J Appl Physiol* 2007; 103: 1929–1941.

38. Smith PL, Wise RA, Gold AR, *et al.* Upper airway pressure-flow relationships in obstructive sleep apnea. *J Appl Physiol* 1988; 64: 789–795.

39. Kirkness JP, Schwartz AR, Schneider H, *et al.* Contribution of male sex, age, and obesity to mechanical instability of the upper airway during sleep. *J Appl Physiol* 2008; 104: 1618–1624.

40. Owens RL, Edwards BA, Sands SA, *et al.* Upper airway collapsibility and patterns of flow limitation at constant end-expiratory lung volume. *J Appl Physiol* 2012; 113: 691–699.

41. Genta PR, Owens RL, Edwards BA, *et al.* Influence of pharyngeal muscle activity on inspiratory negative effort dependence in the human upper airway. *Respir Physiol Neurobiol* 2014; 201: 55–59.

42. Owens RL, Edwards BA, Sands SA, *et al.* The classical Starling resistor model often does not predict inspiratory airflow patterns in the human upper airway. *J Appl Physiol* 2014; 116: 1105–1112.

43. Younes M. Role of respiratory control mechanisms in the pathogenesis of obstructive sleep disorders. *J Appl Physiol* 2008; 105: 1389–1405.

44. Wellman A, Edwards BA, Sands SA, *et al.* A simplified method for determining phenotypic traits in patients with obstructive sleep apnea. *J Appl Physiol* 2013; 114: 911–922.

45. Onal E, Burrows DL, Hart RH, *et al.* Induction of periodic breathing during sleep causes upper airway obstruction in humans. *J Appl Physiol* 1986; 61: 1438–1443.

46. Badr MS, Toiber F, Skatrud JB, *et al.* Pharyngeal narrowing/occlusion during central sleep apnea. *J Appl Physiol* 1995; 78: 1806–1815.

47. Badr MS, Kawak A, Skatrud JB, *et al.* Effect of induced hypocapnic hypopnea on upper airway patency in humans during NREM sleep. *Respir Physiol* 1997; 110: 33–45.

48. Edwards BA, Connolly JG, Campana LM, *et al.* Acetazolamide attenuates the ventilatory response to arousal in patients with obstructive sleep apnea. *Sleep* 2013; 36: 281–285.

49. Eckert DJ, Gandevia SC. The human upper airway: more than a floppy tube. *J Appl Physiol* 2014; 116: 288–290.

50. Saboisky J, Eckert D, Malhotra A. Stable breathing through deeper sleeping. *Thorax* 2010; 65: 95–96.

51. Gleeson K, Zwillich CW, White DP. The influence of increasing ventilatory effort on arousal from sleep. *Am Rev Respir Dis* 1990; 142: 295–300.

52. Ratnavadivel R, Chau N, Stadler D, *et al.* Marked reduction in obstructive sleep apnea severity in slow wave sleep. *J Clin Sleep Med* 2009; 5: 519–524.

53. Ratnavadivel R, Stadler D, Windler S, *et al.* Upper airway function and arousability to ventilatory challenge in slow wave *versus* stage 2 sleep in obstructive sleep apnoea. *Thorax* 2010; 65: 107–112.

54. Jordan AS, Eckert DJ, Catcheside PG, *et al.* Ventilatory response to brief arousal from non-rapid eye movement sleep is greater in men than in women. *Am J Respir Crit Care Med* 2003; 168: 1512–1519.

55. Horner RL, Innes JA, Morrell MJ, *et al.* The effect of sleep on reflex genioglossus muscle activation by stimuli of negative airway pressure in humans. *J Physiol* 1994; 476: 141–151.

56. Fogel RB, Malhotra A, Pillar G, *et al.* Genioglossal activation in patients with obstructive sleep apnea *versus* control subjects. Mechanisms of muscle control. *Am J Respir Crit Care Med* 2001; 164: 2025–2030.

57. Wheatley JR, White DP. The influence of sleep on pharyngeal reflexes. *Sleep* 1993; 16: Suppl. 8, S87–S89.

58. Wheatley JR, Mezzanotte WS, Tangel DJ, *et al.* Influence of sleep on genioglossus muscle activation by negative pressure in normal men. *Am Rev Respir Dis* 1993; 148: 597–605.

59. Stanchina ML, Malhotra A, Fogel RB, *et al.* Genioglossus muscle responsiveness to chemical and mechanical stimuli during non-rapid eye movement sleep. *Am J Respir Crit Care Med* 2002; 165: 945–949.

60. Patil S, Schneider H, Gladmon E, *et al.* Obesity and upper airway mechanical control during sleep. *Am J Respir Crit Care Med* 2004; 169: Suppl., A435.

61. Brown EC, Cheng S, McKenzie DK, *et al.* Respiratory movement of upper airway tissue in obstructive sleep apnea. *Sleep* 2013; 36: 1069–1076.

62. Cheng S, Brown EC, Hatt A, *et al.* Healthy humans with a narrow upper airway maintain patency during quiet breathing by dilating the airway during inspiration. *J Physiol* 2014; 592: 4763–4774.

63. Sands SA, Eckert DJ, Jordan AS, *et al.* Enhanced upper-airway muscle responsiveness is a distinct feature of overweight/obese individuals without sleep apnea. *Am J Respir Crit Care Med* 2014; 190: 930–937.

64. Saboisky JP, Butler JE, Gandevia SC, *et al.* Functional role of neural injury in obstructive sleep apnea. *Front Neurol* 2012; 3: 95.

65. White LH, Bradley TD. Role of nocturnal rostral fluid shift in the pathogenesis of obstructive and central sleep apnoea. *J Physiol* 2013; 591: 1179–1193.

66. Kribbs NB, Pack AI, Kline LR, *et al.* Objective measurement of patterns of nasal CPAP use by patients with obstructive sleep apnea. *Am Rev Respir Dis* 1993; 147: 887–895.

67. Engelman H, Wild MR. Improving CPAP use by patients with the sleep apnoea/hypopnoea syndrome (SAHS). *Sleep Med Rev* 2003; 7: 81–99.

68. Edwards BA, Eckert DJ, McSharry DG, *et al.* Clinical predictors of the respiratory arousal threshold in patients with obstructive sleep apnea. *Am J Respir Crit Care Med* 2014; 190: 1293–1300.

69. Terrill PI, Edwards BA, Nemati S, *et al.* Quantifying the ventilatory control contribution to sleep apnoea using polysomnography. *Eur Respir J* 2014; 45: 408–418.

70. Edwards BA, Sands SA, Eckert DJ, *et al.* Acetazolamide improves loop gain but not the other physiological traits causing obstructive sleep apnoea. *J Physiol* 2012; 590: 1199–1211.

71. Lai J, Bruce EN. Ventilatory stability to transient CO_2 disturbances in hyperoxia and normoxia in awake humans. *J Appl Physiol* 1997; 83: 466–476.

72. Simakajornboon N, Beckerman RC, Mack C, *et al.* Effect of supplemental oxygen on sleep architecture and cardiorespiratory events in preterm infants. *Pediatrics* 2002; 110: 884–888.

73. Reite M, Jackson D, Cahoon RL, *et al.* Sleep physiology at high altitude. *Electroencephalogr Clin Neurophysiol* 1975; 38: 463–471.

74. Nakayama H, Smith CA, Rodman JR, *et al.* Effect of ventilatory drive on carbon dioxide sensitivity below eupnea during sleep. *Am J Respir Crit Care Med* 2002; 165: 1251–1260.

75. Wagenaar M, Teppema L, Berkenbosch A, *et al.* Effect of low-dose acetazolamide on the ventilatory CO_2 response during hypoxia in the anaesthetized cat. *Eur Respir J* 1998; 12: 1271–1277.

76. Eastwood PR, Barnes M, Walsh JH, *et al.* Treating obstructive sleep apnea with hypoglossal nerve stimulation. *Sleep* 2011; 34: 1479–1486.

77. Strollo PJ Jr, Soose RJ, Maurer JT, *et al.* Upper-airway stimulation for obstructive sleep apnea. *N Engl J Med* 2014; 370: 139–149.

78. Grace KP, Hughes SW, Horner RL. Identification of a pharmacological target for genioglossus reactivation throughout sleep. *Sleep* 2014; 37: 41–50.

79. Horner RL, Hughes SW, Malhotra A. State-dependent and reflex drives to the upper airway: basic physiology with clinical implications. *J Appl Physiol* 2014; 116: 325–336.
80. Wirth KJ, Steinmeyer K, Ruetten H. Sensitization of upper airway mechanoreceptors as a new pharmacologic principle to treat obstructive sleep apnea: investigations with AVE0118 in anesthetized pigs. *Sleep* 2013; 36: 699–708.
81. Wang D, Eckert DJ, Grunstein RR. Drug effects on ventilatory control and upper airway physiology related to sleep apnea. *Respir Physiol Neurobiol* 2013; 188: 257–266.
82. Guimaräes KC, Drager LF, Genta PR, *et al.* Effects of oropharyngeal exercises on patients with moderate obstructive sleep apnea syndrome. *Am J Respir Crit Care Med* 2009; 179: 962–966.
83. Puhan MA, Suarez A, Lo Cascio C, *et al.* Didgeridoo playing as alternative treatment for obstructive sleep apnoea syndrome: randomised controlled trial. *BMJ* 2006; 332: 266–270.
84. Xie A, Teodorescu M, Pegelow DF, *et al.* Effects of stabilizing or increasing respiratory motor outputs on obstructive sleep apnea. *J Appl Physiol* 2013; 115: 22–33.
85. Schwartz AR, O'Donnell CP, Baron J, *et al.* The hypotonic upper airway in obstructive sleep apnea: role of structures and neuromuscular activity. *Am J Respir Crit Care Med* 1998; 157: 1051–1057.
86. Sutherland K, Vanderveken OM, Tsuda H, *et al.* Oral appliance treatment for obstructive sleep apnea: an update. *J Clin Sleep Med* 2014; 10: 215–227.
87. Schwartz AR, Schubert N, Rothman W, *et al.* Effect of uvulopalatopharyngoplasty on upper airway collapsibility in obstructive sleep apnea. *Am Rev Respir Dis* 1992; 145: 527–532.
88. Smith PL, Haponik EF, Bleecker ER. The effects of oxygen in patients with sleep apnea. *Am Rev Respir Dis* 1984; 130: 958–963.
89. Martin RJ, Sanders MH, Gray BA, *et al.* Acute and long-term ventilatory effects of hyperoxia in the adult sleep apnea syndrome. *Am Rev Respir Dis* 1982; 125: 175–180.
90. Gold AR, Bleecker ER, Smith PL. A shift from central and mixed sleep apnea to obstructive sleep apnea resulting from low-flow oxygen. *Am Rev Respir Dis* 1985; 132: 220–223.
91. Gold AR, Schwartz AR, Bleecker ER, *et al.* The effect of chronic nocturnal oxygen administration upon sleep apnea. *Am Rev Respir Dis* 1986; 134: 925–929.
92. Tojima H, Kunitomo F, Kimura H, *et al.* Effects of acetazolamide in patients with the sleep apnoea syndrome. *Thorax* 1988; 43: 113–119.
93. Sharp JT, Druz WS, D'Souza V, *et al.* Effect of metabolic acidosis upon sleep apnea. *Chest* 1985; 87: 619–624.
94. Whyte KF, Gould GA, Airlie MA, *et al.* Role of protriptyline and acetazolamide in the sleep apnea/hypopnea syndrome. *Sleep* 1988; 11: 463–472.
95. Sakamoto T, Nakazawa Y, Hashizume Y, *et al.* Effects of acetazolamide on the sleep apnea syndrome and its therapeutic mechanism. *Psychiatry Clin Neurosci* 1995; 49: 59–64.
96. Inoue Y, Takata K, Sakamoto I, *et al.* Clinical efficacy and indication of acetazolamide treatment on sleep apnea syndrome. *Psychiatry Clin Neurosci* 1999; 53: 321–322.
97. Rosenberg R, Roach JM, Scharf M, *et al.* A pilot study evaluating acute use of eszopiclone in patients with mild to moderate obstructive sleep apnea syndrome. *Sleep Med* 2007; 8: 464–470.
98. Heinzer RC, White DP, Jordan AS, *et al.* Trazodone increases arousal threshold in obstructive sleep apnoea. *Eur Respir J* 2008; 31: 1308–1312.
99. Berry RB, Kouchi K, Bower J, *et al.* Triazolam in patients with obstructive sleep apnea. *Am J Respir Crit Care Med* 1995; 151: 450–454.
100. Höijer U, Hedner J, Ejnell H, *et al.* Nitrazepam in patients with sleep apnoea: a double-blind placebo-controlled study. *Eur Respir J* 1994; 7: 2011–2015.
101. Wang D, Marshall NS, Duffin J, *et al.* Phenotyping interindividual variability in obstructive sleep apnoea response to temazepam using ventilatory chemoreflexes during wakefulness. *J Sleep Res* 2011; 20: 526–532.

Support statement: D.J. Eckert is supported by the National Health and Medical Research Council of Australia and holds an R.D. Wright Fellowship (1049814). Both authors have been supported by the US National Institutes of Health.

Disclosures: A. Wellman reports grants from Apnicure, and consultancy fees from Philips Respironics, SOVA and Galleon, outside the submitted work.

Chapter 3

Cancer: insights into biological plausibility

Isaac Almendros[1], David Gozal[1] and Ramon Farré[2,3]

Recently, an increasing number of epidemiological studies has focused on potential associations between cancer and OSA, and are generating intense interest in the field. IH and sleep fragmentation, the two hallmark features of OSA, have been shown to increase tumour growth, invasion and metastasis in mice. However, the potential mechanisms underlying the intersection between cancer and OSA are only now being explored and are, therefore, far from being well understood. This is due, in part, to the multiplicity of sleep disorder phenotypes and also to the myriad of cancers, which will require comprehensive and systematic translational investigations to elucidate specific biological mechanisms that account for the clinical correlates being currently uncovered. In this chapter, the state-of-the-art *in vivo* and *in vitro* published data on the effects of IH and sleep fragmentation in tumour malignancy are presented, and potential mechanistic pathways that may be involved (*e.g.* oxidative stress, inflammation and immunomodulation) are discussed.

In the past decades, OSA has emerged as being causally or epidemiologically associated with a large array of end-organ morbidities affecting different systems [1]. OSA, the most common form of sleep apnoea, is characterised by recurrent obstructions of the UA during sleep, resulting in IH, increased inspiratory efforts, hypercapnia and sleep fragmentation [2]. Most of these features have been extensively investigated and characterised in patients and murine models with the aim to elucidate potential mechanisms underlying the extensive cardiovascular, cognitive and metabolic morbidities of this condition [3, 4]. Recent seminal epidemiological studies have reported that OSA appears to be associated with increased cancer incidence [5–7], aggressiveness [8] and mortality [7, 9]. In these studies, a significant relationship between clinical characteristics of cancer and indices of nocturnal O_2 desaturation in arterial blood emerged, and were consistent with previous tumour biological data indicating that hypoxia operates as a major determinant of processes involving cancer invasion and metastasis [10, 11]. In addition, epidemiological studies focusing on sleep duration or changes in the circadian alignment (*e.g.* shift work), rather than revolving around OSA, have been published in the past decade, and showed that altered sleep patterns can promote higher incidence or adversely affect cancer prognosis [12–26]. In agreement with such relatively scarce epidemiological evidence, a recent study reported increased expression of tumour-associated genes in peripheral

[1]Sections of Pediatric Sleep Medicine and Pediatric Pulmonology, Dept of Pediatrics, Comer Children's Hospital, Pritzker School of Medicine, The University of Chicago, Chicago, IL, USA. [2]Unitat de Biofísica i Bioenginyeria, Facultat de Medicina, Universitat de Barcelona – IDIBAPS, Barcelona, Spain. [3]CIBER de Enfermedades Respiratorias, Madrid, Spain.

Correspondence: Isaac Almendros, Section of Sleep Medicine, Dept of Pediatrics, Biological Sciences Division, The University of Chicago, KCBD, Room 4115D, 900 E. 57th Street, Chicago, IL 60637-1470, USA. E-mail: isaac.almendros@ub.edu

Copyright ©ERS 2015. Print ISBN: 978-1-84984-059-0. Online ISBN: 978-1-84984-060-6. Print ISSN: 2312-508X. Online ISSN: 2312-5098.

ERS Monogr 2015; 67: 24–36. DOI: 10.1183/2312508X.10005514

blood leukocytes from OSA patients. Although the significance of such findings was not explored, treatment of OSA with CPAP reversed most of the alterations in these cancer-related gene networks suggesting a potential role for the immune system in the neoplastic processes affected by the presence of OSA [27]. Taken together, the available data emanating from both clinical and basic research studies to date suggest that IH and sleep disruption may play significant roles in processes such as neoplasia, tumour proliferation, local or remote tumour spreading, and even resistance to therapy.

IH in the tumour microenvironment

The role of tumour hypoxia in cancer biology is one of the most intensively studied phenomena in recent years. It is well known that hypoxia in the tumour microenvironment can promote a more aggressive cancer phenotype, namely increased metastatic potential, reduction of the effectiveness of some treatments and poor prognosis in patients [28–31]. In fact, two main regions are commonly defined within the tumours, each presenting a different hypoxic profile: 1) areas more distant to vessels that are continuously hypoxic, and usually correspond to more necrotic tumour sections; and 2) areas that are closer to newly formed vasculature within the tumour, in which hypoxia may be intermittently present (fig. 1). Indeed, although cells are in closer proximity to the newly formed vessels in these tumoural regions, sufficient O_2 levels are not ensured since tissue oxygenation not only depends on the distance to the vessels, but is also dependent on changes in flow perfusion caused by an aberrant and poorly organised vasculature [32, 33]. Therefore, the oxygenation profile experienced by cells within the tumour, and presumably in the tumour periphery [34], is not constant or homogeneous. Consequently, tumour cells are probably subjected to an erratic pattern of cyclical hypoxia, as recently revealed using arterial oxygen tension (P_aO_2) electrodes in human tumours [35].

The potential effects of the cyclic hypoxic oscillations on tumour behaviour have been explored using both *in vivo* and *in vitro* models, and these studies have uncovered clear evidence that cyclical hypoxia alters tumour malignancy and resistance to conventional

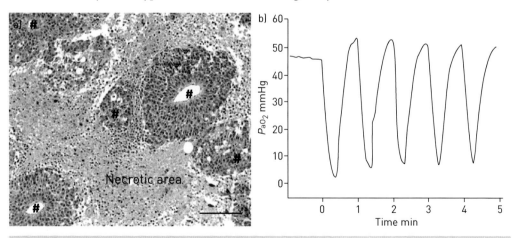

Figure 1. a) Haematoxylin-eosin preparation of a B16F10 tumour illustrates two types of tumour areas manifesting clearly divergent hypoxia/perfusion profiles within the tumour. Areas located far from the vessels (#) are not well perfused and are necrotic. Those next to the vessels show viable tumour cells, and do not show evidence of necrosis. b) Arterial oxygen tension (P_aO_2) measurements reveal that well-perfused areas display substantial O_2 tension swings during IH exposure.

therapy [36]. Some investigators have further shown that acute hypoxia may significantly increase the number of spontaneous microscopic metastases [11, 37, 38]. Moreover, cells pre-exposed to cyclical hypoxia with a frequency pattern similar to that experienced in OSA patients can increase the metastatic potential in a rodent model [11, 39]. In addition, cyclic hypoxia can reduce the effectiveness of some antitumour therapies [39]. These observed changes in biological cancer properties could have major implications in the context of OSA as outlined below.

IH is one of the most extensively studied hallmark features of OSA. When severe OSA is present, a higher frequency of hypoxic events with lower nadir O_2 levels is typically seen. These conditions appear to disable adaptive processes and manifest more pathological outcomes when compared with cyclic hypoxia, in which lower frequency oscillation of O_2 tension and lessened severity of the hypoxic event occur [40]. Furthermore, in some tissues, particularly those with higher metabolic rates such as tumours, IH can induce a state of continuous hypoxia in regions where blood flow is already compromised. Of note, in OSA patients the tumour regions with better blood perfusion will be exposed to IH as a result of the typical recurrent hypoxaemic events that occur throughout the night during sleep (fig. 1). Moreover, the tumour microenvironment is not only subjected to IH, but is also exposed to soluble external factors triggered systemically by IH, which will ultimately reach the tumour site through the systemic circulation. Thus, IH-induced alterations in non-tumoural tissues, which include increased expression and activity of a large network of transcription factors, will ultimately trigger oxidative stress, chronic inflammation and metabolic changes, as well as modulate the immune response [41–46]. The repertoire of tissue-specific responses to IH will ultimately be reflected in the systemic circulation, thereby imposing important implications as far as the tumour environment, especially when considering that well-irrigated regions within the tumour coincide with those regions in which processes such as cancer cell migration and tumour invasion primarily occur. Based on the aforementioned considerations, IH would be expected to change tumour behaviour through a complex interplay of multiple mechanisms reflecting both intra- and extra-tumoural cascades of events.

Recent and overall exploratory data obtained from rodent models of OSA has thus far corroborated these sets of assumptions (fig. 2). Specifically, IH not only increases tumour growth and invasion in two cancer types (melanoma and lung carcinoma) [47–49], but also enhances the metastatic potential of solid cancers when using two different experimental paradigms of lung metastases that rely on intravenous and subcutaneous tumour injections [50, 51]. Thus, the inferences derived from the rodent-based experiments lend biological plausibility to the epidemiological studies in patients with OSA [5–9, 12], while further supporting the putative role of hypoxia, and more specifically IH, in tumour biological processes. As a note of caution, most of these studies were conducted in mice, but were descriptive in nature, even though they clearly showed that IH increased tumour malignancy in a controlled environment that was void of other frequent clinical confounders seen in OSA patients, such obesity or sleep disruption.

Sleep fragmentation and cancer

Several epidemiological studies related to sleep duration and cancer outcomes have started to emerge in recent years [12–26]. For instance, disruption of the normal circadian rhythms may increase the risk of several types of cancer [52–54]. In particular, night shift work has

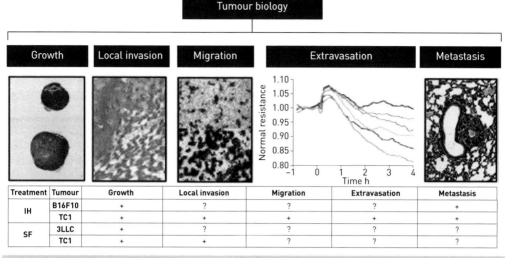

Figure 2. Effects of IH and sleep fragmentation (SF) in tumour biology. The table shows the currently available information on the effects of IH and SF regarding each of the characteristics that define cancer malignancy. Line colours for extravasation refer to the following: black: medium; red: TC1; green: tumour-associated macrophages (TAM) room air (RA); orange: TC1 plus TAMs RA; purple: TAMs IH; grey: TC1 plus TAMs IH. LLC: lewis lung carcinoma.

been associated with an increased prevalence of breast, prostate and colorectal cancers [52–55]. In addition, there is now a well-established "U"-like shaped association between sleep duration and cancer, whereby reductions or prolongations of routine sleep patterns are fraught with increased risk for cancer-related diagnoses or adverse cancer outcomes [13–16, 19–22, 24–26, 54]. However, the potential effects of sleep fragmentation or sleep disruption, as occurs in OSA, have not been explored. To elucidate the potential effects on tumour behaviour of the type of sleep disruption that is frequently observed in OSA patients, a well-established mouse model of sleep fragmentation was employed [56]. Interestingly, application of sleep fragmentation in the context of two syngeneic murine models involving lung epithelial tumour models (TC1 and lewis lung carcinoma) resulted in a two-fold increase in tumour size when compared with sleep controls, with tumours showing markedly increased frequency of invasive features toward the surrounding tissues (fig. 2) [57]. These findings are the first clear evidence of a relationship between sleep disruption mimicking the one experienced by OSA patients and cancer, independently from IH (fig. 3).

Potential mechanisms linking OSA and cancer

Oxidative stress and inflammation

The recurrent O_2 desaturations in arterial blood are translated into P_aO_2 swings in most tissues. The hypoxia/re-oxygenation events have recently been measured in several tissues, including fat, liver, muscle, kidney, testes and cerebral cortex [58–61]. Although some long-term homeostatic responses to IH may be triggered by the oscillating changes in O_2 availability, they are also a potential and important source of reactive oxygen species (ROS). Excessive ROS production is *per se* considered a risk factor of cancer incidence since it can damage proteins, lipids and DNA [62].

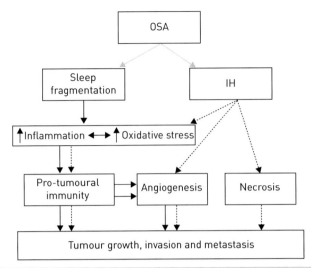

Figure 3. Flow diagram of the current mechanisms proposed for IH and sleep fragmentation on cancer outcomes.

Hypoxia inducible factor (HIF)-1 has been widely studied in OSA and cancer as a pivotal molecule in both diseases [63–66]. This transcriptional factor is composed of two subunits, one which is constitutively expressed and one which is an O_2-regulated subunit [67]. Thus, HIF-1 can be induced by hypoxia as a consequence of HIF prolyl-hydroxylase inhibition, since it uses O_2 as a co-substrate [64, 68]. In addition, the HIF family may participate in some of the processes linking IH to ROS production. For example, those involving the systemic carotid body responses to hypoxia through increases in local ROS production [65], and also through processes linked to the variable and more severe hypoxic environment within the tumour, as suggested by the presence of necrotic areas [47, 48]. Activation of the HIF family, either alone or in conjunction with several other transcriptional pathways, may promote the activation of inflammatory mechanisms or ultimately upregulate the production of downstream products involved in malignant processes within the tumour stroma, including angiogenesis and local immunity. It has also been shown that chronic inflammation is self-perpetuating, and can result in the aberrant activation of several transcriptional pathways that ultimately promote neoplastic transformation and propagation [69]. For example, sustained activation of HIF-1 acts as a regulator of pro-angiogenic genes, such as vascular endothelial growth factor (VEGF), which is also over-expressed in OSA patients [43]. In cancer, VEGF is a key molecule promoting angiogenesis and contributing to tumour growth [70, 71], and is used as a target molecule in some therapeutic strategies [72].

Another well-known redox-sensitive transcription factor is nuclear factor (NF)-κB [73]. Recurrent obstructions in the UA in a rat model of OSA elicited increases in NF-κB expression in lungs and diaphragm [74]. Once in the cell nucleus, NF-κB upregulates the transcription of inflammatory genes including TNF-α, IL-6 and IL-8, as well as other enzymes such cyclooxygenase-2 [75], all of which have been associated with malignant processes. Also, NF-κB has been reported to play an important role in HIF-1α activation, and basal NF-κB activity seems to be required for HIF-1α protein accumulation during hypoxia, both *in vitro* and *in vivo* [76]. Thus, the complex interplay of critical elements that constitutively modulate oncogenic processes can be recapitulated by the IH affecting OSA patients, thereby establishing the biological foundation for more than just a random link between cancer and OSA (fig. 3).

Role of the immune system

The recruitment of immune cells to the tumour has been linked to an exacerbated malignant phenotype [77]. Macrophages are the dominant leukocytes found in the tumour microenvironment, where they have been named tumour-associated macrophages (TAMs). During the initial phases of their recruitment to the tumour, TAMs express inflammatory molecules in response to the tumour and operate as innate immune cells fighting to eradicate the neoplastic elements. However, by virtue of their exposure to the tumour microenvironment, TAMs will alter their "antitumour" phenotype, and will begin to express other molecules facilitating tumour progression. At the two extremes of the spectrum of differentiation of TAMs, the criteria for recognition of the classically activated type 1 macrophage (M1) and the alternatively activated type 2 macrophage (M2) have been clearly established [78]. Basically, pro-inflammatory cytokines released by M1 TAMs act against tumour growth, while the angiogenic properties of M2 TAMs support tumour progression. It is likely that shifts in TAM polarity are induced by the unique characteristics of the tumour microenvironment, including hypoxia [79, 80]. Indeed, the changes induced by hypoxia on the phenotypic characteristics of TAMs include the secretion of mitogenic factors, pro-angiogenic cytokines and immunosuppressive agents [29, 81].

To ascertain the potential effects of IH on TAMs and their role in tumour behaviour, mice were exposed to either room air or IH (90 s at 6% inspiratory oxygen fraction (F_{IO_2}) followed by 21% F_{IO_2}, 20 cycles·h^{-1}) for 12 h·day^{-1}. After 2 weeks, the animals were injected with ×10^5 lung tumour cells (TC1) in the left flank. 28 days later, the mice subjected to IH displayed increased tumour growth and invasion in a similar manner as reported with melanoma cells [49]. Inmunohistological samples revealed that TAMs are a major component of the tumour cellularity, particularly in the periphery of the tumour, suggesting their potential role in the invasion of adjacent tissues. Using quantitative plasma membrane proteomics of TAMs, a reduction of some proteins involved in the interferon response and in antigen processing and presentation emerged in TAMs exposed to IH. Also, cell surface expression of CD86, CD40 (M1 markers), transferrin receptor and CD206 (M2 markers) in TAMs [82, 83] showed a shift from the M1 (antitumour) towards the M2 (pro-tumour) phenotypic spectrum. These findings were also supported by specific *in vitro* assessments. Specifically, TAMs isolated from tumours of mice exposed to IH were able to promote enhanced proliferation, migration, invasion and extravasation processes in naïve tumour cells [49].

Interestingly, similar changes were observed in the TAMs derived from normoxic mice exposed to sleep fragmentation [57]. Tumours from these mice experienced increased growth and invasiveness, as well as increases in the number of TAMs in the periphery of the tumour, along with a shift toward M2 polarisation. Also, TAMs from sleep fragmentation-exposed mice showed higher expression of Toll-like receptor (TLR)4, which seems to mediate the enhanced tumourigenesis, as revealed by the use of knockout mice targeting either TLR4 or its two major downstream signalling pathways (MYD88 and TIR-domain-containing adapter-inducing interferon-β). These findings support the importance of innate immune response on tumour growth, and its disruption by sleep fragmentation exposure. Of note, tumours from mice exposed to sleep fragmentation exhibited increased expression of matrix metalloproteinase (MMP)9 in the tumour boundaries, probably accounting for the increased invasion of surrounding tissues under sleep fragmentation conditions [57].

However, we should emphasise that the malignant properties of the tumour may also be modulated by other immune cells within and surrounding the tumour, such as lymphocytes and immune progenitor cells. As a corollary to such comment, increased recruitment of T-regulatory lymphocytes and myeloid-derived suppressor cells (MDSCs) was observed within the tumours exposed to IH [49]. Both these cells can suppress the immune and inflammatory responses, and thus support tumour growth [84–88]. In addition, the hypoxic microenvironment can modulate MDSC differentiation toward macrophages within the tumour through HIF activation [89].

Metabolic dysfunction

An increased risk for development of the metabolic syndrome has been associated with OSA in both obese adults and children [90–98]. IH can promote dyslipidaemia, which increases lipolysis within the adipose tissue in mice [99]. In addition, higher levels of leptin and adipose tissue inflammation have been observed in response to IH [100]. Adipose tissues may be a key source of inflammatory mediators in OSA due to the stronger sensitivity to inflammation observed in adipocytes in response to IH [101].

In humans, increased visceral fat deposits in OSA patients correlated with the severity of nocturnal IH [102].The increases in adipose tissue deposits are thought to induce a state of chronic low-grade inflammation [103, 104], and are associated with an increased number of macrophages in adipose tissues [105]. To explore the potential effects of sleep fragmentation in adipose tissues and metabolic function, a well-established mouse model of sleep fragmentation was employed [56, 106, 107]. C57BL/6 mice exposed to sleep fragmentation for 8 weeks showed increased weight gain (increased calorie intake in the absence of significant changes in caloric expenditure). Plasma leptin levels were elevated at the end of sleep fragmentation treatment [107]. Furthermore, abdominal magnetic resonance imaging revealed markedly enlarged visceral and subcutaneous adipose tissue depots. Evidence of systemic adipose tissue inflammation elicited by IH and characterised by increased macrophage infiltrates has also been described [108–111]. Cumulatively, IH and sleep fragmentation could act synergistically by expanding adipose tissues in the long-term, in addition to promoting a chronic state of inflammation and macrophage infiltration. In the context of obesity, adipose cells are less well oxygenated due to the expansion of the cell soma and the increase in the O_2 diffusion distance from the surrounding microvasculature. These features could be further exacerbated by the IH regime, thus activating HIF-1 [112] with a subsequent increased expression of IL-6 and leptin [113]. Therefore, both sleep fragmentation and IH can trigger components of the metabolic syndrome by modifying the structural and physiological function of adipose tissues, ultimately leading to insulin resistance, chronic inflammation and altered secretion of adipokines.

The metabolic dysfunction associated with IH or sleep fragmentation could be a potential risk of cancer and could also play a role in modulating tumour malignancy. Obesity is known to increase the risk of several types of neoplasia [114, 115] and enhances tumour growth [47, 116–118]. Although the causes of inflammation in the adipose tissue in response to IH or sleep fragmentation have not been fully delineated, the increased release of IL-6 and leptin is believed to play an important role in carcinogenesis and tumour malignancy [116, 119–121]. For instance, leptin has been considered as a potential mediator of obesity-related cancer, since it induces cancer progression through activation of PI3K, mitogen-activated protein kinase, and signal transducer and activator of transcription 3 pathways [121–123]. Additionally, circulating IL-6 has been correlated with cancer mortality [124, 125], and hypoxia can increase the adipocyte expression of MMPs and VEGF, which are crucial molecules in cancer invasion and angiogenesis [126].

Other potential and yet unexplored mechanisms

To date, the following mechanisms have been identified in the context of continuous hypoxia. Therefore, the possible effects of IH (and sleep fragmentation) still need to be thoroughly examined. However, due to the relative similarity of several of the transcriptional pathways activated by IH and sustained hypoxia, these mechanisms could participate in OSA-associated changes in tumour progression, resistance and malignancy.

Cancer stem cells

Recent studies have reported that cancer stem cells can confer increased tumour resistance to conventional cancer therapies [127], and are associated with poorer cancer prognosis [128]. Low levels of O_2 can increase the cancer stem cell fraction in tumour stroma and promote acquisition of a stem-like state [129, 130]. For example, it has been suggested that hypoxia helps to maintain cancer stem cell populations and re-programmes non-stem cells towards a more stem cell behaviour [131]. These cells can also participate in processes such as angiogenesis, *via* increased secretion of VEGF [132].

Microvesicles

Microvesicles have recently been suggested as a potential mechanism of intercellular communication promoting tumour malignancy. Microvesicles can carry membrane-bound particles such as proteins, mRNAs and microRNAs, all of which may induce changes in the expression of cancer-related regulatory genes within tumour stromal cells, as well as in host cells (*e.g.* endothelial cells). Hypoxia has been shown to increase the release of pro-angiogenic extracellular microvesicles [133–135], a phenomenon that appears to be mediated through the HIF pathway [136]. Recently, it was reported that microvesicle shedding from human breast cancer cells is increased by hypoxia, and that these microvesicles are able to increase focal adhesion formation, invasion and metastasis in non-exposed tumour cells [137].

Conclusion

Although there is increasing epidemiological evidence that OSA may increase cancer incidence and malignancy, the potential mechanisms involved in such human cohort-based observations are far from being completely understood. The deficits in knowledge are undoubtedly due, at least in part, to the vast array of mechanistic pathways involved in oncogenic processes, and similarly triggered by IH and sleep fragmentation. In this setting, both inflammation and oxidative stress seem to play a pivotal role. To date, translational research using OSA models and carried out *in vivo* and *in vitro* has confirmed that IH and sleep fragmentation increase tumour growth, invasion and metastasis. These changes seem to be mediated, at least in part, by modifications within the immune system, more specifically involving TAMs. However, further research is clearly needed to investigate the mechanisms involved in the pathogenesis of each selected aspect of cancer biology and its connection to OSA. In addition, the potential effects of IH and sleep fragmentation, the role of other immune cells and the roles of even less well-explored stromal elements, such as adipocytes, endothelial cells, cancer associated fibroblasts, cancer stem cells and microvesicles, are all *a priori* worthy research directions that should occupy the field in the years to come.

References

1. Punjabi NM. The epidemiology of adult obstructive sleep apnea. *Proc Am Thorac Soc* 2008; 5: 136–143.
2. Arnardottir ES, Mackiewicz M, Gislason T, *et al.* Molecular signatures of obstructive sleep apnea in adults: a review and perspective. *Sleep* 2009; 32: 447–470.
3. Vijayan VK. Morbidities associated with obstructive sleep apnea. *Expert Rev Respir Med* 2012; 6: 557–566.
4. Lavie L. Oxidative stress in obstructive sleep apnea and intermittent hypoxia – Revisited – the bad ugly and good: implications to the heart and brain. *Sleep Med Rev* 2014 [in press DOI: 10.1016/j.smrv.2014.07.003].
5. Chen JC, Hwang JH. Sleep apnea increased incidence of primary central nervous system cancers: a nationwide cohort study. *Sleep Med* 2014; 15: 749–754.
6. Campos-Rodriguez F, Martinez-Garcia MA, Martinez M, *et al.* Association between obstructive sleep apnea and cancer incidence in a large multicenter Spanish cohort. *Am J Respir Crit Care Med* 2013; 187: 99–105.
7. Marshall NS, Wong KK, Cullen SR, *et al.* Sleep apnea and 20-year follow-up for all-cause mortality, stroke, and cancer incidence and mortality in the busselton health study cohort. *J Clin Sleep Med* 2014; 10: 355–362.
8. Martinez-Garcia MA, Martorell-Calatayud A, Nagore E, *et al.* Association between sleep disordered breathing and aggressiveness markers of malignant cutaneous melanoma. *Eur Respir J* 2014; 43: 1661–1668.
9. Nieto FJ, Peppard PE, Young T, *et al.* Sleep-disordered breathing and cancer mortality: results from the Wisconsin Sleep Cohort Study. *Am J Respir Crit Care Med* 2012; 186: 190–194.
10. Lee SL, Rouhi P, Dahl JL, *et al.* Hypoxia-induced pathological angiogenesis mediates tumor cell dissemination, invasion, and metastasis in a zebrafish tumor model. *Proc Natl Acad Sci USA* 2009; 106: 19485–19490.
11. Rofstad EK, Gaustad JV, Egeland TA, *et al.* Tumors exposed to acute cyclic hypoxic stress show enhanced angiogenesis, perfusion and metastatic dissemination. *Int J Cancer* 2010; 127: 1535–1546.
12. Chang WP, Liu ME, Chang WC, *et al.* Sleep apnea and the subsequent risk of breast cancer in women: a nationwide population-based cohort study. *Sleep Med* 2014; 15: 1016–1020.
13. Verkasalo PK, Lillberg K, Stevens RG, *et al.* Sleep duration and breast cancer: a prospective cohort study. *Cancer Res* 2005; 65: 9595–9600.
14. Pinheiro SP, Schernhammer ES, Tworoger SS, *et al.* A prospective study on habitual duration of sleep and incidence of breast cancer in a large cohort of women. *Cancer Res* 2006; 66: 5521–5525.
15. McElroy JA, Newcomb PA, Titus-Ernstoff L, *et al.* Duration of sleep and breast cancer risk in a large population-based case-control study. *J Sleep Res* 2006; 15: 241–249.
16. Kakizaki M, Kuriyama S, Sone T, *et al.* Sleep duration and the risk of breast cancer: the Ohsaki Cohort Study. *Br J Cancer* 2008; 99: 1502–1505.
17. Kakizaki M, Inoue K, Kuriyama S, *et al.* Sleep duration and the risk of prostate cancer: the Ohsaki Cohort Study. *Br J Cancer* 2008; 99: 176–178.
18. Vogtmann E, Levitan EB, Hale L, *et al.* Association between sleep and breast cancer incidence among postmenopausal women in the Women's Health Initiative. *Sleep* 2013; 36: 1437–1444.
19. Jiao L, Duan Z, Sangi-Haghpeykar H, *et al.* Sleep duration and incidence of colorectal cancer in postmenopausal women. *Br J Cancer* 2013; 108: 213–221.
20. Zhang X, Giovannucci EL, Wu K, *et al.* Associations of self-reported sleep duration and snoring with colorectal cancer risk in men and women. *Sleep* 2013; 36: 681–688.
21. Patel SR, Ayas NT, Malhotra MR, *et al.* A prospective study of sleep duration and mortality risk in women. *Sleep* 2004; 27: 440–444.
22. Kripke DF, Garfinkel L, Wingard DL, *et al.* Mortality associated with sleep duration and insomnia. *Arch Gen Psychiatry* 2002; 59: 131–136.
23. Kripke DF, Langer RD, Elliott JA, *et al.* Mortality related to actigraphic long and short sleep. *Sleep Med* 2011; 12: 28–33.
24. Gallicchio L, Kalesan B. Sleep duration and mortality: a systematic review and meta-analysis. *J Sleep Res* 2009; 18: 148–158.
25. Ikehara S, Iso H, Date C, *et al.* Association of sleep duration with mortality from cardiovascular disease and other causes for Japanese men and women: the JACC study. *Sleep* 2009; 32: 295–301.

26. Thompson CL, Larkin EK, Patel S, *et al.* Short duration of sleep increases risk of colorectal adenoma. *Cancer* 2011; 117: 841–847.

27. Gharib SA, Seiger AN, Hayes AL, *et al.* Treatment of obstructive sleep apnea alters cancer-associated transcriptional signatures in circulating leukocytes. *Sleep* 2014; 37: 709–714.

28. Liu Y, Song X, Wang X, *et al.* Effect of chronic intermittent hypoxia on biological behavior and hypoxia-associated gene expression in lung cancer cells. *J Cell Biochem* 2010; 111: 554–563.

29. Lewis C, Murdoch C. Macrophage responses to hypoxia: implications for tumor progression and anti-cancer therapies. *Am J Pathol* 2005; 167: 627–635.

30. Semenza GL. Hypoxia-inducible factors: mediators of cancer progression and targets for cancer therapy. *Trends Pharmacol Sci* 2012; 33: 207–214.

31. Rofstad EK, Galappathi K, Mathiesen B, *et al.* Fluctuating and diffusion-limited hypoxia in hypoxia-induced metastasis. *Clin Cancer Res* 2007; 13: 1971–1978.

32. Kimura H, Braun RD, Ong ET, *et al.* Fluctuations in red cell flux in tumor microvessels can lead to transient hypoxia and reoxygenation in tumor parenchyma. *Cancer Res* 1996; 56: 5522–5528.

33. Dewhirst MW, Kimura H, Rehmus SW, *et al.* Microvascular studies on the origins of perfusion-limited hypoxia. *Br J Cancer Suppl* 1996; 27: S247–S251.

34. Brurberg KG, Benjaminsen IC, Dorum LM, *et al.* Fluctuations in tumor blood perfusion assessed by dynamic contrast-enhanced MRI. *Magn Reson Med* 2007; 58: 473–481.

35. Matsumoto S, Yasui H, Mitchell JB, *et al.* Imaging cycling tumor hypoxia. *Cancer Res* 2010; 70: 10019–10023.

36. Dewhirst MW, Cao Y, Moeller B. Cycling hypoxia and free radicals regulate angiogenesis and radiotherapy response. *Nat Rev Cancer* 2008; 8: 425–437.

37. Toffoli S, Michiels C. Intermittent hypoxia is a key regulator of cancer cell and endothelial cell interplay in tumours. *FEBS J* 2008; 275: 2991–3002.

38. Cairns RA, Kalliomaki T, Hill RP. Acute (cyclic) hypoxia enhances spontaneous metastasis of KHT murine tumors. *Cancer Res* 2001; 61: 8903–8908.

39. Martinive P, Defresne F, Bouzin C, *et al.* Preconditioning of the tumor vasculature and tumor cells by intermittent hypoxia: implications for anticancer therapies. *Cancer Res* 2006; 66: 11736–11744.

40. Almendros I, Wang Y, Gozal D. The polymorphic and contradictory aspects of intermittent hypoxia. *Am J Physiol Lung Cell Mol Physiol* 2014; 307: L129–L140.

41. Lavie L. Intermittent hypoxia: the culprit of oxidative stress, vascular inflammation and dyslipidemia in obstructive sleep apnea. *Expert Rev Respir Med* 2008; 2: 75–84.

42. Gozal D, Kheirandish-Gozal L, Bhattacharjee R, *et al.* C-reactive protein and obstructive sleep apnea syndrome in children. *Front Biosci (Elite Ed)* 2012; 4: 2410–2422.

43. Gozal D, Lipton AJ, Jones KL. Circulating vascular endothelial growth factor levels in patients with obstructive sleep apnea. *Sleep* 2002; 25: 59–65.

44. Hakim F, Wang Y, Zhang S, *et al.* Toll-Like Receptor 4 (TLR4) signaling in Tc1 cell tumor accelerated growth induced by chronic sleep disruption (SD) in mice. *Am J Respir Crit Care Med* 2013; 187: A2300.

45. Lurie A. Inflammation, oxidative stress, and procoagulant and thrombotic activity in adults with obstructive sleep apnea. *Adv Cardiol* 2011; 46: 43–66.

46. Lin QC, Chen LD, Yu YH, *et al.* Obstructive sleep apnea syndrome is associated with metabolic syndrome and inflammation. *Eur Arch Otorhinolaryngol* 2014; 271: 825–831.

47. Almendros I, Montserrat JM, Torres M, *et al.* Obesity and intermittent hypoxia increase tumor growth in a mouse model of sleep apnea. *Sleep Med* 2012; 13: 1254–1260.

48. Almendros I, Montserrat JM, Ramirez J, *et al.* Intermittent hypoxia enhances cancer progression in a mouse model of sleep apnoea. *Eur Respir J* 2012; 39: 215–217.

49. Almendros I, Wang Y, Becker L, *et al.* Intermittent hypoxia-induced changes in tumor-associated macrophages and tumor malignancy in a mouse model of sleep apnea. *Am J Respir Crit Care Med* 2014; 189: 593–601.

50. Almendros I, Montserrat JM, Torres M, *et al.* Intermittent hypoxia increases melanoma metastasis to the lung in a mouse model of sleep apnea. *Respir Physiol Neurobiol* 2013; 186: 303–307.

51. Eubank T, Sherwani S, Peters S, *et al.* Intermittent hypoxia augments melanoma tumor metastases in a mouse model of sleep apnea. *Am J Respir Crit Care Med* 2013; 187: A2302.

52. Truong T, Liquet B, Menegaux F, *et al.* Breast cancer risk, nightwork, and circadian clock gene polymorphisms. *Endocr Relat Cancer* 2014; 21: 629–638.

53. Stevens RG, Brainard GC, Blask DE, *et al.* Breast cancer and circadian disruption from electric lighting in the modern world. *CA Cancer J Clin* 2014; 64: 207–218.

54. Gapstur SM, Diver WR, Stevens VL, *et al.* Work schedule, sleep duration, insomnia, and risk of fatal prostate cancer. *Am J Prev Med* 2014; 46: Suppl. 1, S26–S33.

55. Schernhammer ES, Laden F, Speizer FE, *et al.* Night-shift work and risk of colorectal cancer in the nurses' health study. *J Natl Cancer Inst* 2003; 95: 825–828.

56. Ramesh V, Nair D, Zhang SX, *et al.* Disrupted sleep without sleep curtailment induces sleepiness and cognitive dysfunction *via* the tumor necrosis factor-α pathway. *J Neuroinflammation* 2012; 9: 91.

57. Hakim F, Wang Y, Zhang SX, *et al.* Fragmented sleep accelerates tumor growth and progression through recruitment of tumor-associated macrophages and TLR4 signaling. *Cancer Res* 2014; 74: 1329–1337.

58. Almendros I, Montserrat JM, Torres M, *et al.* Changes in oxygen partial pressure of brain tissue in an animal model of obstructive apnea. *Respir Res* 2010; 11: 3.

59. Almendros I, Farre R, Planas AM, *et al.* Tissue oxygenation in brain, muscle, and fat in a rat model of sleep apnea: differential effect of obstructive apneas and intermittent hypoxia. *Sleep* 2011; 34: 1127–1133.

60. Dalmases M, Torres M, Marquez-Kisinousky L, *et al.* Brain tissue hypoxia and oxidative stress induced by obstructive apneas is different in young and aged rats. *Sleep* 2014; 37: 1249–1256.

61. Torres M, Laguna-Barraza R, Dalmases M, *et al.* Male fertility is reduced by chronic intermittent hypoxia mimicking sleep apnea in mice. *Sleep* 2014; 37: 1757–1765.

62. Marnett LJ. Oxyradicals and DNA damage. *Carcinogenesis* 2000; 21: 361–370.

63. Semenza GL, Prabhakar NR. HIF-1-dependent respiratory, cardiovascular, and redox responses to chronic intermittent hypoxia. *Antioxid Redox Signal* 2007; 9: 1391–1396.

64. Yuan G, Nanduri J, Khan S, *et al.* Induction of HIF-1α expression by intermittent hypoxia: involvement of NADPH oxidase, Ca^{2+} signaling, prolyl hydroxylases, and mTOR. *J Cell Physiol* 2008; 217: 674–685.

65. Peng YJ, Yuan G, Ramakrishnan D, *et al.* Heterozygous HIF-1α deficiency impairs carotid body-mediated systemic responses and reactive oxygen species generation in mice exposed to intermittent hypoxia. *J Physiol* 2006; 577: 705–716.

66. Semenza GL. HIF-1 mediates metabolic responses to intratumoral hypoxia and oncogenic mutations. *J Clin Invest* 2013; 123: 3664–3671.

67. Wang GL, Jiang BH, Rue EA, *et al.* Hypoxia-inducible factor 1 is a basic-helix-loop-helix-PAS heterodimer regulated by cellular O$_2$ tension. *Proc Natl Acad Sci USA* 1995; 92: 5510–5514.

68. Coleman ML, Ratcliffe PJ. Oxygen sensing and hypoxia-induced responses. *Essays Biochem* 2007; 43: 1–15.

69. Bartsch H, Nair J. Chronic inflammation and oxidative stress in the genesis and perpetuation of cancer: role of lipid peroxidation, DNA damage, and repair. *Langenbecks Arch Surg* 2006; 391: 499–510.

70. Eltzschig HK, Carmeliet P. Hypoxia and inflammation. *N Engl J Med* 2011; 364: 656–665.

71. Mittal K, Ebos J, Rini B. Angiogenesis and the tumor microenvironment: vascular endothelial growth factor and beyond. *Semin Oncol* 2014; 41: 235–251.

72. Mittal K, Koon H, Elson P, *et al.* Dual VEGF/VEGFR inhibition in advanced solid malignancies: clinical effects and pharmacodynamic biomarkers. *Cancer Biol Ther* 2014; 15: 975–981.

73. Lavie L. Sleep-disordered breathing and cerebrovascular disease: a mechanistic approach. *Neurol Clin* 2005; 23: 1059–1075.

74. Nacher M, Farre R, Montserrat JM, *et al.* Biological consequences of oxygen desaturation and respiratory effort in an acute animal model of obstructive sleep apnea (OSA). *Sleep Med* 2009; 10: 892–897.

75. Lim JW, Kim H, Kim KH. Nuclear factor-κB regulates cyclooxygenase-2 expression and cell proliferation in human gastric cancer cells. *Lab Invest* 2001; 81: 349–360.

76. Rius J, Guma M, Schachtrup C, *et al.* NF-κB links innate immunity to the hypoxic response through transcriptional regulation of HIF-1α. *Nature* 2008; 453: 807–811.

77. Gozal D, Almendros I, Hakim F. Sleep apnea awakens cancer: a unifying immunological hypothesis. *Oncoimmunology* 2014; 3: e28326.

78. Solinas G, Germano G, Mantovani A, *et al.* Tumor-associated macrophages (TAM) as major players of the cancer-related inflammation. *J Leukoc Biol* 2009; 86: 1065–1073.

79. Ruffell B, Affara NI, Coussens LM. Differential macrophage programming in the tumor microenvironment. *Trends Immunol* 2012; 33: 119–126.

80. Murdoch C, Lewis CE. Macrophage migration and gene expression in response to tumor hypoxia. *Int J Cancer* 2005; 117: 701–708.

81. Obeid E, Nanda R, Fu YX, *et al.* The role of tumor-associated macrophages in breast cancer progression (review). *Int J Oncol* 2013; 43: 5–12.

82. Becker L, Liu NC, Averill MM, *et al.* Unique proteomic signatures distinguish macrophages and dendritic cells. *PLoS One* 2012; 7: e33297.

83. Kadl A, Meher AK, Sharma PR, *et al.* Identification of a novel macrophage phenotype that develops in response to atherogenic phospholipids *via* Nrf2. *Circ Res* 2010; 107: 737–746.

84. Gabrilovich DI, Nagaraj S. Myeloid-derived suppressor cells as regulators of the immune system. *Nat Rev Immunol* 2009; 9: 162–174.

85. Wilke CM, Wu K, Zhao E, *et al.* Prognostic significance of regulatory T cells in tumor. *Int J Cancer* 2010; 127: 748–758.

86. Oleinika K, Nibbs RJ, Graham GJ, *et al.* Suppression, subversion and escape: the role of regulatory T cells in cancer progression. *Clin Exp Immunol* 2013; 171: 36–45.

87.   Lindau D, Gielen P, Kroesen M, *et al.* The immunosuppressive tumour network: myeloid-derived suppressor cells, regulatory T cells and natural killer T cells. *Immunology* 2013; 138: 105–115.

88.   Deng B, Zhu JM, Wang Y, *et al.* Intratumor hypoxia promotes immune tolerance by inducing regulatory T cells *via* TGF-β1 in gastric cancer. *PLoS One* 2013; 8: e63777.

89.   Corzo CA, Condamine T, Lu L, *et al.* HIF-1α regulates function and differentiation of myeloid-derived suppressor cells in the tumor microenvironment. *J Exp Med* 2010; 207: 2439–2453.

90.   Nannapaneni S, Ramar K, Surani S. Effect of obstructive sleep apnea on type 2 diabetes mellitus: a comprehensive literature review. *World J Diabetes* 2013; 4: 238–244.

91.   Coughlin SR, Mawdsley L, Mugarza JA, *et al.* Obstructive sleep apnoea is independently associated with an increased prevalence of metabolic syndrome. *Eur Heart J* 2004; 25: 735–741.

92.   Peled N, Kassirer M, Shitrit D, *et al.* The association of OSA with insulin resistance, inflammation and metabolic syndrome. *Respir Med* 2007; 101: 1696–1701.

93.   Tkacova R, Dorkova Z, Molcanyiova A, *et al.* Cardiovascular risk and insulin resistance in patients with obstructive sleep apnea. *Med Sci Monit* 2008; 14: CR438–CR444.

94.   Bonsignore MR, Borel AL, Machan E, *et al.* Sleep apnoea and metabolic dysfunction. *Eur Respir Rev* 2013; 22: 353–364.

95.   Gozal D, Capdevila OS, Kheirandish-Gozal L. Metabolic alterations and systemic inflammation in obstructive sleep apnea among nonobese and obese prepubertal children. *Am J Respir Crit Care Med* 2008; 177: 1142–1149.

96.   Ryan S, Crinion SJ, McNicholas WT. Obesity and sleep-disordered breathing – when two "bad guys" meet. *QJM* 2014; 107: 949–954.

97.   Drager LF, Togeiro SM, Polotsky VY, *et al.* Obstructive sleep apnea: a cardiometabolic risk in obesity and the metabolic syndrome. *J Am Coll Cardiol* 2013; 62: 569–576.

98.   Trzepizur W, Le Vaillant M, Meslier N, *et al.* Independent association between nocturnal intermittent hypoxemia and metabolic dyslipidemia. *Chest* 2013; 143: 1584–1589.

99.   Drager LF, Jun JC, Polotsky VY. Metabolic consequences of intermittent hypoxia: relevance to obstructive sleep apnea. *Best Pract Res Clin Endocrinol Metab* 2010; 24: 843–851.

100. Reinke C, Bevans-Fonti S, Drager LF, *et al.* Effects of different acute hypoxic regimens on tissue oxygen profiles and metabolic outcomes. *J Appl Physiol (1985)* 2011; 111: 881–890.

101. Taylor CT, Kent BD, Crinion SJ, *et al.* Human adipocytes are highly sensitive to intermittent hypoxia induced NF-κB activity and subsequent inflammatory gene expression. *Biochem Biophys Res Commun* 2014; 447: 660–665.

102. Vgontzas AN, Papanicolaou DA, Bixler EO, *et al.* Sleep apnea and daytime sleepiness and fatigue: relation to visceral obesity, insulin resistance, and hypercytokinemia. *J Clin Endocrinol Metab* 2000; 85: 1151–1158.

103. Bullo M, Garcia-Lorda P, Megias I, *et al.* Systemic inflammation, adipose tissue tumor necrosis factor, and leptin expression. *Obes Res* 2003; 11: 525–531.

104. Ramos EJ, Xu Y, Romanova I, *et al.* Is obesity an inflammatory disease? *Surgery* 2003; 134: 329–335.

105. Weisberg SP, McCann D, Desai M, *et al.* Obesity is associated with macrophage accumulation in adipose tissue. *J Clin Invest* 2003; 112: 1796–1808.

106. Nair D, Zhang SX, Ramesh V, *et al.* Sleep fragmentation induces cognitive deficits *via* nicotinamide adenine dinucleotide phosphate oxidase-dependent pathways in mouse. *Am J Respir Crit Care Med* 2011; 184: 1305–1312.

107. Wang Y, Carreras A, Lee S, *et al.* Chronic sleep fragmentation promotes obesity in young adult mice. *Obesity (Silver Spring)* 2014; 22: 758–762.

108. Fujisaka S, Usui I, Ikutani M, *et al.* Adipose tissue hypoxia induces inflammatory M1 polarity of macrophages in an HIF-1α-dependent and HIF-1α-independent manner in obese mice. *Diabetologia* 2013; 56: 1403–1412.

109. Gharib SA, Khalyfa A, Abdelkarim A, *et al.* Intermittent hypoxia activates temporally coordinated transcriptional programs in visceral adipose tissue. *J Mol Med (Berl)* 2012; 90: 435–445.

110. van den Borst B, Schols AM, de Theije C, *et al.* Characterization of the inflammatory and metabolic profile of adipose tissue in a mouse model of chronic hypoxia. *J Appl Physiol (1985)* 2013; 114: 1619–1628.

111. Poulain L, Thomas A, Rieusset J, *et al.* Visceral white fat remodelling contributes to intermittent hypoxia-induced atherogenesis. *Eur Respir J* 2014; 43: 513–522.

112. Neels JG, Olefsky JM. Inflamed fat: what starts the fire? *J Clin Invest* 2006; 116: 33–35.

113. Wang B, Wood IS, Trayhurn P. Dysregulation of the expression and secretion of inflammation-related adipokines by hypoxia in human adipocytes. *Pflugers Arch* 2007; 455: 479–492.

114. Renehan AG, Tyson M, Egger M, *et al.* Body-mass index and incidence of cancer: a systematic review and meta-analysis of prospective observational studies. *Lancet* 2008; 371: 569–578.

115. Renehan AG, Roberts DL, Dive C. Obesity and cancer: pathophysiological and biological mechanisms. *Arch Physiol Biochem* 2008; 114: 71–83.

116. Brandon EL, Gu JW, Cantwell L, *et al.* Obesity promotes melanoma tumor growth: role of leptin. *Cancer Biol Ther* 2009; 8: 1871–1879.

117. Kanasaki K, Koya D. Biology of obesity: lessons from animal models of obesity. *J Biomed Biotechnol* 2011; 2011: 197636.

118. van Kruijsdijk RC, van der Wall E, Visseren FL. Obesity and cancer: the role of dysfunctional adipose tissue. *Cancer Epidemiol Biomarkers Prev* 2009; 18: 2569–2578.

119. Chang Q, Daly L, Bromberg J. The IL-6 feed-forward loop: a driver of tumorigenesis. *Semin Immunol* 2014; 26: 48–53.

120. Che Q, Liu BY, Wang FY, *et al.* Interleukin 6 promotes endometrial cancer growth through an autocrine feedback loop involving ERK-NF-κB signaling pathway. *Biochem Biophys Res Commun* 2014; 446: 167–172.

121. Jaffe T, Schwartz B. Leptin promotes motility and invasiveness in human colon cancer cells by activating multiple signal-transduction pathways. *Int J Cancer* 2008; 123: 2543–2556.

122. Chen J. Multiple signal pathways in obesity-associated cancer. *Obes Rev* 2011; 12: 1063–1070.

123. Gao J, Tian J, Lv Y, *et al.* Leptin induces functional activation of cyclooxygenase-2 through JAK2/STAT3, MAPK/ ERK, and PI3 K/AKT pathways in human endometrial cancer cells. *Cancer Sci* 2009; 100: 389–395.

124. Il'yasova D, Colbert LH, Harris TB, *et al.* Circulating levels of inflammatory markers and cancer risk in the health aging and body composition cohort. *Cancer Epidemiol Biomarkers Prev* 2005; 14: 2413–2418.

125. Kim S, Keku TO, Martin C, *et al.* Circulating levels of inflammatory cytokines and risk of colorectal adenomas. *Cancer Res* 2008; 68: 323–328.

126. Lolmede K, Durand de SFV, Galitzky J, *et al.* Effects of hypoxia on the expression of proangiogenic factors in differentiated 3T3-F442A adipocytes. *Int J Obes Relat Metab Disord* 2003; 27: 1187–1195.

127. Cojoc M, Mabert K, Muders MH, *et al.* A role for cancer stem cells in therapy resistance: cellular and molecular mechanisms. *Semin Cancer Biol* 2014 [in press DOI: 10.1016/j.semcancer.2014.06.004].

128. Li M, Zhang B, Zhang Z, *et al.* Stem cell-like circulating tumor cells indicate poor prognosis in gastric cancer. *Biomed Res Int* 2014; 2014: 981261.

129. Soeda A, Park M, Lee D, *et al.* Hypoxia promotes expansion of the CD133-positive glioma stem cells through activation of HIF-1α. *Oncogene* 2009; 28: 3949–3959.

130. Keith B, Simon MC. Hypoxia-inducible factors, stem cells, and cancer. *Cell* 2007; 129: 465–472.

131. Heddleston JM, Li Z, McLendon RE, *et al.* The hypoxic microenvironment maintains glioblastoma stem cells and promotes reprogramming towards a cancer stem cell phenotype. *Cell Cycle* 2009; 8: 3274–3284.

132. Eyler CE, Foo WC, LaFiura KM, *et al.* Brain cancer stem cells display preferential sensitivity to Akt inhibition. *Stem Cells* 2008; 26: 3027–3036.

133. Park JE, Tan HS, Datta A, *et al.* Hypoxic tumor cell modulates its microenvironment to enhance angiogenic and metastatic potential by secretion of proteins and exosomes. *Mol Cell Proteomics* 2010; 9: 1085–1099.

134. Svensson KJ, Kucharzewska P, Christianson HC, *et al.* Hypoxia triggers a proangiogenic pathway involving cancer cell microvesicles and PAR-2-mediated heparin-binding EGF signaling in endothelial cells. *Proc Natl Acad Sci USA* 2011; 108: 13147–13152.

135. Kucharzewska P, Christianson HC, Welch JE, *et al.* Exosomes reflect the hypoxic status of glioma cells and mediate hypoxia-dependent activation of vascular cells during tumor development. *Proc Natl Acad Sci USA* 2013; 110: 7312–7317.

136. King HW, Michael MZ, Gleadle JM. Hypoxic enhancement of exosome release by breast cancer cells. *BMC Cancer* 2012; 12: 421.

137. Wang T, Gilkes DM, Takano N, *et al.* Hypoxia-inducible factors and RAB22A mediate formation of microvesicles that stimulate breast cancer invasion and metastasis. *Proc Natl Acad Sci USA* 2014; 111: E3234–E3242.

Support statement: I. Almendros is supported by a Beatriu de Pinós fellowship from Generalitat de Catalunya (2010 BP_A2 00023). D. Gozal is supported by a National Institutes of Health grant (HL-65270). R. Farré is supported by a Ministerio de Ciencia y Competitividad grant (SAF2011-22576).

Disclosures: None declared.

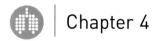

Chapter 4

Cardiovascular disease: pathophysiological mechanisms

Manuel Sánchez-de-la-Torre[1,2], Maria R. Bonsignore[3,4] and Ferran Barbé[1,2]

OSA is a common disease that affects approximately 10% of the middle-aged population and becomes more prevalent with age. It is caused by intermittent and repetitive collapse of the UA during sleep. The main acute physiological consequences of OSA are oxygen desaturation, intrathoracic pressure changes and arousals. OSA is associated with significant cardiovascular morbidity and mortality and is an independent risk factor for CVD. The pathogenesis of CVD in OSA is not completely understood but is likely to be multifactorial, involving a diverse range of closely interrelated and detrimental intermediate mechanisms that predispose patients to atherosclerosis, including oxidative stress, sympathetic activation, inflammation, hypercoagulability, endothelial dysfunction and metabolic dysregulation. IH is considered to lead to increased oxidative stress, systemic inflammation and sympathetic stimulation. Despite the existence of these detrimental mechanisms, there are epidemiological studies that suggest that some protective mechanisms could also be activated in OSA patients. This chapter describes the underlying mechanisms linking OSA with CVD.

OSA has been associated with significant cardiovascular morbidity and mortality and seems to be an independent risk factor for CVD [1, 2]. It should be suspected in hypertensive individuals, especially those with resistant hypertension [3]. Additionally, OSA appears to be associated with stroke [4]. In patients with OSA, CPAP treatment reduces BP, and its effects are related to compliance and baseline BP [3, 5–7].

Underlying mechanisms linking OSA with CVD

The pathogenesis of CVD in OSA is not completely understood but is likely to be multifactorial, involving a diverse range of intermediate mechanisms that predispose patients to atherosclerosis, including oxidative stress, sympathetic activation, inflammation, hypercoagulability, endothelial dysfunction and metabolic dysregulation. Nevertheless, the mechanisms underlying the initiation and aggravation of CVD in OSA have not been fully

[1]Respiratory Dept, Hospital Universitari Arnau de Vilanova and Santa Maria, IRB Lleida, Lleida, Spain. [2]Centro de Investigación Biomédica en Red de Enfermedades Respiratorias (CIBERES), Madrid, Spain. [3]Biomedical Dept of Internal and Specialistic Medicine (DiBiMIS), Cardio-Respiratory Section, University of Palermo, Palermo, Italy. [4]Institute of Biomedicine and Molecular Immunology (IBIM), National Research Council (CNR), Palermo, Italy.

Correspondence: Ferran Barbé, Respiratory Dept, Hospital Univ Arnau de Vilanova, Rovira Roure 80, 25198 Lleida, Spain. E-mail: febarbe.lleida.ics@gencat.cat

elucidated. All these are closely interrelated and manifest simultaneously, linking physiological consequences of OSA with CVD (fig. 1).

Oxidative stress

Oxidative stress is defined as an imbalance between oxidant and antioxidant systems (redox status imbalance). It results in an excessive production of reactive oxygen species (ROS) that can react with and cause damage to lipids, proteins and nucleic acids, which is the pathogenic basis of age-related and chronic diseases such as cancer, CVD, diabetes, chronic inflammation and neurodegenerative disorders. Low or moderate concentrations of ROS act in vital signalling pathways that are essential for repair and survival. Nevertheless, in high quantities, ROS promote inflammation and injury. The hypothesis that IH causes oxidative stress stems from observations that hypoxia and reoxygenation injury triggers an increase in ROS production, mainly during the restoration of tissue oxygenation [8, 9]. Mitochondrial dysfunction is the major source of ROS during ischaemia/reperfusion-associated morbidities.

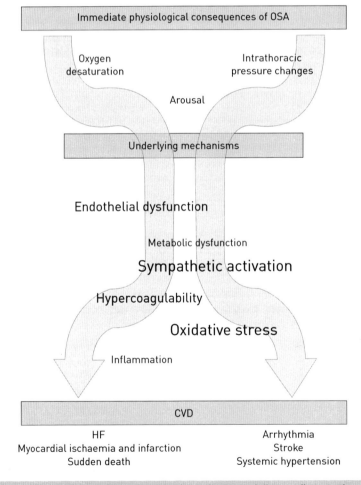

Figure 1. OSA consequences and underlying mechanisms that potentially contribute to the risk of CVD. The main acute physiological consequences of OSA are oxygen desaturation, intrathoracic pressure changes and arousals. Several intermediate mechanisms link OSA with the initiation and progression of CVD. Text size reflects the degree of evidence for the association of the intermediate mechanisms.

Thus, mitochondria are considered a potential target for cardioprotection in acute myocardial ischaemia. Studies conducted on cells in culture, in animal models mimicking OSA and in patients with OSA suggest that IH induces mitochondrial dysfunction, thereby increasing oxidative stress [10, 11].

In the last few years, numerous studies have been performed that implicate oxidative stress in OSA, with the majority of these studies providing indirect evidence based on various markers related to oxidative stress. In a mouse model of OSA consisting of the exposure of the animals to IH, IH caused tissue-specific oxidative stress related to the hypoxic intensity [12]. Additionally, in an animal model, IH exposure causes increased apoptosis of pancreatic β-cells, indicating a critical role of oxidative stress in the regulation of apoptosis. Additionally, antioxidant pre-treatment significantly decreased IH-mediated β-cell apoptosis [13].

Observational and interventional clinical studies have evaluated the effect of IH in oxidative stress in OSA patients, and the majority of the studies that evaluate CPAP treatment show a significant decrease in oxidative stress and an increase in antioxidant capacity. Non-RCTs in patients with OSA have shown increased ROS production in monocyte and granulocyte subpopulations [14], increased isoprostane concentration in exhaled condensate [15], and increased serum malondialdehyde [16] and neutrophil superoxide production [17]. Several authors have reported that CPAP treatment reduces markers of oxidative stress in the saliva, serum and urine [16–22]. Additionally, in children with moderate-to-severe OSA, increased hydrogen peroxide levels have been recently reported in morning exhaled breath condensate [23], which is an indirect index of altered redox status in the respiratory tract. OSA in children was also shown to be associated with increased lipid peroxidation [24].

In addition to the increased ROS production, some researchers have suggested that sleep apnoea might enhance oxidative stress by reducing the antioxidant capacity of the blood [25]. Total antioxidant capacity in OSA was reported to be decreased compared with controls, and low levels of vitamins A and E and of superoxide dismutase were also described [26–29].

The degree of oxidative stress in patients with OSA varies and is uncommon in patients with no comorbidities [14]. Additionally, sex-related differences in susceptibility to oxidative stress have been noted; in experimentally induced oxidative brain injuries in mice, pre-menopausal females had greater protection than age-matched males or ovariectomised age-matched females [30]. This sex-related susceptibility may be related to differences in cardiovascular morbidity associated with OSA. For a comprehensive review of the relationship between oxidative stress and OSA, we strongly recommend the review published by Lavie [9].

Inflammation

The role of inflammation in the development of atherosclerosis is well established, and chronic inflammation has been closely related to the formation and progression of atherosclerosis [31]. ROS and oxidative stress have been implicated in inflammation, and a great number of transcription factors and signalling pathways are modulated by ROS.

OSA seems to be associated with local and systemic inflammation. Snoring in OSA patients could promote local inflammation, by triggering vibration frequencies associated with soft-tissue damage. Histological analysis of tissues from OSA patients undergoing uvulopalatopharyngoplasty showed substantial subepithelial oedema, excessive plasma cell infiltration and reduction in the surface area of connective tissue papillae, which provide anchorage for the epithelium. Polymorphonuclear leukocytes were also increased in nasal lavage fluid of patients with OSA, compared with people without OSA [32]. Additionally, chronic IH induces local inflammation of the rat carotid body *via* functional upregulation of pro-inflammatory cytokine pathways [33]. A recent study demonstrates that in an animal model, OSA induces the development of atrial fibrosis, which may be accounted for by either systemic or local inflammation, or both [34].

The application of IH by modifying oxygen concentration in breathed gas, which is the most widely used model in OSA, is able to induce systemic inflammation. Some settings used in animal models in addition to IH have allowed the application of increased negative intrathoracic pressure swings [35]. These increased inspiratory efforts aggravate the early local inflammatory response triggered by IH alone.

In addition to local inflammation, systemic inflammation is observed in patients with OSA. The activation of redox-sensitive gene expression is suggested by an increase in specific protein products, including inflammatory cytokines. This implies the participation of transcription factors, such as hypoxia-inducible factor-1, activator protein-1 and nuclear factor (NF)-κB. NF-κB is one of the key regulators of inflammation, the immune response and cell survival. Several NF-κB-dependent cytokines are elevated in OSA, mainly inflammatory markers, matrix metalloproteinases and acute phase proteins, as well as endothelial adhesion molecules and vascular cell adhesion molecules [36–40]. NF-κB is highly activated in patients with OSA compared with healthy controls, and CPAP treatment reduces NF-κB activation [31]. Additionally, it has been recently reported that the platelet–lymphocyte ratio, a biomarker of inflammation, is strongly associated with the severity of OSA and CVD in OSA patients [41]. The effect of CPAP treatment on biomarkers of inflammation has been evaluated: CPAP treatment lowered TNF-α and markers of acute inflammation [42], while other inflammatory markers appeared unaffected [43]. Also, no significant difference was found in C-reactive protein, a well-documented inflammatory protein, after CPAP treatment. Other studies did not find any impact of short-term CPAP on inflammatory biomarker concentrations before and after sleep [44]. Recently reported data from the MOSAIC (Multi-centre Obstructive Sleep Apnoea Interventional Cardiovascular) randomised trial, which evaluated the effect of 6 months of CPAP treatment in patients with minimally symptomatic OSA, showed that CPAP did not change any of the markers of systemic inflammation [45].

Obesity is the most common comorbidity and is present in more than half of OSA patients. Adipokines are involved in a range of processes, including immunity and inflammation [46], and several studies have shown that patients with OSA have higher concentrations of pro-inflammatory adipokines than patients without OSA [47]. Pro-inflammatory adipokines seem to contribute substantially to the inflammatory state of obese patients. Obesity is considered a chronic inflammatory condition in itself, and it might be the most important confounding factor in the association between sleep apnoea and inflammation. In fact, it was reported that obesity had a strong association with C-reactive protein but not with OSA [48]. A randomised trial reported no improvement in inflammatory markers after CPAP treatment [49].

Finally, the inflammatory effect of IH is modulated by oestrogens, suggesting sex-related differences in the impact of IH on inflammation [50].

Endothelial dysfunction

The relationship between endothelial dysfunction and CVD is well established. The vascular endothelium is a biologically active, cellular monolayer that lines the entire internal vasculature compartment at the interface between blood and the vessel wall. The vascular endothelium is intimately involved in controlling vasomotor tone and is the main regulator of vascular haemostasis. The endothelium continuously adjusts the balance between vasoconstriction and vasodilatation; if this balance is tilted towards vasoconstriction, endothelial dysfunction occurs, causing damage to the arterial wall. The healthy endothelium produces nitric oxide and is anti-atherogenic through the following mechanisms: favourable paracrine effects on vasodilation; inhibition of leukocyte adhesion, platelet aggregation and coagulation; inhibition of the expression of adhesion molecules, which facilitates the migration of monocytes that transform into macrophages; and promotion of healing *via* endothelial progenitor cells (EPCs) [51].

Endothelial dysfunction is the earliest detectable abnormality that occurs in response to cardiovascular risk factors and can precede or accelerate the development of atherosclerosis. Pre-atherosclerotic modifications include increased intima–media thickness with smooth muscle cell hypertrophy, elastic fibre alterations, mucoid degeneration and leukocyte infiltration in the adventitia and peri-adventitia tunica. The initiation can begin years before clinically manifest vascular disease [52]. A large body of evidence suggests that impaired endothelial function is present in OSA. Increased oxidative stress and lipid peroxidation in OSA was associated with endothelial dysfunction [21, 53] and increased carotid intima–media thickness [54].

EPCs are important to maintain vascular endothelium health, and circulating EPCs are lower than normal in OSA [55–57]. The possible mechanisms underlying the decrease in the number or function of EPCs include a prolonged inflammation response, oxidative stress, increased sympathetic activation, physiological adaptive responses of tissue to hypoxia, reduced EPC mobilisation, EPC apoptosis and functional impairment in untreated OSA [58]. CPAP therapy increased EPC levels to those of control participants when patients adhered to CPAP for more than 4 h daily [55].

Assessment of endothelial function in OSA involves functional evaluation of vascular responses, *i.e.* recording changes in blood flow in response to endothelium-dependent vasodilators or hypoxaemia, quantification of the levels of circulating apoptotic endothelial cells, and measuring the plasma concentrations of various endothelial biomarkers [59]. Several studies have shown indirect evidence of reduced nitric oxide availability and high plasma concentrations of adhesion molecules, suggesting that inflammation and vascular endothelial dysfunction contribute to the development of vascular diseases in patients with OSA [14]. Moreover, increased sympathetic activation and oxidative stress, which are common in OSA patients, might contribute to the development of endothelial dysfunction. Increased oxidative stress promotes the activation of inflammatory pathways that facilitate the recruitment and accumulation of blood cells on the vasculature of the endothelial lining [14, 60].

Although cross-sectional data from population-based studies suggested an association between OSA severity and impaired endothelial function, not all studies confirm this finding independent of other risk factors. Studies evaluating the effect of CPAP treatment on endothelial function also yielded contradictory results. Some studies showed an improvement in endothelium-dependent vasodilatation after CPAP treatment, while other studies did not show this change [61]. It has been reported that effective CPAP therapy (>4 h each night) reverses vascular endothelial dysfunction and inflammation, and enhances endothelial repair capacity [55]. Additionally, it has been shown that CPAP treatment improved endothelial function [21], microvascular disease and nitroglycerin-induced coronary vasodilation [62]. CPAP withdrawal has also been associated with impaired endothelial function [63]. Furthermore, in OSA patients, endothelial dysfunction is proportional to hypoxaemia and is improved by CPAP therapy [64]. The MOSAIC trial recently reported that CPAP treatment improves endothelial function in minimally symptomatic OSA [65]. Nevertheless, other recent RCTs showed that in patients without CVD, CPAP did not modify endothelial function [66].

Overall, OSA appears to directly affect the vascular endothelium by promoting inflammation and oxidative stress while decreasing nitric oxide availability and repair capacity. Therefore, endothelial dysfunction, an established risk factor for CVD, is associated with OSA independent of obesity [67]. Furthermore, CPAP treatment reverses endothelial dysfunction and enhances endothelial repair capacity. Finally, some authors have postulated that there may be sex-related differences in the vulnerability of the vascular endothelium to the adverse effects of OSA. In this way, OSA was independently associated with impaired digital vascular function, impaired conduit, and resistance endothelial function in women only [68, 69]. These suggest that women with sleep disordered breathing may be more vulnerable to early related CVD than are men. For a comprehensive review of the relationship between endothelial function and OSA, the interested reader is referred to Hoyos *et al.* [61].

Sympathetic activity

One of the main underlying mechanisms responsible for the association between OSA and CVD is the sympathetic overactivity. Increased activity of the sympathetic nervous system constricts blood vessels and increases cardiac output [70]. The degree of sympathetic nervous system activation correlates with the severity of the increase in BP and is more pronounced in the context of metabolic diseases such as diabetes, obesity and the metabolic syndrome [71]. Hypoxia and hypercapnia act synergistically to increase sympathetic activity [72], and this effect is especially marked during the apnoeic event. Patients with sleep apnoea have a high frequency of arousals from sleep, which induce a sympathetic burst and vagal withdrawal during each apnoeic episode. Overactivation of central and peripheral chemoreceptors in OSA contributes to the exaggerated sympathetic activity [73]. OSA is tightly linked to hypertension, and the chemoreflex has been implicated as a possible major contributor. Patients with OSA have high sympathetic activity when awake, with further increases in BP and sympathetic activity during sleep [70].

Measurement of sympathetic nerve activity in muscle yields accurate and direct information about sympathetic nerve impulses. Moreover, sympathetic tone can be evaluated by measurement of plasma and urinary catecholamines, a robust biomarker reflecting sympathetic overactivity. In rat models, IH increased catecholamine levels and sympathetic nerve activity [74–76], which appears to be mediated by heightened acute hypoxia sensing *via* the formation of ROS [77, 78]. In normotensive OSA patients, increased urine levels of epinephrine and norepinephrine during both the day and night have been described [79]. CPAP treatment has been noted to result in decreased sympathetic activity [70] and this effect was the greatest in those patients with best CPAP compliance [80, 81]. Several randomised trials have also shown that CPAP treatment reduces sympathetic nervous system activity and attenuates the increased sympathetic tone in OSA patients [82–84], probably contributing to decreased BP after treatment. The significant reduction of sympathetic overactivity is probably one of the main mechanisms explaining the BP reduction in CPAP-treated OSA patients.

Hypercoagulability

One of the possible mechanisms contributing to the initiation and progression of atherosclerosis in OSA is a prothrombotic state due to a haemostatic imbalance between the coagulation and fibrinolysis systems [85]. There is evidence of a hypercoagulability state in patients with OSA, which might contribute to an increased risk of cardiovascular events and an observed peak in sudden death from cardiac causes during the sleeping hours [86]. A vulnerable plaque may rupture when exposed to high shear forces during apnoea-triggered BP peaks. At the time of atherosclerotic plaque rupture, enhanced clotting may accelerate thrombus growth, thereby inducing critical myocardial or cerebral ischaemia [87]. Patients with OSA show a morning increase in plasma fibrinogen concentration and whole blood viscosity, as well as low fibrinolytic activity [88]. Furthermore, studies have reported high levels of coagulation factors XIIa, VIIa and thrombin-antithrombin complex [85]. OSA patients show increased platelet activation and aggregation, although the mechanisms of platelet activation are not completely understood and might be related to increased sympathetic activity [70].

Hypoxaemia and repetitive arousals from sleep combine to produce increased concentrations of epinephrine and norepinephrine, and high levels of circulating catecholamines cause concentration-dependent platelet activation *in vitro* and *in vivo* [89]. The influence of sleep apnoea on the diurnal variations in various haemostatic parameters and markers of endothelial dysfunction has been investigated, showing that day/night variations in the levels of several endothelial markers and haemostatic factors do not differ between patients with sleep apnoea and controls of similar weight. Thus, day/night variations may be dependent on either the obesity index or metabolic dysfunction rather than on sleep apnoea alone [90]. Additionally, a recent RCT showed that CPAP treatment for 3 weeks did not affect day/night rhythm of prothrombotic markers in OSA. Other interventional studies have shown that CPAP treatment reduces coagulability and the risk of thrombosis in patients with OSA, although not all coagulability markers were reduced after CPAP treatment [91–94]. The available data suggest that OSA patients are in a procoagulant state, but the relationship between OSA and individual clotting factors still remains undefined.

Metabolic dysregulation

OSA-related factors such as increased sympathetic activity, sleep fragmentation and IH contribute to the development of metabolic dysregulation [95]. Metabolic syndrome is a cluster of risk factors, including insulin resistance, dyslipidaemia, hypertension and abdominal obesity, that together result in increased cardiovascular risk [96, 97]. Metabolic syndrome is common in patients with OSA, and OSA is frequently found in conditions associated with metabolic abnormalities [98]. Studies show that patients with OSA have higher free fatty acid concentrations than controls, and this could be one of the mechanisms involved in the metabolic complications of OSA [99]. Nevertheless, there is no clear metabolic pattern associated with OSA, and the single components of the metabolic syndrome found in patients with OSA may vary. Independent of adiposity, OSA is associated with impairments of insulin sensitivity, glucose effectiveness, pancreatic β-cell function and dyslipidaemia [100].

There is much debate about whether OSA increases the risk of type 2 diabetes and whether CPAP treatment could reverse insulin resistance. CPAP reduced post-prandial triglycerides and total cholesterol [84]. Several clinical trials, however, have shown a partial or no benefit of CPAP treatment on metabolic components, such as insulin sensitivity, visceral abdominal fat, liver fat or insulin glucose tolerance [101]. Similarly, CPAP treatment does not improve measures of glycaemic control or insulin resistance in men with type 2 diabetes and OSA when compared with sham CPAP [102]. Nevertheless, another study has reported that CPAP treatment rapidly improved insulin sensitivity in non-obese OSA patients [103]. Additionally, an RCT showed that CPAP treatment for 1 week improved insulin sensitivity in males without diabetes and in those with moderate obesity. This improvement appeared to be maintained after 12 weeks of treatment in those with moderate obesity [104]. Because obesity often coexists with OSA, it is not yet clear whether the presence of metabolic disorders is a consequence of OSA or simply reflects the effects of coexisting severe obesity [105]. A recent study showed that in a morbidly obese population with metabolic syndrome, the presence of OSA did not determine any difference in biomarkers related to inflammation and endothelial function, nor did the studied biomarkers allow discrimination between OSA patients with and without metabolic syndrome [106]. It has also been recently reported that the day/night variations in the levels of several metabolic hormones are not influenced by the presence of sleep apnoea [107].

Mechanisms underlying cardiovascular protection in OSA

This chapter has described underlying mechanisms linking OSA with CVD. Despite the existence of these detrimental mechanisms there are epidemiological studies that suggest that some protective mechanisms could also be activated in OSA patients [9]. This is a relevant question from a clinical point of view, since some studies did not find any association of sleep disordered breathing and cardiovascular morbidities [108–112]. Furthermore, there are paradoxical findings on significantly improved post-operative survival of OSA patients [113, 114], as well as on increased survival of elderly patients with mild OSA [115].

ROS exert a vital role in signalling pathways that are essential for repair and survival. In the heart, the increased production of ROS associated with ischaemia/reperfusion is manifested by contractile dysfunction and cell death. Conversely, ROS signalling can contribute to cardioprotection by activating ROS-dependent signalling pathways such as ischaemic preconditioning. In animal models, exposure to mild-to-moderate IH supports the activation of cardio- and neuro-protection. It has been demonstrated that exposure to IH results in increased left ventricular contractility [116] and improved tolerance of the myocardium to ischaemia [117–119]. Also, in these animal models, the decreased infarct size was dependent on the depth and the duration of the IH exposure. These results suggest the existence of dichotomous effects on the heart depending on the IH severity. In some cases, OSA may confer cardio- and neuro-protection by activating the mechanisms of ischaemic preconditioning principally through IH. This is particularly evident in patients with cardiovascular morbidity and concomitant mild-to-moderate OSA [120].

Conclusion

Closely interrelated and detrimental mechanisms link OSA and CVD. The main acute physiological consequences of OSA are oxygen desaturation, intrathoracic pressure changes and arousals. IH is considered to lead to increased oxidative stress, systemic inflammation and sympathetic stimulation. Intrathoracic pressure changes are thought to result in excessive mechanical stress on large arterial walls, and arousals have been related to reflex sympathetic activation associated with recurrent rises in BP. Although the majority of available data support that physiological consequences of OSA increase sympathetic activity, oxidative stress and endothelial dysfunction, there is currently insufficient evidence from well-controlled trials in humans to definitively conclude that OSA is independently associated with systemic inflammation. Also, well-designed studies failed to demonstrate that CPAP alters metabolic or inflammatory markers in OSA. Nevertheless, it has been clearly established that CPAP has a beneficial effect on sympathetic activity, and the impact of CPAP on sympathetic activity is robust across studies and occurs rapidly [121].

Additionally, there have been contradictory results regarding the associations between hypercoagulability and OSA, and between metabolic dysregulation and OSA. Although some authors have demonstrated the association of these damaging mechanisms in OSA patients, others did not show this association, especially for metabolic dysregulation. Because obesity often coexists with OSA, it is not yet clear whether the presence of metabolic disorders is a consequence of OSA or simply reflects the effects of coexisting severe obesity.

Sex-related differences in susceptibility to oxidative stress and in the impact of IH on inflammation have also been demonstrated. Additionally, some authors have proposed that there may be sex-related differences in the vulnerability of the vascular endothelium to the adverse effects of OSA. This sex-related susceptibility could be related to differences in cardiovascular morbidity associated with OSA. Moreover, it will be clinically useful to identify specific phenotypes associated with increased susceptibility to cardiovascular risk, specifically in asymptomatic OSA patients, and to explore the protective mechanism(s) preventing cardiovascular damage in some patients with OSA. Finally, more randomised controlled interventional trials are needed to establish a causal relationship between OSA and some of the proposed mechanisms of vascular damage and to evaluate the effect of other treatments, such as drugs, lifestyle changes and MADs, on the intermediate mechanisms linking OSA with CVD.

References

1. Sánchez-de-la-Torre M, Campos-Rodriguez F, Barbé F. Obstructive sleep apnoea and cardiovascular disease. *Lancet Respir Med* 2013; 1: 61–72.
2. Kohler M, Stradling JR. Mechanisms of vascular damage in obstructive sleep apnea. *Nat Rev Cardiol* 2010; 7: 677–685.
3. Martínez-García MA, Capote F, Campos-Rodriguez F, *et al.* Effect of CPAP on blood pressure in patients with obstructive sleep apnea and resistant hypertension: the HIPARCO randomized clinical trial. *JAMA* 2013; 310: 2407–2415.
4. Loke YK, Brown JW, Kwok CS, *et al.* Association of obstructive sleep apnea with risk of serious cardiovascular events: a systematic review and meta-analysis. *Circ Cardiovasc Qual Outcomes* 2012; 5: 720–728.

5. Durán-Cantolla J, Aizpuru F, Montserrat JM, *et al.* Continuous positive airway pressure as treatment for systemic hypertension in people with obstructive sleep apnoea: randomised controlled trial. *BMJ* 2010; 341: c5991.

6. Barbé F, Durán-Cantolla J, Capote F, *et al.* Long-term effect of continuous positive airway pressure in hypertensive patients with sleep apnea. *Am J Respir Crit Care Med* 2010; 181: 718–726.

7. Lozano L, Tovar JL, Sampol G, *et al.* Continuous positive airway pressure treatment in sleep apnea patients with resistant hypertension: a randomized, controlled trial. *J Hypertens* 2010; 28: 2161–2168.

8. Dean RT, Wilcox I. Possible atherogenic effects of hypoxia during obstructive sleep apnea. *Sleep* 1993; 16: Suppl. 8, S15–S21.

9. Lavie L. Oxidative stress in obstructive sleep apnea and intermittent hypoxia – revisited – the bad ugly and good: implications to the heart and brain. *Sleep Med Rev* 2014 [In press DOI: 10.1016/j.smrv.2014.07.003].

10. Peng YJ, Overholt JL, Kline D, *et al.* Induction of sensory long-term facilitation in the carotid body by intermittent hypoxia: implications for recurrent apneas. *Proc Natl Acad Sci USA* 2003; 100: 10073–10078.

11. McGown AD, Makker H, Elwell C, *et al.* Measurement of changes in cytochrome oxidase redox state during obstructive sleep apnea using near-infrared spectroscopy. *Sleep* 2003; 26: 710–716.

12. Quintero M, Gonzalez-Martin MDC, Vega-Agapito V, *et al.* The effects of intermittent hypoxia on redox status, NF-κB activation, and plasma lipid levels are dependent on the lowest oxygen saturation. *Free Radic Biol Med* 2013; 65: 1143–1154.

13. Fang Y, Zhang Q, Tan J, *et al.* Intermittent hypoxia-induced rat pancreatic β-cell apoptosis and protective effects of antioxidant intervention. *Nutr Diabetes* 2014; 4: e131.

14. Dyugovskaya L, Lavie P, Lavie L. Increased adhesion molecules expression and production of reactive oxygen species in leukocytes of sleep apnea patients. *Am J Respir Crit Care Med* 2002; 165: 934–939.

15. Carpagnano GE, Kharitonov SA, Resta O, *et al.* 8-Isoprostane, a marker of oxidative stress, is increased in exhaled breath condensate of patients with obstructive sleep apnea after night and is reduced by continuous positive airway pressure therapy. *Chest* 2003; 124: 1386–1392.

16. Barceló A, Miralles C, Barbé F, *et al.* Abnormal lipid peroxidation in patients with sleep apnoea. *Eur Respir J* 2000; 16: 644–647.

17. Schulz R, Mahmoudi S, Hattar K, *et al.* Enhanced release of superoxide from polymorphonuclear neutrophils in obstructive sleep apnea. Impact of continuous positive airway pressure therapy. *Am J Respir Crit Care Med* 2000; 162: 566–570.

18. Lavie L, Vishnevsky A, Lavie P. Evidence for lipid peroxidation in obstructive sleep apnea. *Sleep* 2004; 27: 123–128.

19. Tóthová L, Hodosy J, Mucska I, *et al.* Salivary markers of oxidative stress in patients with obstructive sleep apnea treated with continuous positive airway pressure. *Sleep Breath* 2014; 18: 563–570.

20. Del Ben M, Fabiani M, Loffredo L, *et al.* Oxidative stress mediated arterial dysfunction in patients with obstructive sleep apnoea and the effect of continuous positive airway pressure treatment. *BMC Pulm Med* 2012; 12: 36.

21. Jurado-Gámez B, Fernandez-Marin MC, Gómez-Chaparro JL, *et al.* Relationship of oxidative stress and endothelial dysfunction in sleep apnoea. *Eur Respir J* 2011; 37: 873–879.

22. Alonso-Fernández A, García-Río F, Arias MA, *et al.* Effects of CPAP on oxidative stress and nitrate efficiency in sleep apnoea: a randomised trial. *Thorax* 2009; 64: 581–586.

23. Malakasioti G, Alexopoulos E, Befani C, *et al.* Oxidative stress and inflammatory markers in the exhaled breath condensate of children with OSA. *Sleep Breath* 2012; 16: 703–708.

24. Tauman R, Lavie L, Greenfeld M, *et al.* Oxidative stress in children with obstructive sleep apnea syndrome. *J Clin Sleep Med* 2014; 10: 677–681.

25. Simiakakis M, Kapsimalis F, Chaligiannis E, *et al.* Lack of effect of sleep apnea on oxidative stress in obstructive sleep apnea syndrome (OSAS) patients. *PLoS One* 2012; 7: e39172.

26. Sales LV, Bruin VM, D'Almeida V, *et al.* Cognition and biomarkers of oxidative stress in obstructive sleep apnea. *Clinics* 2013; 68: 449–455.

27. Baysal E, Taysi S, Aksoy N, *et al.* Serum paraoxonase, arylesterase activity and oxidative status in patients with obstructive sleep apnea syndrome (OSAS). *Eur Rev Med Pharmacol Sci* 2012; 16: 770–774.

28. Barceló A, Barbé F, de la Peña M, *et al.* Antioxidant status in patients with sleep apnoea and impact of continuous positive airway pressure treatment. *Eur Respir J* 2006; 27: 756–760.

29. Christou K, Moulas AN, Pastaka C, *et al.* Antioxidant capacity in obstructive sleep apnea patients. *Sleep Med* 2003; 4: 225–228.

30. Tamás A, Lubics A, Szalontay L, *et al.* Age and gender differences in behavioral and morphological outcome after 6-hydroxydopamine-induced lesion of the substantia nigra in rats. *Behav Brain Res* 2005; 158: 221–229.

31. Yamauchi M, Tamaki S, Tomoda K, *et al.* Evidence for activation of nuclear factor κB in obstructive sleep apnea. *Sleep Breath* 2006; 10: 189–193.

32. Rubinstein I. Nasal inflammation in patients with obstructive sleep apnea. *Laryngoscope* 1995; 105: 175–177.

33. Lam SY, Liu Y, Ng KM, *et al.* Chronic intermittent hypoxia induces local inflammation of the rat carotid body *via* functional upregulation of proinflammatory cytokine pathways. *Histochem Cell Biol* 2012; 137: 303–317.

34. Ramos P, Rubies C, Torres M, *et al.* Atrial fibrosis in a chronic murine model of obstructive sleep apnea: mechanisms and prevention by mesenchymal stem cells. *Respir Res* 2014; 15: 54.

35. Farré R, Nácher M, Serrano-Mollar A, *et al.* Rat model of chronic recurrent airway obstructions to study the sleep apnea syndrome. *Sleep* 2007; 30: 930–933.

36. Vgontzas AN, Papanicolaou DA, Bixler EO, *et al.* Elevation of plasma cytokines in disorders of excessive daytime sleepiness: role of sleep disturbance and obesity. *J Clin Endocrinol Metab* 1997; 82: 1313–1316.

37. Ciftci TU, Kokturk O, Bukan N, *et al.* The relationship between serum cytokine levels with obesity and obstructive sleep apnea syndrome. *Cytokine* 2004; 28: 87–91.

38. Yokoe T, Minoguchi K, Matsuo H, *et al.* Elevated levels of C-reactive protein and interleukin-6 in patients with obstructive sleep apnea syndrome are decreased by nasal continuous positive airway pressure. *Circulation* 2003; 107: 1129–1134.

39. Ohga E, Nagase T, Tomita T, *et al.* Increased levels of circulating ICAM-1, VCAM-1, and L-selectin in obstructive sleep apnea syndrome. *J Appl Physiol* 1999; 87: 10–14.

40. Ohga E, Tomita T, Wada H, *et al.* Effects of obstructive sleep apnea on circulating ICAM-1, IL-8, and MCP-1. *J Appl Physiol* 2003; 94: 179–184.

41. Koseoglu HI, Altunkas F, Kanbay A, *et al.* Platelet–lymphocyte ratio is an independent predictor for cardiovascular disease in obstructive sleep apnea syndrome. *J Thromb Thrombolysis* 2014 [In press DOI: 10.1007/s11239-014-1103-4].

42. Kobukai Y, Koyama T, Watanabe H, *et al.* Morning pentraxin3 levels reflect obstructive sleep apnea-related acute inflammation. *J Appl Physiol* 2014; 117: 1141–1148.

43. Ryan S, Taylor CT, McNicholas WT. Predictors of elevated nuclear factor-κB-dependent genes in obstructive sleep apnea syndrome. *Am J Respir Crit Care Med* 2006; 174: 824–830.

44. Maeder MT, Strobel W, Christ M, *et al.* Comprehensive biomarker profiling in patients with obstructive sleep apnea. *Clin Biochem* 2014 [In press DOI: 10.1016/j.clinbiochem.2014.09.005].

45. Stradling JR, Craig SE, Kohler M, *et al.* Markers of inflammation: data from the MOSAIC randomised trial of CPAP for minimally symptomatic OSA. *Thorax* 2015; 70: 181–182.

46. Lago F, Dieguez C, Gómez-Reino J, *et al.* Adipokines as emerging mediators of immune response and inflammation. *Nat Clin Pract Rheumatol* 2007; 3: 716–724.

47. Harsch IA, Konturek PC, Koebnick C, *et al.* Leptin and ghrelin levels in patients with obstructive sleep apnoea: effect of CPAP treatment. *Eur Respir J* 2003; 22: 251–257.

48. Guilleminault C, Kirisoglu C, Ohayon MM. C-reactive protein and sleep-disordered breathing. *Sleep* 2004; 27: 1507–1511.

49. Kohler M, Ayers L, Pepperell JC, *et al.* Effects of continuous positive airway pressure on systemic inflammation in patients with moderate to severe obstructive sleep apnoea: a randomised controlled trial. *Thorax* 2009; 64: 67–73.

50. Torres M, Palomer X, Montserrat JM, *et al.* Effect of ovariectomy on inflammation induced by intermittent hypoxia in a mouse model of sleep apnea. *Respir Physiol Neurobiol* 2014; 202: 71–74.

51. Celermajer DS. Reliable endothelial function testing: at our fingertips? *Circulation* 2008; 117: 2428–2430.

52. Ross R. Atherosclerosis – an inflammatory disease. *N Engl J Med* 1999; 340: 115–126.

53. Itzhaki S, Dorchin H, Clark G, *et al.* The effects of 1-year treatment with a Herbst mandibular advancement splint on obstructive sleep apnea, oxidative stress, and endothelial function. *Chest* 2007; 131: 740–749.

54. Monneret D, Pépin JL, Godin-Ribuot D, *et al.* Association of urinary 15-F2t-isoprostane level with oxygen desaturation and carotid intima-media thickness in nonobese sleep apnea patients. *Free Radic Biol Med* 2010; 48: 619–625.

55. Jelic S, Padeletti M, Kawut SM, *et al.* Inflammation, oxidative stress, and repair capacity of the vascular endothelium in obstructive sleep apnea. *Circulation* 2008; 117: 2270–2278.

56. de la Peña M, Barceló A, Barbé F, *et al.* Endothelial function and circulating endothelial progenitor cells in patients with sleep apnea syndrome. *Respiration* 2008; 76: 28–32.

57. Kheirandish-Gozal L, Bhattacharjee R, Kim J, *et al.* Endothelial progenitor cells and vascular dysfunction in children with obstructive sleep apnea. *Am J Respir Crit Care Med* 2010; 182: 92–97.

58. Wang Q, Wu Q, Feng J, *et al.* Obstructive sleep apnea and endothelial progenitor cells. *Patient Prefer Adherence* 2013; 7: 1077–1090.

59. Budhiraja R, Parthasarathy S, Quan SF. Endothelial dysfunction in obstructive sleep apnea. *J Clin Sleep Med* 2007; 3: 409–415.

60. Lavie L. Obstructive sleep apnoea syndrome – an oxidative stress disorder. *Sleep Med Rev* 2003; 7: 35–51.

61. Hoyos CM, Melehan KL, Liu PY, *et al.* Does obstructive sleep apnea cause endothelial dysfunction? A critical review of the literature. *Sleep Med Rev* 2014 [In press DOI: 10.1016/j.smrv.2014.06.003].

62. Nguyen PK, Katikireddy CK, McConnell MV, et al. Nasal continuous positive airway pressure improves myocardial perfusion reserve and endothelial-dependent vasodilation in patients with obstructive sleep apnea. J Cardiovasc Magn Reson 2010; 12: 50.

63. Kohler M, Stoewhas AC, Ayers L, et al. Effects of continuous positive airway pressure therapy withdrawal in patients with obstructive sleep apnea: a randomized controlled trial. Am J Respir Crit Care Med 2011; 184: 1192–1199.

64. Cross MD, Mills NL, Al-Abri M, et al. Continuous positive airway pressure improves vascular function in obstructive sleep apnoea/hypopnoea syndrome: a randomised controlled trial. Thorax 2008; 63: 578–583.

65. Kohler M, Craig S, Pepperell JC, et al. CPAP improves endothelial function in patients with minimally symptomatic OSA: results from a subset study of the MOSAIC trial. Chest 2013; 144: 896–902.

66. Jones A, Vennelle M, Connell M, et al. The effect of continuous positive airway pressure therapy on arterial stiffness and endothelial function in obstructive sleep apnea: a randomized controlled trial in patients without cardiovascular disease. Sleep Med 2013; 14: 1260–1265.

67. Namtvedt SK, Hisdal J, Randby A, et al. Impaired endothelial function in persons with obstructive sleep apnoea: impact of obesity. Heart 2013; 99: 30–34.

68. Randby A, Namtvedt SK, Hrubos-Strøm H, et al. Sex-dependent impact of OSA on digital vascular function. Chest 2013; 144: 915–922.

69. Faulx MD, Larkin EK, Hoit BD, et al. Sex influences endothelial function in sleep-disordered breathing. Sleep 2004; 27: 1113–1120.

70. Somers VK, Dyken ME, Clary MP, et al. Sympathetic neural mechanisms in obstructive sleep apnea. J Clin Invest 1995; 96: 1897–1904.

71. Scherrer U, Randin D, Tappy L, et al. Body fat and sympathetic nerve activity in healthy subjects. Circulation 1994; 89: 2634–2640.

72. Somers VK, Mark AL, Zavala DC, et al. Contrasting effects of hypoxia and hypercapnia on ventilation and sympathetic activity in humans. J Appl Physiol 1989; 67: 2101–2106.

73. Narkiewicz K, van de Borne PJ, Montano N, et al. Contribution of tonic chemoreflex activation to sympathetic activity and blood pressure in patients with obstructive sleep apnea. Circulation 1998; 97: 943–945.

74. Bao G, Randhawa PM, Fletcher EC. Acute blood pressure elevation during repetitive hypocapnic and eucapnic hypoxia in rats. J Appl Physiol 1997; 82: 1071–1078.

75. Greenberg HE, Sica AL, Scharf SM, et al. Expression of c-fos in the rat brainstem after chronic intermittent hypoxia. Brain Res 1999; 816: 638–645.

76. Dick TE, Hsieh YH, Wang N, et al. Acute intermittent hypoxia increases both phrenic and sympathetic nerve activities in the rat. Exp Physiol 2007; 92: 87–97.

77. Arora T, Singh S, Sharma RK. Probiotics: interaction with gut microbiome and antiobesity potential. Nutrition 2013; 29: 591–596.

78. MacFarlane PM, Mitchell GS. Respiratory long-term facilitation following intermittent hypoxia requires reactive oxygen species formation. Neuroscience 2008; 152: 189–197.

79. Marrone O, Riccobono L, Salvaggio A, et al. Catecholamines and blood pressure in obstructive sleep apnea syndrome. Chest 1993; 103: 722–727.

80. Narkiewicz K, Kato M, Phillips BG, et al. Nocturnal continuous positive airway pressure decreases daytime sympathetic traffic in obstructive sleep apnea. Circulation 1999; 100: 2332–2335.

81. Imadojemu VA, Mawji Z, Kunselman A, et al. Sympathetic chemoreflex responses in obstructive sleep apnea and effects of continuous positive airway pressure therapy. Chest 2007; 131: 1406–1413.

82. Kohler M, Pepperell JC, Casadei B, et al. CPAP and measures of cardiovascular risk in males with OSAS. Eur Respir J 2008; 32: 1488–1496.

83. Nelesen RA, Yu H, Ziegler MG, et al. Continuous positive airway pressure normalizes cardiac autonomic and hemodynamic responses to a laboratory stressor in apneic patients. Chest 2001; 119: 1092–1101.

84. Phillips CL, Yee BJ, Marshall NS, et al. Continuous positive airway pressure reduces postprandial lipidemia in obstructive sleep apnea: a randomized, placebo-controlled crossover trial. Am J Respir Crit Care Med 2011; 184: 355–361.

85. von Känel R, Dimsdale JE. Hemostatic alterations in patients with obstructive sleep apnea and the implications for cardiovascular disease. Chest 2003; 124: 1956–1967.

86. Gami AS, Howard DE, Olson EJ, et al. Day-night pattern of sudden death in obstructive sleep apnea. N Engl J Med 2005; 352: 1206–1214.

87. Choi BG, Vilahur G, Ibanez B, et al. Measures of thrombosis and fibrinolysis. Clin Lab Med 2006; 26: 655–678.

88. Rångemark C, Hedner JA, Carlson JT, et al. Platelet function and fibrinolytic activity in hypertensive and normotensive sleep apnea patients. Sleep 1995; 18: 188–194.

89. Larsson PT, Wallén NH, Hjemdahl P. Norepinephrine-induced human platelet activation in vivo is only partly counteracted by aspirin. Circulation 1994; 89: 1951–1957.

90. Barceló A, Piérola J, de la Peña M, *et al.* Day-night variations in endothelial dysfunction markers and haemostatic factors in sleep apnoea. *Eur Respir J* 2012; 39: 913–918.

91. Phillips CL, McEwen BJ, Morel-Kopp MC, *et al.* Effects of continuous positive airway pressure on coagulability in obstructive sleep apnoea: a randomised, placebo-controlled crossover study. *Thorax* 2012; 67: 639–644.

92. von Känel R, Loredo JS, Ancoli-Israel S, *et al.* Association between sleep apnea severity and blood coagulability: treatment effects of nasal continuous positive airway pressure. *Sleep Breath* 2006; 10: 139–146.

93. Robinson GV, Pepperell JC, Segal HC, *et al.* Circulating cardiovascular risk factors in obstructive sleep apnoea: data from randomised controlled trials. *Thorax* 2004; 59: 777–782.

94. Toukh M, Pereira EJ, Falcon BJ, *et al.* CPAP reduces hypercoagulability, as assessed by thromboelastography, in severe obstructive sleep apnoea. *Respir Physiol Neurobiol* 2012; 183: 218–223.

95. Phillips BG, Kato M, Narkiewicz K, *et al.* Increases in leptin levels, sympathetic drive, and weight gain in obstructive sleep apnea. *Am J Physiol Heart Circ Physiol* 2000; 279: H234–H237.

96. Simmons RK, Alberti KG, Gale EA, *et al.* The metabolic syndrome: useful concept or clinical tool? Report of a WHO Expert Consultation. *Diabetologia* 2010; 53: 600–605.

97. Ho JS, Cannaday JJ, Barlow CE, *et al.* Relation of the number of metabolic syndrome risk factors with all-cause and cardiovascular mortality. *Am J Cardiol* 2008; 102: 689–692.

98. Bonsignore MR, Esquinas C, Barceló A, *et al.* Metabolic syndrome, insulin resistance and sleepiness in real-life obstructive sleep apnoea. *Eur Respir J* 2012; 39: 1136–1143.

99. Barceló A, Piérola J, de la Peña M, *et al.* Free fatty acids and the metabolic syndrome in patients with obstructive sleep apnoea. *Eur Respir J* 2011; 37: 1418–1423.

100. Punjabi NM, Beamer BA. Alterations in glucose disposal in sleep-disordered breathing. *Am J Respir Crit Care Med* 2009; 179: 235–240.

101. Weinstock TG, Wang X, Rueschman M, *et al.* A controlled trial of CPAP therapy on metabolic control in individuals with impaired glucose tolerance and sleep apnea. *Sleep* 2012; 35: 617–625B.

102. West SD, Nicoll DJ, Wallace TM, *et al.* Effect of CPAP on insulin resistance and HbA1c in men with obstructive sleep apnoea and type 2 diabetes. *Thorax* 2007; 62: 969–974.

103. Harsch IA, Schahin SP, Radespiel-Tröger M, *et al.* Continuous positive airway pressure treatment rapidly improves insulin sensitivity in patients with obstructive sleep apnea syndrome. *Am J Respir Crit Care Med* 2004; 169: 156–162.

104. Lam JC, Lam B, Yao TJ, *et al.* A randomised controlled trial of nasal continuous positive airway pressure on insulin sensitivity in obstructive sleep apnoea. *Eur Respir J* 2010; 35: 138–145.

105. Sánchez-de-la-Torre M, Mediano O, Barceló A, *et al.* The influence of obesity and obstructive sleep apnea on metabolic hormones. *Sleep Breath* 2012; 16: 649–656.

106. Salord N, Gasa M, Mayos M, *et al.* Impact of OSA on biological markers in morbid obesity and metabolic syndrome. *J Clin Sleep Med* 2014; 10: 263–270.

107. Sánchez-de-la-Torre M, Barceló A, Piérola J, *et al.* Impact of obstructive sleep apnea on the 24-h metabolic hormone profile. *Sleep Med* 2014; 15: 625–630.

108. Mehra R, Principe-Rodriguez K, Kirchner HL, *et al.* Sleep apnea in acute coronary syndrome: high prevalence but low impact on 6-month outcome. *Sleep Med* 2006; 7: 521–528.

109. Marín JM, Carrizo SJ, Kogan I. Obstructive sleep apnea and acute myocardial infarction: clinical implications of the association. *Sleep* 1998; 21: 809–815.

110. Lee CH, Khoo SM, Tai BC, *et al.* Obstructive sleep apnea in patients admitted for acute myocardial infarction. Prevalence, predictors, and effect on microvascular perfusion. *Chest* 2009; 135: 1488–1495.

111. Gottlieb DJ, Yenokyan G, Newman AB, *et al.* Prospective study of obstructive sleep apnea and incident coronary heart disease and heart failure: the Sleep Heart Health Study. *Circulation* 2010; 122: 352–360.

112. Aronson D, Nakhleh M, Zeidan-Shwiri T, *et al.* Clinical implications of sleep disordered breathing in acute myocardial infarction. *PLoS One* 2014; 9: e88878.

113. Mokhlesi B, Hovda MD, Vekhter B, *et al.* Sleep-disordered breathing and postoperative outcomes after bariatric surgery: analysis of the nationwide inpatient sample. *Obes Surg* 2013; 23: 1842–1851.

114. Mokhlesi B, Hovda MD, Vekhter B, *et al.* Sleep-disordered breathing and postoperative outcomes after elective surgery: analysis of the nationwide inpatient sample. *Chest* 2013; 144: 903–914.

115. Lavie P, Lavie L. Unexpected survival advantage in elderly people with moderate sleep apnoea. *J Sleep Res* 2009; 18: 397–403.

116. Naghshin J, McGaffin KR, Witham WG, *et al.* Chronic intermittent hypoxia increases left ventricular contractility in C57BL/6 mice. *J Appl Physiol* 2009; 107: 787–793.

117. Béguin PC, Belaidi E, Godin-Ribuot D, *et al.* Intermittent hypoxia-induced delayed cardioprotection is mediated by PKC and triggered by p38 MAP kinase and Erk1/2. *J Mol Cell Cardiol* 2007; 42: 343–351.

118. Béguin PC, Joyeux-Faure M, Godin-Ribuot D, *et al.* Acute intermittent hypoxia improves rat myocardium tolerance to ischemia. *J Appl Physiol* 2005; 99: 1064–1069.

119. Belaidi E, Béguin PC, Lévy P, *et al*. Prevention of HIF-1 activation and iNOS gene targeting by low-dose cadmium results in loss of myocardial hypoxic preconditioning in the rat. *Am J Physiol Heart Circ Physiol* 2008; 294: H901–H908.
120. Berger S, Aronson D, Lavie P, *et al*. Endothelial progenitor cells in acute myocardial infarction and sleep-disordered breathing. *Am J Respir Crit Care Med* 2013; 187: 90–98.
121. Jullian-Desayes I, Joyeux-Faure M, Tamisier R, *et al*. Impact of obstructive sleep apnea treatment by continuous positive airway pressure on cardiometabolic biomarkers: a systematic review from sham CPAP randomized controlled trials. *Sleep Med Rev* 2014 [In press DOI: 10.1016/j.smrv.2014.07.004].

Support statement: This work was supported by the Fondo de Investigación Sanitaria (grants PI10/02763, PI10/02745 and PI14/01266), the Spanish Respiratory Society (SEPAR) and Associació Lleidatana de Respiratori (ALLER).

Disclosures: None declared.

Acknowledgements: We thank Daniel Sánchez and Ferran B. Miró (Respiratory Dept, Hospital Universitari Arnau de Vilanova and Santa Maria, IRB Lleida, Lleida, Spain) for their contribution to the realisation of the figure.

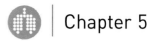
Pathophysiological interactions of OSA, HF and nocturnal fluid redistribution

Owen D. Lyons[1,2] and T. Douglas Bradley[1,2,3]

OSA is highly prevalent in patients with HF. The relationship between OSA and HF is likely to be bi-directional. The presence of OSA leads to exaggerated swings in negative intrathoracic pressure, surges in sympathetic nervous system activity, IH and frequent awakenings, all of which may have adverse cardiovascular consequences and contribute to the progression of HF. Fluid overload, secondary to HF, may lead to increased fluid shift from the legs during sleep. Resulting fluid redistribution to the neck may lead to UA narrowing and increased UA collapsibility that could contribute to the pathogenesis of OSA. In patients with OSA, therapies that reduce leg fluid volume while awake, such as compression stockings and diuretics, or therapies that reduce total body fluid volume at night, such as diuretics and nocturnal dialysis, can attenuate OSA severity. In HF patients with OSA, diuretic therapy leads to increased UA size and attenuation of OSA severity.

Heart failure is a clinical condition, arising from abnormalities in cardiac structure or function that limit cardiac output, activate the sympathetic nervous and renin–angiotensin systems, cause salt and water retention, and increase left ventricular filling pressure, which causes pulmonary congestion and peripheral oedema. These physiological abnormalities are accompanied by physical signs that can include a third and fourth heart sound, enlarged heart, elevated jugular venous pressure, pulmonary crackles, pleural effusions and pedal oedema, which are accompanied by symptoms such as exertional dyspnoea, orthopnoea, paroxysmal nocturnal dyspnoea and fatigue [1]. Approximately 50% of HF patients have predominantly systolic HF with reduced left ventricular ejection fraction (LVEF), while approximately 50% have predominantly diastolic HF with a preserved LVEF [2]. Ischaemic heart disease is the commonest cause of HF but there are many other causes including hypertension, valvular abnormalities, infiltrative diseases of the myocardium, familial cardiomyopathies and heart rhythm disturbances. Despite recent advances in HF therapy, morbidity and mortality remain high [3–6]. Therefore, it is important that underlying conditions that could contribute to disease causation and progression are identified so that novel therapies can be developed. One such condition could be OSA, which is common in patients with either systolic or diastolic HF.

[1]Sleep Research Laboratory of the University Health Network, Toronto Rehabilitation Institute, Toronto, Canada. [2]Centre for Sleep Medicine and Circadian Biology, University of Toronto, Toronto, Canada. [3]Dept of Medicine, University Health Network, Toronto General Hospital, Toronto, Canada.

Correspondence: T. Douglas Bradley, University Health Network, Toronto General Hospital, 9N-943, 200 Elizabeth St, Toronto, ON, M5G 2C4, Canada. E-mail: douglas.bradley@utoronto.ca

Copyright ©ERS 2015. Print ISBN: 978-1-84984-059-0. Online ISBN: 978-1-84984-060-6. Print ISSN: 2312-508X. Online ISSN: 2312-5098.

The vast majority of studies of sleep apnoea in patients with HF concern those with reduced LVEF and predominantly systolic HF and, as a consequence, this chapter focuses on the associations between OSA and systolic HF. In view of the above, this chapter has two main purposes: 1) to discuss the pathogenesis of OSA in systolic HF with a specific focus on the role of fluid overload and nocturnal rostral fluid shift from the legs; and 2) to consider the cardiovascular consequences of OSA and mechanisms by which OSA could play a role in the development and progression of systolic HF.

The presence of systolic HF is usually confirmed, and its severity assessed, by measuring LVEF by echocardiography or other techniques [1]. LVEF is a measure of systolic function: [end diastolic volume−end systolic volume]/end diastolic volume. Significant systolic dysfunction is usually defined as an LVEF ⩽40–45% [7, 8]. LVEF is an important functional variable because it predicts prognosis [9] and because the majority of HF research studies including large clinical trials have used it as diagnostic and inclusion criteria, typically including patients with an LVEF ⩽35% or ⩽45%.

Estimates of the prevalence of systolic HF range from 1% to 2% of the adult population and are increasing, largely due to an ageing population and improved survival from myocardial infarction. For example, prevalence rates of systolic HF in the elderly are much higher: in the USA it is approximately 8.4% in those aged >75 years, while in Europe the prevalence has been reported as 7% in those aged 75–84 years [10, 11]. Until the 1990s, 5-year mortality rates for HF were as high as 70% [3]. Subsequent improvements in the treatment of HF with angiotensin-converting enzyme inhibitors, spironolactone, β-blockers and implantable cardioverter defibrillators have led to improved survival and reduced hospitalisations. Notwithstanding this, 5-year mortality rates remain high [4–6]. The progressive deterioration of systolic function that characterises HF is driven by several key variables including local factors, such as myocyte death, and systemic neurohormonal factors, such as increased sympathetic nervous and renin-angiotensin-aldosterone activity [12, 13]. Interruption of some of these processes forms the basis of effective HF treatment [12, 13].

OSA is characterised by repetitive collapse of the UA during sleep, leading to large swings in negative inspiratory intrathoracic pressure, IH, repetitive arousals and surges of sympathetic nervous system activity (SNA) [14], with consequent cardiovascular [15–17], neurocognitive and metabolic effects [18]. OSA is far more common in fluid retaining conditions, such as end-stage renal disease and HF [19, 20], than in subjects without such conditions. This observation has led to an interest in the role of fluid overload and nocturnal fluid redistribution as a potential mechanism in the pathogenesis of OSA. Fluid retention and overnight rostral fluid shift from the legs may initiate or contribute to the severity of OSA by causing fluid accumulation in the neck, narrowing the pharynx and increasing its propensity to collapse during sleep. It is, however, likely that the relationship between OSA and HF is bi-directional with sodium retention and fluid overload of HF contributing to the development of OSA, and with OSA contributing to the progression of HF [21].

Fluid shift measurement and mechanisms

Measurement

Historically, measurement of body fluid volumes was driven by an interest in changes in plasma volume, and movement of fluid from the intravascular to the extravascular space secondary to postural changes [22–24]. Subsequently, various techniques were developed to measure fluid volumes in specific body segments. These included the water displacement leg volumetric technique that is no longer routinely used [25, 26].

Blood pool scintigraphy involves the intravenous injection of a radio-labelled isotope. The subsequent radiation emitted by this can be measured using a gamma camera and quantified. The quantity of isotope detected by the gamma camera is directly proportional to the intravascular volume in the area being imaged [27, 28]. Repeated measurements post-intervention or post-postural change allows for assessment of changes in the intravascular volume [29, 30]. This technique is a reliable method of detecting fluid changes from a limb or body segment but has the disadvantages of being invasive and involving exposure to radiation [29].

Bio-electrical impedance is a well-validated, noninvasive technique to estimate fluid volume of tissues by measuring their resistance to an electrical current [31, 32]. It is widely used in clinical practice and its applications include measurement of total body fluid volume in end stage renal disease patients, pre- and post-dialysis, and measurement of body composition in patients undergoing nutritional assessment [31, 33]. Based on Ohm's Law, the resistance of a tissue to electric current is inversely related to its fluid content and directly related to its length [33, 34]. Bio-impedance can be used to measure extracellular fluid volume, intracellular fluid volume, total fluid volume, and body composition (fat-free mass and fat mass). It can be used to measure fluid volumes of the whole body or a body segment (*e.g.* the arm, leg or trunk). It has the advantages over other techniques of being noninvasive, portable and providing continuous measurements over time. Because of these advantages, the majority of studies referenced in this chapter have used this technique to measure fluid volumes in human subjects.

Mechanisms

The movement of isotonic fluid between the capillaries (intravascular) and the interstitial (extravascular) space is dictated by the balance of opposing Starling forces that include capillary hydrostatic pressure and oncotic pressure [35]. Postural changes alter hydrostatic pressures leading to significant changes in body fluid distribution between the intravascular and extravascular space [23, 24, 26]. On moving from lying to standing, the hydrostatic pressure of the capillaries in the legs increases from ~10 mmHg to 65–90 mmHg which is far greater than the pressure of 15 mmHg required for fluid movement into the interstitial space [36–38]. On standing, plasma volume decreases by 300–400 mL and leg fluid volume increases by 80–250 mL, due to a combination of venous pooling and fluid movement into the interstitial space [22, 23, 26, 37]. The movement of fluid into the interstitial space by filtration occurs over the first 40 min on standing and then plateaus. This plateauing effect is due to increases in capillary intravascular oncotic pressure, which will tend to maintain fluid within the capillary, and to increases in extravascular tissue pressure which slow the rate of flow of fluid out of the capillaries into the extravascular space [36, 37]. A reversal of this process occurs on changing from standing to lying, with fluid that has accumulated in the interstitium of the legs being rapidly reabsorbed into the intravascular space. On lying down in bed at night, the fluid that has moved back into the intravascular space moves rostrally, due to gravity, into the chest and neck, and leg fluid volumes decrease [39, 40]. These changes are more pronounced in fluid overloaded patients, such as those with HF, who, while standing, have increased venous pressure that causes a large increase in fluid movement into the interstitial space, leading to leg oedema [41]. On lying down, the degree of leg oedema will determine the volume of fluid moving back into the intravascular space. Consequently, in oedematous patients, there is a greater volume of fluid moving from the interstitial spaces of the legs into the intravascular space and a greater degree of fluid redistribution into the chest and neck than in non-oedematous normovolemic subjects [42, 43].

OSA epidemiology and clinical features in HF

Epidemiology

In the original report of the Wisconsin Sleep Cohort Study in 1993, that involved state employees aged 30–60 years, the prevalence of OSA in men and women, respectively, was: 24% and 9% using an AHI cut-off $\geqslant 5$ events·h^{-1}; 15% and 5% using an AHI cut-off $\geqslant 10$ events·h^{-1}; and 9% and 4% using an AHI cut-off $\geqslant 15$ events·h^{-1} [44]. A more recent report of this cohort from 2013 indicated somewhat higher prevalence estimates of sleep apnoea. At an AHI cut-off $\geqslant 15$ events·h^{-1} the prevalence was 10% among 30–49 year-old men, 17% among 50–70 year-old men, 3% among 30–49 year-old women and 9% among 50–70 year-old women [45]. In a cross-sectional analysis of the Sleep Heart Health Study, compromising more than 6000 men and women, the presence of OSA with an AHI $\geqslant 11$ events·h^{-1} conferred a 2.38 relative increase in the likelihood of having HF independent of other risk factors [46]. In a subsequent prospective analysis of the Sleep Heart Health Study that followed 1927 men and 2495 women aged $\geqslant 40$ years and who were free of coronary heart disease and HF at the time of PSG for 8 years, OSA increased the risk of new onset HF in men (adjusted HR 1.13 (95% CI 1.02–1.26) per 10-unit increase in AHI) but not in women and men with an AHI $\geqslant 30$ events·h^{-1} were 58% more likely to develop HF than those with AHI <5 events·h^{-1} [47]. While not conclusive, these relationships support a cause–effect relationship between the presence of OSA and the development of HF. Reported prevalence of OSA among HF patients vary widely; one study using an AHI cut-off of $\geqslant 10$ events·h^{-1} reported a prevalence of 53% [48], while other studies using a cut-off of $\geqslant 15$ events·h^{-1} reported rates of 12%, 15% and 26% [19, 49, 50]. Some of these differences could be due to differing populations in which both men and women [19, 48], or only men were included [49, 50]. In HF patients with preserved LVEF, reported prevalence rates vary depending on the AHI cut-off used to define OSA; one study using an AHI cut-off of $\geqslant 15$ events·h^{-1} reported a prevalence of 11% [51] while two other studies using an AHI cut-off of >5 events·h^{-1} reported prevalence rates of 40% [52] and 62% [53].

Clinical features

Risk factors for OSA in the healthy population, such as older age, male sex and higher BMI are also risk factors for OSA in HF [19]. However, BMI does not appear to play as important a role as a risk factor for OSA in HF as it does in the general population. HF patients have a lower BMI for any given AHI than the general population and the correlation between BMI and AHI is weaker [54]. Therefore, other factors, such as nocturnal rostral fluid shift, as discussed below, appear to play a greater role in the pathogenesis of OSA in HF than in the general population. Among patients with HF, OSA is often accompanied by a history of snoring [55]. However, compared to the general population, HF patients complain of hypersomnolence less often and have lower ESS scores at any given AHI [54]. This is despite the fact that, compared to the general population,

HF patients have longer sleep onset latency and sleep on average 1.3 h less than the general population [54]. One factor that appears to contribute to the lack of hypersomnolence is excessive SNA both during sleep and wakefulness [56, 57]. Both HF and OSA cause sympathetic activation, and the superimposition of OSA on HF causes an additive effect on SNA that is at least partially reversible by treatment of OSA with CPAP [58]. Such elevated SNA appears to counteract the soporific effect of sleep fragmentation by OSA, probably by augmenting alertness *via* adrenergic stimulation of the reticular activating and arousals systems.

Possibly the most important clinical implication of OSA in HF is that it may increase mortality risk. For example, two observational studies have reported that HF patients with untreated, moderate-to-severe OSA have an approximate two-fold increase in all-cause mortality compared to HF patients without sleep apnoea as demonstrated in figure 1 [59, 60]. In both these studies, treatment of OSA by CPAP was associated with a tendency to reduced mortality compared to the untreated OSA groups. In contrast, another observational study did not find a difference in mortality rates in HF patients with and without OSA. However, they did not divide OSA patients into those who were treated or untreated, making interpretation of the results difficult [61].

Pathogenesis of OSA in HF

Obstructive apnoeas and hypopnoeas are caused by complete or partial collapse of the pharynx during sleep. The UA collapses when sleep-related loss in UA dilator muscle tone is superimposed upon a narrow and/or collapsible UA [62, 63]. There are multiple, complex anatomical and physiological factors that predispose collapse of the UA (fig. 2) and their relative role in the pathogenesis of OSA varies from patient to patient. In general, compared to subjects without OSA, patients with OSA have smaller UA cross-sectional area, and higher UA resistance and compliance [64, 65]. The UA is more collapsible when exposed to negative pressure during wakefulness or under passive conditions during sleep

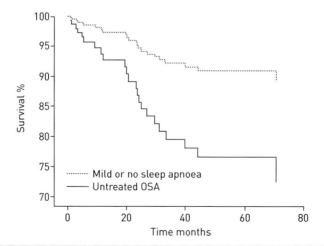

Figure 1. Multivariate Cox proportional hazards survival plots show worse survival for HF patients with untreated OSA (AHI $\geqslant$15 events·h^{-1}; nine (24%) deaths) than those with mild or no sleep apnoea (AHI <15 events·h^{-1}; 14 (12%) deaths) after adjusting for significant confounders (left ventricular ejection fraction, New York Heart Association functional class and age). Hazard ratio 2.81 (p=0.029). Reproduced from [59] with permission from the publisher.

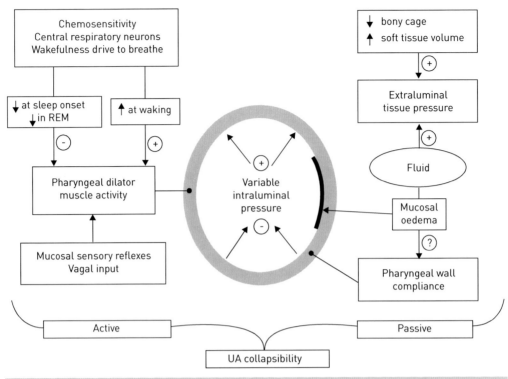

Figure 2. Mechanisms influencing UA collapsibility in the pathogenesis of OSA. A number of dynamic factors, including fluid shift into the neck, determine the active (pharyngeal dilator muscle activity) and passive (intra- and extra-luminal pressure and pharyngeal wall compliance) properties of the UA, which can increase UA collapsibility and lead to UA obstruction and OSA. Reproduced from [43] with permission from the publisher.

[66, 67]. OSA patients are, therefore, more prone than healthy subjects to UA collapse at end-expiration, when neural input to the UA dilators is least [67, 68].

UA narrowing is often due to an increase in surrounding soft tissue owing to muscular hypertrophy, fat or fluid accumulation in the lateral pharyngeal walls. In the neck, expansion of soft tissues laterally and posteriorly is limited by the bony cage of the mandible and cervical spine making it likely that any increase in soft tissue leads to increased pressure medially on the UA lumen. Indeed, in OSA patients, UA narrowing, assessed by magnetic resonance imaging (MRI), is predominantly in the lateral-medial direction rather than in the anterior-posterior direction and UA cross-sectional area is inversely related to thickness of the lateral pharyngeal walls [68, 69]. Furthermore, weight loss in obese subjects increases UA cross-sectional area due to reduced lateral pharyngeal wall thickness [70]. The internal jugular veins lie lateral to the pharynx and their volume and pressure increase on moving from the upright to supine position [71, 72]. Their distension in hypervolemic states, such as renal failure and HF, displaces their lateral walls outwardly, increasing neck circumference. Since neck circumference correlates with AHI, outward expansion of the neck may be accompanied by inward displacement of the lateral pharyngeal walls that could impinge on the UA lumen [73]. Pharyngeal mucosal oedema could result from elevated pressure of the neck veins. In patients with renal failure, both internal jugular vein volume and pharyngeal mucosal water content, assessed by MRI, are related to the AHI suggesting that fluid overload facilitates UA collapse and OSA by contributing to extravascular and intravascular fluid accumulation surrounding the UA [74]. Furthermore, in OSA patients, UA mucosal oedema diminishes with chronic CPAP therapy [74, 75]. Taken together, these data suggest that an increase in soft tissue and/or fluid in the neck lead to an increase in tissue pressure surrounding the UA, which makes it narrower and renders it more collapsible. It is therefore likely that fluid overload in HF patients could contribute to increased neck fluid accumulation with a consequent increase in peripharyngeal tissue pressure and a reduction in UA size.

The initial evidence suggesting a possible link between overnight fluid shift from the legs, changes in UA size and OSA came from a study of men with OSA, in which the authors aimed to determine the effect of changes in central venous pressure on UA cross-sectional area assessed by computed tomography [76]. They used leg elevation to increase and leg tourniquets to decrease venous return from the legs. They showed that at end inspiration, but not at end expiration, there was a significant decrease in both the minimum and mean UA cross-sectional area with leg elevation compared to application of leg tourniquet suggesting that UA size may be influenced by changes in venous blood volume in pharyngeal and neck tissues. However, because they did not assess fluid volumes, fluid movement or central venous pressure, they were unable to demonstrate that changes in neck or peripharyngeal fluid content were causes of change in UA cross-sectional area in response to their interventions.

Subsequently, the effects of rostral fluid shift on UA size and mechanics were investigated in a systematic series of experiments in which application of lower body positive pressure (LBPP), using anti-shock trousers inflated to 40 mmHg, was used to mimic overnight rostral fluid shift by rapidly displacing approximately 300–350 mL of fluid from the legs in nonobese men and women while awake [77, 78]. These changes in fluid volumes are similar to spontaneous overnight rostral fluid shift volumes in patients with sleep apnoea [79]. Leg fluid volume was assessed by bio-electrical impedance, neck circumference by mercury strain gauge, UA cross-sectional area by acoustic pharyngometry, pharyngeal resistance by naso- and hypopharyngeal pressure catheters and pneumotachography, and UA collapsibility by critical closing pressure. Application of LBPP led to increases in neck circumference, pharyngeal airflow resistance and critical closing pressure, and a decrease in UA size indicating that fluid redistributed to the neck and thereby induced narrowing and increased collapsibility of the UA. These data strongly supported the concept that overnight rostral fluid shift from the legs into the neck could induce UA obstruction with obstructive apnoeas and hypopnoeas during sleep [77, 78, 80].

In another series of experiments, the role of spontaneous overnight rostral fluid shift in the pathogenesis of OSA was examined in a variety of patient populations. In the first of these studies involving 23 healthy nonobese men, it was shown that the overnight decrease in leg fluid volume correlated strongly with the overnight change in neck circumference (r= −0.792, p<0.001) and AHI (r=−0.773, p<0.001). In multivariate analysis, which included BMI, the only significant independent correlates of AHI were the overnight changes in leg fluid volume and neck circumference (total model r=0.823, p<0.001) [79]. Significant independent correlates of the overnight change in leg fluid volume were the time spent sitting during the day of the sleep study and age (model r=0.703, p=0.001) [79]. None of these subjects had any clinically detectable leg oedema. These findings favoured a role for overnight fluid redistribution from the legs to the neck in the pathogenesis of OSA in otherwise healthy men. They also suggested that the longer one spends sitting while awake, the more fluid is displaced from the legs overnight, probably because of increased fluid retention in the legs during the day. Older age may also have played a role because the venous valves of the legs become less competent with ageing leading to predisposition of fluid accumulation in the legs while upright. Similar relationships between OSA severity and the degree of overnight fluid volume displacement from the legs were observed in hypertensive patients and those on haemodialysis for renal failure [81, 82].

Regarding patients with HF, YUMINO et al. [42] examined relationships between overnight rostral fluid shift and AHI in patients with either predominantly OSA or predominantly CSA. Among those patients with predominant OSA (⩾50% of apnoeas and hypopnoeas were obstructive), there were strong relationships between the overnight reduction in leg fluid volume and both the overnight increase in neck circumference (r=−0.780, p<0.001) and the AHI (r=−0.881, p<0.001) (fig. 3).

In another study, KASAI et al. [83] examined the effects of LBPP on HF patients with either OSA or CSA. Their findings were intriguing. Among patients with OSA, fluid displacement from the legs by LBPP led to an increase in UA resistance that was accompanied by a reduction in minute volume of ventilation and a consequent increase in arterial carbon dioxide tension ($P\text{CO}_2$). These data indicated that rostral fluid shift from the legs induced a significant degree of UA obstruction while awake, and imply that spontaneous rostral fluid shift from the legs overnight could cause a similar effect and provoke or worsen OSA in HF patients. In contrast, among HF patients with CSA, LBPP had the opposite effects: it reduced UA resistance, increased minute volume of ventilation and reduced $P\text{CO}_2$. These findings indicated that in HF patients with CSA, rostral fluid shift augmented respiratory drive, presumably via fluid accumulation in the lungs, which stimulated pulmonary vagal irritant receptors. Such stimulation probably increased both UA dilator muscle and respiratory pump muscle activity, resulting in a reduction in $P\text{CO}_2$. The authors implied that similar overnight rostral fluid shift could provoke hyperventilation and a fall in $P\text{CO}_2$ below the apnoea threshold that could trigger central apnoeas and provoke or worsen CSA. Taken together the above findings also suggest that nocturnal rostral fluid shift is a common pathophysiological feature of OSA and CSA in HF, but that the pathological manifestation differs according to where fluid accumulates and what receptors are stimulated.

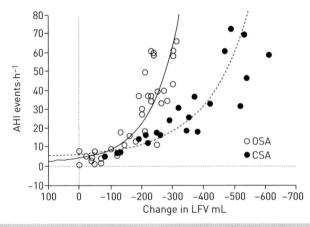

Figure 3. Relationship between overnight change in leg fluid volume (LFV) and AHI in HF patients with either predominantly OSA (r=−0.881, p<0.001) or CSA (r=−0.919, p<0.001). Reproduced from [42] with permission from the publisher.

Among patients with HF, excessive sodium intake can worsen fluid retention and trigger exacerbations of HF [84]. Since fluid retention also appears to play a role in the pathogenesis of OSA in HF, KASAI et al. [85] examined the relationship between dietary sodium intake and both OSA and CSA, which they examined together as sleep apnoea in HF. They found that among HF patients with sleep apnoea, sodium intake was higher than in HF patients without sleep apnoea (3.0±1.2 g *versus* 1.9±0.8 g; p<0.001) and sodium intake was an independent predictor of the AHI (r=0.364, p=0.037) suggesting that fluid retention mediated by sodium intake predisposes to both OSA and CSA [85]. However, measurements of fluid volumes and overnight fluid shift were not made in this study so that a causal relationship between sodium intake and overnight fluid shifts could not be established. Nevertheless, these findings suggest that sodium restriction among HF patients may not only prevent HF exacerbations, but may also reduce severity of OSA.

Further evidence to support the role of fluid overload and fluid shift in the pathogenesis of OSA comes from several interventional studies in which the aim was to alter the degree of fluid shift or the total body fluid volume to determine its effect on OSA. In a study of patients with exacerbations of diastolic HF who had co-existing OSA, BUCCA et al. [86] reported that aggressive diuresis was accompanied by an increase in UA cross-sectional area and a decrease in the AHI by 24%. These findings suggested that UA oedema contributed to severity of OSA [86]. In a randomised trial, REDOLFI et al. [87] reported that in patients with venous insufficiency wearing compression stockings for 1 week led to a 154-mL reduction in the overnight leg fluid volume shift and a 37% reduction in AHI. In patients with nephrotic syndrome, leg oedema and OSA, treatment of the nephrotic syndrome with steroids resolved oedema, reduced total body water and reduced AHI by 50% [88]. In patients with drug resistant hypertension, GADDAM et al.[89] observed that treatment with the aldosterone antagonist and diuretic, spironolactone, for 8 weeks was accompanied by a 50% decrease in the AHI, in association with diuresis and reduced blood pressure.

More recently, KASAI et al. [90] showed that intensified diuretic therapy over a 14-day period in patients with drug resistant hypertension reduced AHI by 16% and the overnight change in leg fluid volume by 26% (p<0.001). In patients with renal failure, following conversion from nocturnal to 24-h continuous ambulatory peritoneal dialysis, in which there was less fluid removal at night, the UA cross-sectional area decreased, tongue volume increased and AHI increased by 55% in association with an increase in total body water [91]. Furthermore, increasing the duration of haemodialysis by converting from conventional to nocturnal haemodialysis has also been shown to alleviate sleep apnoea [92]. While fluid volumes were not measured, it is likely that greater fluid volume removal by nocturnal haemodialysis contributed to the reduction in AHI. Taken together, these data strongly support a role of fluid retention and/or nocturnal rostral fluid shift in the pathogenesis of OSA in a variety of conditions. The extent to which this mechanism is involved probably varies considerably from patient to patient, and may be related to their underlying volume status.

Pathophysiological consequences of OSA in HF

Since a more detailed review of the overall cardiovascular consequences of OSA is provided elsewhere in this *Monograph* [93], this chapter focuses on the cardiovascular consequences of OSA as they relate to HF. Normally, during non-REM sleep, the cardiovascular system is in a state of relaxation [94]. Vagal output increases while SNA, heart rate, cardiac output and systemic vascular resistance all fall [95–97]. While there may be intermittent surges in SNA, heart rate and BP in REM sleep and following spontaneous arousals the mean heart rate and blood pressure during sleep are typically below waking levels [95]. The presence of OSA, however, disrupts this quiescent state: repetitive cycles of apnoeas and hypopnoeas lead to exaggerated swings in negative intrathoracic pressure, surges in SNA and blood pressure, IH and frequent awakenings [14], all of which may have adverse cardiovascular consequences and contribute to the progression of HF [95, 98–100].

Only one small study involving eight HF patients with OSA assessed mean intrathoracic pressure during sleep which was approximately −6−−8 cm H_2O [101]. However, during obstructive apnoeas in HF patients, intrathoracic pressure can become progressively more negative and fall to as low as −80 cmH_2O in an effort to overcome UA occlusion as respiratory drive is augmented by progressive hypoxia and carbon dioxide retention [102, 103].This increases left ventricular transmural pressure (the difference between intracardiac and intrathoracic pressure) and hence afterload [103]. Venous return also increases, which augments right ventricular pre-load, resulting in right ventricular distension and a leftward shift of the interventricular septum during diastole that impedes left ventricular filling [104, 105]. Together, reduced left ventricular preload and increased left ventricular afterload reduce stroke volume and cardiac output [99, 106]. This reduction is more pronounced in patients with HF than in subjects without HF, partly due to the inability of the failing myocardium to generate sufficient contractile force to overcome the increased afterload [103]. Furthermore, left ventricular transmural pressure increases myocardial oxygen demand and reduces coronary blood flow [107]. Coupled with apnoea-related hypoxia, these mechanisms may precipitate myocardial ischaemia and impair cardiac contractility even further [108, 109].

OSA-induced IH and hypercapnia stimulate peripheral and central chemoreceptors, leading to increases in SNA [110, 111]. SNA is further augmented during apnoeas by the elimination of reflex inhibition of SNA by pulmonary stretch receptors [112]. Arousal from sleep at apnoea termination also augments SNA and reduces cardiac vagal activity, which together cause post-apnoeic surges in BP and heart rate [113]. These adverse autonomic effects of OSA are not confined to sleep, since elevated SNA can carry over into wakefulness through as yet to be identified mechanisms [114]. Indeed, treatment of OSA in patients with HF reduces SNA during wakefulness [58]. The long-term consequences of augmented SNA may include cardiac myocyte necrosis and apoptosis, and worsening ventricular dysfunction [94, 115, 116]. Furthermore, in HF patients with OSA, blood pressure levels during sleep can be higher than during wakefulness and can be reduced by treatment of OSA with CPAP [101]. Elevated nocturnal blood pressure, in combination with the mechanisms described above, can contribute to elevated left ventricular afterload, further compromise left ventricular systolic function and, ultimately, increase mortality risk [59].

OSA-induced IH and subsequent post apnoeic reoxygenation may lead to oxidative stress and activation of inflammatory mediators and transcription factors, which may cause vascular endothelial dysfunction. Patients with OSA have increased levels of TNF-α [117, 118], low plasma nitrate and nitrite levels [119, 120] and up-regulation of leukocyte adhesion molecule expression [121]. IH can activate nuclear factor-κβ, an important transcription factor that stimulates several pro-inflammatory pathways, with the potential to cause endothelial dysfunction [122, 123]. It has been shown that compared to subjects without OSA, those with OSA have impaired vascular endothelium-dependent flow-mediated dilation that improves with CPAP therapy [124]. There is evidence that treatment of OSA by CPAP increases nitric oxide activity, reduces levels of inflammatory markers and improves endothelial function [119, 120, 125].

Conclusion

The prevalence of HF is increasing as more people survive myocardial infarction and the population ages. The associated mortality remains high, despite recent advances in treatment. Similarly, the prevalence of OSA is increasing as obesity rates rise and the population ages [45, 126]. There is a large overlap of OSA and HF and, indeed, OSA appears to be more prevalent in HF patients than in the general population. There are two possible reasons why OSA is so common in HF: 1) OSA contributes to the causation of HF; and 2) fluid overload secondary to HF can cause increased rostral fluid shift from the legs during sleep and thereby contribute to the pathogenesis of OSA. Consequently, there is potential for a vicious cycle to arise whereby pre-existing OSA can contribute to the development and progression of HF, while fluid retention secondary to HF can contribute to the development of OSA. Further elucidation of the pathophysiological mechanisms involved in this vicious cycle could lead to novel therapies targeting fluid overload and overnight rostral fluid shift in reducing severity of OSA and HF. Conversely, direct treatment of OSA by, for example, PAP devices, could lead to reduced morbidity and mortality in HF. Large scale, long-term randomised trials will be required to test this important possibility.

References

1. McMurray JJ, Adamopoulos S, Anker SD, et al. ESC Guidelines for the diagnosis and treatment of acute and chronic heart failure 2012: the Task Force for the Diagnosis and Treatment of Acute and Chronic Heart Failure 2012 of the European Society of Cardiology. Developed in collaboration with the Heart Failure Association (HFA) of the ESC. Eur Heart J 2012; 33: 1787–1847.
2. Owan TE, Hodge DO, Herges RM, et al. Trends in prevalence and outcome of heart failure with preserved ejection fraction. N Engl J Med 2006; 355: 251–259.
3. Levy D, Kenchaiah S, Larson MG, et al. Long-term trends in the incidence of and survival with heart failure. N Engl J Med 2002; 347: 1397–1402.
4. Effect of enalapril on survival in patients with reduced left ventricular ejection fractions and congestive heart failure. The SOLVD Investigators. N Engl J Med 1991; 325: 293–302.
5. Effect of metoprolol CR/XL in chronic heart failure: Metoprolol CR/XL randomised intervention trial in congestive heart failure (MERIT-HF). Lancet 1999; 353: 2001–2007.
6. Pitt B, Zannad F, Remme WJ, et al. The effect of spironolactone on morbidity and mortality in patients with severe heart failure. Randomized Aldactone Evaluation Study Investigators. N Engl J Med 1999; 341: 709–717.
7. Remme WJ, Swedberg K, Task Force for the Diagnosis and Treatment of Chronic Heart Failure, et al. Guidelines for the diagnosis and treatment of chronic heart failure. Eur Heart J 2001; 22: 1527–1560.
8. Raymond I, Pedersen F, Steensgaard-Hansen F, et al. Prevalence of impaired left ventricular systolic function and heart failure in a middle aged and elderly urban population segment of Copenhagen. Heart 2003; 89: 1422–1429.
9. Nelson GR, Cohn PF, Gorlin R. Prognosis in medically-treated coronary artery disease: influence of ejection fraction compared to other parameters. Circulation 1975; 52: 408–412.
10. Redfield MM, Jacobsen SJ, Burnett JC Jr, et al. Burden of systolic and diastolic ventricular dysfunction in the community: appreciating the scope of the heart failure epidemic. JAMA 2003; 289: 194–202.
11. Mosterd A, Hoes AW, de Bruyne MC, et al. Prevalence of heart failure and left ventricular dysfunction in the general population: the Rotterdam Study. Eur Heart J 1999; 20: 447–455.
12. Shah AM, Mann DL. In search of new therapeutic targets and strategies for heart failure: recent advances in basic science. Lancet 2011; 378: 704–712.
13. McMurray JJ. Clinical practice. Systolic heart failure. N Engl J Med 2010; 362: 228–238.
14. Ryan CM, Bradley TD. Pathogenesis of obstructive sleep apnea. J Appl Physiol 2005; 99: 2440–2450.
15. Bradley TD, Floras JS. Obstructive sleep apnoea and its cardiovascular consequences. Lancet 2009; 373: 82–93.

16.   Marin JM, Carrizo SJ, Vicente E, et al. Long-term cardiovascular outcomes in men with obstructive sleep apnoea-hypopnoea with or without treatment with continuous positive airway pressure: an observational study. Lancet 2005; 365: 1046–1053.

17.   Peppard PE, Young T, Palta M, et al. Prospective study of the association between sleep-disordered breathing and hypertension. N Engl J Med 2000; 342: 1378–1384.

18.   Jordan AS, McSharry DG, Malhotra A. Adult obstructive sleep apnoea. Lancet 2014; 383: 736–747.

19.   Yumino D, Wang H, Floras JS, et al. Prevalence and physiological predictors of sleep apnea in patients with heart failure and systolic dysfunction. J Card Fail 2009; 15: 279–285.

20.   Kimmel PL, Miller G, Mendelson WB. Sleep apnea syndrome in chronic renal disease. Am J Med 1989; 86: 308–314.

21.   Kasai T, Floras JS, Bradley TD. Sleep apnea and cardiovascular disease: a bidirectional relationship. Circulation 2012; 126: 1495–1510.

22.   Thompson WO, Alper JM, Thompson PK. The effect of posture upon the velocity of blood flow in man. J Clin Invest 1928; 5: 605–609.

23.   Thompson WO, Thompson PK, Dailey ME. The effect of posture upon the composition and volume of the blood in man. J Clin Invest 1928; 5: 573–604.

24.   Waterfield RL. The effects of posture on the circulating blood volume. J Physiol 1931; 72: 110–120.

25.   Thulesius O, Norgren L, Gjores JE. Foot-volumetry, a new method for objective assessment of edema and venous function. VASA 1973; 2: 325–329.

26.   Waterfield RL. The effect of posture on the volume of the leg. J Physiol 1931; 72: 121–131.

27.   Manyari DE, Wang Z, Cohen J, et al. Assessment of the human splanchnic venous volume-pressure relation using radionuclide plethysmography. Effect of nitroglycerin. Circulation 1993; 87: 1142–1151.

28.   Hirakawa S, Ohsumi Y, Gotoh K, et al. Volume-pressure relations of the human pulmonary "venous" system studied by radionuclide angiocardiography and passive leg elevation, with special reference to the effect of nitroglycerin. Jpn Circ J 1986; 50: 303–314.

29.   Baccelli G, Pacenti P, Terrani S, et al. Scintigraphic recording of blood volume shifts. J Nuclear Med 1995; 36: 2022–2031.

30.   Manyari DE, Malkinson TJ, Robinson V, et al. Acute changes in forearm venous volume and tone using radionuclide plethysmography. Am J Physiol 1988; 255: H947–H952.

31.   Zhu F, Kuhlmann MK, Kotanko P, et al. A method for the estimation of hydration state during hemodialysis using a calf bioimpedance technique. Physiol Meas 2008; 29: S503–S516.

32.   Demura S, Sato S, Kitabayashi T. Percentage of total body fat as estimated by three automatic bioelectrical impedance analyzers. J Physiol Anthropol Appl Human Sci 2004; 23: 93–99.

33.   Kyle UG, Bosaeus I, De Lorenzo AD, et al. Bioelectrical impedance analysis – part I: review of principles and methods. Clin Nutr 2004; 23: 1226–1243.

34.   Jaffrin MY, Morel H. Body fluid volumes measurements by impedance: a review of bioimpedance spectroscopy (BIS) and bioimpedance analysis (BIA) methods. Med Eng Phys 2008; 30: 1257–1269.

35.   Starling EH. On the absorption of fluids from the connective tissue spaces. J Physiol 1896; 19: 312–326.

36.   Krogh A, Landis EM, Turner AH. The movement of fluid through the human capillary wall in relation to venous pressure and to the colloid osmotic pressure of the blood. J Clin Invest 1932; 11: 63–95.

37.   Youmans JB, Wells HS, Donley D, et al. The effect of posture (standing) on the serum protein concentration and colloid osmotic pressure of blood from the foot in relation to the formation of edema. J Clin Invest 1934; 13: 447–459.

38.   Levick JR, Michel CC. The effects of position and skin temperature on the capillary pressures in the fingers and toes. J Physiol 1978; 274: 97–109.

39.   Avasthey P, Wood EH. Intrathoracic and venous pressure relationships during responses to changes in body position. J Appl Physiol 1974; 37: 166–175.

40.   Terada N, Takeuchi T. Postural changes in venous pressure gradients in anesthetized monkeys. Am J Physiol 1993; 264: H21–H25.

41.   Guyton AC. Interstitial fluid pressure. II. Pressure-volume curves of interstitial space. Circ Res 1965; 16: 452–460.

42.   Yumino D, Redolfi S, Ruttanaumpawan P, et al. Nocturnal rostral fluid shift: a unifying concept for the pathogenesis of obstructive and central sleep apnea in men with heart failure. Circulation 2010; 121: 1598–1605.

43.   White LH, Bradley TD. Role of nocturnal rostral fluid shift in the pathogenesis of obstructive and central sleep apnoea. J Physiol 2013; 591: 1179–1193.

44.   Young T, Palta M, Dempsey J, et al. The occurrence of sleep-disordered breathing among middle-aged adults. N Engl J Med 1993; 328: 1230–1235.

45.   Peppard PE, Young T, Barnet JH, et al. Increased prevalence of sleep-disordered breathing in adults. Am J Epidemiol 2013; 177: 1006–1014.

46.   Shahar E, Whitney CW, Redline S, et al. Sleep-disordered breathing and cardiovascular disease: cross-sectional results of the Sleep Heart Health Study. Am J Respir Crit Care Med 2001; 163: 19–25.

47.   Gottlieb DJ, Yenokyan G, Newman AB, et al. Prospective study of obstructive sleep apnea and incident coronary heart disease and heart failure: the sleep heart health study. Circulation 2010; 122: 352–360.

48. Ferrier K, Campbell A, Yee B, et al. Sleep-disordered breathing occurs frequently in stable outpatients with congestive heart failure. Chest 2005; 128: 2116–2122.

49. Javaheri S. Sleep disorders in systolic heart failure: a prospective study of 100 male patients. The final report. Int J Cardiol 2006; 106: 21–28.

50. Vazir A, Hastings PC, Dayer M, et al. A high prevalence of sleep disordered breathing in men with mild symptomatic chronic heart failure due to left ventricular systolic dysfunction. Eur J Heart Fail 2007; 9: 243–250.

51. Sekizuka H, Osada N, Miyake F. Sleep disordered breathing in heart failure patients with reduced versus preserved ejection fraction. Heart Lung Circ 2013; 22: 104–109.

52. Bitter T, Faber L, Hering D, et al. Sleep-disordered breathing in heart failure with normal left ventricular ejection fraction. Eur J Heart Fail 2009; 11: 602–608.

53. Herrscher TE, Akre H, Overland B, et al. High prevalence of sleep apnea in heart failure outpatients: even in patients with preserved systolic function. J Card Fail 2011; 17: 420–425.

54. Arzt M, Young T, Finn L, et al. Sleepiness and sleep in patients with both systolic heart failure and obstructive sleep apnea. Arch Intern Med 2006; 166: 1716–1722.

55. Bitter T, Westerheide N, Hossain SM, et al. Symptoms of sleep apnoea in chronic heart failure – results from a prospective cohort study in 1,500 patients. Sleep Breath 2012; 16: 781–791.

56. Taranto Montemurro L, Floras JS, Picton P, et al. Relationship of heart rate variability to sleepiness in patients with obstructive sleep apnea with and without heart failure. J Clin Sleep Med 2014; 10: 271–276.

57. Taranto Montemurro L, Floras JS, Millar PJ, et al. Inverse relationship of subjective daytime sleepiness to sympathetic activity in patients with heart failure and obstructive sleep apnea. Chest 2012; 142: 1222–1228.

58. Usui K, Bradley TD, Spaak J, et al. Inhibition of awake sympathetic nerve activity of heart failure patients with obstructive sleep apnea by nocturnal continuous positive airway pressure. J Am Coll Cardiol 2005; 45: 2008–2011.

59. Wang H, Parker JD, Newton GE, et al. Influence of obstructive sleep apnea on mortality in patients with heart failure. J Am Coll Cardiol 2007; 49: 1625–1631.

60. Jilek C, Krenn M, Sebah D, et al. Prognostic impact of sleep disordered breathing and its treatment in heart failure: an observational study. Eur J Heart Fail 2011; 13: 68–75.

61. Roebuck T, Solin P, Kaye DM, et al. Increased long-term mortality in heart failure due to sleep apnoea is not yet proven. Eur Respir J 2004; 23: 735–740.

62. Bradley TD, Brown IG, Grossman RF, et al. Pharyngeal size in snorers, nonsnorers, and patients with obstructive sleep apnea. N Engl J Med 1986; 315: 1327–1331.

63. Remmers JE, deGroot WJ, Sauerland EK, et al. Pathogenesis of upper airway occlusion during sleep. J Appl Physiol 1978; 44: 931–938.

64. Stauffer JL, Zwillich CW, Cadieux RJ, et al. Pharyngeal size and resistance in obstructive sleep apnea. Am Rev Respir Dis 1987; 136: 623–627.

65. Brown IG, Bradley TD, Phillipson EA, et al. Pharyngeal compliance in snoring subjects with and without obstructive sleep apnea. Am Rev Respir Dis 1985; 132: 211–215.

66. Suratt PM, McTier RF, Wilhoit SC. Collapsibility of the nasopharyngeal airway in obstructive sleep apnea. Am Rev Respir Dis 1985; 132: 967–971.

67. Younes M. Contributions of upper airway mechanics and control mechanisms to severity of obstructive apnea. Am J Respir Crit Care Med 2003; 168: 645–658.

68. Schwab RJ, Gefter WB. Anatomical factors: insights from imaging studies. In: Pack AI, ed. Sleep apnea: pathogenesis, diagnosis and treatment. New York, Marcel Dekker, 2002; pp. 1–31.

69. Rodenstein DO, Dooms G, Thomas Y, et al. Pharyngeal shape and dimensions in healthy subjects, snorers, and patients with obstructive sleep apnoea. Thorax 1990; 45: 722–727.

70. Schwab RJ, Pasirstein M, Pierson R, et al. Identification of upper airway anatomic risk factors for obstructive sleep apnea with volumetric magnetic resonance imaging. Am J Respir Crit Care Med 2003; 168: 522–530.

71. Cirovic S, Walsh C, Fraser WD, et al. The effect of posture and positive pressure breathing on the hemodynamics of the internal jugular vein. Aviat Space Environ Med 2003; 74: 125–131.

72. Lobato EB, Florete OG Jr, Paige GB, et al. Cross-sectional area and intravascular pressure of the right internal jugular vein during anesthesia: effects of Trendelenburg position, positive intrathoracic pressure, and hepatic compression. J Clin Anesth 1998; 10: 1–5.

73. Davies RJ, Stradling JR. The relationship between neck circumference, radiographic pharyngeal anatomy, and the obstructive sleep apnoea syndrome. Eur Respir J 1990; 3: 509–514.

74. Elias RM, Chan CT, Paul N, et al. Relationship of pharyngeal water content and jugular volume with severity of obstructive sleep apnea in renal failure. Nephrol Dial Transplant 2013; 28: 937–944.

75. Ryan CF, Lowe AA, Li D, et al. Magnetic resonance imaging of the upper airway in obstructive sleep apnea before and after chronic nasal continuous positive airway pressure therapy. Am Rev Respir Dis 1991; 144: 939–944.

76. Shepard JW Jr, Pevernagie DA, Stanson AW, et al. Effects of changes in central venous pressure on upper airway size in patients with obstructive sleep apnea. Am J Respir Crit Care Med 1996; 153: 250–254.

77.   Chiu KL, Ryan CM, Shiota S, et al. Fluid shift by lower body positive pressure increases pharyngeal resistance in healthy subjects. Am J Respir Crit Care Med 2006; 174: 1378–1383.

78.   Shiota S, Ryan CM, Chiu KL, et al. Alterations in upper airway cross-sectional area in response to lower body positive pressure in healthy subjects. Thorax 2007; 62: 868–872.

79.   Redolfi S, Yumino D, Ruttanaumpawan P, et al. Relationship between overnight rostral fluid shift and obstructive sleep apnea in nonobese men. Am J Respir Crit Care Med 2009; 179: 241–246.

80.   Su MC, Chiu KL, Ruttanaumpawan P, et al. Lower body positive pressure increases upper airway collapsibility in healthy subjects. Respir Physiol Neurobiol 2008; 161: 306–312.

81.   Friedman O, Bradley TD, Chan CT, et al. Relationship between overnight rostral fluid shift and obstructive sleep apnea in drug-resistant hypertension. Hypertension 2010; 56: 1077–1082.

82.   Elias RM, Bradley TD, Kasai T, et al. Rostral overnight fluid shift in end-stage renal disease: relationship with obstructive sleep apnea. Nephrol Dial Transplant 2012; 27: 1569–1573.

83.   Kasai T, Motwani SS, Yumino D, et al. Contrasting effects of lower body positive pressure on upper airways resistance and partial pressure of carbon dioxide in men with heart failure and obstructive or central sleep apnea. J Am Coll Cardiol 2013; 61: 1157–1166.

84.   Arcand J, Ivanov J, Sasson A, et al. A high-sodium diet is associated with acute decompensated heart failure in ambulatory heart failure patients: a prospective follow-up study. Am J Clin Nutr 2011; 93: 332–337.

85.   Kasai T, Arcand J, Allard JP, et al. Relationship between sodium intake and sleep apnea in patients with heart failure. J Am Coll Cardiol 2011; 58: 1970–1974.

86.   Bucca CB, Brussino L, Battisti A, et al. Diuretics in obstructive sleep apnea with diastolic heart failure. Chest 2007; 132: 440–446.

87.   Redolfi S, Arnulf I, Pottier M, et al. Effects of venous compression of the legs on overnight rostral fluid shift and obstructive sleep apnea. Respir Physiol Neurobiol 2011; 175: 390–393.

88.   Tang SC, Lam B, Lam JC, et al. Impact of nephrotic edema of the lower limbs on obstructive sleep apnea: gathering a unifying concept for the pathogenetic role of nocturnal rostral fluid shift. Nephrol Dial Transplant 2012; 27: 2788–2794.

89.   Gaddam K, Pimenta E, Thomas SJ, et al. Spironolactone reduces severity of obstructive sleep apnoea in patients with resistant hypertension: a preliminary report. J Hum Hypertens 2010; 24: 532–537.

90.   Kasai T, Bradley TD, Friedman O, et al. Effect of intensified diuretic therapy on overnight rostral fluid shift and obstructive sleep apnoea in patients with uncontrolled hypertension. J Hypertens 2014; 32: 673–680.

91.   Tang SC, Lam B, Lai AS, et al. Improvement in sleep apnea during nocturnal peritoneal dialysis is associated with reduced airway congestion and better uremic clearance. Clin J Am Soc Nephrol 2009; 4: 410–418.

92.   Hanly PJ, Pierratos A. Improvement of sleep apnea in patients with chronic renal failure who undergo nocturnal hemodialysis. N Engl J Med 2001; 344: 102–107.

93.   Sánchez-de-la-Torre M, Bonsignore MR, Barbé F. Cardiovascular disease: pathophysiological mechanisms. In: Pépin J-L, Barbé F, eds. Obstructive Sleep Apnoea. ERS Monogr 2015; 67: 37–50.

94.   Bradley TD, Floras JS. Sleep apnea and heart failure: Part I: obstructive sleep apnea. Circulation 2003; 107: 1671–1678.

95.   Somers VK, Dyken ME, Mark AL, et al. Sympathetic-nerve activity during sleep in normal subjects. N Engl J Med 1993; 328: 303–307.

96.   Khatri IM, Freis ED. Hemodynamic changes during sleep. J Appl Physiol 1967; 22: 867–873.

97.   Van de Borne P, Nguyen H, Biston P, et al. Effects of wake and sleep stages on the 24-h autonomic control of blood pressure and heart rate in recumbent men. Am J Physiol 1994; 266: H548–H554.

98.   Tilkian AG, Guilleminault C, Schroeder JS, et al. Hemodynamics in sleep-induced apnea. Studies during wakefulness and sleep. Ann Intern Med 1976; 85: 714–719.

99.   Tolle FA, Judy WV, Yu PL, et al. Reduced stroke volume related to pleural pressure in obstructive sleep apnea. J Appl Physiol 1983; 55: 1718–1724.

100. Daly PA, Sole MJ. Myocardial catecholamines and the pathophysiology of heart failure. Circulation 1990; 82: Suppl. 2, I35–I43.

101. Tkacova R, Rankin F, Fitzgerald FS, et al. Effects of continuous positive airway pressure on obstructive sleep apnea and left ventricular afterload in patients with heart failure. Circulation 1998; 98: 2269–2275.

102. Malone S, Liu PP, Holloway R, et al. Obstructive sleep apnoea in patients with dilated cardiomyopathy: effects of continuous positive airway pressure. Lancet 1991; 338: 1480–1484.

103. Bradley TD, Hall MJ, Ando S, et al. Hemodynamic effects of simulated obstructive apneas in humans with and without heart failure. Chest 2001; 119: 1827–1835.

104. Stoohs R, Guilleminault C. Cardiovascular changes associated with obstructive sleep apnea syndrome. J Appl Physiol 1992; 72: 583–589.

105. Brinker JA, Weiss JL, Lappe DL, et al. Leftward septal displacement during right ventricular loading in man. Circulation 1980; 61: 626–633.

106. Parker JD, Brooks D, Kozar LF, *et al.* Acute and chronic effects of airway obstruction on canine left ventricular performance. *Am J Respir Crit Care Med* 1999; 160: 1888–1896.

107. Scharf SM, Graver LM, Balaban K. Cardiovascular effects of periodic occlusions of the upper airways in dogs. *Am Rev Respir Dis* 1992; 146: 321–329.

108. Scharf SM, Bianco JA, Tow DE, *et al.* The effects of large negative intrathoracic pressure on left ventricular function in patients with coronary artery disease. *Circulation* 1981; 63: 871–875.

109. Franklin KA, Nilsson JB, Sahlin C, *et al.* Sleep apnoea and nocturnal angina. *Lancet* 1995; 345: 1085–1087.

110. Somers VK, Mark AL, Zavala DC, *et al.* Contrasting effects of hypoxia and hypercapnia on ventilation and sympathetic activity in humans. *J Appl Physiol* 1989; 67: 2101–2106.

111. Bradley TD, Tkacova R, Hall MJ, *et al.* Augmented sympathetic neural response to simulated obstructive apnoea in human heart failure. *Clin Sci* 2003; 104: 231–238.

112. Somers VK, Mark AL, Zavala DC, *et al.* Influence of ventilation and hypocapnia on sympathetic nerve responses to hypoxia in normal humans. *J Appl Physiol* 1989; 67: 2095–2100.

113. Horner RL, Brooks D, Kozar LF, *et al.* Immediate effects of arousal from sleep on cardiac autonomic outflow in the absence of breathing in dogs. *J Appl Physiol* 1995; 79: 151–162.

114. Spaak J, Egri ZJ, Kubo T, *et al.* Muscle sympathetic nerve activity during wakefulness in heart failure patients with and without sleep apnea. *Hypertension* 2005; 46: 1327–1332.

115. Kaye DM, Lambert GW, Lefkovits J, *et al.* Neurochemical evidence of cardiac sympathetic activation and increased central nervous system norepinephrine turnover in severe congestive heart failure. *J Am Coll Cardiol* 1994; 23: 570–578.

116. Cohn JN, Levine TB, Olivari MT, *et al.* Plasma norepinephrine as a guide to prognosis in patients with chronic congestive heart failure. *N Engl J Med* 1984; 311: 819–823.

117. Minoguchi K, Tazaki T, Yokoe T, *et al.* Elevated production of tumor necrosis factor-alpha by monocytes in patients with obstructive sleep apnea syndrome. *Chest* 2004; 126: 1473–1479.

118. Vgontzas AN, Papanicolaou DA, Bixler EO, *et al.* Elevation of plasma cytokines in disorders of excessive daytime sleepiness: role of sleep disturbance and obesity. *J Clin Endocrinol Metab* 1997; 82: 1313–1316.

119. Alonso-Fernandez A, Garcia-Rio F, Arias MA, *et al.* Effects of CPAP on oxidative stress and nitrate efficiency in sleep apnoea: a randomised trial. *Thorax* 2009; 64: 581–586.

120. Ip MS, Lam B, Chan LY, *et al.* Circulating nitric oxide is suppressed in obstructive sleep apnea and is reversed by nasal continuous positive airway pressure. *Am J Respir Crit Care Med* 2000; 162: 2166–2171.

121. Dyugovskaya L, Lavie P, Lavie L. Increased adhesion molecules expression and production of reactive oxygen species in leukocytes of sleep apnea patients. *Am J Respir Crit Care Med* 2002; 165: 934–939.

122. Drager LF, Polotsky VY, Lorenzi-Filho G. Obstructive sleep apnea: an emerging risk factor for atherosclerosis. *Chest* 2011; 140: 534–542.

123. Ryan S, Taylor CT, McNicholas WT. Selective activation of inflammatory pathways by intermittent hypoxia in obstructive sleep apnea syndrome. *Circulation* 2005; 112: 2660–2667.

124. Ip MS, Tse HF, Lam B, *et al.* Endothelial function in obstructive sleep apnea and response to treatment. *Am J Respir Crit Care Med* 2004; 169: 348–353.

125. Ryan S, Taylor CT, McNicholas WT. Predictors of elevated nuclear factor-kappaB-dependent genes in obstructive sleep apnea syndrome. *Am J Respir Crit Care Med* 2006; 174: 824–830.

126. Webber L, Divajeva D, Marsh T, *et al.* The future burden of obesity-related diseases in the 53 WHO European-Region countries and the impact of effective interventions: a modelling study. *BMJ Open* 2014; 4: e004787.

Support statement: Supported by the Canadian Institutes of Health Research operating grant MOP-82731. O. D. Lyons was supported by a Canadian Thoracic Society/European Respiratory Society Peter Macklem Joint Research Fellowship, and by the Joseph M. West Family Memorial Fund Postgraduate Research Award. T.D. Bradley was supported by the Clifford Nordal Chair in Sleep Apnea and Rehabilitation Research.

Disclosures: None declared.

Chapter 6

Women and pregnancy

Francisco Campos-Rodríguez[1], Maria J. Masdeu-Margalef[2] and
Miguel Ángel Martinez-García[3,4]

OSA is a common disorder with sex differences with respect to prevalence, clinical complaints and pathophysiology. Despite these differences, most of the research on OSA has been conducted in studies with a large predominance of men, so the consequences and appropriate treatment of this sleep disorder in women have rarely been addressed.

Recent data suggest that women with OSA may have greater quality of life impairment than their counterparts. The association between OSA and cardiovascular consequences is controversial, but recent observational studies have shown an increased incidence of severe cardiovascular outcomes and mortality in women with OSA. Treatment with CPAP may play a role in reversing this excess cardiovascular risk in women.

The physiological changes of pregnancy may predispose females to develop OSA. OSA during pregnancy has been associated with increased risk of adverse maternal and fetal outcomes. CPAP may play a role in protecting against these consequences, but more research in this field is still needed.

The belief that OSA is a disease primarily affecting men, combined with distinct referral symptoms in women, has ensured that it has long been overlooked in women. There are also sex differences in pathophysiology, polysomnographic findings OSA severity and, maybe, in consequences such as functional status, cardiovascular outcomes and therapeutic options. Unfortunately, most research on OSA outcomes and treatment relies on male cohorts and their results may not be directly applicable to women. Recent studies in women suggest that OSA may pose an increased risk of cardiovascular and functional outcomes in women, and that CPAP therapy may offset this risk.

Pregnancy is a transient condition that may increase the risk of developing or aggravating pre-existing OSA. IH and sleep fragmentation associated with OSA may lead to adverse maternal and fetal outcomes, such as pre-eclampsia, gestational diabetes, preterm delivery, caesarean delivery and low birth weight. However, research in this area is still in the initial phase.

Prevalence

OSA is a frequent condition characterised by repetitive episodes of UA obstruction during sleep that provokes sleep fragmentation and oxygen desaturation. Women have consistently

[1]Sleep-Disordered Breathing Unit, Respiratory Dept, Hospital Universitario de Valme, Seville, Spain. [2]Respiratory Dept and Sleep Center, Hospital de Sabadell, Corporacio Sanitària Parc Tauli, Barcelona, Spain. [3]Pneumology Service, Hospital Universitario y Politécnico La Fe, Valencia, Spain. [4]CIBER de enfermedades respiratorias, Bunyoles, Spain.

Correspondence: Francisco Campos-Rodríguez, Sleep-Disordered Breathing Unit, Respiratory Dept, Hospital Universitario de Valme, 41014, Seville, Spain. E-mail: fracamrod@gmail.com

been reported to have a lower prevalence of this sleep disorder than men, with a male/female ratio of 2:1 to 5:1 [1–4]. Although the prevalence of OSA in women has traditionally been reported to be ~2–3%, updated estimates from the Wisconsin Sleep Cohort have increased the prevalence of moderate-to-severe OSA (AHI $\geqslant$15 events·h^{-1}) to 6% in women in the general population [5]. Another recent Swedish study, including updated criteria for the definition of a hypopnoea, reported a 20% prevalence of moderate-to-severe OSA in women aged 20–70 years [6]. Despite increasing prevalence, the clear sex difference raises the question of whether women manifest OSA differently from men, or whether they may be protected by a distinct pathophysiology (table 1).

Clinical features

It has been postulated that women do not manifest the classical symptoms of OSA as plainly as men do (table 1). However, population-based cohorts have found that the prevalence of

Table 1. Sex differences in prevalence, pathophysiology and clinical manifestations of OSA

	Men	Women
Prevalence of AHI $\geqslant$15 events·h^{-1}	13%	6%
Typical age of diagnosis	40–60 years	50–60 years (usually at an older age than men)
Referral complaints	Typical triad: snoring, breathing pauses and hypersomnolence	Atypical symptoms: depression, anxiety, insomnia, headache and fatigue
EDS	Stronger association with OSA	Weaker association with OSA ESS not validated in women
Prevalence of depression	12–25%	35–38%
Presence of partner during sleep interview	Common	Less common
		Under-reporting of useful objective symptoms
Physician awareness	High	Low
Obesity	Common	Common, women are usually more obese than men
	Central obesity	Peripheral obesity
UA	More collapsible: larger but longer UA	Less collapsible: lower passive critical value of positive end-expiratory pressure than men
Sex hormones	Small role	Large role Progesterone/oestrogen protect against OSA Menopause increases OSA risk
Polysomnographic profile	Men have more severe OSA	Milder OSA severity in women
	Men have more positional and less stage-dependent OSA than women	Clustering of respiratory events in REM sleep
	Men have higher AHI than women in non-REM sleep	Partial upper airway obstruction more common than in men

typical symptoms such as snoring and breathing pauses are similar in both sexes [2, 7]. Women usually come to clinical interviews alone, so it is probable that symptoms witnessed by their partner, such as snoring and apnoeic events, may be under reported [8, 9]. Other researchers have suggested that the characteristics of snoring may differ from men to women, which may also have an impact on clinical suspicion [10]. More importantly, women, unlike men, more frequently present with "atypical" symptoms, such as depression, anxiety, insomnia, headache and fatigue [1, 11–15]. This different presentation, rather than any real differences in symptoms, coupled with a low awareness among physicians, may lead to delayed recognition of the disease and underdiagnosis.

EDS, one of the hallmarks of OSA, appears to have very poor predictive value in women. In the Wisconsin Sleep Cohort, EDS was reported in ~20% of women without OSA and was twice as common as in men [7]. Furthermore, the ESS, a common tool used to subjectively measure EDS, has not been validated in women. BALDWIN et al. [16] observed that the ESS was a more sensitive measure of subjective sleepiness in males than in females, and recent data from the Wisconsin Sleep Cohort showed that OSA was not associated with increased subjective or objective sleepiness in women [17].

Pathophysiology and polysomnographic characteristics

The UA seems to be less collapsible in women than in men, thus contributing to a lower prevalence of OSA. Although the cross-sectional area of the UA is larger in men than in women, it is also longer and, therefore, more collapsible [18–20]. KIRKNESS et al. [21] compared 30 males and 30 females matched for AHI, BMI and age, and found that the age-adjusted passive critical value of positive end-expiratory pressure was 1.9±0.9 cmH$_2$O lower in women compared to men.

Women with OSA are usually more obese than males, although it seems that fat distribution, rather than BMI, may be more important in determining the risk of OSA. Men tend to show a higher proportion of central body fat, including both visceral adiposity and upper body fat, as opposed to peripheral obesity in women [9, 22, 23]. Using computed tomography, KRITIKOU et al. [24] have reported that visceral adiposity is the primary type of fat associated with OSA in males, whereas in females it is global adiposity. MAZZUCA et al. [25] studied 423 men and 105 women with suspected OSA and found that BMI and waist circumference explained 30.2% of AHI variability in men, while in women hip and neck circumference explained 33.9% of AHI variability.

There is controversy as to whether women have different respiratory control stability than men. Some studies suggest that ventilatory stability in men may be more susceptible to the influence of chemical factors than women [26–28]. However, JORDAN et al. [29] noted that in both AHI- and BMI-matched men and women with OSA, loop gain did not differ significantly between sexes, suggesting that respiratory control stability was less important than UA collapsibility in the pathogenesis of the disease.

Hormones play a key role in the pathogenesis of OSA in women. There is strong evidence that menopause increases the risk of developing OSA 3.5- to 4-fold [30–32]. In fact, OSA is uncommon in pre-menopausal women, but the prevalence of this sleep disorder increases after the menopause and catches up with that of men of a similar age. Different mechanisms have been proposed to explain how hormones would affect the propensity of female sex towards OSA. Sexual hormones may affect the distribution of body fat, the UA dilatory muscle function and central and neural respiratory control mechanisms [33–35].

This lower propensity to airway collapse is translated to the polysomnographic profile. Several studies have consistently reported a milder OSA severity in women compared to men of similar age [3, 36, 37]. In women, respiratory events tend to cluster during REM sleep [3, 38, 39]. In contrast, men have more severe OSA which is more position dependent and less stage dependent. Although the severity of OSA based on the AHI is milder in women, some researchers have reported that women may be more prone to suffer from UA resistance syndrome or partial UA obstruction than men [40–42].

Consequences of OSA in women

Given the aforementioned differences in prevalence, severity, pathogenesis and clinical manifestations of OSA, it can be speculated that there may also be sex differences regarding the health consequences of this sleep disorder. Unfortunately, there is a dearth of data on this topic and, since few studies have been specifically designed to address the impact of OSA in women, most of our knowledge is supported by studies conducted predominantly or exclusively in men, whose results may not apply to women.

Noncardiovascular consequences

Several studies concur that women show a greater impairment in quality of life than men with similar OSA severity. GREENBERG-DOTAN et al. [43] compared 289 women and 289 men with OSA matched for age, BMI and AHI, and found that women had lower perceived health status and a lower Functional Outcomes of Sleep Questionnaire score than men. Other studies with smaller sample sizes have also reported a lower functional status, greater mood disturbance and poorer neurobehavioral performance compared to men [44, 45]. Depression and anxiety are very common complaints in this population and, in some series, up to 35% of women with OSA have depression or take psychoactive medication [9, 12, 15, 45–47]. Sexual dysfunction has also been reported in women with OSA [48, 49].

YAFFE et al. [50] followed 298 elderly women for an average of 4.7 years and found that women with moderate-to-severe OSA (AHI $\geqslant$15 events·h^{-1}) were more likely to develop cognitive impairment or dementia (adjusted OR 1.85, 95% CI 1.11–3.08) compared to those without the sleep disorder. MACEY et al. [51] used magnetic resonance imaging to measure axonal structural integrity in 30 patients with OSA and 50 controls and found sex differences in white matter structural integrity, with females being more affected than males. It is not yet known whether these structural changes provoke different neuropsychological symptoms or whether they simply reflect different consequences of OSA in the brains of men and women.

This impairment in quality of life, mood and cognitive performance is reflected in an increased use of health resources and work disability. A case–control study in 218 OSA patients and 218 controls matched for age and sex showed that women consumed more than twice the healthcare resources of men [52]. Similarly, another study observed that, compared to men with OSA, health costs for women with OSA were 1.3 times higher, and multivariate analysis showed that antipsychotic and anxiolytic drugs were one of the independent predictors for "most costly" OSA women (OR 2.3, 95% CI 1.2–4.4) [43]. OSA in women has also been associated with increased risk of lost work days due to work disability, compared to control women (RR 1.80, 95% CI 1.43–2.28) [53].

Intermediate mechanisms of cardiovascular injury

Endothelial function has been found to be more impaired in women than in men with OSA. Faulx et al. [54] analysed 82 men and 111 women and observed that flow-mediated vasodilation was significantly lower in women with an AHI $\geqslant$15 events·h^{-1} than in those with an AHI <15 events·h^{-1} (p<0.005). Additionally, peak blood flow decreased significantly with increasing AHI. These relationships were exclusive to women, and were not found in men with OSA. Randby et al. [55] have recently confirmed that OSA was independently associated with impaired digital vascular function in women only, and that this association was independent of the menopausal status. It has also been reported that women with OSA may show a blunted heart rate response when subjected to autonomic challenges, increased markers of systemic inflammation, and a delayed normalisation of C-reactive protein with CPAP treatment [56–59].

The association between OSA and hypertension in women is a matter of controversy (table 2). In a population-based case–control study composed of 161 hypertensive and 183 normotensive subjects, Hedner et al. [60] found an independent association between severe OSA (AHI >30 events·h^{-1}) and hypertension in men (OR 2.6, 95% CI 1.6–5.1) but not in women (OR 0.7, 95% CI 0.3–1.6). Two other retrospective studies have reported that the AHI was independently associated with higher DBP and with an increase in the evening-morning BP differences only in men [61, 62]. Another study found a different hypertension risk associated with OSA only in very obese men [65]. In a very recent study, however, Pedrosa et al. [63] analysed 277 consecutive perimenopausal women using 24-h BP monitoring and home polygraphy and observed that women with an AHI $\geqslant$15 events·h^{-1} had higher awake and nocturnal BP (both systolic and diastolic) than those without OSA (AHI <5 events·h^{-1}). Furthermore, the AHI and ODI were independently associated with 24-h SBP in a multivariate analysis. In agreement with these data, Sforza et al. [12] reported that sex was associated with hypertension in a prospective cohort of 641 elderly community dwellers. Females showed increased hypertension risk (OR 1.52, 95% CI 1.00–2.30) and increased 24-h SBP (OR 1.03, 95% CI 1.00–1.5) compared to males. Finally, data from the collaborative European Sleep Apnoea Database, which analysed 7646 men and 3303 women, observed that AHI and ODI had similar effects on prevalent hypertension in both men and women. In logistic regression analysis stratified by sex, ODI was independently associated with prevalent hypertension, while AHI was not [64].

Very few studies have addressed the association between OSA and glucose metabolism in women (table 2). Theorell-Haglow et al. [66] analysed 400 females from the general population with full PSG and observed that the AHI was independently associated with increased fasting insulin levels, and that low nocturnal minimal saturation predicted decreased insulin sensitivity. In a 16-year follow-up study of 31 women and 137 men from a clinical setting, OSA defined as an ODI $\geqslant$30 events·h^{-1} was an independent predictor of incident self-reported diabetes mellitus in women (OR 11.78, 95% CI 1.14–121.7), but not in men (OR 1.58, 95% CI 0.55–4.58) [67]. In contrast, a recent study comparing 18 women with OSA to 21 controls failed to replicate these findings [68]. Insulin resistance measured

Table 2. Studies analysing the association between hypertension, diabetes mellitus and serious cardiovascular consequences of OSA in women

First author [ref.]	Study characteristics	Quality of evidence	Measures	Key findings
HEDNER [60]	161 hypertensive and 183 normotensive subjects aged >40 years (174 males, 170 females) from the general population studied with ambulatory home PSG	Case–control study	Office BP was measured	An association between an AHI $\geq$30 events·h^{-1} and hypertension was found in males (OR 2.6, 95% CI 1.4–5.1) but not in females (OR 0.7, 95% CI 0.3–1.6)
LEE [61]	348 men and 112 women diagnosed with OSA by PSG	Retrospective study	Office BP was measured	In men, AHI significantly predicted the high BP group (OR 1.019, 95% CI 1.007–1.031) and the high DBP group (OR 1.026, 95% CI 1.015–1.017), but not the high SBP group, in the multiple logistic regression adjusted for confounders In women, AHI did not significantly predict the high BP, DBP or SBP group in the multivariate analysis
LAVIE-NEVO [62]	1566 men (870 nonhypertensive and 696 hypertensive) and 443 women (258 nonhypertensive and 185 hypertensive) studied by PSG for suspected OSA	Retrospective study	Office BP was measured twice in the evening and twice in the morning to evaluate evening morning differences	In men with OSA, morning BP tended to be higher than evening BP and an increasing severity of OSA was linearly associated with an increase in the morning relative to the evening BP values In women, increasing AHI was not associated with a linear increase in the evening-morning BP differences
PEDROSA [63]	277 consecutive perimenopausal women underwent home respiratory polygraphy	Observational cohort study	24-h BP monitoring and pulse wave velocity were used to evaluate BP and arterial stiffness, respectively	Women with an AHI $\geq$15 events·h^{-1} had a higher prevalence of hypertension, were prescribed more medications for hypertension, had higher awake BP (both systolic and diastolic), higher nocturnal BP (both systolic and diastolic) and more arterial

Continued

Table 2. Continued

First author [ref.]	Study characteristics	Quality of evidence	Measures	Key findings
				stiffness compared to those without OSA (AHI <5 events·h⁻¹).
				AHI and ODI were independently and positively associated with 24-h SBP in the multivariate analysis (β=1.28 (95% CI 0.28–2.29), p=0.01 and β=1.30 (95% CI 0.06–2.54), p=0.04 for AHI and ODI, respectively)
				Only ODI was independently associated with arterial stiffness when adjusted for confounders (β=0.22 (95% CI 0.03–0.40), p=0.02)
TKACOVA [64]	7646 men and 3303 women from a multicenter European sample underwent either respiratory polygraphy or PSG	Cross-sectional cohort study	Prevalent hypertension was scored if a subject had prior diagnosis of hypertension by the referring physician or was taking antihypertensive medication	AHI and ODI had similar effects on prevalent hypertension in both men and women. In the logistic regression analysis stratified by sex, ODI, but not AHI, was independently associated with prevalent hypertension in women (β=0.78 (OR 2.18, 95% CI 1.31–3.62), p=0.002 for the highest compared to the lowest ODI quartile)
SFORZA [12]	379 females and 262 males from the general population underwent home respiratory polygraphy	Prospective cohort study	24-h BP was measured	In the multiple logistic regression analysis adjusted for confounders, women showed increased hypertension risk (OR 1.52, 95% CI 1.00–2.30) and increased 24-h SBP (OR 1.03, 95% CI 1.00–1.5) compared to males
MOHSENIN [65]	529 men and 207 women with OSA and 154 males and 161 women without OSA (control)	Cross-sectional cohort study	Prevalent hypertension was scored if a subject had prior diagnosis of hypertension or was	Sex was not significantly associated with prevalent hypertension (OR for men compared to women 1.16, 95% CI 0.84–1.59). When the results were stratified by BMI quartiles, men were at higher risk of

Continued

Table 2. Continued

First author [ref.]	Study characteristics	Quality of evidence	Measures	Key findings
	Subjects underwent an attended PSG		taking antihypertensive medication	prevalent hypertension compared to women only at the highest quartile of BMI [38–94 kg·m^{-2}] (adjusted OR 1.82, 95% CI 1.01–3.20)
THEORELL-HAGLOW [66]	400 females from the general population underwent PSG	Cross-sectional cohort study	Fasting blood sampling and insulin sensitivity index were assessed	After adjusting for confounders, the AHI was associated with increased fasting and 2-h insulin levels (95% CI 0.14–0.99 and 95% CI 0.28–6.47, respectively). After adjusting for confounders, nocturnal minimal saturation was independently associated with decreased insulin sensitivity
CELEN [67]	31 women and 137 men from a clinical setting Patients underwent a respiratory polygraphy, but OSA diagnosis was based on a total number of oxygen desaturations ≥30	Longitudinal observational study, each subject was followed up for 16 years	New onset type 2 diabetes mellitus was assessed by a questionnaire	The incidence of type 2 diabetes mellitus was 24.9% in patients with OSA compared with 10.8% in non-OSA subjects (p=0.020), with higher incidence in women with OSA than men (50% versus 19.1%) After adjustment for confounders, OSA was independently associated with incident diabetes in women (OR 11.78, 95% CI 1.14–121.7) but not in men (OR 1.58, 95% CI 0.55–4.58)
KRITIKOU [68]	77 subjects (38 middle-aged males and post-menopausal females with OSA and 39 male and female controls) underwent an attended PSG	Case–control study	IL-6, TNF receptor-1, leptin, adiponectin, hsCRP, fasting glucose and insulin levels were assessed	No significant difference in TNF receptor-1, HOMA index, leptin or adiponectin was detected in women with OSA compared to control women without OSA
GOTTLIEB [69]	1927 men and 2495 women aged ≥40 years from the general	Prospective longitudinal epidemiological	Incident CHD and HF were assessed Information was	Compared to women without OSA (AHI <5 events·h^{-1}), those with severe OSA (AHI ≥30 events·h^{-1}) did not show increased risk of

Continued

Table 2. Continued

First author [ref.]	Study characteristics	Quality of evidence	Measures	Key findings
	population with no history of CHD or HF All subjects underwent in-home PSG	study, median follow-up of 8.7 years	obtained from hospital and physician office records	CHD (HR 0.40, 95% CI 0.12–1.27) or HF (HR 1.19, 95% CI 0.56–2.52) in the fully adjusted model After adjustment for multiple risk factors, OSA was a significant predictor of incident CHD only in men aged <70 years of age (adjusted HR 1.10 (95% CI 1.00–1.21) per 10-unit increase in AHI)
REDLINE [70]	2462 men and 2960 women aged ⩾40 years from the general population with no history of stroke All subjects underwent in-home PSG	Prospective longitudinal epidemiological study, median follow-up of 8.7 years	Incident stroke was assessed Information was obtained from hospital and physician records	Compared to women at the lowest AHI quartile (<4.05), those at the highest AHI quartile (>19.13) did not show increased risk of stroke (HR 1.21, 95% CI 0.65–2.24) in the fully adjusted analysis Compared to men at the lowest AHI quartile, those at the highest AHI quartile showed increased risk of stroke (HR 2.86, 95% CI 1.10–7.39) in the fully adjusted analysis
PUNJABI [71]	2959 men and 3335 women aged ⩾40 years from the general population All subjects underwent in-home PSG	Prospective longitudinal epidemiological study, median follow-up of 8.2 years	All-cause mortality was evaluated Information was obtained from multiple concurrent sources	Compared to subjects without OSA (AHI <5 events·h⁻¹), those with severe OSA (AHI ⩾30 events·h⁻¹) showed increased mortality risk (HR 1.46, 95% CI 1.14–1.86) in the fully adjusted analysis Compared to women without OSA (AHI <5 events·h⁻¹), those with severe OSA (AHI ⩾30 events·h⁻¹) did not show increased mortality risk (HR 1.40, 95% CI 0.89–2.22) in the fully adjusted model
CHANG [72]	29 961 patients with OSA (22 574 men and 7387 women) and a control	Retrospective, longitudinal, case–control study	Incidence of stroke was investigated A universal insurance	In stratified analysis, both women and men with OSA had greater risk of stroke than the non-OSA controls (adjusted HR 1.44, 95% CI

Continued

Table 2. Continued

First author [ref.]	Study characteristics	Quality of evidence	Measures	Key findings
	cohort of 119 844 subjects without OSA (90 296 men and 29 548 women) matched for age and sex. OSA was diagnosed by PSG		claims database was used to identify the study population and patients diagnosed with OSA, as well as new-onset stroke	1.20–1.72, and HR 1.21, 95% CI 1.01–1.24, respectively) Women aged <35 years showed the highest stroke risk (adjusted HR 4.90, 95% CI 1.93–12.4), this risk decreased with age, and those aged >65 years did not show any association with stroke (adjusted HR 1.02, 95% CI 0.78–1.33) The role of CPAP was not assessed

hsCRP: high-sensitivity C-reactive protein; CHD: coronary heart disease; HOMA: Homeostasis Model Assessment.

by the homeostatic model assessment index did not differ in women with and without OSA (3.35±0.40 *versus* 3.59±0.37, p=0.69).

Association between OSA and serious cardiovascular outcomes in women

There is growing evidence that severe OSA (AHI $\geqslant$30 events·h^{-1}) is a risk factor for serious cardiovascular outcomes. This evidence rests, however, on series composed exclusively or predominantly of males, or on others in which the effect of sex has not been properly assessed [71–80] (fig. 1).

The Sleep Heart Health Study (SHHS), a population-based study that enrolled more than 5000 individuals, about 50% of them women, analysed the association between OSA and incident stroke and coronary heart disease (CHD) after an average follow-up of 8 years. In stratified analyses by sex, the researchers could not find any association between severe OSA and incident stroke or CHD in women (HR 1.21 (95% CI 0.65–2.24) and HR 0.40 (95% CI 0.12–1.27), respectively) [69, 70]. However, these results may have been biased by the very low prevalence of severe OSA in this cohort, which accounted for only 3% of all the women sampled. In the only prospective study that has investigated the role of OSA in a large clinical cohort of women, CAMPOS-RODRIGUEZ et al. [81] followed 967 women referred for suspected OSA for 6.8 years and found that the untreated OSA group (AHI $\geqslant$10 events·h^{-1}) showed a greater incidence rate of a composite outcome of stroke or CHD than a control group without OSA (AHI <10 events·h^{-1}) (2.19 *versus* 0.54 per 100 person-years; p<0.0005) (fig. 2). In a multivariate analysis, an independent association was shown between untreated OSA and increased incidence of stroke or CHD, compared to non-OSA women (adjusted HR 2.76, 95% CI 1.35–5.62) [81]. In stratified analyses by age, the association between the untreated OSA group and incident stroke or CHD was limited to women aged <65 years. Interestingly, when the two types of events were assessed separately, untreated OSA retained an association with stroke (HR 6.44, 95% CI 1.46–28.3), but not with CHD (HR 1.77, 95% CI 0.76–4.09). Concurrent with these findings, CHANG

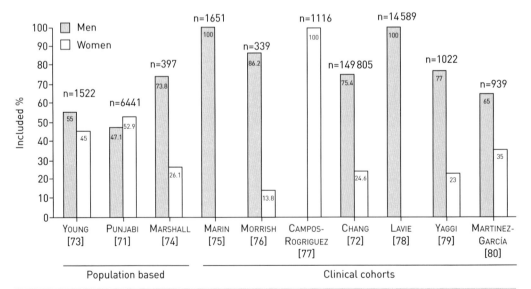

Figure 1. Proportion of women and men included in studies investigating serious cardiovascular outcomes associated with OSA.

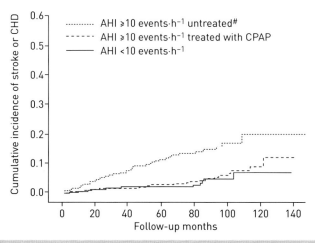

Figure 2. Kaplan–Meier curves showing the cumulative incidence of either stroke or coronary heart disease (CHD) in 967 women studied for suspicion of OSA and followed for a median of 6.8 years. #: cumulative incidence of stroke or CHD was significantly higher in women with AHI ≥10 events·h−1 and untreated compared to those with AHI <10 events·h−1 (p<0.0005). Reproduced and modified from [81] with permission from the publisher.

et al. [72] used a universal insurance claims database to identify a group of 29 961 OSA patients in Taiwan and compared the sex- and age-specific stroke risk with a control cohort without OSA. They found that women with OSA (AHI ≥5 events·h^{-1}) had significantly higher stroke risk compared to women without OSA (adjusted HR 1.44, 95% CI 1.20–1.72), and also that the effects of OSA on stroke risk decreased with age, peaking in women aged <35 years (adjusted HR 4.90, 95% CI 1.93–12.4) and disappearing in those aged >65 years (adjusted HR 1.02, 95% CI 0.78–1.33).

With regards to mortality, the SHHS did not show any association between OSA and overall mortality in women, not even in severe OSA patients (adjusted HR 1.40, 95% CI 0.89–2.22) [71]. In contrast, a prospective Spanish clinical cohort of 1116 women studied for OSA and followed for an average of 6 years found that those with untreated, severe OSA (AHI ≥30 events·h^{-1}) had increased cardiovascular mortality risk (adjusted HR 3.50, 95% CI 1.23–9.98) than women with an AHI <10 events·h^{-1} [81].

Treatment of OSA in women

Non-PAP treatment

Weight loss can reduce OSA severity, but according to some studies it might have a greater impact in men than in women [82]. Bariatric surgery is an effective treatment in morbidly obese patients, and a recent meta-analysis has shown that weight reduction after surgery decreased the AHI by 38.2 events·h^{-1} (95% CI 31.9–44.4) [83]. However, in most of the studies included in the meta-analysis the number of women was either very small or unreported.

MADs are an alternative to CPAP therapy in patients with mild-to-moderate OSA, or in those who do not tolerate CPAP. One large prospective study has assessed the effect of

MADs on 490 men and 120 women with OSA [84]. Women were 2.4 times more likely (95% CI 1.19–4.87) to achieve treatment success than men, with mild OSA being the strongest predictor of success. There were no sex differences in the tolerability of the device in this study.

The role of hormone-replacement therapy (HRT) has been investigated in post-menopausal women with OSA. BIXLER et al. [31] observed that the risk of having OSA in post-menopausal women treated with HRT was similar to that of pre-menopausal women (OR 0.9, 95% CI 0.1–5.8), whereas post-menopausal women without HRT showed a higher prevalence of OSA (OR 4.3, 95% CI 1.1–17.3). In addition, the SHHS also found that the prevalence of OSA was significantly lower in women aged ≥50 years undergoing HRT (OR 0.55, 95% CI 0.41–0.75) [85]. However, other studies have yielded conflicting results [86–88]. The inconsistent evidence and the increased risks of breast cancer and cardiovascular diseases associated with HRT have precluded its recommendation as a first-line treatment in post-menopausal women with OSA.

PAP treatment

CPAP is the treatment of choice for symptomatic OSA patients and those with high cardiovascular risk [89]. CPAP has been shown to effectively reverse the clinical complaints and some of the cardiovascular outcomes associated with OSA. However, most of this research has been conducted in males so CPAP recommendations in women are unclear [75, 90–92].

YE et al. [44] compared CPAP effectiveness in functional status, daytime sleepiness, mood disturbance and neurobehavioral performance in 152 men and 24 women with severe OSA. After 3 months of CPAP treatment, functional status and symptoms significantly improved for both men and women, despite greater baseline impairment in women (table 3). BANNO et al. [93] analysed 414 women with OSA treated with CPAP or weight loss counselling and found an increase in fees of $123.43±25.01 in the 2 years before diagnosis and a reduction of fees of $37.96±21.35 in the 2 years after diagnosis (p<0.0001). Furthermore, the number of clinic visits in women with OSA increased in the 2 years before diagnosis by 2.32±0.43 and decreased over the next 2 years by 1.48±0.42 visits (p<0.0001). MORRISH et al. [76] retrospectively analysed 292 men and 47 women diagnosed with OSA and treated with CPAP and found that women had a 3.44 greater mortality risk than men, but these differences disappeared when the results were adjusted for confounding variables.

Data from the aforementioned large Spanish cohort suggest that adequate CPAP therapy is necessary to reduce cardiovascular outcomes associated with OSA. Women with OSA who used CPAP for at least 4 h per day on average had a risk of cardiovascular mortality and serious incident cardiovascular events similar to that of a control group without OSA (adjusted HR 0.55 (95% CI 0.17–1.74) and adjusted HR 0.91 (95% CI 0.43–1.95), respectively) [77, 81]. Furthermore, an independent association between the number of hours of CPAP use and reduced incidence of cardiovascular events and mortality was observed in both studies, suggesting that greater adherence would be associated with lower incidence of cardiovascular outcomes.

The effectiveness of CPAP therapy greatly depends on consistent use [94]. However, the influence of sex on CPAP adherence has not been clarified and several studies have

Table 3. Studies analysing the role of CPAP treatment in women

First author [ref.]	Study characteristics	Quality of evidence	Type of treatment	Key findings
Ye [44]	152 men and 24 women with OSA Sex differences in response to CPAP were examined with respect to functional status, daytime sleepiness, mood disturbance, apnoea symptoms and neurobehavioral performance	Prospective, observational study	CPAP treatment for 3 months	CPAP treatment significantly improved functional status and relieved OSA symptoms for both men and women. There was no significant difference between sexes in response to CPAP treatment, and sex differences in CPAP adherence were not observed
Banno [93]	414 women with OSA and 1404 matched women from the general population Healthcare use 2 years after diagnosis was analysed in women with OSA	Retrospective, observational cohort study	322 women were treated with CPAP and 92 were only recommended weight loss	There was an increase in fees of $123.43±$25.01 in the 2 years before diagnosis and a reduction in fees of $37.96±$21.35 in the 2 years after diagnosis (p<0.0001) The number of clinic visits increased in the 2 years before diagnosis by 2.32±0.43 and decreased over the next 2 years by 1.48±0.42 (p<0.0001).
Morrish [76]	292 men and 47 women with OSA The study compared the mortality risk in both sexes	Retrospective study	All patients were treated with CPAP	Mortality risk was comparable in men and women with OSA treated with CPAP when the results were adjusted for several confounders, including the Charlson score (OR 0.95, 95% CI 0.39–2.29)
Campos-Rodriguez [77]	1116 women referred for OSA suspicion Cardiovascular mortality was investigated in different OSA groups	Prospective, observational study	278 non-OSA control group (AHI <10 events·h⁻¹), 155 women with mild-moderate OSA (AHI 10–30 events·h⁻¹) with CPAP, 421 with severe OSA (AHI >30 events·h⁻¹) with CPAP, 167 with untreated mild-moderate OSA and 95 with untreated severe OSA Median follow-up 72 months	Compared to the control group without OSA, women with untreated severe OSA had an increased cardiovascular mortality risk (adjusted HR 3.50, 95% CI 1.23–9.98) Women with untreated mild-to-moderate OSA had a similar mortality risk compared with the non-OSA control group (adjusted HR 1.60, 95% CI 0.52–4.90) Compared to the control group without OSA, women with severe OSA treated with CPAP had a similar mortality risk to the control group (HR 0.55, 95% CI 0.17–1.74)

Continued

Table 3. Continued

First author [ref.]	Study characteristics	Quality of evidence	Type of treatment	Key findings
				CPAP compliance measured in hours per day was independently associated with lower cardiovascular mortality risk (HR 0.72, 95% CI 0.63–0.83)
CAMPOS-RODRIGUEZ [81]	967 women referred for OSA suspicion, free of previous stroke and CHD Incidence of a composite outcome of stroke or CHD was investigated in different OSA groups	Prospective, observational study	258 non-OSA control group (AHI <10 events·h⁻¹), 441 women with OSA (AHI ⩾10 events·h⁻¹) treated with CPAP and 268 with untreated OSA (AHI ⩾10 events·h⁻¹) Median follow-up 6.8 years	Compared to the control group without OSA, women with untreated OSA had an increased incidence of stroke or CHD (adjusted HR 2.76, 95% CI 1.35–5.62) When the type of cardiovascular event was separately assessed, untreated OSA showed a stronger association with incident of stroke (adjusted HR 6.44, 95% CI 1.46–28.3) than with CHD (adjusted HR 1.77, 95% CI 0.76–4.09) In stratified analyses by age, the association between the untreated OSA group and incident of stroke or CHD was limited to women aged <65 years Compared to the control group without OSA, women treated with CPAP showed a similar risk of the composite outcome (HR 0.91, 95% CI 0.43–1.95)

CHD: coronary heart disease.

reported conflicting results. Female sex has been identified as a risk factor for both inadequate and good CPAP compliance, whereas other studies have not found sex to be a predictive factor for adherence [95–98]. Campos-Rodriguez *et al.* [47] prospectively followed a cohort of 708 women with OSA who started CPAP therapy and found that the probability of still being on CPAP at 5 years was 82.8%, and the median CPAP use was 6 (IQR 4–7) h·day^{-1}. Psychoactive medication and increasing age were identified as independent predictors of CPAP dropout.

OSA in pregnancy

Pathophysiology and prevalence

The physiological changes of pregnancy may either predispose females to develop OSA or protect against it [99–103]. Some of these factors are depicted in figure 3.

The prevalence of OSA in pregnancy has not been systematically evaluated, because the majority of studies have relied on symptom-based diagnosis rather than objective polysomnographic recordings [31, 99, 104, 105]. A recent prospective study using overnight PSG has estimated that the overall OSA prevalence in the general obstetric population was 8.4% in the first trimester and 19.7% in the third trimester [106]. In this study, AHI was found to increase throughout pregnancy and, by the third trimester, 26.7 and 4.8% of the women had mild and moderate-to-severe OSA, respectively. Greater baseline BMI and maternal age increased the risk for third trimester OSA.

The incidence of OSA in this population is unknown, since studies do not separate new-onset OSA cases favoured by this transient state from long-term OSA already present before pregnancy.

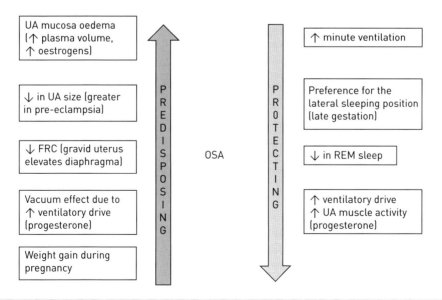

Figure 3. Factors that may predispose and protect against OSA during pregnancy.

OSA and adverse maternal and fetal outcomes

OSA during pregnancy has been associated with increased risk of adverse maternal and fetal outcomes, including gestational hypertension, pre-eclampsia, gestational diabetes, preterm delivery, neonatal intensive care unit admissions, caesarean delivery and low birth weight (table 4) [105, 108, 110–118]. On the other hand, pre-eclampsia might also be a predisposing factor to develop OSA during pregnancy, through excessive fluid retention, rostral fluid shift and UA oedema. One recent meta-analysis including 21 observational studies found that maternal OSA was significantly associated with gestational hypertension/pre-eclampsia (pooled adjusted OR 2.34, 95% CI 1.60–3.09) and gestational diabetes (OR 1.86, 95% CI 1.30–2.42) [119]. In contrast with these data, a prospective cohort study in 105 pregnant women did not observe any associations between OSA and subsequent development of gestational hypertension, pre-eclampsia, gestational diabetes, preterm delivery or low birth weight [106]. Other studies have also reported a lack of association between OSA or snoring and growth restriction or evidence of abnormal fetal heart rate response associated with obstructive events or desaturations [114, 120, 121].

One explanation for these conflicting findings is that pre-existing OSA may represent a greater hazard for adverse outcomes during pregnancy, compared to incident gestational OSA. Nevertheless, research in this area is very scarce, as has been highlighted in a recent review [122]. Large-scale, prospective cohort studies are needed to further elucidate the relationship between maternal OSA and adverse pregnancy outcomes [119].

Treatment

Changes in sleep position, moderate weight gain and alcohol avoidance should be advised during pregnancy.

Few studies with small sample sizes have addressed the safety and effectiveness of CPAP therapy in pregnant women with OSA. One study in 12 women reported good CPAP compliance and improvements in sleepiness and fatigue scales [123]. A small, randomised controlled study in women with risk factors for pre-eclampsia who were treated with CPAP in early pregnancy showed improved BP control compared with an untreated group [124]. Similarly, 1 night of CPAP treatment was shown to improve SBP and DBP in 11 women with severe pre-eclampsia and UA flow limitation, but not OSA, compared to a non-treatment night [107]. A RCT of 24 women with pre-eclampsia and 15 pregnant controls showed that CPAP minimised the reduction in cardiac output associated with sleep in pregnant women with pre-eclampsia [109]. However, these findings need to be confirmed in larger trials before CPAP therapy can be widely recommended. Pressure requirements may slightly increase by 1–2 cmH_2O during the course of the pregnancy [99].

Conclusion

OSA is a common and relatively overlooked disorder in women. The lower prevalence compared to men may be attributed to underdiagnosis due to non-typical clinical presentation, but also to a different pathophysiology and a less collapsible UA. These aforementioned disparities suggest that there may also be sex differences in health, functional and cardiovascular outcomes. Unfortunately, little attention has been paid to these topics and most research related to OSA relies on male populations. This lack of

Table 4. Studies using objective sleep recordings to characterise sleep disordered breathing with reported maternal/infant outcomes

References	Study design	OSA diagnosis	Key findings
EDWARDS [107]	Case–control study: 25 pre-eclampsia, 17 controls	Full overnight PSG	Partial upper airway obstruction during sleep in women with pre-eclampsia was associated with increments in BP, the use of nasal CPAP reduced BP
CONNOLLY [108]	Case–control study: 15 pre-eclampsia/15 controls from each trimester	In-hospital overnight limited PSG	Women with pre-eclampsia had a prolonged pattern of flow limitation without associated oxygen desaturation. SBP and DBP were significantly higher in the pre-eclampsia group but all groups showed a significant fall in BP during sleep
BLYTON [109]	RCT: 24 pre-eclampsia/15 controls	Full overnight PSG	Sleep-induced decrements in heart rate, stroke volume and cardiac output in women with pre-eclampsia with further increments in total peripheral resistance. Cardiac output during sleep was correlated with fetal birth weight Treatment of women with pre-eclampsia with CPAP minimised reductions in cardiac output and increments in total peripheral resistance were also reduced
YINON [110]	Case–control study: 17 pre-eclampsia/25 controls	Nocturnal sleep study using Watch PAT 100	Women with pre-eclampsia had a significantly higher RDI and more impaired endothelial function than controls
SAHIN [111]	Prospective cohort study: 4 OSA/31 non-OSA	Full overnight PSG	Lower Apgar scores in neonates of women with OSA. Fetal heart decelerations accompanying maternal desaturation. Neonates of women diagnosed with OSA had lower mean Apgar scores and birth weights compared with neonates of women without OSA
CHAMPAGNE [112]	Case–control study: 17 gestational hypertension/33 frequency matched controls	Overnight unattended portable PSG	Females with hypertensive pregnancies had higher mean AHI compared with normotensive pregnant females (38.6±36.7 versus 18.2±12.2). The odds ratio for the presence of OSA given the presence of gestational hypertension was 7.5 (95% CI 3.5–16.2), based on a

Continued

Table 4. Continued

References	Study design	OSA diagnosis	Key findings
Louis [113]	Retrospective cohort study: 57 OSA/114 obese and normal weight controls	Full overnight PSG	logistic regression model with adjustment for maternal age, gestational age, pre-pregnancy BMI, prior pregnancies and previous live births OSA patients had more pre-eclampsia and preterm delivery
Olivarez [114]	Prospective cohort study: 20 OSA/80 non-OSA	Full overnight PSG	In pregnancy, the Berlin questionnaire poorly predicts OSA Compared with PSG, sensitivity and specificity by Berlin screening was 35% and 63.8%, respectively No association was observed between fetal heart rate abnormalities and OSA parameters
Reid [115]	Cross-sectional study: 34 gestational hypertension/26 controls	Full overnight PSG	Women with gestational hypertension had a significantly higher frequency of OSA than healthy women with uncomplicated pregnancies of similar gestational age (53% and 12%, respectively; p<0.001)
Chen [116]	Case–control study: 791 with OSA diagnostic codes/4746 controls	Full overnight PSG	Pregnant women with OSA had increased risk of having low birth weight, preterm birth, and small for gestational age infants, cesarean section and pre-eclampsia compared with pregnant women without OSA
Facco [117]	Retrospective cross-sectional study: 145 pregnant women	Full overnight PSG	Increasing severity of OSA was associated with an increasing risk of a composite adverse pregnancy outcomes including pregnancy-related hypertension, gestational diabetes and preterm birth (18.1% AHI <5 events·h^{-1}, 23.5% AHI 5–14.9 events·h^{-1}, 38.5% AHI ⩾15 events·h^{-1}; p=0.038) Obese women with moderate-to-severe OSA had the highest rate of adverse pregnancy outcomes (41.7%)
Pien [106]	Prospective cohort study: 145 pregnant women	Full overnight PSG	There were no significant associations between first or third trimester AHI, OSA or change in AHI and gestational hypertension, pre-eclampsia, preterm delivery or low birth weight babies

reliable information in women precludes the development of specific protocols tailored to the characteristics of this population, leading physicians to treat women according to male criteria. Recent studies suggest that OSA may impair health status and increase the risk of serious cardiovascular consequences in women. CPAP therapy may be effective to counter these adverse outcomes, provided that adherence is adequate. The evidence is still sparse, however, and there is still a long way to go. High-quality trials involving large samples of women are needed to confirm these findings.

Pregnancy may either predispose or protect against OSA, although it seems that OSA prevalence increases throughout pregnancy. OSA may increase the risk of adverse maternal outcomes and, less clearly, fetal outcomes. CPAP may play a role in protecting against these outcomes, but more research is needed.

References

1. Young T, Palta M, Dempsey J, et al. The occurrence of sleep-disordered breathing among middle-aged adults. N Engl J Med 1993; 328: 1230–1235.
2. Redline S, Kump K, Tishler PV, et al. Gender differences in sleep disordered breathing in a community-based sample. Am J Respir Crit Care Med 1994; 149: 722–726.
3. O'Connor C, Thornley KS, Hanly PJ. Gender differences in the polysomnographic features of obstructive sleep apnea. Am J Respir Crit Care Med 2000; 161: 1465–1472.
4. Durán J, Esnaola S, Rubio R, et al. Obstructive sleep apnea-hypopnea and related clinical features in a population-based sample of subjects aged 30 to 70 yr. Am J Respir Crit Care Med 2001; 163: 685–689.
5. Peppard PE, Young T, Barnet JH, et al. Increased prevalence of sleep-disordered breathing in adults. Am J Epidemiol 2013; 177: 1006–1014.
6. Franklin KA, Sahlin C, Stenlund H, et al. Sleep apnoea is a common occurrence in females. Eur Respir J 2013; 41: 610–615.
7. Young T, Hutton R, Finn L, et al. The gender bias in sleep apnea diagnosis. Are women missed because they have different symptoms? Arch Intern Med 1996; 156: 2445–2451.
8. Jordan AS, McEvoy RD. Gender differences in sleep apnea: epidemiology, clinical presentation and pathogenic mechanisms. Sleep Med Rev 2003; 7: 377–389.
9. Quintana-Gallego E, Carmona-Bernal C, Capote F, et al. Gender differences in obstructive sleep apnea syndrome: a clinical study of 1166 patients. Respir Med 2004; 98: 984–989.
10. De Silva S, Abeyratne UR, Hukins C. Impact of gender on snore-based obstructive sleep apnea screening. Physiol Meas 2012; 33: 587–601.
11. Chervin RD. Sleepiness, fatigue, tiredness, and lack of energy in obstructive sleep apnea. Chest 2000; 118: 372–379.
12. Sforza E, Chouchou F, Collet P, et al. Sex differences in obstructive sleep apnoea in an elderly French population. Eur Respir J 2011; 37: 1137–1143.
13. Ye L, Pien GW, Weaver TE. Gender differences in the clinical manifestation of obstructive sleep apnea. Sleep Med 2009; 10: 1075–1084.
14. Shepertycky MR, Banno K, Kryger MH. Differences between men and women in the clinical presentation of patients diagnosed with obstructive sleep apnea syndrome. Sleep 2005; 28: 309–314.
15. Valipour A, Lothaller H, Rauscher H, et al. Gender-related differences in symptoms of patients with suspected breathing disorders in sleep: a clinical population study using the sleep disorders questionnaire. Sleep 2007; 30: 312–319.
16. Baldwin CM, Kapur VK, Holberg CJ, et al. Associations between gender and measures of daytime somnolence in the Sleep Heart Health Study. Sleep 2004; 27: 305–311.
17. Morrell MJ, Finn L, McMillan A, et al. The impact of ageing and sex on the association between sleepiness and sleep disordered breathing. Eur Respir J 2012; 40: 386–393.
18. Mohsenin V. Gender differences in the expression of sleep-disordered breathing: role of upper airway dimensions. Chest 2001; 120: 1442–1447.
19. Ronen O, Malhotra A, Pillar G. Influence of gender and age on upper-airway length during development. Pediatrics 2007; 120: e1028–e1034.
20. Malhotra A, Huang Y, Fogel RB, et al. The male predisposition to pharyngeal collapse: importance of airway length. Am J Respir Crit Care Med 2002; 166: 1388–1395.

21. Kirkness JP, Schwartz AR, Schneider H, *et al.* Contribution of male sex, age, and obesity to mechanical instability of the upper airway during sleep. *J Appl Physiol* 2008; 104: 1618–1624.

22. Simpson L, Mukherjee S, Cooper MN, *et al.* Sex differences in the association of regional fat distribution with the severity of obstructive sleep apnea. *Sleep* 2010; 33: 467–474.

23. Harada Y, Oga T, Chihara Y, *et al.* Differences in associations between visceral fat accumulation and obstructive sleep apnea by sex. *Ann Am Thorac Soc* 2014; 11: 383–391.

24. Kritikou I, Basta M, Tappouni R, *et al.* Sleep apnoea and visceral adiposity in middle-aged male and female subjects. *Eur Respir J* 2013; 41: 601–609.

25. Mazzuca E, Battaglia S, Marrone O, *et al.* Gender-specific anthropometric markers of adiposity, metabolic syndrome and visceral adiposity index (VAI) in patients with obstructive sleep apnea. *J Sleep Res* 2014; 23: 13–21.

26. Regensteiner JG, Woodard WD, Hagerman DD, *et al.* Combined effects of female hormones and metabolic rate on ventilatory drives in women. *J Appl Physiol* 1989; 66: 808–813.

27. Zhou XS, Shahabuddin S, Zahn BR, *et al.* Effect of gender on the development of hypocapnic apnea/hypopnea during NREM sleep. *J Appl Physiol* 2000; 89: 192–199.

28. Sin DD, Jones RL, Man GC. Hypercapnic ventilatory response in patients with and without obstructive sleep apnea: do age, gender, obesity, and daytime $PaCO_2$ matter? *Chest* 2000; 117: 454–459.

29. Jordan AS, Wellman A, Edwards JK, *et al.* Respiratory control stability and upper airway collapsibility in men and women with obstructive sleep apnea. *J Appl Physiol* 2005; 99: 2020–2027.

30. Young T, Finn L, Austin D, *et al.* Menopausal status and sleep-disordered breathing in the Wisconsin Sleep Cohort Study. *Am J Respir Crit Care Med* 2003; 167: 1181–1185.

31. Bixler EO, Vgontzas AN, Lin HM, *et al.* Prevalence of sleep-disordered breathing in women: effects of gender. *Am J Respir Crit Care Med* 2001; 163: 608–613.

32. Dancey DR, Hanly PJ, Soong C, *et al.* Impact of menopause on the prevalence and severity of sleep apnea. *Chest* 2001; 120: 151–155.

33. Lin CM, Davidson TM, Ancoli-Israel S. Gender differences in obstructive sleep apnea and treatment implications. *Sleep Med Rev* 2008; 12: 481–496.

34. Block AJ, Wynne JW, Boysen PG. Sleep-disordered breathing and nocturnal oxygen desaturation in postmenopausal women. *Am J Med* 1980; 69: 75–79.

35. Trémollieres FA, Pouilles JM, Ribot CA. Relative influence of age and menopause on total and regional body composition changes in postmenopausal women. *Am J Obstet Gynecol* 1996; 175: 1594–1600.

36. Pavlova MK, Duffy JF, Shea SA. Polysomnographic respiratory abnormalities in asymptomatic individuals. *Sleep* 2008; 31: 241–248.

37. Gabbay IE, Lavie P. Age- and gender-related characteristics of obstructive sleep apnea. *Sleep Breath* 2012; 16: 453–460.

38. Koo BB, Patel SR, Strohl K, *et al.* Rapid eye movement-related sleep-disordered breathing: influence of age and gender. *Chest* 2008; 134: 1156–1161.

39. Campos-Rodríguez F, Fernández-Palacín A, Reyes-Núñez N, *et al.* Características clínicas y polisomnograficas del síndrome de apneas durante el sueño localizado en la fase REM [Clinical and polysomnographic features of rapid-eye-movement-specific sleep-disordered breathing]. *Arch Bronconeumol* 2009; 45: 330–334.

40. Guilleminault C, Black JE, Palombini L, *et al.* A clinical investigation of obstructive sleep apnea syndrome (OSAS) and upper airway resistance syndrome (UARS) patients. *Sleep Med* 2000; 1: 51–56.

41. Anttalainen U, Polo O, Saaresranta T. Is 'MILD' sleep-disordered breathing in women really mild? *Acta Obstet Gynecol Scand* 2010; 89: 605–611.

42. Anttalainen U, Polo O, Vahlberg T, *et al.* Women with partial upper airway obstruction are not less sleepy than those with obstructive sleep apnea. *Sleep Breath* 2013; 17: 873–876.

43. Greenberg-Dotan S, Reuveni H, Simon-Tuval T, *et al.* Gender differences in morbidity and health care utilization among adult obstructive sleep apnea patients. *Sleep* 2007; 30: 1173–1180.

44. Ye L, Pien GW, Ratcliffe SJ, *et al.* Gender differences in obstructive sleep apnea and treatment response to continuous positive airway pressure. *J Clin Sleep Med* 2009; 5: 512–518.

45. Sampaio R, Pereira MG, Winck JC. Psychological morbidity, illness representations, and quality of life in female and male patients with obstructive sleep apnea syndrome. *Psychol Health Med* 2012; 17: 136–149.

46. Wahner-Roedler DL, Olson EJ, Narayanan S, *et al.* Gender-specific differences in a patient population with obstructive sleep apnea-hypopnea syndrome. *Gend Med* 2007; 4: 329–338.

47. Campos-Rodriguez F, Martinez-García MA, Reyes-Nuñez N, *et al.* Long-term continuous positive airway pressure compliance in females with obstructive sleep apnoea. *Eur Respir J* 2013; 42: 1255–1262.

48. Petersen M, Kristensen E, Berg S, *et al.* Sexual function in female patients with obstructive sleep apnea. *J Sex Med* 2011; 8: 2560–2568.

49. Subramanian S, Bopparaju S, Desai A, *et al.* Sexual dysfunction in women with obstructive sleep apnea. *Sleep Breath* 2010; 14: 59–62.

50. Yaffe K, Laffan AM, Harrison SL, *et al.* Sleep-disordered breathing, hypoxia, and risk of mild cognitive impairment and dementia in older women. *JAMA* 2011; 306: 613–619.

51. Macey PM, Kumar R, Yan-Go FL, *et al.* Sex differences in white matter alterations accompanying obstructive sleep apnea. *Sleep* 2012; 35: 1603–1613.

52. Tarasiuk A, Greenberg-Dotan S, Brin YS, *et al.* Determinants affecting health-care utilization in obstructive sleep apnea syndrome patients. *Chest* 2005; 128: 1310–1314.

53. Sjösten N, Vahtera J, Salo P, *et al.* Increased risk of lost workdays prior to the diagnosis of sleep apnea. *Chest* 2009; 136: 130–136.

54. Faulx MD, Larkin EK, Hoit BD, *et al.* Sex influences endothelial function in sleep-disordered breathing. *Sleep* 2004; 27: 1113–1120.

55. Randby A, Namtvedt SK, Hrubos-Strøm H, *et al.* Sex-dependent impact of OSA on digital vascular function. *Chest* 2013; 144: 915–922.

56. Macey PM, Kumar R, Woo MA, *et al.* Heart rate responses to autonomic challenges in obstructive sleep apnea. *PLoS One* 2013; 8: e76631.

57. Ljunggren M, Lindahl B, Theorell-Haglöw J, *et al.* Association between obstructive sleep apnea and elevated levels of type B natriuretic peptide in a community-based sample of women. *Sleep* 2012; 35: 1521–1527.

58. Svensson M, Venge P, Janson C, *et al.* Relationship between sleep-disordered breathing and markers of systemic inflammation in women from the general population. *J Sleep Res* 2012; 21: 147–154.

59. Mermigkis C, Bouloukaki I, Mermigkis D, *et al.* CRP evolution pattern in CPAP-treated obstructive sleep apnea patients. Does gender play a role? *Sleep Breath* 2012; 16: 813–819.

60. Hedner J, Bengtsson-Boström K, Peker Y, *et al.* Hypertension prevalence in obstructive sleep apnoea and sex: a population-based case–control study. *Eur Respir J* 2006; 27: 564–570.

61. Lee YJ, Jeong DU. Obstructive sleep apnea syndrome is associated with higher diastolic blood pressure in men but not in women. *Am J Hypertens* 2014; 27: 325–330.

62. Lavie-Nevo K, Pillar G. Evening-morning differences in blood pressure in sleep apnea syndrome: effect of gender. *Am J Hypertens* 2006; 19: 1064–1069.

63. Pedrosa RP, Barros IM, Drager LF, *et al.* OSA is common and independently associated with hypertension and increased arterial stiffness in consecutive perimenopausal women. *Chest* 2014; 146: 66–72.

64. Tkacova R, McNicholas WT, Javorsky M, *et al.* Nocturnal intermittent hypoxia predicts prevalent hypertension in the European Sleep Apnoea Database cohort study. *Eur Respir J* 2014; 44: 931–941.

65. Mohsenin V, Yaggi HK, Shah N, *et al.* The effect of gender on the prevalence of hypertension in obstructive sleep apnea. *Sleep Med* 2009; 10: 759–762.

66. Theorell-Haglow J, Berne C, Janson C, *et al.* Obstructive sleep apnoea is associated with decreased insulin sensitivity in females. *Eur Respir J* 2008; 31: 1054–1060.

67. Celen YT, Hedner J, Carlson J, *et al.* Impact of gender on incident diabetes mellitus in obstructive sleep apnea: a 16-year follow-up. *J Clin Sleep Med* 2010; 6: 244–250.

68. Kritikou I, Basta M, Vgontzas AN, *et al.* Sleep apnoea, sleepiness, inflammation and insulin resistance in middle-aged males and females. *Eur Respir J* 2014; 43: 145–155.

69. Gottlieb DJ, Yenokyan G, Newman AB, *et al.* Prospective study of obstructive sleep apnea and incident coronary heart disease and heart failure: the Sleep Heart Health Study. *Circulation* 2010; 122: 352–360.

70. Redline S, Yenokyan G, Gottlieb DJ, *et al.* Obstructive sleep apnea-hypopnea and incident stroke: the sleep heart health study. *Am J Respir Crit Care Med* 2010; 182: 269–277.

71. Punjabi NM, Caffo BS, Goodwin JL, *et al.* Sleep-disordered breathing and mortality: a prospective cohort study. *PLoS Med* 2009; 6: e1000132.

72. Chang CC, Chuang HC, Lin CL, *et al.* High incidence of stroke in young women with sleep apnea syndrome. *Sleep Med* 2014; 15: 410–414.

73. Young T, Finn L, Peppard PE, *et al.* Sleep disordered breathing and mortality: eighteen-year follow-up of the Wisconsin sleep cohort. *Sleep* 2008; 31: 1071–1078.

74. Marshall NS, Wong KK, Cullen SR, *et al.* Sleep apnea and 20-year follow-up for all-cause mortality, stroke, and cancer incidence and mortality in the busselton health study cohort. *J Clin Sleep Med* 2014; 10: 355–362.

75. Marin JM, Carrizo SJ, Vicente E, *et al.* Long-term cardiovascular outcomes in men with obstructive sleep apnoea-hypopnoea with or without treatment with continuous positive airway pressure: an observational study. *Lancet* 2005; 365: 1046–1053.

76. Morrish E, Shneerson JM, Smith IE. Why does gender influence survival in obstructive sleep apnoea? *Respir Med* 2008; 102: 1231–1236.

77. Campos-Rodriguez F, Martinez-García MA, de la Cruz-Moron I, *et al.* Cardiovascular mortality in women with obstructive sleep apnea with or without continuous positive airway pressure treatment: a cohort study. *Ann Intern Med* 2012; 156: 115–122.

78. Lavie P, Lavie L, Herer P. All-cause mortality in males with sleep apnoea syndrome: declining mortality rates with age. *Eur Respir J* 2005; 25: 514–520.

79. Yaggi HK, Concato J, Kernan WN, *et al.* Obstructive sleep apnea as a risk factor for stroke and death. *N Engl J Med* 2005; 353: 2034–2041.

80. Martínez-García M-A, Campos-Rodríguez F, Catalán-Serra P, *et al.* Cardiovascular mortality in obstructive sleep apnea in the elderly: role of long-term continuous positive airway pressure treatment: a prospective observational study. *Am J Respir Crit Care Med* 2012; 186: 909–916.

81. Campos-Rodriguez F, Martinez-García MA, Reyes-Nuñez N, *et al.* Role of sleep apnea and continuous positive airway pressure therapy in the incidence of stroke or coronary heart disease in women. *Am J Respir Crit Care Med* 2014; 189: 1544–1550.

82. Newman AB, Foster G, Givelber R, *et al.* Progression and regression of sleep-disordered breathing with changes in weight: the Sleep Heart Health Study. *Arch Intern Med* 2005; 165: 2408–2413.

83. Greenburg DL, Lettieri CJ, Eliasson AH. Effects of surgical weight loss on measures of obstructive sleep apnea: a meta-analysis. *Am J Med* 2009; 122: 535–542.

84. Marklund M, Stenlund H, Franklin KA. Mandibular advancement devices in 630 men and women with obstructive sleep apnea and snoring: tolerability and predictors of treatment success. *Chest* 2004; 125: 1270–1278.

85. Shahar E, Redline S, Young T, *et al.* Hormone replacement therapy and sleep-disordered breathing. *Am J Respir Crit Care Med* 2003; 167: 1186–1192.

86. Manber R, Kuo TF, Cataldo N, *et al.* The effects of hormone replacement therapy on sleep-disordered breathing in postmenopausal women: a pilot study. *Sleep* 2003; 26: 163–168.

87. Cistulli PA, Barnes DJ, Grunstein RR, *et al.* Effect of short-term hormone replacement in the treatment of obstructive sleep apnoea in postmenopausal women. *Thorax* 1994; 49: 699–702.

88. Saaresranta T, Polo-Kantola P, Rauhala E, *et al.* Medroxyprogesterone in postmenopausal females with partial upper airway obstruction during sleep. *Eur Respir J* 2001; 18: 989–995.

89. Indications and standards for use of nasal continuous positive pressure (CPAP) in sleep apnea syndromes. American Thoracic Society. Official statement adopted March 1944. *Am J Respir Crit Care Med* 1994; 150: 1738–1745.

90. Barbé F, Durán-Cantolla J, Sánchez-de-la-Torre M, *et al.* Effect of continuous positive airway pressure on the incidence of hypertension and cardiovascular events in nonsleepy patients with obstructive sleep apnea: a randomized controlled trial. *JAMA* 2012; 307: 2161–2168.

91. Gay P, Weaver T, Loube D, *et al.* Evaluation of positive airway pressure treatment for sleep related breathing disorders in adults. *Sleep* 2006; 29: 381–401.

92. Jenkinson C, Davies RJ, Mullins R, *et al.* Comparison of therapeutic and subtherapeutic nasal continuous positive airway pressure for obstructive sleep apnoea: a randomised prospective parallel trial. *Lancet* 1999; 353: 2100–2105.

93. Banno K, Manfreda J, Walld R, *et al.* Healthcare utilization in women with obstructive sleep apnea syndrome 2 years after diagnosis and treatment. *Sleep* 2006; 29: 1307–1311.

94. Weaver TE, Maislin G, Dinges DF, *et al.* Relationship between hours of CPAP use and achieving normal levels of sleepiness and daily functioning. *Sleep* 2007; 30: 711–719.

95. Pelletier-Fleury N, Rakotonanahary D, Fleury B. The age and other factors in the evaluation of compliance with nasal continuous positive airway pressure for obstructive sleep apnea syndrome. A Cox's proportional hazard analysis. *Sleep Med* 2001; 2: 225–232.

96. Sin DD, Mayers I, Man GC, *et al.* Long-term compliance rates to continuous positive airway pressure in obstructive sleep apnea: a population-based study. *Chest* 2002; 121: 430–435.

97. Collen J, Lettieri C, Kelly W, *et al.* Clinical and polysomnographic predictors of short-term continuous positive airway pressure compliance. *Chest* 2009; 135: 704–709.

98. Kohler M, Smith D, Tippett V, *et al.* Predictors of long-term compliance with continuous positive airway pressure. *Thorax* 2010; 65: 829–832.

99. Bourjeily G, Ankner G, Mohsenin V. Sleep-disordered breathing in pregnancy. *Clin Chest Med* 2011; 32: 175–189.

100. Pien GW, Schwab RJ. Sleep disorders during pregnancy. *Sleep* 2004; 27: 1405–1417.

101. Izci B, Vennelle M, Liston WA, *et al.* Sleep-disordered breathing and upper airway size in pregnancy and post-partum. *Eur Respir J* 2006; 27: 321–327.

102. Morong S, Hermsen B, de Vries N. Sleep-disordered breathing in pregnancy: a review of the physiology and potential role for positional therapy. *Sleep Breath* 2014; 18: 31–37.

103. Young T, Finn L, Palta M. Chronic nasal congestion at night is a risk factor for snoring in a population-based cohort study. *Arch Intern Med* 2001; 161: 1514–1519.

104. Bourjeily G, Raker CA, Chalhoub M, *et al.* Pregnancy and fetal outcomes of symptoms of sleep-disordered breathing. *Eur Respir J* 2010; 36: 849–855.

105. Louis J, Auckley D, Miladinovic B, *et al.* Perinatal outcomes associated with obstructive sleep apnea in obese pregnant women. *Obstet Gynecol* 2012; 120: 1085–1092.

106. Pien GW, Pack AI, Jackson N, *et al.* Risk factors for sleep-disordered breathing in pregnancy. *Thorax* 2014; 69: 371–377.

107. Edwards N, Blyton DM, Kirjavainen T, *et al.* Nasal continuous positive airway pressure reduces sleep-induced blood pressure increments in preeclampsia. *Am J Respir Crit Care Med* 2000; 162: 252–257.
108. Connolly G, Razak AR, Hayanga A, *et al.* Inspiratory flow limitation during sleep in pre-eclampsia: comparison with normal pregnant and nonpregnant women. *Eur Respir J* 2001; 18: 672–676.
109. Blyton DM, Sullivan CE, Edwards N. Reduced nocturnal cardiac output associated with preeclampsia is minimized with the use of nocturnal nasal CPAP. *Sleep* 2004; 27: 79–84.
110. Yinon D, Lowenstein L, Suraya S, *et al.* Pre-eclampsia is associated with sleep-disordered breathing and endothelial dysfunction. *Eur Respir J* 2006; 27: 328–333.
111. Sahin FK, Koken G, Cosar E, *et al.* Obstructive sleep apnea in pregnancy and fetal outcome. *Int J Gynaecol Obstet* 2008; 100: 141–146.
112. Champagne K, Schwartzman K, Opatrny L, *et al.* Obstructive sleep apnoea and its association with gestational hypertension. *Eur Respir J* 2009; 33: 559–565.
113. Louis JM, Auckley D, Sokol RJ, *et al.* Maternal and neonatal morbidities associated with obstructive sleep apnea complicating pregnancy. *Am J Obstet Gynecol* 2010; 202: 261.
114. Olivarez SA, Maheshwari B, McCarthy M, *et al.* Prospective trial on obstructive sleep apnea in pregnancy and fetal heart rate monitoring. *Am J Obstet Gynecol* 2010; 202: 552.
115. Reid J, Skomro R, Cotton D, *et al.* Pregnant women with gestational hypertension may have a high frequency of sleep disordered breathing. *Sleep* 2011; 34: 1033–1038.
116. Chen YH, Kang JH, Lin CC, *et al.* Obstructive sleep apnea and the risk of adverse pregnancy outcomes. *Am J Obstet Gynecol* 2012; 206: 136.
117. Facco FL, Liu CS, Cabello AA, *et al.* Sleep-disordered breathing: a risk factor for adverse pregnancy outcomes? *Am J Perinatol* 2012; 29: 277–282.
118. Louis JM, Mogos MF, Salemi JL, *et al.* Obstructive sleep apnea and severe maternal-infant morbidity/mortality in the United States, 1998–2009. *Sleep* 2014; 37: 843–849.
119. Pamidi S, Pinto LM, Marc I, *et al.* Maternal sleep-disordered breathing and adverse pregnancy outcomes: a systematic review and metaanalysis. *Am J Obstet Gynecol* 2014; 210: 52.e1–52.e14.
120. Pérez-Chada D, Videla AJ, O'Flaherty ME, *et al.* Snoring, witnessed sleep apnoeas and pregnancy-induced hypertension. *Acta Obstet Gynecol Scand* 2007; 86: 788–792.
121. Yin TT, Williams N, Burton C, *et al.* Hypertension, fetal growth restriction and obstructive sleep apnoea in pregnancy. *Eur J Obstet Gynecol Reprod Biol* 2008; 141: 35–38.
122. August EM, Salihu HM, Biroscak BJ, *et al.* Systematic review on sleep disorders and obstetric outcomes: scope of current knowledge. *Am J Perinatol* 2013; 30: 323–334.
123. Guilleminault C, Kreutzer M, Chang JL. Pregnancy, sleep disordered breathing and treatment with nasal continuous positive airway pressure. *Sleep Med* 2004; 5: 43–51.
124. Poyares D, Guilleminault C, Hachul H, *et al.* Pre-eclampsia and nasal CPAP: part 2. Hypertension during pregnancy, chronic snoring, and early nasal CPAP intervention. *Sleep Med* 2007; 9: 15–21.

Disclosures: **None declared.**

Chapter 7

Elderly patients

Frédéric Roche, David Hupin, Magali Saint-Martin and Emilia Sforza

Ageing substantially increases the incidence of OSA. However, the disease remains underdiagnosed despite the rising costs of healthcare that the lack of support can cause. In middle-aged adults, EDS, CVD, depression, accelerated cognitive decline and traffic accidents should prompt screening and an evaluation of the severity of OSA. Although OSA in the elderly seems to have a lower impact on mortality than it does in middle-aged adults, the risk of stroke and new-onset hypertension appears to increase in elderly patients. In addition, the presence of CSA must prompt a thorough heart disease assessment, even in the elderly. Both elderly and middle-aged symptomatic OSA patients derive equivalent benefits from CPAP treatment. In the future, epidemiological as well as interventional studies should be carried out in elderly patients, whose number will increase hugely in the coming years.

In the last two decades, the percentage of people aged over 60 years has increased more quickly than any other age group worldwide, as a result of longer life expectancy and the success of public health policies and socioeconomic development. From a medical point of view, a greater effort has been taken to maximise the health and functional ability of older people to achieve "active ageing". In parallel, extensive studies have been performed to assess factors that may affect active ageing, such as metabolic, vascular and neuropsychological factors, and sleep disorders, such as insomnia and OSA. The latter is a clinical entity characterised by repeated pharyngeal collapse during sleep, inducing apnoea, decreasing oxygen saturation and increasing arterial carbon dioxide tension. To restore pharyngeal patency, patients experience recurrent arousal from sleep, which activates the sympathetic nervous system and results in sleep fragmentation. These acute changes contribute to the increased risk of cardiovascular, metabolic and diurnal consequences, such as EDS, cognitive disturbances and poor quality of life. The link between OSA and ageing is now well defined and expressed by the age-related physiological changes inducing a progressive rise in the prevalence of OSA in the elderly.

Several reviews have been performed regarding the clinical aspects of OSA in middle-aged subjects or in the elderly with various diseases. As a consequence, controversial data are present in the literature about OSA in community and clinical samples. In this chapter, we will examine the clinical aspects of OSA in the elderly, focusing on the diurnal consequences and the prognostic implications, to better assess the morbidity and mortality risks in the elderly, as well as the treatment requirements.

Dept of Clinical Physiology and Exercise, Pole NOL, CHU and Faculty of Medicine of Saint-Étienne, UJM and COMUE of Lyon-Saint-Étienne, Saint-Étienne, France.

Correspondence: Frédéric Roche, Dept of Clinical Physiology, EFCR, CHU Nord, Level 6, F-42055 Saint-Étienne Cedex 2, France. E-mail: frederic.roche@univ-st-etienne.fr

Copyright ©ERS 2015. Print ISBN: 978-1-84984-059-0. Online ISBN: 978-1-84984-060-6. Print ISSN: 2312-508X. Online ISSN: 2312-5098.

Screening and diagnosis of OSA

The current gold standard diagnostic tool in clinical practice for assessing OSA, particularly in the elderly, is PSG, as it allows for a more accurate diagnosis of OSA and other age-related sleep disturbances. However, only a minority of patients at risk for OSA have access to PSG, owing to its technical requirements, labour-intensive procedures and cost. Due to increasing demand, a good alternative for diagnosing OSA is a portable respiratory monitoring system that is known for its accuracy, easy management and lower cost [1] and also as a valid tool for the diagnosis of OSA [2] in clinical settings and in the elderly [3], for whom oxymetry could represent a simple alternative for the detection of OSA [4].

From an epidemiological point of view, an efficient pre-selection procedure with an inexpensive and accurate method of screening, such as dedicated questionnaires, can be conveniently incorporated into diagnosis and follow-up studies in the elderly. However, the Berlin questionnaire was found to be insufficiently accurate among the elderly [5], and the STOP-Bang questionnaire, although a more accurate alternative questionnaire, remains to be validated in the elderly [6].

Epidemiology of OSA in the elderly

Prevalence studies conducted over the past decade have demonstrated that up to 5% of adults in western countries are likely to have undiagnosed OSA. When we consider the severity of the disease, stratified according to the AHI, the estimated prevalence ranges from 3% to 28% for mild cases (AHI 5–15 events·h^{-1}) and from 1% to 14% for moderate to severe cases (AHI >15 events·h^{-1}). When only the studies that included in-laboratory PSG conducted on large samples are considered, the results of cohorts in Wisconsin (USA) [7], Pennsylvania (USA) [8, 9] and Spain [10] and those from the Sleep Heart Health Study [11] demonstrated that one out of every five adults suffers from OSA. In large communities with older populations aged 65–90 years, 81% had an AHI >5 events·h^{-1}, 44% and 32% being mild and moderate cases, respectively, and 24% had an AHI >40 events·h^{-1} [12].

Progression of OSA with ageing

Whereas there are considerable prevalence data from western countries, little is known about OSA incidence and progression (*i.e.* the worsening of illness over a given time interval). Data from an 8-year follow-up study of 282 participants in the Wisconsin Sleep Cohort Study show a significant increase in the AHI over this period, the progression being significantly greater in older subjects [13]. A similar trend was found in the Cleveland Family Study [14] with a 5-year increase in the AHI from 2±1.4 to 6.2±7.9 events·h^{-1}. Significant predictors of the rise were obesity, CVD and diabetes. These data confirm previous results in small clinical samples showing that in mild cases of OSA the progression and deterioration of the disease is less [15–17] compared with severe cases [18]. Few data are available in elderly populations that have generally been described as having stable or even improving disease states that are not completely explained by changes in weight or by the baseline OSA severity [19].

In community-dwelling older adults (age 65–95 years), 81% of participants had an AHI >5 events·h^{-1}, with prevalence rates of 44% for an AHI >20 events·h^{-1} and 24% for an AHI >40 events·h^{-1} [20]. Furthermore, in older adults examined in the Sleep Heart Health

Study, the authors found that among subjects aged 60–69 years, 32% had an AHI between 5 and 14 events·h^{-1} and 19% had an AHI >15 events·h^{-1} [21]. This trend in elderly subjects may be explained by the physiological changes in the anatomy or functioning of the UA [22] or by other medical disorders, such as diabetes, hypertension and CVD.

A higher prevalence of OSA in the elderly does not necessarily mean that physiological changes associated with ageing cause an increase in the OSA incidence rate. Some data suggest that OSA in the elderly may be a condition distinct from that in middle-aged people, as suggested by the increase in central or mixed apnoeas related to sleep instability and the reduction of snoring with age [9, 10].

Interestingly, in all of the above-mentioned epidemiological studies, the proportion of subjects with an AHI >15 events·h^{-1} was approximately 1.7-fold higher in older subjects (60–99 years), suggesting that a threshold of an AHI >15 events·h^{-1} might better differentiate the older population with and without OSA [23].

The effect of sex

Sex seems to affect the incidence of the disease, as OSA is more prevalent in males, with a male:female ratio of 8–10:1 in clinical studies and approximately 2:1 or 3:1 in epidemiological studies [24]. The reason for the reduced susceptibility to OSA in females is not entirely clear, and many factors have been proposed, such as the UA shape, the craniofacial morphology and hormonal changes [25], as well as exposure to other risk factors in men, such as fat deposition, smoking and alcohol intake. The most probable explanation is that there are clear sex differences in the UA shape and genioglossus muscle activity during the awake state [26]. Several papers have reported that females with OSA are less likely to show the classic symptoms of OSA [27], such as snoring, apnoea and sleepiness, and they more frequently report fatigue, depression and anxiety. Moreover, they have a lower AHI frequently confined to REM sleep [28]. In the elderly, similar to middle-aged cases, females more frequently complain of depression, anxiety and psychotropic treatment [29], supporting the hypothesis that the psychological profile is related more to a sex phenotype than to OSA itself. Interestingly, the prevalence of OSA in the older sample was quite similar in men and women, stressing the need to assess the risk for OSA in older females.

The effect of obesity

Obesity has long been known to be associated with OSA, and BMI correlates positively with the severity of the disease. To explain sex differences in the relationship between OSA and obesity, the hypothesis of possible differences in fat distribution has been proposed [30–32], although waist and neck circumference are better markers for OSA than BMI [33]. This was confirmed by an earlier analysis of the Wisconsin Sleep Cohort Study [21], which found that the waist/hip ratio and neck girth, rather than BMI, may be considered risk factors for developing OSA in both sexes.

It is well known that men classically have more android (upper body) *versus* gynoid (lower body) fat compared with women. Moreover, obese men with OSA have a significant greater amount of visceral fat than BMI-matched controls, with the indices of OSA positively correlated with visceral fat but not with BMI or subcutaneous fat. In another study of 749 volunteers with a median age of 67 years undergoing dual-energy X-ray absorptiometry, the authors found that in the elderly the central fat mass plays a role only in severe OSA cases, stressing the weak role of central fat mass on OSA occurrence [34].

The diurnal consequences of OSA in the elderly

Cognitive functions

Although the prevalence of OSA increases with age, there is still a debate on whether OSA is associated with the greater susceptibility to cognitive dysfunction in older populations, which generally experience a physiological cognitive decrease and an increase in the prevalence of OSA. An initial epidemiological study has not revealed any evidence of a dose–response relationship between the AHI and cognitive functions in a cohort of 837 men and 923 women over 60 years old, with respect to attentional, memory and executive functions [35]. Studies performed on sleep clinic patients have found conflicting results, with some data confirming a link between AHI, hypoxaemia and cognitive dysfunction [36] and others not [37]. The severity of the disease seems to play a key role in cognitive decline, and older patients are more likely to have cognitive deficits in attention and executive functions when the AHI is >30 events·h^{-1} [38]. In a prospective study conducted among 289 women aged 82 years with mild cognitive impairment and dementia, the authors demonstrated that older women with OSA had an increased risk of developing mild cognitive impairment or dementia after 5 years [39]. When treated, patients without [40] or with mild dementia [41] have slower cognitive deterioration, emphasising the link between cognitive decline and OSA.

The causal model proposed for cognitive dysfunction in OSA [42] suggests that sleep disruption and hypoxaemia induce chemical and structural central nervous system injuries that in turn lead to dysfunction in the prefrontal regions [43] and, consequently, significant executive dysfunction. However, SAINT MARTIN et al. [44] recently showed that after 8 years of follow-up, the presence of OSA in the elderly without neurological or vascular dysfunction was associated with a slight but significant decline in the attentional domain only (p=0.01) and was without changes in the executive and memory functions over time. Moreover, the effects were small, accounting for 4–7% of the variance without a significant effect of the AHI and hypoxaemia, suggesting that OSA alone does not contribute to a severe cognitive decline in OSA cases.

Interestingly, recent data have underlined the link between cognition and the autonomic nervous system, as assessed by the contributing role of heart rate variability [45] and baroreflex sensitivity [46]. A link has been reported between cognitive performances and the lower power spectral density of the heart rate variability, i.e. parasympathetic tone markers, in older adults [47]. These data open the way to evaluate the potential role of other factors on cognitive impairment, apart from hypoxaemia and sleep fragmentation [48].

Sleepiness

An important consequence of OSA is EDS, which has been related to increased numbers of driving accidents [49, 50] and reduced quality of life [51]. Despite the controversy about the validation of the ESS in the elderly, for whom some questions, e.g. driving and falling asleep at crossroads, cannot be completed according to some studies [52, 53], the ESS may be considered useful to assess subjective sleepiness in the elderly.

The most frequent mechanisms that lead to EDS in OSA patients include the severity of the OSA, as indicated by the AHI [54], nocturnal hypoxaemia [55, 56], sleep fragmentation [57, 58] and enhanced sympathetic tone [59]. The few available epidemiological data from elderly populations [60, 61] stress the effects of poor sleep, sex and medication. More recent studies in elderly men [62] and women [63] aged 76–83 years from the Osteoporotic Fractures Study, with an AHI of approximately 17 events·h^{-1}, demonstrated a small effect of AHI, hypoxaemia and total sleep time on EDS, without linearity between the AHI and sleepiness, as well as the severity of sleepiness and the degree of sleep disruption and sleep fragmentation [64]. Therefore, other factors are implicated in EDS [65, 66], particularly in the elderly, for whom compensatory mechanisms such as physical and social activity and the correction of mood disorders may act to prevent sleepiness.

An interesting question that should be considered is whether the presence of OSA, EDS and sleep disturbances contribute to increased risks of falling in older populations. A few studies have been performed suggesting relationships between the risk of falling and OSA-related EDS (in a small sample [67]) and sleep disturbances [68].

Metabolic and cardiovascular consequences of OSA in the elderly

Metabolic syndrome

In patients with metabolic syndrome, the prevalence of moderate to severe OSA is very high (60%). Few data are available in elderly populations. In the PROOF-SYNAPSE cohort study (806 subjects with a mean age of 68.5 years), 9.8% of cases met the criteria for metabolic syndrome, with a similar prevalence in men and women. Assoumou et al. [69] found that after adjusting for confounders, such as obesity and sex, the oxyhaemoglobin desaturation index was independently associated with glycaemia (p<0.0001), hypertension (p=0.002) and triglyceride levels (p=0.02), without an effect of EDS or sleep duration.

Autonomic nervous system activation

In patients with OSA, disruptions of autonomic activity have been described [70] and are now recognised to contribute to cardiovascular risk in the elderly [71]. While the mechanism explaining this association remains unclear, we found that autonomic activation might be considered to be a marker for new-onset hypertension [72]. Diurnal baroreflex control alteration is also associated with sleep-related autonomic overactivity in the elderly [73] and increases the incidence of cardiovascular complications in elderly OSA patients. Moreover, when we consider sleep-related autonomic overactivity indices, as detected by monitoring of pulse transit time [74], the density of these phasic sympathetic activations in the elderly are clearly better associated with SBP loads than other classical parameters of nocturnal recordings [75]. In addition, these recurrent sympathetic arousals from sleep, i.e. autonomic arousals, seem to contribute to hypertension, increased vascular resistance and altered endothelial functioning [76, 77].

Hypertension

In an elderly community-based population [78], severe OSA (AHI >30 events·h^{-1}) was associated with a significant 5-mmHg increase in diurnal and nocturnal SBP and with a nocturnal 3-mmHg increase in the DBP. Systolic and diastolic hypertension were more frequently found in subjects with moderate (AHI 15–30 events·h^{-1}) or severe OSA (AHI >30 events·h^{-1}), with the degree of hypoxaemia (defined as the time that arterial oxygen saturation was <90%) as the major contributing factor.

An interesting finding is that in an elderly population [79], severe untreated OSA patients had a great and independent risk for the development of hypertension, and the OSA-related hypertension remains an independent risk factor for hypertension after excluding confounders, such as age and obesity, in a large clinical Spanish cohort [80]. During the follow-up of this cohort, the authors found a persistent dose–response relationship between the severity of OSA and the cumulative incidence of hypertension. In contrast, HAAS et al. [81] did not find a relationship between AHI and hypertension in subjects older than 60 years; however, patients with CVD were included in this study, which probably led to underestimation of the strength of the association between OSA and hypertension.

CVD

All of the study populations, including clinical and community-based studies, have reported a significant positive association between OSA and an increased risk of developing CVD [82]. Although OSA occurs in approximately 20% of older adults, the relationship between OSA and CVD in this group is not well established. Reports from the Sleep Heart Health Study indicated no significant association between OSA and coronary heart disease among participants ≥70 years old [83]. In a prospective study [84], snoring was associated with EDS and resulted in a significantly increased hazard ratio (HR) for CVD events (HR 1.46, 95% CI 1.03–2.08; p=0.035) after adjusting for confounding factors. A limitation of this study is that AHI was not measured, and it is likely that the association between snoring and EDS might suggest an analysis restricted to severe cases [85]. In a community-dwelling population >75 years old, JOHANSSON et al. [86] found that while OSA does not appear to be associated with CVD, subjects with CSA had increased risk of CVD and impaired systolic function that induced a higher mortality rate.

Carotid atherosclerosis

Prospective data from the Wisconsin Sleep Cohort indicated that an AHI >20 events·h^{-1} was associated with a four-fold increase in the risk of stroke during a 4-year follow-up period [87]. In contrast to middle-aged samples, the presence of carotid lesions was similar in older subjects with and without OSA. Finally, despite a positive association between the presence of carotid atherosclerosis and AHI, male sex, metabolic variables and hypertension may play key roles in cerebrovascular risk, even in severe cases of OSA [88].

We have to remember that ageing is associated with several changes in cardiovascular structure and functioning. This is confirmed by the presence of asymptomatic carotid arteriosclerosis in the elderly aged >65 years, and human ageing in itself [89] is the main determinant responsible for arterial wall changes and arterial stiffness [90].

Cerebral white matter changes

A recent Korean study has provided evidence for a relationship between OSA and white matter changes [91]. The mean AHI and the prevalence of OSA were higher in the groups with white matter changes, and individuals with moderate to severe OSA had a two-fold increased risk of exhibiting white matter changes, even after adjusting for covariates. Other studies have also reported a significant correlation between subclinical cerebrovascular diseases and moderate to severe OSA [92, 93]. Based on their findings, some authors have concluded that OSA may have a detrimental effect in target organ damage. However, the specific roles of sex and hypertension in the relationship between OSA and white matter changes need to be elucidated [94].

Risk of stroke

The effect of OSA on the incidence of stroke has been evaluated according to population-based, clinic-based and community-based studies. A meta-analysis reviewed 10 studies focusing on this clinical topic [95]. The pooled relative risk (95% CI) for individuals with moderate to severe OSA compared with the reference group was 2.02 (1.40–2.90). An adjustment was made for age in all of these studies. It is of note that the studies on elderly populations showed individually concordant increased incidental risks of fatal or nonfatal stroke in patients with OSA [96, 97]. The high percentage of women included in the previously published studies could preclude extending the conclusion of this meta-analysis to elderly men.

Mortality and OSA in the elderly

All-cause and cardiovascular mortality

In middle-aged people, OSA is associated with an increased cardiovascular mortality [95, 98–101] related to cyclic oxygen desaturations followed by rapid re-oxygenation, causing oxidative stress, inflammation and sympathetic overactivation. GE et al. [102] conducted a meta-analysis to investigate whether OSA is an independent predictor for future cardiovascular and all-cause mortality. Six studies including 11 932 patients were identified and analysed. The pooled HR (95% CI) of all-cause mortality was 1.19 (1.00–1.41) for moderate OSA and reached 1.90 (1.29–2.81) for severe OSA. The pooled HR (95% CI) of cardiovascular mortality was 1.40 (0.77–2.53) for moderate OSA and 2.65 (1.82–3.85) for severe OSA. Under CPAP treatment, treated patients had the same cardiovascular mortality rate as healthy subjects (HR 0.82, 95% CI 0.50–1.33), suggesting that severe OSA is a strong independent predictor for future cardiovascular and all-cause mortality and that CPAP treatment reduces the mortality risk. A limit of this meta-analysis is the variability of data concerning age and sex among the different studies, which does not allow for a specific estimation of the risk of morbidity and mortality in the elderly.

In a Swedish study including 331 community-dwelling elderly subjects aged 71–87 years undergoing polygraphic recording, the authors found that 55% had OSA at baseline, which had no significant impact on the all-cause and cardiovascular mortality after 7 years of follow-up [86, 103]. Conversely, CSA significantly increased the risk for all-cause (p=0.002) and cardiovascular mortality (p=0.018) by more than two-fold. After adjusting for CVD, diabetes and the N-terminal pro-brain natriuretic peptide, the association between CSA and mortality lost significance. With increasing age, AHI and the related hypoxaemic dips may become less severe and could explain these results [8]. Another possible explanation could be that OSA causes more cardiovascular deaths during adult life [104]. For the high mortality risk in CSA subjects, it could be proposed that the presence of impaired left ventricular systolic function associated with unrecognised right ventricular dysfunction enhanced the mortality rate in the elderly [105].

Cancer mortality

In a recently published retrospective study, the authors suggest that the positive association between OSA severity and increased cancer mortality could be limited to patients aged <65 years, whereas no association was shown in elderly patients [106]. One possible explanation for the presence of this association in younger patients only is the ischaemic preconditioning hypothesis [107], which was previously discussed in the context of CVD. Older survivors with a long-term IH challenge could develop compensatory mechanisms to counteract intermittent tissue hypoxia, resulting in lower mortality from cancer.

Treatment of OSA in the elderly

In middle-aged patients with AHI $\geqslant$15 events·h^{-1} and EDS, CPAP therapy produces significant and cost-efficient improvements in daytime sleepiness [108, 109]. However, the need for dedicated trials in other patient groups, such as the elderly, has been mentioned. Reducing sleepiness may be of importance in elderly OSA patients, as improved attentional capacity could delay cognitive dysfunction [110] and prevent traffic accidents [111, 112]. However, the risk reduction may be smaller in older OSA patients because a protective effect of chronic IH has been proposed as an adaptive mechanism in the elderly. A recent randomised study demonstrated that in older people with OSA associated with EDS (n=278), CPAP reduces sleepiness as observed in adults and is marginally more cost-effective over 12 months compared with the classical best supportive care [113]. Thus, CPAP is much more effective in patients with a higher baseline EDS and/or with greater CPAP duration.

Adherence to CPAP treatment in the elderly has been discussed, especially in the case of complaints about cognitive functions or the loss of independence. In the few studies available, compliance did not seem different from that of younger patients [114]. The two main factors associated with good adherence are the severity of daytime symptoms and patient education. Compared with young subjects with similar disease severity, *i.e.* equivalent AHI, older cases may require titration at lower CPAP levels than younger patients [115]. Finally, adherence to CPAP will be even better when it is framed as regular therapeutic monitoring and tailored advice is given based on side-effects [116, 117].

Conclusion

There is now convincing evidence that OSA in elderly populations is an independent factor for diurnal consequences similar to those described in middle-aged populations. However, the elderly have a different clinical phenotype and do not complain of the classical symptoms, such as snoring, sleepiness, fatigue, nocturia and napping. Moreover, cognitive dysfunction, mood disorders and reduced quality of life are frequently explained in clinical practice as symptoms of ageing in itself or related to other somatic or psychological diseases, inducing an underestimation of sleep disorders. We can alert general practitioners that these symptoms may reflect the presence of OSA in elderly patients, which once assessed and treated, may reduce these symptoms and prevent the occurrence of metabolic and cardiovascular morbidity and mortality and reduce healthcare utilisation compared with patients without OSA [118]. In contrast to the first published studies testing the acceptance of CPAP in the elderly, we can say that as a consequence of the improvement of the technical support, CPAP therapy is better tolerated even in very old populations, and it has a significant impact on the overall quality of life and functioning by preventing the high risk of morbidity and mortality.

References

1. Oliveira MG, Garbuio S, Treptow EC, et al. The use of portable monitoring for sleep apnea diagnosis in adults. *Expert Rev Respir Med* 2014; 8: 123–132.
2. Collop NA, Anderson WM, Boehlecke B, et al. Clinical guidelines for the use of unattended portable monitors in the diagnosis of obstructive sleep apnea in adult patients. Portable Monitoring Task Force of the American Academy of Sleep Medicine. *J Clin Sleep Med* 2007; 3: 737–747.
3. Johansson P, Alehagen U, Svanborg E, et al. Sleep disordered breathing in an elderly community-living population: relationship to cardiac function, insomnia symptoms and daytime sleepiness. *Sleep Med* 2009; 10: 1005–1011.
4. Mazière S, Pépin JL, Siyanko N, et al. Usefulness of oximetry for sleep apnea screening in frail hospitalized elderly. *J Am Med Dir Assoc* 2014; 15: 447.e9–447.e14.
5. Sforza E, Chouchou F, Pichot V, et al. Is the Berlin questionnaire a useful tool to diagnose obstructive sleep apnea in the elderly? *Sleep Med* 2011; 12: 142–146.
6. Silva GE, Vana KD, Goodwin JL, et al. Identification of patients with sleep disordered breathing: comparing the four-variable screening tool, STOP, STOP-Bang, and Epworth Sleepiness Scales. *J Clin Sleep Med* 2011; 7: 467–472.
7. Young T, Palta M, Dempsey J, et al. The occurrence of sleep-disordered breathing among middle-aged adults. *N Engl J Med* 1993; 328: 1230–1235.
8. Bixler EO, Vgontzas AN, Ten Have T, et al. Effects of age on sleep apnea in men: I. Prevalence and severity. *Am J Respir Crit Care Med* 1998; 157: 144–148.
9. Bixler EO, Vgontzas AN, Lin HM, et al. Prevalence of sleep-disordered breathing in women: effects of gender. *Am J Respir Crit Care Med* 2001; 163: 608–613.
10. Duran J, Esnaola S, Rubio R, et al. Obstructive sleep apnea-hypopnea and related clinical features in a population-based sample of subjects aged 30 to 70 yr. *Am J Respir Crit Care Med* 2001; 163: 685–689.
11. Quan SF, Howard BV, Iber C, et al. The Sleep Heart Health Study: design, rationale, and methods. *Sleep* 1997; 20: 1077–1085.
12. Roepke SK, Ancoli-Israel S. Sleep disorders in the elderly. *Indian J Med Res* 2010; 131: 302–310.
13. Ancoli-Israel S, Gehrman P, Kripke DF, et al. Long-term follow-up of sleep disordered breathing in older adults. *Sleep Med* 2001; 2: 511–516.
14. Redline S, Larkin E, Schluchter M, et al. Incidence of sleep disordered breathing (SBD) in a population-based sample. *Sleep* 2001; 24: Suppl. 1, A294.
15. Svanborg E, Larsson H. Development of nocturnal respiratory disturbance in untreated patients with obstructive sleep apnea syndrome. *Chest* 1993; 104: 340–343.
16. Pendlebury S, Pépin JL, Veale D, et al. Natural evolution of moderate sleep apnoea syndrome: significant progression over a mean of 17 months. *Thorax* 1997; 52: 872–878.
17. Lindberg E, Elmasry A, Gislason T, et al. Evolution of sleep apnea syndrome in sleepy snorers: a population-based prospective study. *Am J Respir Crit Care Med* 1999; 159: 2024–2027.
18. Sforza E, Addati G, Cirignotta F, et al. Natural evolution of sleep apnoea syndrome: a five year longitudinal study. *Eur Respir J* 1994; 7: 1765–1770.
19. Sforza E, Gauthier M, Crawford-Achour E, et al. A 3-year longitudinal study of sleep disordered breathing in the elderly. *Eur Respir J* 2012; 40: 665–672.
20. Ancoli-Israel S, Kripke DF, Klauber MR, et al. Sleep-disordered breathing in community-dwelling elderly. *Sleep* 1991; 14: 486–495.
21. Young T, Shahar E, Nieto FJ, et al. Predictors of sleep-disordered breathing in community-dwelling adults: the Sleep Heart Health Study. *Arch Intern Med* 2002; 162: 893–900.
22. Eikermann M, Jordan AS, Chamberlin NL, et al. The influence of aging on pharyngeal collapsibility during sleep. *Chest* 2007; 131: 1702–1709.
23. Pavlova MK, Duffy JF, Shea SA. Polysomnographic respiratory abnormalities in asymptomatic individuals. *Sleep* 2008; 31: 241–248.

24. Sforza E, Chouchou F, Collet P, *et al.* Sex differences in obstructive sleep apnoea in an elderly French population. *Eur Respir J* 2011; 37: 1137–1143.

25. Popovic RM, White DP. Upper airway muscle activity in normal women: influence of hormonal status. *J Appl Physiol* 1998; 84: 1055–1062.

26. Schwab RJ. Sex differences and sleep apnoea. *Thorax* 1999; 54: 284–285.

27. Collop NA, Adkins D, Phillips BA. Gender differences in sleep and sleep-disordered breathing. *Clin Chest Med* 2004; 25: 257–268.

28. Koo BB, Dostal J, Ioachimescu O, *et al.* The effects of gender and age on REM-related sleep-disordered breathing. *Sleep Breath* 2008; 12: 259–264.

29. Saint Martin M, Sforza E, Barthélémy JC, *et al.* Sleep perception in non-insomniac healthy elderly: a 3-year longitudinal study. *Rejuvenation Res* 2014; 17: 11–18.

30. Yeo SE, Hays NP, Dennis RA, *et al.* Fat distribution and glucose metabolism in older, obese men and women. *J Gerontol A Biol Sci Med Sci* 2007; 62: 1393–1401.

31. Vgontzas AN, Papanicolaou DA, Bixler EO, *et al.* Sleep apnea and daytime sleepiness and fatigue: relation to visceral obesity, insulin resistance, and hypercytokinemia. *J Clin Endocrinol Metab* 2000; 85: 1151–1158.

32. Lim YH, Choi J, Kim KR, *et al.* Sex-specific characteristics of anthropometry in patients with obstructive sleep apnea: neck circumference and waist-hip ratio. *Ann Otol Rhinol Laryngol* 2014; 123: 517–523.

33. Peppard PE, Ward NR, Morrell MJ. The impact of obesity on oxygen desaturation during sleep-disordered breathing. *Am J Respir Crit Care Med* 2009; 180: 788–793.

34. Degache F, Sforza E, Dauphinot V, *et al.* Relation of central fat mass to obstructive sleep apnea in the elderly. *Sleep* 2013; 36: 501–507.

35. Boland LL, Shahar E, Iber C, *et al.* Measures of cognitive function in persons with varying degrees of sleep-disordered breathing: the Sleep Heart Health Study. *J Sleep Res* 2002; 11: 265–272.

36. Cohen-Zion M, Stepnowsky C, Marler, *et al.* Changes in cognitive function associated with sleep disordered breathing in older people. *J Am Geriatr Soc* 2001; 49: 1622–1627.

37. Phillips BA, Berry DT, Schmitt FA, *et al.* Sleep-disordered breathing in the healthy elderly. Clinically significant? *Chest* 1992; 101: 345–349.

38. Aloia MS, Arnedt JT, Davis JD, *et al.* Neuropsychological sequelae of obstructive sleep apnea-hypopnea syndrome: a critical review. *J Int Neuropsychol Soc* 2004; 10: 772–785.

39. Yaffe K, Laffan AM, Harrison SL, *et al.* Sleep-disordered breathing, hypoxia, and risk of mild cognitive impairment and dementia in older women. *JAMA* 2011; 306: 613–619.

40. Aloia MS, Ilniczky N, Di Dio P, *et al.* Neuropsychological changes and treatment compliance in older adults with sleep apnea. *J Psychosom Res* 2003; 54: 71–76.

41. Ancoli-Israel S, Palmer BW, Cooke JR, *et al.* Cognitive effects of treating obstructive sleep apnea in Alzheimer's disease: a randomized controlled study. *J Am Geriatr Soc* 2008; 56: 2076–2081.

42. Gozal D. CrossTalk proposal: the intermittent hypoxia attending severe obstructive sleep apnoea does lead to alterations in brain structure and function. *J Physiol* 2013; 591: 379–381.

43. Beebe DW, Gozal D. Obstructive sleep apnea and the prefrontal cortex: towards a comprehensive model linking nocturnal upper airway obstruction to daytime cognitive and behavioral deficits. *J Sleep Res* 2002; 11: 1–16.

44. Saint Martin M, Sforza E, Roche F, *et al.* Sleep breathing disorders and cognitive function in the elderly: an 8-year follow-up study. The Proof-Synapse Cohort. *Sleep* 2014 [In press PII: sp-00345-13].

45. Zeki Al Hazzouri A, Haan MN, Deng Y, *et al.* Reduced heart rate variability is associated with worse cognitive performance in elderly Mexican Americans. *Hypertension* 2014; 63: 181–187.

46. Szili-Török T, Kálmán J, Paprika D, *et al.* Depressed baroreflex sensitivity in patients with Alzheimer's and Parkinson's disease. *Neurobiol Aging* 2001; 22: 435–438.

47. Saint Martin M, Sforza E, Thomas-Anterion C, *et al.* Baroreflex sensitivity, vascular risk factors, and cognitive function in a healthy elderly population: the PROOF cohort. *J Am Geriatr Soc* 2013; 61: 2096–2102.

48. Daulatzai MA. Pathogenesis of cognitive dysfunction in patients with obstructive sleep apnea: a hypothesis with emphasis on the nucleus tractus solitarius. *Sleep Disord* 2012; 2012: 251096.

49. George CF. Sleep. 5: Driving and automobile crashes in patients with obstructive sleep apnoea/hypopnoea syndrome. *Thorax* 2004; 59: 804–807.

50. Krieger J, McNicholas WT, Levy P, *et al.* Public health and medicolegal implications of sleep apnoea. *Eur Respir J* 2002; 20: 1594–1609.

51. Baldwin CM, Griffith KA, Nieto FJ, *et al.* The association of sleep-disordered breathing and sleep symptoms with quality of life in the Sleep Heart Health Study. *Sleep* 2001; 24: 96–105.

52. Spira AP, Beaudreau SA, Stone KL, *et al.* Reliability and validity of the Pittsburgh Sleep Quality Index and the Epworth Sleepiness Scale in older men. *J Gerontol A Biol Sci Med Sci* 2012; 67: 433–439.

53. Beaudreau SA, Spira AP, Stewart A, *et al.* Validation of the Pittsburgh Sleep Quality Index and the Epworth Sleepiness Scale in older black and white women. *Sleep Med* 2012; 13: 36–42.

54. Gottlieb DJ, Whitney CW, Bonekat WH, *et al.* Relation of sleepiness to respiratory disturbance index: the Sleep Heart Health Study. *Am J Respir Crit Care Med* 1999; 159: 502–507.

55. BaHammam A. Excessive daytime sleepiness in patients with sleep-disordered breathing. *Eur Respir J* 2008; 31: 685–686.

56. Uysal A, Liendo C, McCarty DE, *et al.* Nocturnal hypoxemia biomarker predicts sleepiness in patients with severe obstructive sleep apnea. *Sleep Breath* 2014; 18: 77–84.

57. Guilleminault C, Partinen M, Quera-Salva MA, *et al.* Determinants of daytime sleepiness in obstructive sleep apnea. *Chest* 1988; 94: 32–37.

58. Colt HG, Haas H, Rich GB. Hypoxemia *vs* sleep fragmentation as cause of excessive daytime sleepiness in obstructive sleep apnea. *Chest* 1991; 100: 1542–1548.

59. Donadio V, Liguori R, Vetrugno R, *et al.* Daytime sympathetic hyperactivity in OSAS is related to excessive daytime sleepiness. *J Sleep Res* 2007; 16: 327–332.

60. Whitney CW, Enright PL, Newman AB, *et al.* Correlates of daytime sleepiness in 4578 elderly persons: the Cardiovascular Health Study. *Sleep* 1998; 21: 27–36.

61. Redline S, Kirchner HL, Quan SF, *et al.* The effects of age, sex, ethnicity, and sleep-disordered breathing on sleep architecture. *Arch Intern Med* 2004; 164: 406–418.

62. Kezirian EJ, Harrison SL, Ancoli-Israel S, *et al.* Behavioral correlates of sleep-disordered breathing in older men. *Sleep* 2009; 32: 253–261.

63. Kezirian EJ, Harrison SL, Ancoli-Israel S, *et al.* Behavioral correlates of sleep-disordered breathing in older women. *Sleep* 2007; 30: 1181–1188.

64. Roehrs T, Zorick F, Wittig R, *et al.* Predictors of objective level of daytime sleepiness in patients with sleep-related breathing disorders. *Chest* 1989; 95: 1202–1206.

65. Wesensten NJ, Balkin TJ, Belenky G. Does sleep fragmentation impact recuperation? A review and reanalysis. *J Sleep Res* 1999; 8: 237–245.

66. Kingshott RN, Engleman HM, Deary IJ, *et al.* Does arousal frequency predict daytime function? *Eur Respir J* 1998; 12: 1264–1270.

67. Onen F, Higgins S, Onen SH. Falling-asleep-related injured falls in the elderly. *J Am Med Dir Assoc* 2009; 10: 207–210.

68. Stone KL, Blackwell TL, Ancoli-Israel S, *et al.* Sleep disturbances and risk of falls in older community-dwelling men: the outcomes of Sleep Disorders in Older Men (MrOS Sleep) Study. *J Am Geriatr Soc* 2014; 62: 299–305.

69. Assoumou HG, Gaspoz JM, Sforza E, *et al.* Obstructive sleep apnea and the metabolic syndrome in an elderly healthy population: the SYNAPSE cohort. *Sleep Breath* 2012; 16: 895–902.

70. Chouchou F, Pichot V, Barthélémy JC, *et al.* Cardiac sympathetic modulation in response to apneas/hypopneas through heart rate variability analysis. *PLoS One* 2014; 9: e86434.

71. Leung RS. Sleep-disordered breathing: autonomic mechanisms and arrhythmias. *Prog Cardiovasc Dis* 2009; 51: 324–338.

72. Dauphinot V, Barthélémy JC, Pichot V, *et al.* Autonomic activation during sleep and new-onset ambulatory hypertension in the elderly. *Int J Cardiol* 2012; 155: 155–159.

73. Crawford-Achour E, Roche F, Pichot V, *et al.* Sleep-related autonomic overactivity in a general elderly population and its relationship to cardiovascular regulation. *Heart Vessels* 2014 [In press DOI: 10.1007/s00380-014-0573-9].

74. Chouchou F, Sforza E, Celle S, *et al.* Pulse transit time in screening sleep disordered breathing in an elderly population: the PROOF-SYNAPSE study. *Sleep* 2011; 34: 1051–1059.

75. Chouchou F, Pichot V, Pépin JL, *et al.* Sympathetic overactivity due to sleep fragmentation is associated with elevated diurnal systolic blood pressure in healthy elderly subjects: the PROOF-SYNAPSE study. *Eur Heart J* 2013; 34: 2122–2131.

76. Pépin JL, Tamisier R, Baguet JP, *et al.* Arterial health is related to obstructive sleep apnea severity and improves with CPAP treatment. *Sleep Med Rev* 2013; 17: 3–5.

77. Hijmering ML, Stroes ES, Olijhoek J, *et al.* Sympathetic activation markedly reduces endothelium-dependent, flow-mediated vasodilation. *J Am Coll Cardiol* 2002; 39: 683–688.

78. Roche F, Pépin JL, Achour-Crawford E, *et al.* At 68 years, unrecognised sleep apnoea is associated with elevated ambulatory blood pressure. *Eur Respir J* 2012; 40: 649–656.

79. Guillot M, Sforza E, Achour-Crawford E, *et al.* Association between severe obstructive sleep apnea and incident arterial hypertension in the older people population. *Sleep Med* 2013; 14: 838–842.

80. Marin JM, Agusti A, Villar I, *et al.* Association between treated and untreated obstructive sleep apnea and risk of hypertension. *JAMA* 2012; 307: 2169–2176.

81. Haas DC, Foster GL, Nieto FJ, *et al.* Age-dependent associations between sleep-disordered breathing and hypertension: importance of discriminating between systolic/diastolic hypertension and isolated systolic hypertension in the Sleep Heart Health Study. *Circulation* 2005; 111: 614–621.

82. Wang X, Ouyang Y, Wang Z, *et al.* Obstructive sleep apnea and risk of cardiovascular disease and all-cause mortality: a meta-analysis of prospective cohort studies. *Int J Cardiol* 2013; 169: 207–214.

83. Gottlieb DJ, Yenokyan G, Newman AB, *et al.* Prospective study of obstructive sleep apnea and incident coronary heart disease and heart failure: the Sleep Heart Health Study. *Circulation* 2010; 122: 352–360.

84. Endeshaw Y, Rice TB, Schwartz AV, *et al.* Snoring, daytime sleepiness, and incident cardiovascular disease in the health, aging, and body composition study. *Sleep* 2013; 36: 1737–1745.

85. Newman AB, Spiekerman CF, Enright P, *et al.* Daytime sleepiness predicts mortality and cardiovascular disease in older adults. The Cardiovascular Health Study Research Group. *J Am Geriatr Soc* 2000; 48: 115–123.

86. Johansson P, Alehagen U, Svanborg E, *et al.* Clinical characteristics and mortality risk in relation to obstructive and central sleep apnoea in community-dwelling elderly individuals: a 7-year follow-up. *Age Ageing* 2012; 41: 468–474.

87. Arzt M, Young T, Finn L, *et al.* Association of sleep-disordered breathing and the occurrence of stroke. *Am J Respir Crit Care Med* 2005; 172: 1447–1451.

88. Sforza E, Boissier C, Saint Martin M, *et al.* Carotid artery atherosclerosis and sleep disordered breathing in healthy elderly subjects: the Synapse cohort. *Sleep Med* 2013; 14: 66–70.

89. Ascher E, DePippo P, Salles-Cunha S, *et al.* Carotid screening with duplex ultrasound in elderly asymptomatic patients referred to a vascular surgeon: is it worthwhile? *Ann Vasc Surg* 1999; 13: 164–168.

90. Bortolotto LA, Hanon O, Franconi G, *et al.* The aging process modifies the distensibility of elastic but not muscular arteries. *Hypertension* 1999; 34: 889–892.

91. Kim H, Yun CH, Thomas RJ, *et al.* Obstructive sleep apnea as a risk factor for cerebral white matter change in a middle-aged and older general population. *Sleep* 2013; 36: 709–715.

92. Minoguchi K, Yokoe T, Tazaki T, *et al.* Silent brain infarction and platelet activation in obstructive sleep apnea. *Am J Respir Crit Care Med* 2007; 175: 612–617.

93. Nishibayashi M, Miyamoto M, Miyamoto T, *et al.* Correlation between severity of obstructive sleep apnea and prevalence of silent cerebrovascular lesions. *J Clin Sleep Med* 2008; 4: 242–247.

94. Schulz UG, Mason RH, Craig SE, *et al.* Leukoaraiosis on MRI in patients with minimally symptomatic obstructive sleep apnoea. *Cerebrovasc Dis* 2013; 35: 363–369.

95. Dong JY, Zhang YH, Qin LQ. Obstructive sleep apnea and cardiovascular risk: meta-analysis of prospective cohort studies. *Atherosclerosis* 2013; 229: 489–495.

96. Martínez-García MA, Campos-Rodríguez F, Catalán-Serra P, *et al.* Cardiovascular mortality in obstructive sleep apnea in the elderly: role of long-term continuous positive airway pressure treatment: a prospective observational study. *Am J Respir Crit Care Med* 2012; 186: 909–916.

97. Munoz R, Duran-Cantolla J, Martínez-Vila E, *et al.* Severe sleep apnea and risk of ischemic stroke in the elderly. *Stroke* 2006; 37: 2317–2321.

98. Marin JM, Carrizo SJ, Vicente E, *et al.* Long-term cardiovascular outcomes in men with obstructive sleep apnoea-hypopnoea with or without treatment with continuous positive airway pressure: an observational study. *Lancet* 2005; 365: 1046–1053.

99. Punjabi NM, Caffo BS, Goodwin JL, *et al.* Sleep-disordered breathing and mortality: a prospective cohort study. *PLoS Med* 2009; 6: e1000132.

100. Young T, Finn L, Peppard PE, *et al.* Sleep disordered breathing and mortality: eighteen-year follow-up of the Wisconsin sleep cohort. *Sleep* 2008; 31: 1071–1078.

101. Marshall NS, Wong KK, Liu PY, *et al.* Sleep apnea as an independent risk factor for all-cause mortality: the Busselton Health Study. *Sleep* 2008; 31: 1079–1085.

102. Ge X, Han F, Huang Y, *et al.* Is obstructive sleep apnea associated with cardiovascular and all-cause mortality? *PLoS One* 2013; 8: e69432.

103. Johansson P, Alehagen U, Ulander M, *et al.* Sleep disordered breathing in community dwelling elderly: associations with cardiovascular disease, impaired systolic function, and mortality after a six-year follow-up. *Sleep Med* 2011; 12: 748–753.

104. Lavie P, Lavie L. Unexpected survival advantage in elderly people with moderate sleep apnoea. *J Sleep Res* 2009; 18: 397–403.

105. Javaheri S, Shukla R, Zeigler H, *et al.* Central sleep apnea, right ventricular dysfunction, and low diastolic blood pressure are predictors of mortality in systolic heart failure. *J Am Coll Cardiol* 2007; 49: 2028–2034.

106. Martínez-García MA, Campos-Rodriguez F, Durán-Cantolla J, *et al.* Obstructive sleep apnea is associated with cancer mortality in younger patients. *Sleep Med* 2014; 15: 742–748.

107. Lavie L, Lavie P. Ischemic preconditioning as a possible explanation for the age decline relative mortality in sleep apnea. *Med Hypotheses* 2006; 66: 1069–1073.

108. Tan MC, Ayas NT, Mulgrew A, *et al.* Cost-effectiveness of continuous positive airway pressure therapy in patients with obstructive sleep apnea-hypopnea in British Columbia. *Can Respir J* 2008; 15: 159–165.

109. Mar J, Rueda JR, Durán-Cantolla J, *et al.* The cost-effectiveness of nCPAP treatment in patients with moderate-to-severe obstructive sleep apnoea. *Eur Respir J* 2003; 21: 515–522.

110. Sforza E, Roche F. Sleep apnea syndrome and cognition. *Front Neurol* 2012; 3: 87.

111. Yamamoto H, Akashiba T, Kosaka N, *et al.* Long-term effects nasal continuous positive airway pressure on daytime sleepiness, mood and traffic accidents in patients with obstructive sleep apnoea. *Respir Med* 2000; 94: 87–90.
112. Ward KL, Hillman DR, James A, *et al.* Excessive daytime sleepiness increases the risk of motor vehicle crash in obstructive sleep apnea. *J Clin Sleep Med* 2013; 9: 1013–1021.
113. McMillan A, Bratton DJ, Faria R, *et al.* Continuous positive airway pressure in older people with obstructive sleep apnoea syndrome (PREDICT): a 12-month, multicentre, randomised trial. *Lancet Respir Med* 2014; 2: 804–812.
114. Russo-Magno P, O'Brien A, Panciera T, *et al.* Compliance with CPAP therapy in older men with obstructive sleep apnea. *J Am Geriatr Soc* 2001; 49: 1205–1211.
115. Weaver TE, Chasens ER. Continuous positive airway pressure treatment for sleep apnea in older adults. *Sleep Med Rev* 2007; 11: 99–111.
116. McDaid C, Durée KH, Griffin SC, *et al.* A systematic review of continuous positive airway pressure for obstructive sleep apnoea-hypopnoea syndrome. *Sleep Med Rev* 2009; 13: 427–436.
117. Russell T, Duntley S. Sleep disordered breathing in the elderly. *Am J Med* 2011; 124: 1123–1126.
118. Diaz K, Faverio P, Hospenthal A, *et al.* Obstructive sleep apnea is associated with higher healthcare utilization in elderly patients. *Ann Thorac Med* 2014; 9: 92–98.

Disclosures: F. Roche has received grants to his institution from VitalAire, Elia Medical and ALLP, and payment for lectures from Philips Healthcare, for activities outside the submitted work.

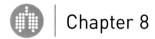

Chapter 8

Bariatric surgery

Sheila Sivam[1,3], Camilla M. Hoyos[1], Brendon J. Yee[1,3], Craig L. Phillips[1,2] and Ronald R. Grunstein[1,3]

OSA is more prevalent in the obese. Bariatric surgery is an effective method to reduce and maintain longer-term weight loss. The additional benefits of weight loss on comorbidities associated with obesity, such as cardiovascular risk factors and cancer, as well as relative reduction in death has resulted in the increased popularity of bariatric surgery in the obese population. Many trials demonstrate a greater beneficial effect of bariatric surgery over lifestyle modification for weight loss, as well as for OSA severity and metabolic outcomes. However, this is not a universal finding. Despite significant reductions in OSA severity, very few patients are cured of OSA following bariatric surgery hence post-operative polysomnography may be necessary prior to cessation of CPAP. Furthermore, ongoing diet and behavioural modification is necessary to maintain the significant weight loss achieved with bariatric surgery.

In 2008, it was estimated by the World Health Organization that 21% of the world population were overweight and about 500 million of these individuals were classified as obese [1]. OSA is more prevalent in the obese population, defined as having a BMI $\geqslant 30$ kg·m^{-2}. The odds ratio of developing OSA increases by 1.14 (95% CI 1.10–1.19) with each unit increase in BMI, where sleep disordered breathing was defined by an AHI of at least 10 events·h^{-1} [2]. Classically, the estimated prevalence of OSA in the general population is ~4% of males and ~2% of females, with OSA defined by an AHI >5 events·h^{-1}. By comparison, obese adults have a significantly higher prevalence of OSA with values as high as 42–48% and 8–38% in men and women, respectively [3, 4]. The increasing prevalence of obesity is reflected in more recent population estimates suggesting that ~55% of men and ~20% of women are at high risk of OSA [5]. Severe obesity is also increasing in adolescents and is associated with premature death [6]. However, less than half of morbidly obese teenagers have OSA [7].

Of the many risk factors for developing OSA which include male sex, age, genetic predisposition (familial and ethnic), cranio-facial anatomical differences, menopause and obesity, it is obesity that has been consistently identified as the strongest predisposing factor in both population- and clinic-based studies [4, 8–12]. A number of mechanisms have been postulated to result in OSA in obese subjects. Increased body weight can alter normal UA

[1]Sleep & Circadian Research Group, Woolcock Institute of Medical Research and NHMRC Centre for Integrated Research for Understanding of Sleep (CIRUS), University of Sydney, Sydney, Australia.. [2]Department of Respiratory and Sleep Medicine, Royal North Shore Hospital, St Leonard's, Sydney, Australia. [3]Department of Respiratory and Sleep Medicine, Royal Prince Alfred Hospital, Camperdown, Sydney, Australia.

Correspondence: Sheila Sivam, Sleep & Circadian Research Group, Woolcock Institute of Medical Research, PO Box M77, Missenden Road, NSW 2050, Australia. E-mail: sheila.sivam@sydney.edu.au

function during sleep. Increased parapharyngeal fat deposition as well as a change in neural compensation and stability of the respiratory control centres can reduce airway patency and increase collapsibility. In addition, a reduction in lung volume caused by abdominal adiposity can reduce UA traction and increase collapsibility [13, 14].

Bariatric surgery is an effective method to reduce and maintain longer-term weight loss compared with lifestyle modification [15–18]. North American and European clinical guidelines for the management of obesity all recommend consideration of bariatric surgery for class III (BMI 40 $kg \cdot m^{-2}$) and class II (BMI 35 $kg \cdot m^{-2}$) obesity, in individuals with comorbidities who are unable to lose weight despite attempting with conventional measures [19–21].The additional benefits of weight loss on comorbidities associated with obesity, cardiovascular risk factors and the incidence of cancer as well as its relative reduction in death has resulted in the increased popularity of bariatric surgery in the obese population [22–25]. The term "metabolic" surgery has also been used to reflect the beneficial metabolic effects, including improved glycemic control in type 2 diabetes mellitus, with surgical weight loss [26].

While there are many surgical techniques, the four main categories are gastric bypass surgery (principally Roux-en-Y variations), adjustable gastric banding, vertical band gastroplasty and sleeve gastrectomy. Mechanisms of weight loss with these procedures include restriction of food intake, stimulation of nerves or hormones that suppress hunger and delay of digestion and absorption of food. Less common procedures include biliopancreatic diversion or duodenal switch, biliary intestinal bypass, ilieogastrotomy and jejunoileal bypass. In a recent updated systematic review and meta-analysis, complication rates associated with bariatric surgery ranged from 10% to 17%; however, mortality associated with surgery was generally low (0.08–0.35%) [27]. This review also revealed that while gastric bypass surgery was more effective in weight loss outcomes than sleeve gastrectomy and adjustable gastric banding, it generated more adverse events. A more recent 3 year follow up analysis compared sleeve gastrectomy and gastric bypass surgery and showed no major differences in surgical complications; however, the study may not have been adequately powered to detect a modest difference [28].

Higher reoperation rates and less substantial weight loss were observed with adjustable gastric banding although it was the safer procedure with lower mortality and complication rates [27]. In obese patients with co-morbid OSA, a variety of procedures outlined above were utilised including in a recently published randomised controlled trial [29] and a multitude of controlled non-randomised trials [30–35] including the Swedish Obese Subjects (SOS) study which now includes 20-year follow-up data [25, 36] and several case series.

It is also important to highlight the fact that morbidly obese patients with OSA may be at a higher risk for post-operative complications when undergoing surgical procedures requiring general anaesthetic. Use of CPAP should be considered in the perioperative period to reduce such complications and shorten length of hospital stay [37]. High-dependency unit support rather than intensive care resources are often sufficient for laparascopic procedures [38].

In a prospective, multicentre observational study of patients undergoing bariatric surgery, the 30-day composite endpoint which included death, venous thromboembolism, operative re-intervention or no discharge at 30 days, occurred in 4.1% of patients and included 0.3% mortality [39]. A history of OSA, deep vein thrombosis/venous thromboembolism and an excessively high BMI of 70 $kg \cdot m^{-2}$, increased the estimated percentage of participants with the composite endpoint to over 10% compared with 3% for patients with a BMI in the 50s, without a history of OSA and venous thromboembolism.

This chapter examines the current evidence on the effects of bariatric surgery in OSA. Its concurrent impact on OSA, weight loss and metabolic derangements will be highlighted. This is not an exhaustive systematic review but we have preferentially included studies higher in the evidence-based hierarchy.

Effects of bariatric surgery

Uncontrolled observational studies

Weight loss
Of the publications with 25 or more subjects (table 1), most studies reported a significant reduction in BMI after bariatric surgery ranging from 9 to 24 $kg \cdot m^{-2}$ [32, 34, 35, 40–46]. The most substantial reduction was observed in the MARTI-VALERI et al. [42] study with a cohort of 30 subjects, who were followed up for 12 months after Roux-en-Y gastric bypass surgery. This group had a mean reduction in weight of 62 kg, where the mean pre-operative weight was 145 kg. Most other studies which reported weight change revealed a significant decrease (26–49 kg) amongst their subjects after surgery (table 1). In 2014, a study by RAVESLOOT et al. [44] demonstrated changes in BMI and weight at two post-operative intervals. At 7.7 months, 110 subjects showed a mean reduction in BMI of 9 $kg \cdot m^{-2}$ and weight loss of 26 kg. 50 participants from this group with persisting OSA were randomly invited to have a second follow up at 16.9 months. The group's mean BMI fell from 45 $kg \cdot m^{-2}$ at baseline to 36.7 $kg \cdot m^{-2}$ at 7.7 months and 35 $kg \cdot m^{-2}$ at 16.9 months. Weight decreased from 130.2 kg to 106.6 kg at 7.7 months and dropped further at 16.9 months to 102.1 kg. This study demonstrates that although rapid weight loss is achieved within the first 8 months, continued albeit less dramatic weight loss can be expected at 1 year or more after the initial surgery. Three additional studies did not provide pre- and post-surgery BMI and/or weights [47–49].

OSA severity
With this impact on weight reduction, it is not surprising that a significant reduction in AHIs were observed the aforementioned studies (table 2). The study by MARTI-VALERI et al. [42] which produced the largest fall in mean BMI and weight loss, demonstrated a reduction in the RDI of 46 events·h^{-1} (AHI fell from 63 to 17 events·h^{-1}). Overall, the group OSA severity improved from severe to moderate OSA 12 months after bariatric surgery, where the mean BMI changed from 57 to 37 $kg \cdot m^{-2}$. The largest fall in AHI was demonstrated by CHARUZI et al. [48]. While BMI and post-surgery actual weight was not recorded for the 47 subjects in the study, excess body weight in this group declined from 117.4 kg to 44.4 kg at a mean of 10.5 weeks after surgery with a parallel reduction in AHI of 52 events·h^{-1} (60 events·h^{-1} compared with 8 events·h^{-1}). At a mean follow up period of 7 years after surgery, 42 participants had a mean weight of 102 kg compared with 139 kg pre-surgery. While their weight was still lower than that prior to surgery, patients had regained a substantial amount of weight from their mean excess body weight loss of 73 kg at 10.5 months. Six subjects from this group underwent PSG at this second follow-up visit and expectedly showed an increase in AHI from 12 events·h^{-1} at the first post-weight loss visit to 34 events·h^{-1}. These values are still lower than the pre-operative AHI of 60 events·h^{-1}; however, it is clear from this study that ongoing diet and behavioural modification will be necessary if patients are to maintain weight loss that was initially

Table 1. Observational studies: body mass index, weight loss and metabolic effects with bariatric surgery

First author [ref.]	Subjects n Total	Subjects n Male	Age years	Follow-up months	Surgery type	BMI kg·m⁻² Pre-surgery	BMI kg·m⁻² Post-surgery	Weight kg Pre-surgery	Weight kg Post-surgery	Metabolic effects
HAINES [32]	101	NR	NR	11 (6–42)	RYGB	56	38[#]	NR	NR	NR
RAO [34]	46	NR	36	13±20	LAGB	45.2	30[#]	111	70.9[#]	Number with HT decreased from 31 to 21 (p=0.05)
RASHEID [35]	100	21	46	6	Gastric bypass	62	40	NR	NR	NR
DIXON [40]	25	17	44	17.7	LAGB	52.7	37.2[#]	NR	105[#]	↓ Waist circumference[#]; ↓ FBG[#]; ↑ QUICKI[#]; ↓ HbA1c[#]; ↓ insulin[#]; ↓ triglycerides[#]; ↑ HDL[#]; ↓ metabolic syndrome[#]; ~ BP; ~ total cholesterol; ~ LDL
KRIEGER [41]	30	10	44	12	LAGB	47.2	35.6[#]	NR	NR	↓ Leptin[#]; ~ Ghrelin, ~ BP
MARTI-VALERI [42]	30	8	44	12	RYGB	56.5	32.1[#]	145	83[#]	↓ DM[#]; ↓ HT[#]
POTOI [43]	35	6	44	12	RYGB, LAGB	51.3	39.9[#]	139	109[#]	NR
RAVESLOOT [44]	110	37	NR	7.7	LAGB, RYGB, sleeve gastrectomy	45.4	36.3[#]	132.5	106.4[#]	NR
RAVESLOOT [44]	50	17	NR	7.1 / 16.9	LAGB, RYGB, sleeve gastrectomy	45.0	36.7[#] / 35.0[#]	130.2	106.6[#] / 102.1[#]	NR
SUGERMAN [45]	63	NR	NR	54	RYGB, VBG, HG	56	37[#]	166	110[#]	NR
VALENCIA-FLORES [46]	29	13	40	13.7	RYGB, VBG	56.5	39.2[#]	140	NR	↓ waist circumference[#]
CHARUZI [47]	46	39	42	6	RYGB, VBG	NR	NR	139	NR	NR
CHARUZI [48]	47	44	41	10.5	RYGB, VBG	NR NR	NR	139	NR	NR
	42	37	48	86				NR	102	NR
VARELA [49]	56	20	46	12	RYGB	49	NR	NR	NR	NR

NR: not reported; RYGB: Roux-en-Y gastric bypass; LAGB: laparoscopic adjustable gastric banding; HT: hypertension; ↑: increase; ~: no change; ↓: decrease; FBG: fasting blood glucose; QUICKI: quantitative insulin sensitivity check index; HbA1c: haemoglobin A1c; HDL: high-density lipoprotein; BP: blood pressure; LDL: low-density lipoprotein; DM: diabetes mellitus; VBG: Vertical banded gastroplasty; HG: Horizontal gastroplasty. Follow-up time is presented as mean, except HAINES [32] [median (range)], RAO [34] [mean±SD] and RASHEID [35] [median]. [#]: significant change from baseline.

Table 2. Observational studies: bariatric surgery and OSA severity

First author [ref.]	Subjects n		Age years	Follow-up months	Surgery type	AHI events·h^{-1}		ODI events·h^{-1}	
	Total	Male				Pre-surgery	Post-surgery	Pre-surgery	Post-surgery
HAINES [32]	101	NR	NR	11 (6–42)	RYGB	51	15[#]	NR	NR
RAO [34]	46	NR	36	13±20	LAGB	38	13[#]	NR	NR
RASHEID [35]	100	21	46	6 (median)	Gastric bypass	56	23	NR	NR
DIXON [40]	25	17	45	17.7	LAGB	61	13[#]	NR	NR
KRIEGER [41]	30	10	44	12	LAGB	34	19[#]	NR	NR
MARTI-VALERI [42]	30	8	44	12	RYGB	63	17[#]	NR	NR
POITOI [43]	35	6	44	12	RYGB, LAGB	24	10[#]	26.9	10.8[#]
RAVESLOOT [44]	110	37	NR	7.7	LAGB, RYGB, sleeve gastrectomy	39	15[#]	28.3	11.8[#]
RAVESLOOT [44]	50	17	NR	7.7 16.9	LAGB, RYGB, sleeve gastrectomy	49.1	22.7[#] 17.4[#]	37.7	17.6[#] 14.9[#]
SUGERMAN [45]	40	NR	NR	54	RYGB, VBG, HG	64	26[#]	NR	NR
VALENCIA-FLORES [46]	29	13	40	13.7	RYGB, VBG	54	14[#]	NR	NR
CHARUZI [47]	46			6	RYGB, VBG	58	36	NR	NR
CHARUZI [48]	47	NR	NR	10.5	RYGB,VBG	60	8[#]	NR	NR
VARELA [49]	56	20	46	12	RYGB	35	NR	NR	NR

[#]: Significant change from baseline. NR: not reported; RYGB: Roux-en-Y gastric bypass; LAGB: laparoscopic adjustable gastric banding; VBG: Vertical banded gastroplasty; HG: Horizontal gastroplasty.

achieved 5 weeks after surgery at 2.5 years and beyond. The study by RAVESLOOT et al. [44] with two follow-up intervals with PSG within a period of 1.5 years, demonstrated a similar maintenance or continued modest reductions in weight and AHI in the short term (mean ±SD 16.9±4.3 months; table 2) [44].

One study compared patients undergoing either gastric banding or gastric bypass surgery (n=12) to patients receiving CPAP (n=15) in a non-randomised controlled study. There was a substantial reduction in BMI in the surgical group compared to a small gain in the CPAP group (−11 versus 1 kg·m^{-2}). However, the CPAP group had a larger reduction in AHI at 6 months with a reduction from severe OSA to mild or no OSA (−31 events·h^{-1}) but on CPAP compared with a reduction in the surgical group from moderate OSA to mild OSA (−8 events·h^{-1}) [50] that were not using CPAP.

Controlled studies

Weight loss
The largest controlled prospective cohort (Swedish Obese Subjects) study involved 1592 individuals undergoing surgery and 1430 controls [51]. The study was not randomised as the ethics committees in Sweden did not approve randomisation into surgical or control groups. Three surgical techniques were utilised in the surgery group which included laparoscopic-adjustable gastric banding, Roux-en-Y gastric bypass and vertical banded gastroplasty. Control subjects received routine obesity management including dietary advice, physical training, low calorie diets, and behaviour modification however there was no attempt to standardise treatment in this group. As a result, some patients received

sophisticated lifestyle interventions and behaviour modification while others received no intervention [36]. No anti-obesity drugs were registered in Sweden during the study period. At the 2 year follow up, the surgical group had a substantial reduction in BMI of 10 kg·m^{-2} with no change in the controls [52]. The mean weight loss in the surgery cohort was 27 kg, which corresponded to 23% of their weight at baseline.

Another non-randomised controlled trial by FREDHEIM et al. [53] (comparing bariatric surgery to lifestyle modification in a population where 63% of participants had OSA, also demonstrated a significant reduction in weight and BMI at 1 year. In contrast to the previous SOS study, improvements were observed after both Roux-en-Y gastric bypass surgery and lifestyle modification [53]. However, the effectiveness of surgery in weight reduction was still approximately three-fold higher than intensive lifestyle modification. The lifestyle group underwent a 1-year programme at a single rehabilitation centre with four intermittent stays, one lasting 2 weeks and three lasting 1 week each. A multidisciplinary approach was also utilised by engaging nutritionists, physiotherapists, medical doctors and trained nurses. Motivational interviewing and client centred counselling style were also undertaken to invoke behavioural change. Hence the authors underscored the need to not underestimate the effects of intensive lifestyle intervention on the remission of OSA.

In 2012, DIXON et al., [29] published the first randomised controlled trial comparing laparoscopic adjustable gastric banding surgery (n=30) with lifestyle modification (n=30) over a 2-year period in OSA patients. The conventional lifestyle intervention arm involved a multipronged approach, similar to the intensive lifestyle intervention programme established by FREDHEIM et al. [53] but utilised very low energy diet (VLED) and did not have dedicated inpatient admissions. This programme encouraged walking and 200 min·week^{-1} of structured aerobic and resistance activity, dietary advice which included a planned daily deficit of 500 kcal from estimated energy requirements and used VLED with provided meal replacements (Optifast; Nestle Australia, Sydney, Australia) particularly at the start of the trial and intermittently thereafter. The surgical arm was provided with 2 weeks of VLED to reduce the liver size prior to banding. The management of OSA, intensity, and nature of the lifestyle programmes were common to both groups. Surgery resulted in a five-fold greater reduction in weight compared with the lifestyle group.

OSA severity
No sleep studies were performed in the SOS study; however, there was a reduction in partner reported apnoea events by 16% compared with controls (1%) (table 3). Patients in the surgical group also reported less persistence of both snoring and daytime sleepiness compared with the control group [52].

The study by FREIDHEM et al. [51] demonstrated a significant reduction at 1 year in AHI and ODI in both surgery and lifestyle modification groups. Similar to weight, improvements in AHI with surgery was up to three-fold higher compared with intensive lifestyle modification. Despite the five-fold increase in weight loss in the surgical group, the single randomised controlled trial on this issue by DIXON et al. [29] surprisingly failed to demonstrate a significant difference in AHI with surgery compared to lifestyle modification despite there being only a modest change in weight in the latter group (5.1 kg). In addition, an interval analysis at 1 year demonstrated an attenuated benefit on AHI beyond the first 8–10% or 10 kg of weight loss in both groups with substantial inter-individual variability in responses. For example, some individuals showed no reduction in AHI with ~40 kg weight loss whilst others with similar weight loss showed falls in AHI of 75 events·h^{-1}. These unexpected results indicate that the relationship between OSA severity and weight loss is not as strong as was initially suggested by prior non-randomised controlled and observational studies. Given this great variability in inter-individual responses, it is possible that this study was underpowered to detect between group differences in reducing OSA over 2 years. Finally, both groups demonstrated a reduction in daytime sleepiness as measured by ESS score and symptoms of depression. However, it is important to note that very few patients were cured of OSA in either group with the average AHI remaining in the severe category ($\geqslant$30 events·h^{-1}). This highlights the need for post-operative PSGs to determine whether CPAP treatment can be stopped.

In a meta-analysis which included 16 944 patients, of whom 2399 had sleep disordered breathing, OSA resolved in 85.7% (95% CI 79.2%–92.2%) of patients after bariatric surgery [54]. For the entire group, independent of co-morbidities, surgery reduced BMI by 14 kg·m^{-2}, mean excess weight by 61.2% (95% CI 58.1%–64.4%) and absolute weight by 39.7 kg (37.2–42.2 kg). However, a more recent meta-analysis of 12 studies specifically focussed on OSA and representing 342 patients, only showed a reduction in mean AHI to moderately severe OSA after bariatric surgery. The baseline AHI of 55 events·h^{-1} (95% CI 49.0–60.3) was reduced to 16 events·h^{-1} (95% CI 12.6–19.0) after surgery. This incomplete resolution of OSA occurred despite a mean reduction in BMI of 18 kg·m^{-2} and underscores the likely need for continued OSA treatment after surgery [55].

CPAP and weight loss

Many studies have examined the role of OSA in promoting obesity through hypothesised mechanisms related to hormonal and activity changes [56]. Although there is good rationale to support this, several randomised controlled trials that have investigated the use of CPAP on abdominal fat have found no significant change in obesity measures [57, 58]. Surprisingly, a more recent large RCT with 1015 patients demonstrated modest weight gain associated with CPAP use over a 6 month period compared with participants using a sham device [59]. The greatest weight gain was found in those most compliant with CPAP. However the weight gain may reflect a gain in muscle rather than fat mass [60] and, if true, would support an important role for OSA treatment during weight loss. Indeed, a recent smaller randomised trial by CHIRINOS et al. [61] showed no significant decline in body weight in patients using CPAP alone compared with a loss in weight in those receiving a weight loss intervention alone or weight loss combined with CPAP [61]. Although the latter two groups achieved similar weight loss (−6.8 kg and −7 kg, respectively), there was a tendency for patients receiving combined weight loss and CPAP to show greater metabolic improvements (see below). It is therefore plausible that combinational therapy involving surgical weight loss and effective OSA treatment may substantially enhance fat loss and metabolic improvements however there are no studies that have specifically examined this.

Pharmaceutical therapies and more detailed lifestyle intervention studies for weight loss are outlined in their respective chapters.

Metabolic effects

Of the surgical weight loss studies in patients with OSA described above, the largest uncontrolled study demonstrated a reduction in the number of subjects with hypertension, defined as a BP above 140/90 mmHg, with 10 patients able to discontinue anti-hypertensive

Table 3. Comparative studies

First author [ref.]	Design	Age	Follow-up	ΔBMI kg·m⁻²	ΔWeight kg	ΔAHI events·h⁻¹	ΔODI events·h⁻¹	Metabolic effects
DIXON [29]	Randomised controlled trial							No between-group differences in BP, FBG, FPI, lipids, anti-hypertensive, DM and lipid-lowering medication use
	LAGB (n=30)	47	2 years	−9.7	−27.8$^{\#}$	−25.5$^{\#}$	NR	
	Lifestyle Modification (n=30)	50		−1.5	−5.1	−14.0$^{\#}$	NR	
BAKKER [50]	Non-randomised controlled							
	CPAP (n=15)	48	6 months	1	NR	−31$^{\#}$	NR	NR
	Surgery (n=12)	43		−11$^{\#}$	NR	−8$^{\#}$	NR	
GRUNSTEIN [52]	Non-randomised controlled							
	RYGB,VBG, LAGB (n=1592)	47	2 years	−10 Unchanged	−27 Unchanged	Not performed	Not performed	↓ DM; ↓ Triglycerides
	Lifestyle Modification (n=1430)	48						
FREDHEIM [53]	Non-randomised controlled							
	RYGB (n=74)	51	1 year	−14.0	−42.0	−21.6	−22.9	NR
	Lifestyle Modification (n=59)	47		−4.2$^{\#}$	−12.1*	−8.8$^{\#}$	−5.6$^{\#}$	

#: significant change from baseline. FBG: fasting blood glucose; FPI: fasting plasma insulin; DM: diabetes mellitus; LAGB: laparoscopic adjustable gastric banding; NR: not reported; RYGB: Roux-en-Y gastric bypass; VGB: vertical banded gastroplasty; HG: horizontal gastroplasty; ↓: decrease.

medications [34]. Similar improvements were revealed in other studies [29, 42]; however, one study [41] did not reflect similar improvements in blood pressure despite a similar duration of follow up and study population size [41, 42].

In 2012, a randomised, unblinded, single-centre study showed that bariatric surgery plus 12 months of medical therapy resulted in a significant improvement in glycaemic control compared with intensive medical therapy alone, in 150 obese patients with type II diabetes mellitus [26]. OSA was not quantified with PSG in this study. Much like the improvements demonstrated in the general bariatric population, uncontrolled [29, 42] and controlled [52] studies in patients with OSA also revealed better glycaemic control and insulin sensitivity. Triglyceride levels also decreased significantly in these studies [40, 52] although total cholesterol and low density lipoprotein did not [40]. The single RCT in this population with a 2-year follow up period showed equivalent reductions in haemoglobin A1c, plasma insulin levels and resting heart rate after both surgery and a conventional weight loss programme. This occurred despite a five-fold greater weight loss in the surgery patients [29]. While patients in the surgery group tended to have a greater reduction in AHI (-25.5 versus -14.0 events·h^{-1}), the difference was not statistically significant and ultimately, both groups continued to display persistent severe OSA (39.5 versus 43.2 events·h^{-1} respectively). Of note, only 50% of participants were good CPAP users (>4 h^{-1} of use each night) at 2 years. In this context, CHIRINOS et al. [61] assessed metabolic improvements at 6 months in three groups assigned to either weight loss alone, CPAP alone or weight loss and CPAP combined. Weight loss was achieved through a dietary programme. Although, not statistically different from weight loss alone, the improvements in metabolic markers with the combination therapy of weight loss and CPAP tended to be greater. CPAP alone failed to improve any health component. This finding suggests that metabolic improvements that accompany weight loss (either by surgery or dietary means) may be maximised if the underlying OSA is also effectively treated during weight loss.

For detailed reviews on OSA and metabolic syndrome as well as cardiovascular consequences of OSA, please refer to the relevant chapters.

Cost effectiveness

In the general bariatric surgery population, a 6-year observational study of 29820 BlueCross BlueShield Health Insurance plan members matched 1:1 with a comparison non-surgical group who had similar obesity-associated comorbidities showed that while the surgical group incurred higher healthcare-related expenditure in the second and third years, subsequent years demonstrated similar costs between groups. The bariatric surgery group had lower prescription and outpatient costs but higher overall inpatient expenditure [62]. Long-term healthcare-related expenses were higher in all bariatric surgery groups independent of the type of procedure. In an expanded Centers for Disease Control and Prevention–RTI International Diabetes Cost-Effectiveness Model incorporating bariatric surgery, while bariatric surgery increased cost, this was accompanied by an increase in quality-adjusted life-years (QALY) [63]. Similar increases in healthcare resources in the initial post-operative years were demonstrated in a 20-year Swedish Obese Subjects study follow-up. After the initial 6 years, there were no significant differences in inpatient and non-primary care outpatient visits. In addition, pharmaceutical costs in the surgical group were lower from years 7 to 20, compared with controls [64]. While bariatric surgery improved QALY, the increased initial expenditure warrants future cost-effectiveness studies with a focus on healthcare use in patients with OSA. It will allow us to determine the effectiveness and efficiency of CPAP use in the moderate and severely obese population as well as its impact on various obesity related comorbidities compared with bariatric surgery. The societal effect of either modality on workplace productivity, health economics and road safety would also be informative. In summary, surgery does appear to be more costly but results in improved quality of life. Future studies comparing bariatric surgery with and without concurrent CPAP use in subjects with OSA may be helpful to determine if combining surgical weight loss with OSA treatment offers any additional economic benefit as a result of superior metabolic improvements [61].

Conclusion

Bariatric surgery reduces weight and OSA severity and has the added benefit on metabolic consequences of obesity related comorbidities including type II diabetes mellitus. Larger randomised studies are still necessary to definitively compare the effects of bariatric surgery with intensive lifestyle modification programmes. These studies will need to include the cost–benefit analysis of bariatric surgery and the resource intensive lifestyle programmes, some of which include inpatient admissions. Ongoing diet and behavioural programmes are necessary to maintain the initial dramatic weight loss achieved by bariatric surgery. Significant weight loss may not result in complete resolution of OSA. Post-surgery polysomnograms and treatment for OSA may still be indicated after bariatric surgery to control the clinical symptoms of OSA and to prevent the known deleterious cardio-metabolic effect of untreated OSA.

References

1. Courcoulas AP. Progress in filling the gaps in bariatric surgery. *JAMA* 2012; 308: 1160–1161.
2. Tishler PV, Larkin EK, Schluchter MD, *et al.* Incidence of sleep-disordered breathing in an urban adult population: the relative importance of risk factors in the development of sleep-disordered breathing. *JAMA* 2003; 289: 2230–2237.
3. Lee W, Nagubadi S, Kryger MH, *et al.* Epidemiology of obstructive sleep apnea: a population-based perspective. *Expert Rev Respir Med* 2008; 2: 349–364.
4. Young T, Palta M, Dempsey J, *et al.* The occurrence of sleep-disordered breathing among middle-aged adults. *New Engl J Med* 1993; 328: 1230–1235.
5. Adams RJ, Piantadosi C, Appleton SL, *et al.* Investigating obstructive sleep apnoea: will the health system have the capacity to cope? A population study. *Aust Health Rev* 2012; 36: 424–429.
6. Fitzgerald DA, Baur L. Bariatric surgery for severely obese adolescents. *Paediatr Respir Rev* 2014; 15: 227–230.
7. Koeck ES, Barefoot LC, Hamrick M, *et al.* Predicting sleep apnea in morbidly obese adolescents undergoing bariatric surgery. *Surg Endosc* 2014; 28: 1146–1152.
8. Young T, Peppard PE, Gottlieb DJ. Epidemiology of obstructive sleep apnea: a population health perspective. *Am J Respir Crit Care Med* 2002; 165: 1217–1239.
9. Bearpark H, Elliott L, Grunstein R, *et al.* Snoring and sleep apnea. A population study in Australian men. *Am J Respir Crit Care Med* 1995; 151: 1459–1465.
10. Grunstein R, Wilcox I, Yang TS, *et al.* Snoring and sleep apnoea in men: association with central obesity and hypertension. *Int J Obes Relat Metab Disord* 1993; 17: 533–540.
11. Jennum P, Sjol A. Snoring, sleep apnoea and cardiovascular risk factors: the MONICA II Study. *Int J Epidemiol* 1993; 22: 439–444.
12. Olson LG, King MT, Hensley MJ, *et al.* A community study of snoring and sleep-disordered breathing. Health outcomes. *Am J Respir Crit Care Med* 1995; 152: 717–720.
13. Carter R, 3rd, Watenpaugh DE. Obesity and obstructive sleep apnea: or is it OSA and obesity? *Pathophysiology* 2008; 15: 71–77.
14. Fogel RB, Malhotra A, White DP. Sleep. 2: pathophysiology of obstructive sleep apnoea/hypopnoea syndrome. *Thorax* 2004; 59: 159–163.

15. Avenell A, Broom J, Brown TJ, *et al.* Systematic review of the long-term effects and economic consequences of treatments for obesity and implications for health improvement. *Health Technol Assess* 2004; 8: 1–182.

16. Lara MD, Kothari SN, Sugerman HJ. Surgical management of obesity: a review of the evidence relating to the health benefits and risks. *Treat Endocrinol* 2005; 4: 55–64.

17. Marsk R, Naslund E, Freedman J, *et al.* Bariatric surgery reduces mortality in Swedish men. *Brit J Surg* 2010; 97: 877–883.

18. McTigue KM, Harris R, Hemphill B, *et al.* Screening and interventions for obesity in adults: summary of the evidence for the U.S. Preventive Services Task Force. *Ann Intern Med* 2003; 139: 933–949.

19. Gastrointestinal surgery for severe obesity. *Consensus statement/NIH Consensus Development Conference National Institutes of Health Consensus Development Conference* 1991; 9: 1–20.

20. Tsigos C, Hainer V, Basdevant A, *et al.* Management of obesity in adults: European clinical practice guidelines. *Obes Facts* 2008; 1: 106–116.

21. Obesity: preventing and managing the global epidemic. Report of a WHO consultation. *World Health Organization Technical Report Series* 2000; 894: i–xii, 1–253.

22. Buchwald H, Oien DM. Metabolic/bariatric surgery Worldwide 2008. *Obes Surg* 2009; 19: 1605–1611.

23. Buchwald H, Oien DM. Metabolic/bariatric surgery worldwide 2011. *Obes Surg* 2013; 23: 427–436.

24. Sjostrom L, Gummesson A, Sjostrom CD, *et al.* Effects of bariatric surgery on cancer incidence in obese patients in Sweden (Swedish Obese Subjects Study): a prospective, controlled intervention trial. *Lancet Oncol* 2009; 10: 653–662.

25. Sjostrom L, Narbro K, Sjostrom CD, *et al.* Effects of bariatric surgery on mortality in Swedish obese subjects. *N Engl J Med* 2007; 357: 741–752.

26. Schauer PR, Kashyap SR, Wolski K, *et al.* Bariatric surgery versus intensive medical therapy in obese patients with diabetes. *N Engl J Med* 2012; 366: 1567–1576.

27. Chang SH, Stoll CR, Song J, *et al.* The effectiveness and risks of bariatric surgery: an updated systematic review and meta-analysis, 2003–2012. *JAMA Surg* 2014; 149: 275–287.

28. Schauer PR, Bhatt DL, Kirwan JP, *et al.* Bariatric surgery versus intensive medical therapy for diabetes--3-year outcomes. *N Engl J Med* 2014; 370: 2002–2013.

29. Dixon JB, Schachter LM, O'Brien PE, *et al.* Surgical vs conventional therapy for weight loss treatment of obstructive sleep apnea: a randomized controlled trial. *JAMA* 2012; 308: 1142–1149.

30. Dixon JB, Schachter LM, O'Brien PE. Sleep disturbance and obesity: changes following surgically induced weight loss. *Arch Intern Med* 2001; 161: 102–106.

31. Fritscher LG, Canani S, Mottin CC, *et al.* Bariatric surgery in the treatment of obstructive sleep apnea in morbidly obese patients. *Respiration* 2007; 74: 647–652.

32. Haines KL, Nelson LG, Gonzalez R, *et al.* Objective evidence that bariatric surgery improves obesity-related obstructive sleep apnea. *Surgery* 2007; 141: 354–358.

33. Lettieri CJ, Eliasson AH, Greenburg DL. Persistence of obstructive sleep apnea after surgical weight loss. *J Clin Sleep Med* 2008; 4: 333–338.

34. Rao A, Tey BH, Ramalingam G, *et al.* Obstructive sleep apnoea (OSA) patterns in bariatric surgical practice and response of OSA to weight loss after laparoscopic adjustable gastric banding (LAGB). *Ann Acad Med Singap* 2009; 38: 587–587.

35. Rasheid S, Banasiak M, Gallagher SF, *et al.* Gastric bypass is an effective treatment for obstructive sleep apnea in patients with clinically significant obesity. *Obes Surg* 2003; 13: 58–61.

36. Sjostrom L, Lindroos AK, Peltonen M, *et al.* Lifestyle, diabetes, and cardiovascular risk factors 10 years after bariatric surgery. *N Engl J Med* 2004; 351: 2683–2693.

37. Proczko MA, Stepaniak PS, de Quelerij M, *et al.* STOP-Bang and the effect on patient outcome and length of hospital stay when patients are not using continuous positive airway pressure. *J Anesth* 2014 [In press DOI: 10.1007/s00540-014-1848-0].

38. Shearer E, Magee CJ, Lacasia C, *et al.* Obstructive sleep apnea can be safely managed in a level 2 critical care setting after laparoscopic bariatric surgery. *Surg Obes Relat Dis* 2013; 9: 845–849.

39. Flum DR, Belle SH, King WC, *et al.* Perioperative safety in the longitudinal assessment of bariatric surgery. *N Engl J Med* 2009; 361: 445–454.

40. Dixon JB, Schachter LM, O'Brien PE. Polysomnography before and after weight loss in obese patients with severe sleep apnea. *Int J Obes* 2005; 29: 1048–1054.

41. Krieger AC, Youn H, Modersitzki F, *et al.* Effects of laparoscopic adjustable gastric banding on sleep and metabolism: a 12-month follow-up study. *Int J Gen Med* 2012; 5: 975–981.

42. Marti-Valeri C, Sabate A, Masdevall C, Improvement of associated respiratory problems in morbidly obese patients after open Roux-en-Y gastric bypass. *Obes Surg* 2007; 17: 1102–1110.

43. Poitou C, Coupaye M, Laaban JP, *et al.* Serum amyloid A and obstructive sleep apnea syndrome before and after surgically-induced weight loss in morbidly obese subjects. *Obes Surg* 2006; 16: 1475–1481.

44. Ravesloot MJ, Hilgevoord AA, van Wagensveld BA, *et al.* Assessment of the effect of bariatric surgery on obstructive sleep apnea at two postoperative intervals. *Obes Surg* 2014; 24: 22–31.

45. Sugerman HJ, Fairman RP, Sood RK, *et al.* Long-term effects of gastric surgery for treating respiratory insufficiency of obesity. *Am J Clin Nutr* 1992; 55: Suppl. 2, 597S–601S.

46. Valencia-Flores M, Orea A, Herrera M, *et al.* Effect of bariatric surgery on obstructive sleep apnea and hypopnea syndrome, electrocardiogram, and pulmonary arterial pressure. *Obes Surg* 2004; 14: 755–762.

47. Charuzi I, Fraser D, Peiser J, *et al.* Sleep apnea syndrome in the morbidly obese undergoing bariatric surgery. *Gastroenterology Clin North Am* 1987; 16: 517–519.

48. Charuzi I, Lavie P, Peiser J, *et al.* Bariatric surgery in morbidly obese sleep-apnea patients: short- and long-term follow-up. *Am J Clin Nutr* 1992; 55: Suppl. 2, 594S–596S.

49. Varela JE, Hinojosa MW, Nguyen NT. Resolution of obstructive sleep apnea after laparoscopic gastric bypass. *Obes Surg* 2007; 17: 1279–1282.

50. Bakker JP, Balachandran JS, Tecilazich F, *et al.* Pilot study of the effects of bariatric surgery and continuous positive airway pressure treatment on vascular function in obese subjects with obstructive sleep apnoea. *Intern Med J* 2013; 43: 993–998.

51. Sjostrom L, Larsson B, Backman L, *et al.* Swedish obese subjects (SOS). Recruitment for an intervention study and a selected description of the obese state. *Int J Obes Relat Metab Disord* 1992; 16: 465–479.

52. Grunstein RR, Stenlof K, Hedner JA, *et al.* Two year reduction in sleep apnea symptoms and associated diabetes incidence after weight loss in severe obesity. *Sleep* 2007; 30: 703–710.

53. Fredheim JM, Rollheim J, Sandbu R, *et al.* Obstructive sleep apnea after weight loss: a clinical trial comparing gastric bypass and intensive lifestyle intervention. *J Clin Sleep Med* 2013; 9: 427–432.

54. Buchwald H, Estok R, Fahrbach K, *et al.* Weight and type 2 diabetes after bariatric surgery: systematic review and meta-analysis. *Am J Med* 2009; 122: 248–256.

55. Greenburg DL, Lettieri CJ, Eliasson AH. Effects of surgical weight loss on measures of obstructive sleep apnea: a meta-analysis. *Am J Med* 2009; 122: 535–542.

56. Hamilton GS, Naughton MT. Impact of obstructive sleep apnoea on diabetes and cardiovascular disease. *Med J Aust* 2013; 199: S27–S30.

57. Sivam S, Phillips CL, Trenell MI, *et al.* Effects of 8 weeks of continuous positive airway pressure on abdominal adiposity in obstructive sleep apnoea. *Eur Respir J* 2012; 40: 913–918.

58. Hoyos CM, Killick R, Yee BJ, *et al.* Cardiometabolic changes after continuous positive airway pressure for obstructive sleep apnoea: a randomised sham-controlled study. *Thorax* 2012; 67: 1081–1089.

59. Quan SF, Budhiraja R, Clarke DP, *et al.* Impact of treatment with continuous positive airway pressure (CPAP) on weight in obstructive sleep apnea. *J Clin Sleep Med* 2013; 9: 989–993.

60. Hoyos CM, Phillips CL, Grunstein RR. From couch potato to gym junkie--CPAP may not be the answer. *J Clin Sleep Med* 2014; 10: 473–474.

61. Chirinos JA, Gurubhagavatula I, Teff K, *et al.* CPAP, weight loss, or both for obstructive sleep apnea. *N Engl J Med* 2014; 370: 2265–2275.

62. Maciejewski ML, Arterburn DE. Cost-effectiveness of bariatric surgery. *JAMA* 2013; 310: 742–743.

63. Hoerger TJ, Zhang P, Segel JE, *et al.* Cost-effectiveness of bariatric surgery for severely obese adults with diabetes. *Diabetes Care* 2010; 33: 1933–1939.

64. Neovius M, Narbro K, Keating C, *et al.* Health care use during 20 years following bariatric surgery. *JAMA* 2012; 308: 1132–1141.

Disclosures: **None declared.**

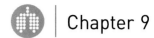

Chapter 9

Children

Hui-Leng Tan[1], David Gozal[2] and Leila Kheirandish-Gozal[2]

In this chapter, we highlight salient differences in both the aetiology and pathophysiology of OSA in children compared with adults, and will document their clinical management implications. The aetiology of paediatric OSA is usually the confluence of multifactorial elements including anatomical factors (*e.g.* enlarged adenoids and tonsils) that promote intrinsic UA narrowing and factors that contribute to UA collapsibility (*e.g.* UA inflammation and altered neurological reflexes). Adenotonsillectomy remains the mainstay of treatment but medical anti-inflammatory therapies such as nasal steroids and leukotriene antagonists are gaining wider acceptance in the treatment of mild OSA. OSA morbidities primarily involve the neurocognitive, cardiovascular and metabolic systems. However, the phenotypic variance of paediatric OSA is only partially explained by its severity, such that a combination of genetic and environmental factors is likely to be an important contributor, opening the door for implementation of genomic and proteomic approaches to enable future personalised diagnosis and management.

In 1889, Dr William Hill published an article in the *British Medical Journal* titled "On some causes of backwardness and stupidity in children: and the relief of these symptoms in some instances by naso-pharyngeal scarifications" [1]. At a time when knowledge on sleep disorders was virtually nonexistent, Dr Hill summarised his observations of a group of developmentally challenged children who "frequently evince marked inability to fix their attention on their lessons or work for any length of time" and were "nearly all mouth-breathers, night snorers and the victims, *inter alia*, of some form of nasal or pharyngeal obstruction". Dr Hill further depicted the "often remarkable" relief afforded by nasopharyngeal scarifications.

From initial reports such as this, the evidence has now accumulated to show that paediatric OSA is one of the most common causes of sleep disordered breathing in children, with a reported prevalence ranging from 1% to 5%, with these figures primarily reflecting the nature of the population studied and the stringency of the diagnostic criteria being employed [2, 3]. Peak prevalence occurs between the ages of 2 and 8 years, and similar to the OSA seen in the adult population, paediatric OSA is characterised by intermittent obstruction of the UA, with resultant IH, hypercarbia, increase in respiratory effort, pronounced intrathoracic pressure changes and sleep fragmentation [4]. However, the developmental trajectories in anatomy and neural networks in childhood mean that there are significant differences in its aetiology, pathophysiology and consequences [5], necessitating different interventions from those usually undertaken in adult patients.

[1]Dept of Paediatric Respiratory Medicine, Royal Brompton Hospital, London, UK. [2]Sections of Pediatric Sleep Medicine and Pediatric Pulmonology, Dept of Pediatrics, Comer Children's Hospital, Pritzker School of Medicine, The University of Chicago, Chicago, IL, USA.

Correspondence: Leila Kheirandish-Gozal, Section of Pediatric Sleep Medicine, Dept of Pediatrics, Pritzker School of Medicine, The University of Chicago, 5841 S. Maryland Avenue/MC2117, Chicago, IL 60637-1470, USA. E-mail: lgozal@peds.bsd.uchicago.edu

Aetiology

The aetiology of paediatric OSA is often arbitrarily divided into factors that result in a reduction in UA calibre and those that promote UA collapsibility. In reality, as with most medical conditions, OSA in children is multifactorial and a combination of factors is often present in the majority of children.

Anatomical factors

Adenotonsillar hypertrophy is by far the most common cause of paediatric OSA. Magnetic resonance imaging (MRI) of the UA revealed that the size of the adenoids and tonsils is significantly increased in children with OSA compared with matched controls, concomitant with smaller UA volumes [6]. However, the exact mechanisms and potential antecedents underlying this follicular lymphoid proliferation and hyperplasia of the tonsils and adenoids remain poorly understood. When tonsillar tissues from children with OSA were cultured in vitro, the proliferative rates of CD3$^+$, CD4$^+$ and CD8$^+$ cells were increased when compared to those isolated from children with recurrent tonsillitis [7, 8]. Furthermore, increased expression of the pro-inflammatory cytokines TNF-α, IL-6, and IL-1α was apparent. It is likely that respiratory viruses and possibly recurrent vibration of the UA wall may promote localised inflammation and consequent increased UA collapsibility. Indeed, increased exhaled breath condensate levels of leukotriene B$_4$ and cysteinyl leukotrienes along with increased neutrophilia have been reported to be higher in children with OSA [9, 10]. Notably, children with OSA also have hypertrophy/hyperplasia of lymphoid tissues in other regions of the airway as well as in the deep cervical lymph nodes [11]. UA tract perturbations such as prominence of the inferior nasal turbinates, middle-ear effusions and opacification of the sinuses have also been described [12], suggesting that OSA may reflect the presence of a broader inflammatory disorder affecting the airway as a whole [13].

Other anatomical factors include small or retropositioned mandible, large or retropositioned tongue, mid-face hypoplasia and increased pharyngeal fat pads, particularly in obese children. Thus, conditions commonly associated with OSA include children with craniofacial syndromes (e.g. Treacher Collins syndrome, Crouzon's syndrome, Apert's syndrome, Pierre Robin sequence, achondroplasia, trisomy 21 and Beckwith–Wiedemann syndrome). Children with mucopolysaccharidoses often have narrower airways due to excessive mucopolysaccharide deposition in the UA and have a higher prevalence of OSA. Afro-Caribbean ethnicity, sickle cell disease and obesity are also frequent and important risk factors [14].

Based on aforementioned considerations, adenotonsillectomy is currently the first-line therapy for children with OSA [4]. However, while the majority of children improve following this procedure, a significant proportion will have residual OSA [15]. Furthermore, the severity of OSA as indicated by the AHI is not strongly correlated with airway volume or adenotonsillar size [6], suggesting interplay with other factors.

Increased UA collapsibility

The presence of UA inflammation and altered neurological reflexes involving respiratory control of UA muscles emerge as the most prominent driver leading to increased UA collapsibility. Examples of the former include allergic rhinitis and asthma, while cerebral palsy, neuromuscular disorders and myelomeningocoele are some examples of the latter.

A useful paradigm for understanding UA instability is to model the UA as a Starling resistor, *i.e.* a tube with a collapsible segment. Under conditions of flow limitation, the maximum inspiratory airflow is determined by the pressure changes upstream (nasal) to a collapsible locus of the UA and is relatively independent of the downstream (tracheal) pressure generated by the diaphragm. Collapse occurs when the pressure outside the collapsible segment is greater than that within the segment and this has been termed the critical closing pressure (Pcrit). Pcrit is thus an objective measure of airway collapsibility. MARCUS *et al.* [16] determined Pcrit in children who were asleep by plotting the maximal inspiratory airflow against the level of negative nasal pressure applied *via* a nasal mask and found that Pcrit was less negative in children with OSA than in those with primary snoring or healthy children. In other words, children with OSA have demonstrably more collapsible UA during sleep. During wakefulness, active neural processes preserve UA patency (children will rarely snore when they are awake). However, the application of local anaesthetic to the pharyngeal introitus can remove these compensatory processes, such that noninvasive measures of UA dynamics before and after local anaesthetic application provide highly sensitive and specific predictions in the detection of children with moderate-to-severe OSA [17].

OSA and inflammation

There is increasing evidence that OSA can promote the activation and propagation of systemic inflammatory responses. Elevation of pro-inflammatory cytokines such as IL-6, interferon-γ and TNF-α have all been reported in children with OSA (albeit inconsistently), as have reduced levels of the anti-inflammatory cytokine IL-10 [18, 19]. Microarray analyses of RNA from peripheral leukocytes of children with OSA revealed the coordinated recruitment of functionally relevant gene clusters involved in the regulation and propagation of inflammatory pathways and the inflammasome [20]. A potential mechanism responsible for the initiation of inflammation may reside in molecular events in specific genes. For example, the promoter region of the *FOXP3* gene, which controls the transcriptional fate and differentiation of lymphocytes into regulatory T-cells (Tregs), exhibits severity-dependent increases in methylation in paediatric OSA [21]. Such epigenetic alterations were subsequently linked to reduced numbers and impaired function of Tregs in the peripheral blood of children with OSA [22], a significant finding considering the major role Tregs play in the suppression of inflammation. Differentially orchestrated responses of various tissues to perturbations induced by OSA may interact with environmental and genetic factors to elicit a spectrum of inflammatory phenotypes linked to end-organ morbidities [23].

OSA and obesity

With the current obesity epidemic, the demographics of paediatric OSA appear to be changing. Although several decades ago, the prototypical child with OSA was one with adenotonsillar hypertrophy and failure to thrive, a large proportion of children currently being diagnosed with OSA are obese. The NANOS study, a cross-sectional, prospective, multicentre study that aimed to assess the contributions of obesity and adenotonsillar hypertrophy to paediatric OSA, found that 46.6% of obese children in the community who were otherwise healthy had an obstructive AHI of >1 event·h^{-1} total sleep time (TST) [24]. Although all of the pathophysiological mechanisms described above remain applicable in the context of obesity, it is likely that other factors unique to obese children are operational as well. Indeed, obese children with OSA seem to preferentially resemble the adult OSA phenotype, and therefore often manifest more prominent daytime sleepiness symptoms and less prominent adenotonsillar hypertrophy [25, 26]. However, when MRI-volumetric approaches were used to compare the UA of obese children with and without OSA, the size of the UA lymphoid tissues and parapharyngeal fat pads was increased in those with OSA [27]. Fatty infiltrates within compartments of UA structures and the neck probably contribute to UA narrowing and increased pharyngeal collapsibility. Central obesity also reduces the FRC of the lungs due to abdominal visceral fat impinging on the chest cavity, limiting diaphragmatic descent, particularly when supine; in addition, thoracic fat weighing on the chest wall can effectively decrease lung compliance, leading to hypoventilation, atelectasis and ventilation/perfusion mismatch. The reduced lung volumes may decrease airway stiffness by reducing the tracheal tethering effect, further increasing the risk of UA collapse during sleep [28]. All these factors probably explain the lower success rate of adenotonsillectomy in obese children with OSA.

A reciprocal interaction between obesity and OSA has also been postulated. Leptin, a key hormonal regulator of appetite and metabolism that is predominantly secreted by adipocytes, promotes satiety and reduces food intake. Another important hormone, ghrelin, is an orexigenic hormone secreted in the gut. OSA can induce leptin resistance and increase ghrelin levels, both of which can potentiate obesogenic behaviours, in particular, the intake of high-calorie "comfort" foods [29]. OSA can also cause EDS and fatigue, both of which are likely to reduce the participation in and commitment to physical activity. The low-grade inflammatory responses induced by OSA could further interact and potentiate the underlying inflammation due to obesity, thereby exacerbating their corresponding morbidities [30].

Certainly, monocyte chemoattractant protein 1 and plasminogen activator inhibitor 1 levels have recently been shown to be significantly higher in obese OSA children than their BMI-matched controls [31]. In a subset of children with moderate-to-severe OSA, IL-6 levels were also significantly higher than children who were obese but did not have OSA.

Consequences of OSA

Neurocognitive and behavioural consequences

Childhood is a time of remarkable physical and cognitive growth, development and maturation: any effect of OSA on learning, behaviour or neurocognition can have considerable impact on the child's ability to fulfil their potential. There have been numerous studies reporting the association between OSA and neurocognitive and behavioural morbidity [32–35]. One of the first seminal papers to highlight the potential causative links between OSA and its detrimental consequences on academic performance was a prospective study looking at 297 first-grade children whose school performance was in the lowest 10% of their class. Screening for OSA revealed that an excessive proportion had the condition. Compellingly, the children who were treated for OSA showed significant academic improvements in their school grades the subsequent year while children who had OSA but were not treated failed to improve academically [36]. Impairments in executive functioning have also been reported: the Tucson Children's Assessment of Sleep Apnea Study (TuCASA) identified a negative correlation between AHI and immediate recall, full-scale intelligence quotient (IQ), performance IQ and mathematics achievements, while nocturnal hypoxaemia adversely affected nonverbal skills [37]. Children with OSA took longer and needed more learning opportunities to learn a pictorially based short- and long-term declarative memory test [38].

Event-related potential recordings revealed altered temporal trajectories and localisation patterns during an attention task in children with OSA [39, 40]. There is now intriguing preliminary functional MRI evidence that OSA influences cognitive and empathetic processing: children with OSA with preserved cognitive abilities show greater activity in the regions of the brain implicated in cognitive control, conflict monitoring and attentional allocation in order to perform tasks at the same level as children without OSA, suggesting they either require greater neural recruitment or are using alternative strategies, or a combination thereof [41]. Furthermore, when viewing empathy-eliciting scenarios, children with more severe OSA displayed less activity in the left amygdala.

OSA and habitual snoring have also been associated with hyperactivity, difficulty in concentrating, attention deficits and impulsivity. Recent 5-year follow-up results from TuCASA revealed that youths with untreated OSA exhibited hyperactivity, had attention problems and aggressive behaviours, lower social competencies, poorer communication and/or diminished adaptive skills [42]. It is important to consider OSA as a differential diagnosis when investigating a child with attention deficit hyperactivity disorder, as some children may have been misdiagnosed.

Notwithstanding such considerations, not all children with OSA exhibit cognitive or behavioural deficits. Furthermore, although improvements in learning and behaviour have been reported following treatment of OSA, in the first ever therapeutic RCT of paediatric OSA, the Childhood Adenotonsillectomy Trial (CHAT), no changes in cognitive function emerged after treatment, although there were improvements in symptoms, behaviour and quality of life [43]. It is important to note that the children studied in this trial only had mild OSA with no significant oxygen desaturations, children younger than 5 years were excluded and the follow-up period was relatively short at 7 months, therefore restricting the generalisation of these findings.

Susceptibility modifiers, both genetic and environmental, probably play a role in phenotypic expression: differences in systemic inflammatory responses as reported by plasma C-reactive protein (CRP) levels differentiate children with similar OSA severity who do and do not exhibit cognitive deficits [44]; genetic variants in NADPH oxidase 2, insulin-like growth factor 1 and apolipoprotein E are some of the candidates thus far identified as affecting neurocognitive consequences in children with OSA [45–47]. Neurocognitive morbidity seems to be closely related to vascular dysfunction, suggesting mechanisms of pathogenesis may be similar in both [48].

Cardiovascular consequences

Pulmonary hypertension, and the resultant cor pulmonale if left untreated, is one of the most serious cardiovascular consequences of OSA [49]. Fortunately, it is not commonly seen. Children with OSA tend to exhibit more subtle evidence of cardiovascular dysfunction such as dysregulation of BP, cardiac remodelling and endothelial dysfunction. AMIN *et al.* [50] found that children with OSA had evidence of BP deregulation: significantly greater mean BP variability during wakefulness and sleep, higher night/day SBP ratio, and marked reductions in nocturnal dipping of the mean BP were identified. In fact, children with OSA had night/day SBP ratios that surpassed the established cut-off ratios of 0.899 for females and 0.9009 for males, both of which are known to increase the risk for cardiovascular morbidity in adults.

Furthermore, children with OSA exhibit increases in morning BP surges, BP load and 24-h ambulatory BP compared with healthy controls. These differences were associated with left ventricular remodelling [51–53]. The evidence of left ventricular strain and reduced contractility reported may be due to effects on brain natriuretic peptide (BNP), which is released by cardiac myocytes in response to cardiac wall distension. Greater overnight changes in BNP levels have been demonstrated in children with moderate-to-severe OSA compared with mild OSA and controls, which is probably related to the more frequent and pronounced negative intrathoracic pressure swings seen in more severe OSA [54]. It remains unclear whether these left ventricular changes are reversible or whether they indicate a group of susceptible individuals at risk of more adverse CVD during adulthood.

In comparison with weight-matched children without OSA, children with OSA have diminished exercise performance due to reduced cardiac output and oxygen consumption at peak exercise capacity [55]. These findings were associated with the frequency of respiratory-related arousals, the severity of hypoxia and heart rate during sleep. Minute ventilation and ventilatory responses to exercise were not affected.

Endothelial dysfunction is believed to be a precursor to atherosclerosis. Assessment of post-occlusive hyperaemic responses in children using various methodologies, such as flow-mediated dilation, pulse arterial tonometry and laser-Doppler reperfusion kinetics, has consistently revealed significant impairments in endothelial function in children with OSA compared with controls [56–58]. Furthermore, although the majority of these children demonstrated resolution of the endothelial dysfunction following treatment with adenotonsillectomy, a subgroup who had a strong family history of CVD did not show the anticipated normalisation [56, 59], suggesting that the effects of OSA in a genetically susceptible subset of children may persist for unknown periods of time, potentially into adulthood. The severity of endothelial dysfunction is greater in children with both obesity and OSA compared with either condition in isolation, suggesting the convergence of the deleterious consequences of obesity and OSA [60–64]. It should be emphasised that not every child with OSA manifests endothelial dysfunction: a potential explanation for this variance in endothelial phenotype may reside in the intrinsic ability to recruit endothelial progenitors to the circulation *via* the release of stromal-derived factor 1 [57, 65].

CRP, an acute-phase reaction protein, is recognised as a robust and independent predictor of cardiovascular morbidity [66]. It has been postulated that CRP may even participate directly in atheromatous lesion formation through reduction of nitric oxide synthesis and induction of the expression of adhesion molecules in endothelial cells [67]. Increased CRP levels have been demonstrated in children with OSA, correlate with severity of the disease and decrease following effective treatment [68–70]. Once again, not all children with OSA have raised CRP levels, as the interplay of genetic variants in the IL-6 and CRP genes, as well as environmental factors, plays an important role [71]. However, we would surmise that the children in whom CRP levels are elevated constitute a higher-risk group for the development of long-term cardiovascular complications. Indeed, markers of vascular injury and endothelial activation, such as adhesion molecules, myeloid-related protein 8/14, fatty acid-binding protein and circulating microparticles, have all been shown to be elevated in children with OSA and are associated with the presence of endothelial dysfunction [72–75].

Metabolic consequences

Although in adult cohorts, OSA has been identified as an important risk factor for insulin resistance and dyslipidaemia, the evidence in children is less robust. Factors such as pubertal status and the concurrent presence of obesity may explain some of the conflicting results. Sleep fragmentation and IH have been associated with decreased insulin sensitivity in obese adolescent boys [76, 77]. Another study involving predominantly post-pubertal adolescents demonstrated strong associations between OSA and the metabolic syndrome, as well as with individual metabolic parameters such as fasting insulin and homeostatic model assessment (HOMA) [78]. In younger children, OSA has been shown to be associated with reduced insulin sensitivity only when obesity was concurrently present and effective treatment of OSA ameliorated HOMA in these children [79–81]. Interestingly, when highly sensitive bioinformatic approaches and gene pathway analyses were employed in conjunction with transcriptomic microarrays in children with primary snoring, alterations in insulin homeostatic mechanisms emerged [82], suggesting that even mild perturbations in sleep may impose subclinical changes in peripheral tissue insulin receptor sensitivity.

Paediatric OSA has also been implicated in elevations of low-density lipoprotein cholesterol with concomitant decreases in high-density lipoprotein cholesterol in both obese and non-obese children [81, 83]. Significant improvements in lipid profile were observed in all children after treatment of OSA.

End-organ morbidity in the context of metabolic deregulation has been described in obese snoring children, particularly those with OSA and/or metabolic dysfunction, as evidenced by elevated serum liver enzymes [84]. Treatment of the OSA resulted in improvement in these levels in the majority of the patients. Two recent studies examined obese children with biopsy-proven nonalcoholic fatty liver disease (NAFLD) [85, 86] and in 60%, OSA/ nocturnal hypoxaemia was present. The presence and severity of OSA was associated with the presence of NAFLD, liver fibrosis and NAFLD activity score independent of BMI, abdominal adiposity, metabolic syndrome and insulin resistance, while the percentage of time with oxygen saturation ⩽90% correlated with increased intrahepatic leukocytes, activated Kupffer cells, and circulating markers of hepatocyte apoptosis and fibrogenesis.

Excessive daytime sleepiness

In contrast to adults, EDS manifesting as falling asleep involuntarily is infrequently reported in children, and tends to become manifest in the more severe and/or obese patients. Children with OSA do have higher ESS scores compared to controls (8.1±4.9 *versus* 5.3±3.9), even though many still score within the normal range [87]. Objective measurements of EDS using the Multiple Sleep Latency Test have shown that children with OSA have severity-dependent shortening of their sleep latencies [88]. Interestingly, the magnitude of sleep latency reduction is associated with measures of systemic inflammation, such as plasma TNF-α levels, which is modulated by polymorphisms in the TNF-α gene [89].

Nocturnal enuresis

A higher prevalence of nocturnal enuresis has been reported in children with OSA [90, 91]. It has been postulated that this may be due to the dampening effects of OSA on arousal responses to changes in bladder pressure or due to elevated BNP levels, which impact on the renin–angiotensin pathway, vasopressin, and excretion of sodium and water [92].

Healthcare utilisation

Children with OSA have been reported to have increased healthcare utilisation compared with their peers, with more hospital visits and more medication prescriptions, predominantly for respiratory infections [93, 94]. Admittedly, association does not equate to causation, and the explanation may be that children who have more contact with healthcare professionals are more likely to be screened and thus diagnosed with OSA, or children who have recurrent upper respiratory tract infections are at higher risk of OSA. However, following treatment of OSA by adenotonsillectomy, healthcare utilisation was significantly reduced to the extent that total annual health care costs were reduced by a third [95]. These findings have also since been confirmed in another population-based cohort [96].

Diagnosis

The current gold standard for diagnosis of OSA in the USA and Australia is an overnight, in-laboratory PSG study [97, 98]. In Europe, a significant proportion of sleep units perform respiratory polygraphy [99–101]. Sleep studies provide an objective quantification of disturbances in respiratory parameters and sleep patterns, allowing the stratification of patients into differential disease severities, thereby enabling clinicians to tailor clinical management accordingly. The current accepted practice has consisted in the use of an arbitrary cut-off for AHI corresponding to more than three standard deviations beyond the mean of the normative AHI in healthy children. Most, if not all, clinicians would agree that a child with an AHI >5 event·h^{-1} TST requires treatment and that a child with an AHI <1 event·h^{-1} TST does not have significant OSA. However, there is no international consensus with regard to therapy, particularly when AHI fall between these two arbitrary values. Some algorithms have recently been proposed that recognise the importance of treating the patient and not just the values obtained from the sleep study [102, 103]. In addition to PSG-derived measures, these algorithms incorporate factors such as the severity of symptoms, risk factors and the presence of any OSA-related morbidity, and may therefore provide a more coherent, clinically pertinent and applicable approach to the diagnosis and prioritisation of treatment.

Treatment

Adenotonsillectomy is the first-line therapy for paediatric OSA for children with adenotonsillar hypertrophy and is, overall, an effective treatment. However, a large, multicentre, retrospective study showed that although the majority of children have marked AHI improvements following adenotonsillectomy, residual OSA is still frequent and clinically significant in a relatively large subset, particularly in children who were obese, who had severe OSA before surgery (AHI >20 events·h^{-1} TST), older children (those aged

>7 years) and in those with bronchial asthma. Similar findings have been reported in other studies and additional risk factors for residual OSA have been identified, including high Mallampati score, African-American ethnicity, and children with craniofacial anomalies, chromosomal defects and neuromuscular disease (including trisomy 21, achondroplasia, Prader–Willi syndrome and Pierre Robin syndrome). Clinicians should be aware that 1) specific protocols may need to be set in place so that the subset of children at high risk of residual OSA undergoes post-surgical sleep studies and 2) recurrence or persistence of OSA symptoms post-adenotonsillectomy warrants re-evaluation. Some ear, nose and throat surgeons advocate tonsillotomy as an alternative to tonsillectomy, claiming reduced post-operative pain resulting in an earlier return to normal diet and activity, with similar outcomes, but the jury is still out as to the universal validity of such findings [104, 105].

In children who manifest residual OSA after adenotonsillectomy, those who do not have significantly enlarged UA lymphadenoid tissues or those who opt not to undergo surgery, PAP therapy in the form of CPAP or BPAP is recommended. The goal is to maintain patency of the airway throughout the respiratory cycle, improve FRC and decrease the work of breathing. Pressure requirements vary from patient to patient so individual titration is required [106]. The main potential side-effects include local skin pressure effects from the mask, discomfort from air leaks and drying of the oronasal mucosa [107]. Adherence can be a major challenge [108–112] and can be improved by behavioural modification techniques, which are time and labour intensive, often requiring admission to the in-patient service, and needing *a priori* engagement with the child and family [113].

A possible alternative to mask-based PAP is high-flow oxygen *via* a nasal cannula (HFNC). Most HFNC experience derives from its use in acute respiratory distress but there has been one study that looked at 12 patients with OSA. The reduction in AHI was comparable to that of CPAP, leading the authors to postulate that HFNC may be a gentler, kinder alternative to CPAP [114].

In terms of medical therapy, there has been considerable interest in anti-inflammatory agents, particularly leukotriene receptor antagonists such as montelukast and intranasal steroids, in the treatment of paediatric OSA [115]. Tonsils from children with OSA have been shown to express increased levels of leukotriene receptors 1 and 2 compared with tonsils from children with recurrent tonsillitis [116]. The application of leukotriene antagonists to an *in vitro* cell culture system of tonsillar tissues from children with OSA elicited dose-dependent reductions in cell proliferation, and reductions in the secretion of the cytokines TNF-α, IL-6 and IL-12 [117]. In an open-label intervention study where children with mild OSA received montelukast for 16 weeks, significant reductions in adenoid size and respiratory-related sleep disturbances occurred [118]. A recent double-blind, randomised, placebo-controlled trial has further confirmed these findings [119]. Similarly, the application of steroids to *in vitro* cell cultures of tonsillar tissue resulted in decreased proliferation, increased apoptosis, and reduction in the secretion of the pro-inflammatory cytokines IL-6, IL-8 and TNF-α [120]. A randomised cross-over trial of 6 weeks' treatment with intranasal budesonide for mild OSA showed reductions in the severity of OSA, as well as in the size of adenoidal tissues [121]. Importantly, discontinuation of therapy for 8 weeks did not promote the occurrence of rebound symptoms. Intranasal fluticasone has also shown similar results [122]. Use of both montelukast and nasal budesonide for 12 weeks in children who had residual mild OSA after adenotonsillectomy led to significant improvements in AHI, nadir oxygen saturation and respiratory arousal index [123]. A recent large, retrospective review of anti-inflammatory outcomes in children also suggested that this combination was an effective alternative to adenotonsillectomy, particularly in younger and non-obese children with mild OSA [124].

Considering the recent CHAT findings in which normalisation of PSG findings in a large number of children in the watchful-waiting group occurred [43], along with an absence of significant cognitive decline, it is legitimate to propose that medical management and reassessment after a period of observation in children with mild OSA may be a valid therapeutic option. Studies examining the desirable optimal duration of treatment, long-term outcomes, combinatorial approaches and criteria for patient selection for optimal outcomes are therefore critically needed.

In selected patient populations, some orthodontic procedures such as rapid maxillary expansion have been proposed to be efficacious [125, 126]. Procedures such as tongue-base suspension and uvulopalatopharyngoplasty have also been studied in children with cerebral palsy and OSA [127]. Recently, the use of more comprehensive assessments and interventions including myofacial re-education has been advocated in a series of uncontrolled studies [128]. In complex or persistent cases of OSA, sleep endoscopy may enable identification of the exact level of obstruction in the child, thus facilitating site-specific surgical therapy [129].

The use of nasal EPAP (NEPAP) devices has been recently advanced as an alternative treatment for OSA [130]. NEPAP devices are essentially a mechanical valve that is applied to each nostril. It has low inspiratory resistance but high expiratory resistance, which results in positive pressure during exhalation, thus splinting the UA and reducing collapsibility on subsequent inspiration. The study was performed in 14 teenagers and results were promising, with improvement in the obstructive apnoea index in the group as a whole. However, it is important to note that considerable individual variability was observed: three patients did not improve and two actually worsened. Clearly, more research is needed.

Future developments

PSGs undoubtedly provide an objective measure of sleep disturbance. However, if we were to critically appraise it as a diagnostic test, it not only is costly but also requires an overnight stay, and is time and labour intensive with regard to set-up and scoring. More importantly perhaps is that PSGs are poorly predictive of OSA-associated morbidities. Some children with primary snoring already display neurocognitive or cardiovascular sequelae despite a normal sleep study. Conversely, not every child fulfilling PSG criteria for OSA manifests end-organ morbidity. Surely, a simpler test to determine which children to treat and how to provide optimal treatment on an individual basis is critically needed. In this context, "omics" technologies and new bioinformatic approaches may be a possible way forward. Proteomic approaches have revealed that paediatric OSA is associated with specific and consistent alterations in certain clusters of urinary proteins [131]. Increased levels of the urinary catecholamines adrenaline and noradrenaline have been described, which are probably secondary to increased sympathetic activity from the episodic hypoxaemia and arousals caused by OSA [132]. Overnight changes in the levels of three other neurotransmitters (increases in γ-aminobutyric acid, and decreases in taurine and β-phenylethylamine) appeared to differentiate children with OSA with neurocognitive deficits from those who were protected from such morbid consequences of OSA. With the use of genomic and proteomic approaches, there is also emerging, preliminary data on exosomal microRNAs as potential biomarkers of cardiovascular risk in children with OSA [133]. Thus, it is likely that coordinated combinatorial approaches will soon emerge to tailor the diagnosis and treatment to the individual patient.

Conclusion

Significant progress has occurred since the publication of Hill's article back in 1889 [1]. We now have a much better understanding of the aetiology and resultant morbidity of paediatric OSA, and a greater range of therapies. However, there are still many fundamental questions that remain unanswered: in particular, a detailed understanding of the mechanisms underlying the pathogenesis of the disease and factors influencing the phenotypic variability such as to enable their accurate prediction. Such knowledge is critical to formulate novel biomarkers and individualised therapies, and permit the implementation of personalised medicine. Until these mechanisms are better understood, the mainstay of treatment as outlined by Dr Hill, *i.e.* adenotonsillectomy, will remain the same. Hill's article concludes "The stupid looking lazy child who frequently suffers from headache at school, breathes through his mouth instead of his nose, snores and is restless at night, and wakes up with a dry mouth in the morning, is well worthy of the solicitous attention of the school medical officer". While one would hope most children in this day would not be thus labelled, and would have been diagnosed and treated well before such severe sequelae developed, it is still a prescient reminder of the importance of early diagnosis and prompt effective treatment.

References

1. Hill W. On some causes of backwardness and stupidity in children: and the relief of these symptoms in some instances by naso-pharyngeal scarifications. *Br Med J* 1889; 2: 711–712.
2. Bixler EO, Vgontzas AN, Lin HM, *et al.* Sleep disordered breathing in children in a general population sample: prevalence and risk factors. *Sleep* 2009; 32: 731–736.
3. Rosen CL, Larkin EK, Kirchner HL, *et al.* Prevalence and risk factors for sleep-disordered breathing in 8- to 11-year-old children: association with race and prematurity. *J Pediatr* 2003; 142: 383–389.
4. Marcus CL, Brooks LJ, Draper KA, *et al.* Diagnosis and management of childhood obstructive sleep apnea syndrome. *Pediatrics* 2012; 130: 576–584.
5. Kheirandish-Gozal L, Gozal D, eds. Sleep Disordered Breathing in Children. 1st Edn. Berlin, Springer Science, 2012.
6. Arens R, McDonough JM, Costarino AT, *et al.* Magnetic resonance imaging of the upper airway structure of children with obstructive sleep apnea syndrome. *Am J Respir Crit Care Med* 2001; 164: 698–703.
7. Kim J, Bhattacharjee R, Dayyat E, *et al.* Increased cellular proliferation and inflammatory cytokines in tonsils derived from children with obstructive sleep apnea. *Pediatr Res* 2009; 66: 423–428.
8. Serpero LD, Kheirandish-Gozal L, Dayyat E, *et al.* A mixed cell culture model for assessment of proliferation in tonsillar tissues from children with obstructive sleep apnea or recurrent tonsillitis. *Laryngoscope* 2009; 119: 1005–1010.
9. Goldbart AD, Krishna J, Li RC, *et al.* Inflammatory mediators in exhaled breath condensate of children with obstructive sleep apnea syndrome. *Chest* 2006; 130: 143–148.
10. Li AM, Hung E, Tsang T, *et al.* Induced sputum inflammatory measures correlate with disease severity in children with obstructive sleep apnoea. *Thorax* 2007; 62: 75–79.
11. Parikh SR, Sadoughi B, Sin S, *et al.* Deep cervical lymph node hypertrophy: a new paradigm in the understanding of pediatric obstructive sleep apnea. *Laryngoscope* 2013; 123: 2043–2049.
12. Arens R, Sin S, Willen S, *et al.* Rhino-sinus involvement in children with obstructive sleep apnea syndrome. *Pediatr Pulmonol* 2010; 45: 993–998.
13. Gozal D. Pediatric OSA: a case for "United We Stand" in the way of a breath. *Pediatr Pulmonol* 2010; 45: 1151–1152.

14. Sheldon S, Kryger M, Ferber R, *et al.* Principles and Practice of Pediatric Sleep Medicine. 2nd Edn. Philadelphia, Elsevier, 2014.

15. Bhattacharjee R, Kheirandish-Gozal L, Spruyt K, *et al.* Adenotonsillectomy outcomes in treatment of obstructive sleep apnea in children: a multicenter retrospective study. *Am J Respir Crit Care Med* 2010; 182: 676–683.

16. Marcus CL, McColley SA, Carroll JL, *et al.* Upper airway collapsibility in children with obstructive sleep apnea syndrome. *J Appl Physiol* 1994; 77: 918–924.

17. Gozal D, Burnside MM. Increased upper airway collapsibility in children with obstructive sleep apnea during wakefulness. *Am J Respir Crit Care Med* 2004; 169: 163–167.

18. Gozal D. Sleep, sleep disorders and inflammation in children. *Sleep Med* 2009; 10: Suppl. 1, S12–S16.

19. Gozal D, Serpero LD, Sans Capdevila O, *et al.* Systemic inflammation in non-obese children with obstructive sleep apnea. *Sleep Med* 2008; 9: 254–259.

20. Khalyfa A, Capdevila OS, Buazza MO, *et al.* Genome-wide gene expression profiling in children with non-obese obstructive sleep apnea. *Sleep Med* 2009; 10: 75–86.

21. Kim J, Bhattacharjee R, Khalyfa A, *et al.* DNA methylation in inflammatory genes among children with obstructive sleep apnea. *Am J Respir Crit Care Med* 2012; 185: 330–338.

22. Tan HL, Gozal D, Wang Y, *et al.* Alterations in circulating T-cell lymphocyte populations in children with obstructive sleep apnea. *Sleep* 2013; 36: 913–922.

23. Kheirandish-Gozal L, Gozal D. Genotype-phenotype interactions in pediatric obstructive sleep apnea. *Respir Physiol Neurobiol* 2013; 189: 338–343.

24. Alonso-Alvarez ML, Cordero-Guevara JA, Teran-Santos J, *et al.* Obstructive sleep apnea in obese community-dwelling children: the NANOS study. *Sleep* 2014; 37: 943–949.

25. Gozal D, Kheirandish-Gozal L. The obesity epidemic and disordered sleep during childhood and adolescence. *Adolesc Med State Art Rev* 2010; 21: 480–490.

26. Dayyat E, Kheirandish-Gozal L, Gozal D. Childhood obstructive sleep apnea: one or two distinct disease entities? *Sleep Med Clin* 2007; 2: 433–444.

27. Nandalike K, Shifteh K, Sin S, *et al.* Adenotonsillectomy in obese children with obstructive sleep apnea syndrome: magnetic resonance imaging findings and considerations. *Sleep* 2013; 36: 841–847.

28. Tauman R, Gozal D. Obstructive sleep apnea syndrome in children. *Expert Rev Respir Med* 2011; 5: 425–440.

29. Spruyt K, Sans Capdevila O, Serpero LD, *et al.* Dietary and physical activity patterns in children with obstructive sleep apnea. *J Pediatr* 2010; 156: 724–730.

30. Bhattacharjee R, Kim J, Kheirandish-Gozal L, *et al.* Obesity and obstructive sleep apnea syndrome in children: a tale of inflammatory cascades. *Pediatr Pulmonol* 2011; 46: 313–323.

31. Gileles-Hillel A, Alonso-Alvarez ML, Kheirandish-Gozal L, *et al.* Inflammatory markers and obstructive sleep apnea in obese children: the NANOS study. *Mediators Inflamm* 2014; 2014: 605280.

32. Chervin RD, Ruzicka DL, Giordani BJ, *et al.* Sleep-disordered breathing, behavior, and cognition in children before and after adenotonsillectomy. *Pediatrics* 2006; 117: e769–e778.

33. Wei JL, Bond J, Mayo MS, *et al.* Improved behavior and sleep after adenotonsillectomy in children with sleep-disordered breathing: long-term follow-up. *Arch Otolaryngol Head Neck Surg* 2009; 135: 642–646.

34. Friedman BC, Hendeles-Amitai A, Kozminsky E, *et al.* Adenotonsillectomy improves neurocognitive function in children with obstructive sleep apnea syndrome. *Sleep* 2003; 26: 999–1005.

35. Montgomery-Downs HE, Crabtree VM, Gozal D, *et al.* Cognition, sleep and respiration in at-risk children treated for obstructive sleep apnoea. *Eur Respir J* 2005; 25: 336–342.

36. Gozal D. Sleep-disordered breathing and school performance in children. *Pediatrics* 1998; 102: 616–620.

37. Kaemingk KL, Pasvogel AE, Goodwin JL, *et al.* Learning in children and sleep disordered breathing: findings of the Tucson Children's Assessment of Sleep Apnea (TuCASA) prospective cohort study. *J Int Neuropsychol Soc* 2003; 9: 1016–1026.

38. Kheirandish-Gozal L, De Jong MR, Spruyt K, *et al.* Obstructive sleep apnoea is associated with impaired pictorial memory task acquisition and retention in children. *Eur Respir J* 2010; 36: 164–169.

39. Barnes ME, Huss EA, Garrod KN, *et al.* Impairments in attention in occasionally snoring children: an event-related potential study. *Dev Neuropsychol* 2009; 34: 629–649.

40. Barnes ME, Gozal D, Molfese DL, *et al.* Attention in children with obstructive sleep apnoea: an event-related potentials study. *Sleep Med* 2012; 13: 368–377.

41. Kheirandish-Gozal L, Yoder K, Kulkarni R, *et al.* Preliminary functional MRI neural correlates of executive functioning and empathy in children with obstructive sleep apnea. *Sleep* 2014; 37: 587–592.

42. Perfect MM, Archbold K, Goodwin JL, *et al.* Risk of behavioral and adaptive functioning difficulties in youth with previous and current sleep disordered breathing. *Sleep* 2013; 36: 517–525B.

43. Marcus CL, Moore RH, Rosen CL, *et al.* A randomized trial of adenotonsillectomy for childhood sleep apnea. *N Engl J Med* 2013; 368: 2366–2376.

44. Gozal D, Crabtree VM, Sans Capdevila O, *et al.* C-reactive protein, obstructive sleep apnea, and cognitive dysfunction in school-aged children. *Am J Respir Crit Care Med* 2007; 176: 188–193.

45. Gozal D, Khalyfa A, Capdevila OS, *et al.* Cognitive function in prepubertal children with obstructive sleep apnea: a modifying role for NADPH oxidase p22 subunit gene polymorphisms? *Antioxid Redox Signal* 2012; 16: 171–177.

46. Gozal D, Sans Capdevila O, McLaughlin Crabtree V, *et al.* Plasma IGF-1 levels and cognitive dysfunction in children with obstructive sleep apnea. *Sleep Med* 2009; 10: 167–173.

47. Gozal D, Capdevila OS, Kheirandish-Gozal L, *et al.* APOE ε4 allele, cognitive dysfunction, and obstructive sleep apnea in children. *Neurology* 2007; 69: 243–249.

48. Gozal D, Kheirandish-Gozal L, Bhattacharjee R, *et al.* Neurocognitive and endothelial dysfunction in children with obstructive sleep apnea. *Pediatrics* 2010; 126: e1161–e1167.

49. Bhattacharjee R, Kheirandish-Gozal L, Pillar G, *et al.* Cardiovascular complications of obstructive sleep apnea syndrome: evidence from children. *Prog Cardiovasc Dis* 2009; 51: 416–433.

50. Amin RS, Carroll JL, Jeffries JL, *et al.* Twenty-four-hour ambulatory blood pressure in children with sleep-disordered breathing. *Am J Respir Crit Care Med* 2004; 169: 950–956.

51. Amin R, Somers VK, McConnell K, *et al.* Activity-adjusted 24-hour ambulatory blood pressure and cardiac remodeling in children with sleep disordered breathing. *Hypertension* 2008; 51: 84–91.

52. Amin RS, Kimball TR, Kalra M, *et al.* Left ventricular function in children with sleep-disordered breathing. *Am J Cardiol* 2005; 95: 801–804.

53. Nisbet LC, Yiallourou SR, Walter LM, *et al.* Blood pressure regulation, autonomic control and sleep disordered breathing in children. *Sleep Med Rev* 2014; 18: 179–189.

54. Goldbart AD, Levitas A, Greenberg-Dotan S, *et al.* B-type natriuretic peptide and cardiovascular function in young children with obstructive sleep apnea. *Chest* 2010; 138: 528–535.

55. Evans CA, Selvadurai H, Baur LA, *et al.* Effects of obstructive sleep apnea and obesity on exercise function in children. *Sleep* 2014; 37: 1103–1110.

56. Gozal D, Kheirandish-Gozal L, Serpero LD, *et al.* Obstructive sleep apnea and endothelial function in school-aged non obese children: effect of adenotonsillectomy. *Circulation* 2007; 116: 2307–2314.

57. Kheirandish-Gozal L, Bhattacharjee R, Kim J, *et al.* Endothelial progenitor cells and vascular dysfunction in children with obstructive sleep apnea. *Am J Respir Crit Care Med* 2010; 182: 92–97.

58. Kheirandish-Gozal L, Etzioni T, Bhattacharjee R, *et al.* Obstructive sleep apnea in children is associated with severity-dependent deterioration in overnight endothelial function. *Sleep Med* 2013; 14: 526–531.

59. Kheirandish-Gozal L, Bhattacharjee R, Gozal D, *et al.* Autonomic alterations and endothelial dysfunction in pediatric obstructive sleep apnea. *Sleep Med* 2010; 11: 714–720.

60. Bhattacharjee R, Kim J, Alotaibi WH, *et al.* Endothelial dysfunction in children without hypertension: potential contributions of obesity and obstructive sleep apnea. *Chest* 2012; 141: 682–691.

61. Bhattacharjee R, Alotaibi WH, Kheirandish-Gozal L, *et al.* Endothelial dysfunction in obese non-hypertensive children without evidence of sleep disordered breathing. *BMC Pediatr* 2010; 10: 8.

62. Dayyat E, Kheirandish-Gozal L, Sans Capdevila O, *et al.* Obstructive sleep apnea in children: relative contributions of body mass index and adenotonsillar hypertrophy. *Chest* 2009; 136: 137–144.

63. Gozal D, Kheirandish-Gozal L. Childhood obesity and sleep: relatives, partners, or both? – a critical perspective on the evidence. *Ann NY Acad Sci* 2012; 1264: 135–141.

64. Gozal D, Kheirandish-Gozal L. Cardiovascular morbidity in obstructive sleep apnea: oxidative stress, inflammation, and much more. *Am J Respir Crit Care Med* 2008; 177: 369–375.

65. Kheirandish-Gozal L, Farre R. The injury theory, endothelial progenitors, and sleep apnea. *Am J Respir Crit Care Med* 2013; 187: 5–7.

66. Pearson TA, Mensah GA, Alexander RW, *et al.* Markers of inflammation and cardiovascular disease: application to clinical and public health practice: A statement for healthcare professionals from the Centers for Disease Control and Prevention and the American Heart Association. *Circulation* 2003; 107: 499–511.

67. Pasceri V, Willerson JT, Yeh ET, *et al.* Direct proinflammatory effect of C-reactive protein on human endothelial cells. *Circulation* 2000; 102: 2165–2168.

68. Kheirandish-Gozal L, Capdevila OS, Tauman R, *et al.* Plasma C-reactive protein in non obese children with obstructive sleep apnea before and after adenotonsillectomy. *J Clin Sleep Med* 2006; 2: 301–304.

69. Ingram DG, Matthews CK. Effect of adenotonsillectomy on C-reactive protein levels in children with obstructive sleep apnea: a meta-analysis. *Sleep Med* 2013; 14: 172–176.

70. Li AM, Chan MH, Yin J, *et al.* C-reactive protein in children with obstructive sleep apnea and the effects of treatment. *Pediatr Pulmonol* 2008; 43: 34–40.

71. Kaditis AG, Gozal D, Khalyfa A, *et al.* Variants in C-reactive protein and IL-6 genes and susceptibility to obstructive sleep apnea in children: a candidate-gene association study in European American and Southeast European populations. *Sleep Med* 2014; 15: 228–235.

72. Bhushan B, Khalyfa A, Spruyt K, *et al.* Fatty-acid binding protein 4 gene polymorphisms and plasma levels in children with obstructive sleep apnea. *Sleep Med* 2011; 12: 666–671.

73. Kim J, Bhattacharjee R, Kheirandish-Gozal L, et al. Circulating microparticles in children with sleep disordered breathing. Chest 2011; 140: 408–417.

74. Kim J, Bhattacharjee R, Snow AB, et al. Myeloid-related protein 8/14 levels in children with obstructive sleep apnoea. Eur Respir J 2010; 35: 843–850.

75. O'Brien LM, Serpero LD, Tauman R, et al. Plasma adhesion molecules in children with sleep-disordered breathing. Chest 2006; 129: 947–953.

76. Lesser DJ, Bhatia R, Tran WH, et al. Sleep fragmentation and intermittent hypoxemia are associated with decreased insulin sensitivity in obese adolescent Latino males. Pediatr Res 2012; 72: 293–298.

77. Oliveira FM, Tran WH, Lesser D, et al. Autonomic and metabolic effects of OSA in childhood obesity. Conf Proc IEEE Eng Med Biol Soc 2010; 2010: 6134–6137.

78. Redline S, Storfer-Isser A, Rosen CL, et al. Association between metabolic syndrome and sleep-disordered breathing in adolescents. Am J Respir Crit Care Med 2007; 176: 401–408.

79. Tauman R, O'Brien LM, Ivanenko A, et al. Obesity rather than severity of sleep-disordered breathing as the major determinant of insulin resistance and altered lipidemia in snoring children. Pediatrics 2005; 116: e66–e73.

80. Kaditis AG, Alexopoulos EI, Damani E, et al. Obstructive sleep-disordered breathing and fasting insulin levels in non obese children. Pediatr Pulmonol 2005; 40: 515–523.

81. Gozal D, Capdevila OS, Kheirandish-Gozal L. Metabolic alterations and systemic inflammation in obstructive sleep apnea among non obese and obese prepubertal children. Am J Respir Crit Care Med 2008; 177: 1142–1149.

82. Khalyfa A, Gharib SA, Kim J, et al. Peripheral blood leukocyte gene expression patterns and metabolic parameters in habitually snoring and non-snoring children with normal polysomnographic findings. Sleep 2011; 34: 153–160.

83. Zong J, Liu Y, Huang Y, et al. Serum lipids alterations in adenoid hypertrophy or adenotonsillar hypertrophy children with sleep disordered breathing. Int J Pediatr Otorhinolaryngol 2013; 77: 717–720.

84. Kheirandish-Gozal L, Sans Capdevila O, Kheirandish E, et al. Elevated serum aminotransferase levels in children at risk for obstructive sleep apnea. Chest 2008; 133: 92–99.

85. Sundaram SS, Sokol RJ, Capocelli KE, et al. Obstructive sleep apnea and hypoxemia are associated with advanced liver histology in pediatric nonalcoholic fatty liver disease. J Pediatr 2014; 164: 699–706.

86. Nobili V, Cutrera R, Liccardo D, et al. Obstructive sleep apnea syndrome affects liver histology and inflammatory cell activation in pediatric nonalcoholic fatty liver disease, regardless of obesity/insulin resistance. Am J Respir Crit Care Med 2014; 189: 66–76.

87. Melendres MC, Lutz JM, Rubin ED, et al. Daytime sleepiness and hyperactivity in children with suspected sleep-disordered breathing. Pediatrics 2004; 114: 768–775.

88. Gozal D, Serpero LD, Kheirandish-Gozal L, et al. Sleep measures and morning plasma TNF-α levels in children with sleep-disordered breathing. Sleep 2010; 33: 319–325.

89. Khalyfa A, Serpero LD, Kheirandish-Gozal L, et al. TNF-α gene polymorphisms and excessive daytime sleepiness in pediatric obstructive sleep apnea. J Pediatr 2011; 158: 77–82.

90. Weider DJ, Hauri PJ. Nocturnal enuresis in children with upper airway obstruction. Int J Pediatr Otorhinolaryngol 1985; 9: 173–182.

91. Jeyakumar A, Rahman SI, Armbrecht ES, et al. The association between sleep-disordered breathing and enuresis in children. Laryngoscope 2012; 122: 1873–1877.

92. Sans Capdevila O, Crabtree VM, Kheirandish-Gozal L, et al. Increased morning brain natriuretic peptide levels in children with nocturnal enuresis and sleep-disordered breathing: a community-based study. Pediatrics 2008; 121: e1208–e1214.

93. Reuveni H, Simon T, Tal A, et al. Health care services utilization in children with obstructive sleep apnea syndrome. Pediatrics 2002; 110: 68–72.

94. Tarasiuk A, Greenberg-Dotan S, Simon-Tuval T, et al. Elevated morbidity and health care use in children with obstructive sleep apnea syndrome. Am J Respir Crit Care Med 2007; 175: 55–61.

95. Tarasiuk A, Simon T, Tal A, et al. Adenotonsillectomy in children with obstructive sleep apnea syndrome reduces health care utilization. Pediatrics 2004; 113: 351–356.

96. Tsou YA, Lin CC, Lai CH, et al. Does adenotonsillectomy really reduced clinic visits for pediatric upper respiratory tract infections? A national database study in Taiwan. Int J Pediatr Otorhinolaryngol 2013; 77: 677–681.

97. Wise MS, Nichols CD, Grigg-Damberger MM, et al. Executive summary of respiratory indications for polysomnography in children: an evidence-based review. Sleep 2011; 34: 389–398.

98. Aurora RN, Zak RS, Karippot A, et al. Practice parameters for the respiratory indications for polysomnography in children. Sleep 2011; 34: 379–388.

99. Luz Alonso-Alvarez M, Canet T, Cubell-Alarco M, et al. Documento de consenso del síndrome de apneas-hipopneas durante el sueño en niños (versión completa) [Consensus document on sleep apnea-hypopnea syndrome in children (full version)]. Arch Bronconeumol 2011; 47: Suppl. 5, 2–18.

100. Thurnheer R, Bloch KE, Laube I, et al. Respiratory polygraphy in sleep apnoea diagnosis. Report of the Swiss respiratory polygraphy registry and systematic review of the literature. Swiss Med Wkly 2007; 137: 97–102.

101. Royal College of Paediatrics and Child Health, Working Party on Sleep Physiology and Respiratory Control Disorders in Childhood. Standards for Services for Children with Disorders of Sleep. London, RCPCH, 2009.

102. Kaditis A, Kheirandish-Gozal L, Gozal D. Algorithm for the diagnosis and treatment of pediatric OSA: a proposal of two pediatric sleep centers. *Sleep Med* 2012; 13: 217–227.

103. Gozal D, Kheirandish-Gozal L. New approaches to the diagnosis of sleep-disordered breathing in children. *Sleep Med* 2010; 11: 708–713.

104. Cantarella G, Viglione S, Forti S, *et al.* Comparing postoperative quality of life in children after microdebrider intracapsular tonsillotomy and tonsillectomy. *Auris Nasus Larynx* 2012; 39: 407–410.

105. Ericsson E, Lundeborg I, Hultcrantz E. Child behavior and quality of life before and after tonsillotomy *versus* tonsillectomy. *Int J Pediatr Otorhinolaryngol* 2009; 73: 1254–1262.

106. Marcus CL. Concerns regarding the pediatric component of the AASM clinical guidelines for the manual titration of positive airway pressure in patients with obstructive sleep apnea. *J Clin Sleep Med* 2008; 4: 607–609.

107. Liner LH, Marcus CL. Ventilatory management of sleep-disordered breathing in children. *Curr Opin Pediatr* 2006; 18: 272–276.

108. DiFeo N, Meltzer LJ, Beck SE, *et al.* Predictors of positive airway pressure therapy adherence in children: a prospective study. *J Clin Sleep Med* 2012; 8: 279–286.

109. King MS, Xanthopoulos MS, Marcus CL. Improving positive airway pressure adherence in children. *Sleep Med Clin* 2014; 9: 219–234.

110. Marcus CL, Beck SE, Traylor J, *et al.* Randomized, double-blind clinical trial of two different modes of positive airway pressure therapy on adherence and efficacy in children. *J Clin Sleep Med* 2012; 8: 37–42.

111. Marcus CL, Rosen G, Ward SL, *et al.* Adherence to and effectiveness of positive airway pressure therapy in children with obstructive sleep apnea. *Pediatrics* 2006; 117: e442–e451.

112. Sawyer AM, Gooneratne NS, Marcus CL, *et al.* A systematic review of CPAP adherence across age groups: clinical and empiric insights for developing CPAP adherence interventions. *Sleep Med Rev* 2011; 15: 343–356.

113. Koontz KL, Slifer KJ, Cataldo MD, *et al.* Improving pediatric compliance with positive airway pressure therapy: the impact of behavioral intervention. *Sleep* 2003; 26: 1010–1015.

114. McGinley B, Halbower A, Schwartz AR, *et al.* Effect of a high-flow open nasal cannula system on obstructive sleep apnea in children. *Pediatrics* 2009; 124: 179–188.

115. Kheirandish-Gozal L, Kim J, Goldbart AD, *et al.* Novel pharmacological approaches for treatment of obstructive sleep apnea in children. *Expert Opin Investig Drugs* 2013; 22: 71–85.

116. Goldbart AD, Goldman JL, Li RC, *et al.* Differential expression of cysteinyl leukotriene receptors 1 and 2 in tonsils of children with obstructive sleep apnea syndrome or recurrent infection. *Chest* 2004; 126: 13–18.

117. Dayyat E, Serpero LD, Kheirandish-Gozal L, *et al.* Leukotriene pathways and *in vitro* adenotonsillar cell proliferation in children with obstructive sleep apnea. *Chest* 2009; 135: 1142–1149.

118. Goldbart AD, Goldman JL, Veling MC, *et al.* Leukotriene modifier therapy for mild sleep-disordered breathing in children. *Am J Respir Crit Care Med* 2005; 172: 364–370.

119. Goldbart AD, Greenberg-Dotan S, Tal A. Montelukast for children with obstructive sleep apnea: a double-blind, placebo-controlled study. *Pediatrics* 2012; 130: e575–e580.

120. Kheirandish-Gozal L, Serpero LD, Dayyat E, *et al.* Corticosteroids suppress *in vitro* tonsillar proliferation in children with obstructive sleep apnoea. *Eur Respir J* 2009; 33: 1077–1084.

121. Kheirandish-Gozal L, Gozal D. Intranasal budesonide treatment for children with mild obstructive sleep apnea syndrome. *Pediatrics* 2008; 122: e149–e155.

122. Brouillette RT, Manoukian JJ, Ducharme FM, *et al.* Efficacy of fluticasone nasal spray for pediatric obstructive sleep apnea. *J Pediatr* 2001; 138: 838–844.

123. Kheirandish L, Goldbart AD, Gozal D. Intranasal steroids and oral leukotriene modifier therapy in residual sleep-disordered breathing after tonsillectomy and adenoidectomy in children. *Pediatrics* 2006; 117: e61–e66.

124. Kheirandish-Gozal L, Bhattacharjee R, Bandla HP, *et al.* Antiinflammatory therapy outcomes for mild OSA in children. *Chest* 2014; 146: 88–95.

125. Guilleminault C, Monteyrol PJ, Huynh NT, *et al.* Adeno-tonsillectomy and rapid maxillary distraction in pre-pubertal children, a pilot study. *Sleep Breath* 2011; 15: 173–177.

126. Pirelli P, Saponara M, Guilleminault C. Rapid maxillary expansion in children with obstructive sleep apnea syndrome. *Sleep* 2004; 27: 761–766.

127. Hartzell LD, Guillory RM, Munson PD, *et al.* Tongue base suspension in children with cerebral palsy and obstructive sleep apnea. *Int J Pediatr Otorhinolaryngol* 2013; 77: 534–537.

128. Guilleminault C, Huang YS, Monteyrol PJ, *et al.* Critical role of myofascial reeducation in pediatric sleep-disordered breathing. *Sleep Med* 2013; 14: 518–525.

129. Lin AC, Koltai PJ. Sleep endoscopy in the evaluation of pediatric obstructive sleep apnea. *Int J Pediatr* 2012; 2012: 576719.

130. Kureshi SA, Gallagher PR, McDonough JM, *et al.* Pilot study of nasal expiratory positive airway pressure devices for the treatment of childhood obstructive sleep apnea syndrome. *J Clin Sleep Med* 2014; 10: 663–669.

131. Becker L, Kheirandish-Gozal L, Peris E, *et al.* Contextualised urinary biomarker analysis facilitates diagnosis of paediatric obstructive sleep apnoea. *Sleep Med* 2014; 15: 541–549.
132. Kheirandish-Gozal L, McManus CJ, Kellermann GH, *et al.* Urinary neurotransmitters are selectively altered in children with obstructive sleep apnea and predict cognitive morbidity. *Chest* 2013; 143: 1576–1583.
133. Khalyfa A, Gozal D. Exosomal miRNAs as potential biomarkers of cardiovascular risk in children. *J Transl Med* 2014; 12: 162.

Support statement: L. Kheirandish-Gozal and D. Gozal are supported by US National Institutes of Health grant HL-65270.

Disclosures: None declared.

Chapter 10

OHS: definition, diagnosis, pathophysiology and management

Juan Fernando Masa[1,2], Jean Paul Janssens[3], Jean Christian Borel[4,5,6,7] and Jean-Louis Pépin[5,6,7]

Obesity hypoventilation syndrome (OHS) is defined as a combination of obesity (BMI ≥ 30 kg·m^{-2}), daytime hypercapnia (arterial carbon dioxide tension ≥ 45 mmHg) and sleep disordered breathing after ruling out other disorders that may cause alveolar hypoventilation. OHS is a chronic condition associated with impairments of body structures or functions, leading to a decrease in daily life activities, a lack of social participation, and high risk of hospitalisation and death. Despite its severity, OHS is largely underdiagnosed. This chapter discusses the definition, epidemiology, physiopathology and treatment modalities. Clinicians should adapt treatment modalities, aiming to improve the specific impairments, dysfunctions and handicaps of each OHS patient. From this perspective, the three main strategies available are nocturnal PAP therapies (NIV/CPAP), body weight loss strategies and rehabilitation.

O besity hypoventilation syndrome (OHS) is defined as the combination of obesity (BMI ≥ 30 kg·m^{-2}), daytime hypercapnia (arterial carbon dioxide tension (PaCO$_2$) ≥ 45 mmHg) and various types of sleep disordered breathing after ruling out other disorders that may cause alveolar hypoventilation (obstructive or restrictive pulmonary diseases, chest wall disorders, neuromuscular diseases, severe hypothyroidism and congenital central hypoventilation syndrome) [1]. 70–90% of patients with OHS also have OSA syndrome (OSAS) [2, 3] while 10–15% of sleep apnoea patients referred to the sleep laboratory have diurnal hypercapnia and can be classified as having OHS [4].

This definition, based on a single measurement of PaCO$_2$, is considered by some authors as too restrictive and may miss early stages of OHS when hypoventilation remains limited to the sleep period [5]. It has been proposed to add the presence of an arterial base excess >3 mmol·L^{-1} or a standard bicarbonate concentration >27 mmol·L^{-1} in the absence of another cause of metabolic alkalosis to the definition [6]. Although metabolic alkalosis is often difficult to exclude in obese patients with comorbidities and on-going treatments, the high sensitivity of bicarbonate in detecting OHS can alert clinicians to search for it [7]. Further studies are needed to better validate the appropriate threshold of bicarbonate that would clearly define OHS in ambulatory obese subjects.

[1]Pulmonary Division, San Pedro de Alcantara Hospital, Caceres, Spain. [2]CIBER de enfermedades respiratorias (CIBERES), Madrid, Spain. [3]Service de Pneumologie, Hôpital Cantonal Universitaire, Geneva, Switzerland. [4]AGIR á dom Association, Meylan, France. [5]Grenoble Alpes University, HP2 Laboratory, Grenoble, France. [6]INSERM U1042, Grenoble, France. [7]Clinique Universitaire de Physiologie et Sommeil, Pôle Thorax et Vaisseaux, Hôpital A. Michallon, Grenoble, France.

Correspondence: Jean-Louis Pépin, Laboratoire EFCR, CHU de Grenoble, BP217X, 38043 Grenoble cedex 09, France. E-mail: jpepin@chu-grenoble.fr

Copyright ©ERS 2015. Print ISBN: 978-1-84984-059-0. Online ISBN: 978-1-84984-060-6. Print ISSN: 2312-508X. Online ISSN: 2312-5098.

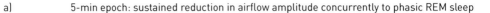

a)   5-min epoch: sustained reduction in airflow amplitude concurrently to phasic REM sleep

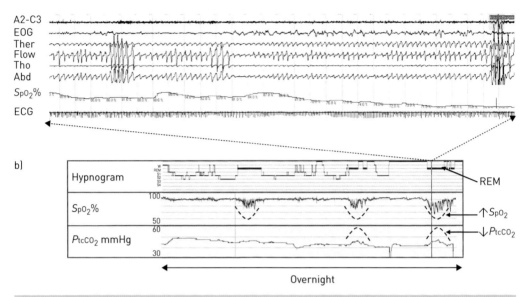

Figure 1. Polysomnographic pattern of REM sleep hypoventilation. a) 5-min epoch. A2-C3: electroencephalogram; SpO_2: blood oxygen saturation measured by pulse oximetry; Tho: thoracic movements; Abd: abdominal movements; Ther: bucconasal thermistor; Flow: nasal pressure; EOG: electro-oculogram. b) Overnight hypnogram: transcutaneous carbon dioxide tension ($PtcCO_2$) trends clearly depict a significant increase in $PtcCO_2$ during REM sleep concurrently to a sustained oxygen desaturation. The trend of variation is more important than absolute value. Reproduced from [11] with permission from the authors.

Diagnosis

The aforementioned definition is applicable to stable patients; two thirds of OHS cases are diagnosed in this situation. The clinical presentation differs slightly from the classical patient referred to the sleep laboratory for suspicion of a sleep breathing disorder. These patients are more likely to have class III obesity, to complain of severe sleepiness and to exhibit multimorbid conditions including right HF [8, 9]. PSG shows prolonged apnoeas, hypopnoeas and/or episodes of severe continuous desaturation during REM sleep suggestive of REM sleep hypoventilation. Adding transcutaneous carbon dioxide tension ($PtcCO_2$) monitoring to PSG is helpful to confirm the presence of episodes of sleep hypoventilation [10] (fig. 1).

One third of OHS patients are diagnosed when hospitalised for acute respiratory failure [12–15]. Furthermore, Carrillo et al. [16] recently reported that about two-thirds of patients admitted to an intensive care unit (ICU) for acute hypercapnic respiratory failure (AHRF) due to obesity hypoventilation had already been admitted for similar episodes of AHRF but had not been treated by home noninvasive ventilation (NIV) or CPAP after their first episode. This highlights that OHS is underdiagnosed or that the diagnosis is dramatically delayed [17]. A better awareness of OHS and systematic screening for hypercapnia or elevated bicarbonates in patients with obesity is desirable, particularly in primary care settings and obesity clinics.

Epidemiology

Although the overall prevalence of OHS has never been directly assessed in the general population, it is currently estimated that OHS concerns 3.7 out of 1000 persons in the US population [18]. Prevalence of OHS has been reported in patients referred to sleep clinics for suspected sleep disordered breathing [3, 9], in patients already diagnosed with OSA [4, 19–21] and in a cohort of hospitalised obese patients [22]. It is estimated between 10% and 20% in patients referred to sleep laboratories, and reaches 20–30% in patients already diagnosed with OSA and in hospitalised, obese adult subjects. There is a linear relationship between obesity, as expressed by BMI, and OHS prevalence [3, 4, 22]. Over the past decade, the general progression of obesity seems to have stabilised in the USA [23]. However, extreme obesity among adults is still increasing [24, 25]. Thus, it can be anticipated that both prevalence and incidence of OHS will increase in forthcoming years.

Socioeconomic consequences and mortality of OHS

Direct health costs (*i.e.* general practitioners' services, hospital services and medications) per year of an OHS patient can reach twice those of an OSA patient [26] or an obese eucapnic patient [8] and about six times the expenses of an age-, sex- and socioeconomic status-matched control subject [26]. This health cost burden is a corollary of a lower labour income and employment rate in OHS patients than in patients with OSA or control subjects [26]. Beyond these social consequences, OHS patients have a higher risk of death compared with eucapnic obese individuals, particularly when they are left untreated [14, 17, 22].

Pathophysiology

Daytime hypoventilation in obese patients results from the conjunction of several factors that interact to overwhelm the compensatory mechanisms of carbon dioxide homeostasis.

Respiratory mechanics

A decrease in lung volumes (vital capacity, total lung capacity and FRC) has been reported as a determinant of daytime hypercapnia in obese patients [3, 4, 21, 27, 28]. This restriction is associated with decreases in total respiratory system compliance and lung compliance [29], and with an increase in work of breathing [30–32]. The decrease in lung volume is usually related to fat mass, and intrathoracic and abdominal fat distribution [33, 34]. These fat deposits could have direct mechanical effects on respiratory function by impeding diaphragm motion, and changing the balance of elastic recoil between the chest wall and lung. Another possible mechanism may involve the low-grade inflammation associated with excess visceral and intrathoracic adiposity that might induce specific muscle impairment [35, 36].

Respiratory muscle function

Although studies have shown that weight loss improves the strength/endurance of respiratory muscles [37, 38], the question of whether there is inspiratory muscle weakness in OHS is still debated. OHS patients are able to temporarily correct hypoventilation by voluntarily hyperventilating [21]. Additionally, in OHS patients, during spontaneous breathing [32] and hypercapnia-induced hyperventilation [39], trans-diaphragmatic pressure has been documented as higher or at least equivalent to values reported in obese eucapnic patients. Taken together, these results suggest that muscle function may be only slightly impaired but cannot cope with the overload imposed on the respiratory system. The underlying causes of respiratory muscle dysfunction that may co-exist in OHS include inflammation [35, 36] and somatotopic axis impairment [40]. Further studies are needed to explore respiratory muscle structure and function in OHS in detail.

Sleep disordered breathing

It is largely recognised that most OHS patients suffer from an OSAS [41] and its severity is a key component in the development of diurnal hypoventilation [42]. The pattern of sleep apnoea also contributes to this hypoventilation, with two mechanisms involved: 1) the mean duration of apnoea and hypopnoea is increased with a reduced duration of inter-apnoea ventilation [43]; and 2) there is insufficient post-event ventilatory compensation [44].

Another type of sleep respiratory abnormality encountered in patients with OHS is central hypoventilation, which is characterised by a sustained reduction in ventilation associated with a constant or reduced respiratory drive [45, 46]. Hypoventilation is more pronounced during REM sleep [45] and the severity of REM sleep hypoventilation is associated with a blunted awake ventilatory response to carbon dioxide [46].

Ventilatory drive

NORMAN et al. [47] proposed a computational model that unifies acute hypercapnia during sleep breathing events with chronic sustained hypoventilation during wakefulness. In this model, the persistence of an elevated bicarbonate concentration after the sleep period (characterised by repetitive, acute hypercapnic events), possibly due to either an alteration of renal excretion or a reduction in ventilatory drive (or both), further blunts ventilatory response to carbon dioxide, which in turn increases $PaCO_2$.

Another hypothesis, evoked as a possible mechanism of alteration in ventilator drive, is the participation of neurohumoural agents such as the adipokine leptin, a powerful ventilatory stimulant [48]. This hypothesis is supported by animal studies. However, in humans, congenital leptin deficiency exists but is very rare [49]. In obese subjects, circulating leptin levels are often higher than in nonobese subjects [50]. These results suggest that a central resistance to leptin may occur in obesity and particularly in OHS. A possible mechanism for this central resistance could be deficient leptin transport through the blood–brain barrier [51, 52].

Management

OHS is a chronic condition associated with impairments of body structures (UA and respiratory muscles) or body functions (control of breathing, sleep, cardiovascular and metabolic), decrease in activities and a lack of social participation [11] (fig. 2). Clinicians should adapt treatment modalities, aiming to improve the specific impairments, dysfunctions and handicaps of each OHS patient. From this perspective, the three main strategies available to clinicians are PAP therapies (CPAP and/or NIV), body weight loss strategies and rehabilitation.

PAP therapies

PAP therapies (CPAP and/or NIV) represent the first-line therapy for sleep breathing disorders. The choice of nocturnal CPAP versus NIV is often based on the underlying sleep-related respiratory abnormality encountered.

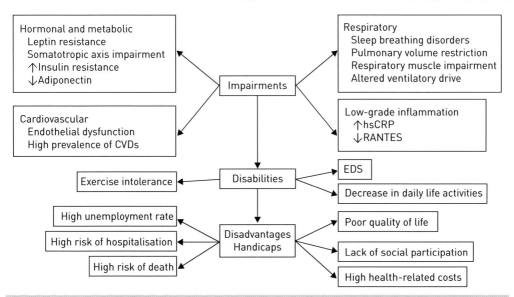

Figure 2. Obesity hypoventilation syndrome: a chronic condition observed through the prism of the International Classification of Functioning. Reproduced from [11] with permission from the authors. hsCRP: high-sensitivity C-reactive protein; RANTES: regulated on activation, normal T-cell expressed and secreted.

Impact of NIV on clinical and functional outcomes

Nonrandomised studies have reported improvement in clinical symptoms and reduction in PaCO$_2$ in OHS patients treated with NIV [14, 46, 53–58]. A randomised study allocated 37 OHS patients with mild hypercapnia to either NIV or a control group and found significant improvement for the NIV group in PaCO$_2$ and bicarbonates, but not in arterial oxygen tension (PaO$_2$) [59]. Adherence to NIV is essential to obtain optimal results and may explain differences in results between studies. Two studies analysed the relationship between improvement in daytime PaCO$_2$ and adherence [60, 61] and showed that an adherence for more than 4 h per day is required. Other respiratory functional tests (spirometry or static volumes) improved with NIV in two randomised studies [59, 61] and in some clinical series [53–55] but results are not consistent across studies [14, 62]. There is no clear explanation for these differences, although the level of IPAP or EPAP, type of ventilatory mode, compliance and degree of obesity may be interesting issues to be investigated. MURPHY et al. [61] suggested that NIV can increase daytime physical activity measured by actigraphy and potentially favour weight loss. However, this study included patients both in a stable state and post-acute respiratory failure. Patients post-acute respiratory failure were likely to have low physical activity at baseline and an improvement in activity was expected after 3 months of recovery. A significant increase in 6-min walking distance has also been reported after NIV treatment in association with a significant reduction in pulmonary artery SBP [63, 64].

After 6 months of NIV, pulmonary artery SBP, measured by echocardiography, decreased in patients with previous pulmonary hypertension [63]. These favourable changes may be caused by the daytime respiratory functional improvement, the prevention of obstructive events and hypoventilation during sleep rather than a direct effect on the pre- and post-load of the right ventricle.

Although NIV is mainly applied during sleep, there are few studies assessing the impact of NIV on sleep parameters. One randomised [59] and two nonrandomised studies [46, 65] showed an improvement in sleep quality, an important reduction in AHI and arterial oxygen saturation (S_{aO_2}), and improvements in P_{tcCO_2} [65].

Overall, studies have found an improvement in health-related quality of life (HRQoL) with NIV [8, 13, 15, 57]. This is mainly due to the suppression of sleep breathing disorders and associated symptoms.

Impact of CPAP on clinical and functional outcomes

Despite the fact that CPAP was used earlier than NIV to treat OHS [66], there are fewer studies assessing its efficacy. "Nonresponders" to CPAP are classically more obese (BMI >40 kg·m^{-2}), with a higher P_{aCO_2}, a lower P_{aO_2} and more severe oxygen desaturation during the night [67–69]. CPAP adherence is again crucial to achieve treatment goals [60]. One open study compared the improvement in daytime P_{aCO_2} with CPAP and NIV treatments, after selecting patients with predominantly nocturnal central hypoventilation to be treated by NIV and those with predominantly obstructive events to use CPAP [70]. The daytime P_{aCO_2} improved similarly in both groups, emphasising the role of predominant obstructive events as a predictor of CPAP treatment success in OHS. In the only RCT available in the field, similar results were observed when comparing the efficacy of CPAP and NIV on P_{aCO_2} in 36 OHS patients [71]. However, this study excluded patients with persistent desaturations on CPAP, who are supposedly good candidates for NIV. Therefore, although large studies comparing CPAP to NIV in patients with and without severe obstructive sleep apnoea–hypopnoea syndrome (OSAHS) are lacking, it seems reasonable to use CPAP as first line therapy for OHS with severe OSAHS without REM hypoventilation and NIV for other OHS patients (fig. 3). HRQoL seems to improve slightly more with NIV than with CPAP [71, 72] but this remains to be confirmed in larger studies.

Long-term results of CPAP and NIV

There are no randomised studies comparing long term results of NIV *versus* either CPAP or a control group. In clinical series, P_{aO_2} and P_{aCO_2} improvements with NIV were maintained after 12 [54] and 54 months [14]. Two longitudinal studies observed reductions in hospitalisation days after NIV treatment [56] or both CPAP and NIV treatments [8]. In addition, there was a significant linear reduction in physician visits and fees. Therefore, NIV and CPAP can reduce the high economic burden of OHS [8, 15] although more specific cost-effectiveness studies are required.

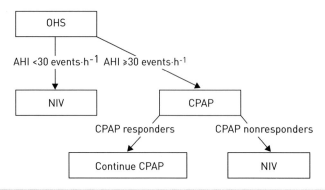

Figure 3. Obesity hypoventilation syndrome (OHS) management algorithm. NIV: noninvasive ventilation.

A nonrandomised study including 28 OHS patients under NIV found that mortality in compliant *versus* noncompliant patients was 1% and 37%, respectively [14]. In a retrospective cohort of 126 OHS patients treated chronically with NIV, mortality at 18 months was reduced to 3% [53]. Overall, NIV reduces mortality in adherent OHS patients in comparison with untreated patients [17].

Titration and settings

The usual CPAP titration protocol increases pressure to remove apnoea, hypopnoea, flow limitation and snoring [73] (fig. 4). Because OHS patients are generally more obese than OSA patients, effective CPAP pressure is expected to be higher in OHS than in OSA patients [60]. It has been proposed [71, 74] to continue to increase pressure when persistent desaturations remain after suppression of obstructive events. The goal here is to increase FRC and try to reduce REM hypoventilation. Further studies are needed to demonstrate whether increasing CPAP pressure beyond the level required for suppressing obstructive events is really effective in reducing nocturnal hypoventilation. Studies comparing the efficacy and cost-effectiveness of CPAP titration under PSG to simplified procedures (*i.e.* respiratory polygraphy or oximetry plus PtcCO$_2$) are also lacking.

Recently, guidelines for nocturnal NIV titration were published by the American Academic of Sleep Medicine (AASM) [75] recommending PSG for implementing NIV, although there is no convincing evidence supporting the systematic use of PSG for NIV titration in OHS. Oximetry and probably PtcCO$_2$ may represent a first approach [76], at least in a group of patients. Accordingly, in the literature, many studies used nocturnal oximetry and PtcCO$_2$ to refine NIV settings [61], and only two [59, 71] used PSG titration to improve hypoventilation and eliminate obstructive events. Two protocols can be used to increase EPAP and IPAP (fig. 5). Usually, EPAP is adjusted to suppress apnoeas and hypopnoeas while IPAP aims to correct hypoventilation [59, 71, 77]. The "default" ventilator mode presently used for OHS in most centres is bilevel pressure support ventilation in a spontaneous (S) or spontaneous/timed (S/T) mode. However, it has been previously shown that volume-cycled ventilators are also efficient for stabilising OHS patients after hypercapnic respiratory failure [57, 67, 78]. There is a controversy regarding the use of an

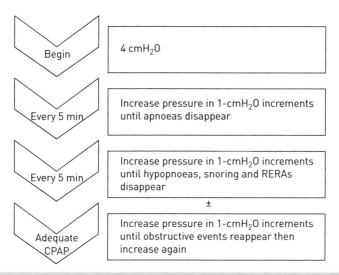

Figure 4. CPAP titration protocol. RERA: respiratory effort-related arousal.

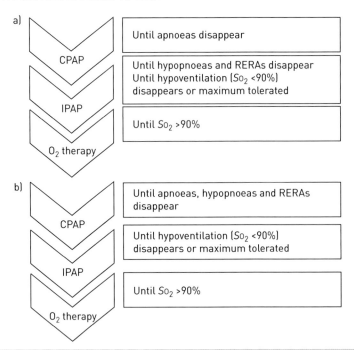

Figure 5. Protocols for noninvasive ventilation titration (BPAP). RERA: respiratory effort-related arousal; So_2: oxygen saturation.

S *versus* an S/T mode. The AASM recommends using bilevel pressure support in S mode as a default modality [75] unless a significant number of central events are present. Conversely, CONTAL *et al.* [79] found, in OHS patients under long-term NIV, that switching to an S mode generated a high number of central events. Earlier studies in healthy subjects had also shown that positive pressure ventilation generated a high number of central events with an S than with an S/T mode [80]. It is generally admitted, at least in Europe, that a high back-up rate is the most appropriate setting for OHS. Rise time is adjusted according to patient comfort; inspiratory time is set to provide an inspiratory/expiratory time ratio between 1/1 and 1/1.5; and the cycling criterion is set as a low of peak inspiratory flow, compensating for the tendency of pressure-cycled ventilators to cycle prematurely under restrictive conditions [81]. Under NIV, asynchronies between the patient and ventilator may occur. Patient–ventilator asynchronies can have a negative impact on sleep quality or correction of hypoventilation [82, 83]. This justifies a systematic overnight monitoring under NIV with the aim of adjusting ventilator settings and interface to suppress abnormal residual events [76, 84]. Future studies should be dedicated to demonstrating the benefits of correcting patient–ventilator asynchronies, the cost-effectiveness of simpler titration procedures than PSG or to validating automatic titration by bilevel ventilators outside the sleep laboratory.

Volume-targeting mode
Over recent years, several ventilator manufacturers have developed a "volume-targeting" option, which aims to guarantee that the ventilator provides a pre-set minimal tidal volume (V_T) (monitored continuously by a built-in pneumotachograph), despite position-related changes in respiratory compliance or sleep-related events. Two studies in OHS showed that volume-targeted ventilation might slightly improve the correction of nocturnal hypoventilation compared with conventional bilevel pressure support; in one of these

studies, this was at the expense of a lesser quality of sleep [65, 85], as variations in pressure might induce microarousals. One prospective RCT of 46 patients over a 3-month period [61] did not find any difference between volume targeting and conventional bilevel pressure support in terms of correction of alveolar hypoventilation or HRQoL. The clinical relevance of this option has, thus, yet to be clarified, and should presently be restricted for selected cases with residual periods of nocturnal hypoventilation after having optimised conventional settings [86].

Acute-on-chronic exacerbation

One of the most common presentations of OHS is an acute-on-chronic exacerbation with respiratory acidosis leading to admission to an ICU [15]. CPAP has virtually no place in this clinical situation. Prompt initiation of NIV, without sleep study confirmation, is indicated and reduces the need for invasive mechanical ventilation and probably mortality [87]. Due to the presence of associated comorbid conditions [13], OHS patients in acute-on-chronic exacerbation may develop haemodynamic instability that, added to acute respiratory failure, requires ICU monitoring. During PAP therapy, careful observation and monitoring of the level of consciousness, vital signs, SaO_2 and arterial blood gases (ABGs) are the standard of care [87]. NIV can be initiated with an EPAP of 6–8 cmH_2O to re-open and stabilise the UA. EPAP should then be increased until SaO_2 oscillations (IH) disappear during sleep. IPAP is gradually increased until an acceptable level of steady-state oxygen saturation (>90%) is achieved. If the patient continues to have persistent hypoxaemia despite the delivery of high pressure to eliminate hypoventilation, oxygen should be administered through the mask. The use of oxygen without NIV should be discouraged. At least two RCTs, in OHS in the stable condition, demonstrate that oxygen causes worsening hypercapnia [88, 89]. Even breathing moderate concentrations supplemental oxygen for 20 min worsened hypercapnia, and induced acidaemia due to hypoventilation and a worsening of the deadspace volume/VT ratio [89]. Respiratory stimulants can theoretically increase respiratory drive and improve daytime hypercapnia, but the data and clinical usefulness are extremely limited [1].

Non-PAP treatment modalities

Although NIV is a major component of the treatment of OHS, it does not treat the underlying cause of OHS, i.e. obesity, and has no direct impact on the multiple comorbidities associated with obesity. In addition, NIV may fail or be poorly tolerated. It is therefore important to explore other therapeutic options for OHS, such as surgical or nonsurgical weight reduction, exercise, respiratory stimulants or use of oxygen, which may either enhance the benefits of NIV or, to some extent, provide an alternative in case of failure or intolerance to NIV.

Weight reduction

At least two large trials suggested that medical treatment alone yields results that are far below those of surgical approaches in obese subjects with a BMI above 35 $kg·m^{-2}$, without providing detailed information on the prevalence of OHS or on ABGs in the populations studied [90, 91]. Indeed, there is a general consensus that obese subjects with a BMI >40 $kg·m^{-2}$ in whom nonsurgical approaches have failed or subjects with a BMI >35 $kg·m^{-2}$ and weight-related comorbidities are candidates for bariatric surgery. Common surgical procedures include vertical banded gastroplasty (VBG), adjustable gastric banding, Roux-en-Y gastric bypass (RYGBP) and biliopancreatic diversion with or without duodenal switch. RYGBP appears to provide the best results for long-term weight loss [91]. Associated mortality and morbidity are low in expert centres: a large Swedish study reported a 30-day death rate of 0.3% and occurrence of a major adverse event in 4.3% of patients undergoing a RYGBP [90].

A few authors have studied the impact of bariatric surgery on OSAHS and OHS. SUGERMAN et al. [92] analysed the outcome of patients with morbid obesity and respiratory failure who underwent bariatric surgery. In a subset of 40 patients with pre- and post-surgery PSGs, AHI decreased very significantly from mean±SD 64±39 events·h^{-1} (baseline), to 33 ±27 events·h^{-1} (after 1 year) and 32±32 events·h^{-1} (last visit). For patients for whom ABG were available, PaCO$_2$ also decreased significantly from baseline (53±9 mmHg) to last visit (47±12 mmHg). Of the 38 patients with OHS, 29 (76%) became asymptomatic 5.8 ±2.4 years after surgery.

BOONE et al. [93] followed 35 obese patients with OSAHS with or without OHS undergoing VBG. Use of CPAP decreased from 24 (68%) to eight (22%) subjects studied after VBG. In OSAHS patients, AHI dropped from 45±11 events· h^{-1} at baseline to 12±6 events· h^{-1} after surgery. PaCO$_2$ also decreased from 55±4 to 41±3 Torr after VBG.

In another study by MARTI-VALERI et al. [94], 30 morbidly obese patients on either CPAP or NIV underwent RYGBP. 1 year after the procedure, hypoxaemia, hypercapnia, spirometry and PSG results had all significantly improved, and treatment with PAP (CPAP or NIV) was required in only 14% of patients.

A recent, uncontrolled Italian study [95] described 102 morbidly obese patients undergoing "malabsorptive" biliodigestive surgery, of whom 16 (15.7%) had OHS and 22 (21.7%) OSAHS. Weight loss ranged from 45% to 64% of baseline after 3–5 years. Post-operatively, no patient fulfilled the criteria for OHS and only two patients required CPAP for residual OSAHS.

Bariatric surgery is thus not only associated with a very significant weight reduction but is also effective in decreasing OSAHS and OHS, and is considered a "metabolic surgery" in as much as it impacts on comorbidities and morbimortality [96]. Clinicians must, however, be aware of the time course of weight loss after bariatric surgery, with a maximal weight loss often reached 1 year after surgery and a possible relapse after a few years of follow-up. In addition, objective measurements (ABGs and sleep studies) are important as symptomatic improvements after surgery may not necessarily be corroborated by normalisation of AHI or ABGs.

Exercise and rehabilitation programmes
Although patients with OHS have a relatively preserved functional capacity compared with patients with other indications for long term NIV, their exercise tolerance is, on average, lower than that of obese eucapnic patients with OSAHS [97, 98]. They also often have a very limited social activity and lack motivation regarding rehabilitation programmes [26, 99]. The implementation of NIV could be an appropriate time to initiate a rehabilitation programme as nocturnal NIV itself may increase exercise tolerance [100]. Modalities of exercise training in this population require further studies. For instance, in patients who hypoventilate during exercise, NIV during exercise training may increase performance and efficacy of training [101–103]. Combining respiratory muscle training with a low-calorie diet and a physical activity programme may improve dyspnoea and exercise capacity more than physical activity and diet alone [104]. Finally, home-based neuromuscular electrical stimulation might help morbidly obese patients to return to at least a minimal level of physical activity.

Respiratory stimulants for OHS

Certain substances have been studied as possible adjuncts or alternatives to CPAP or NIV. A Cochrane review of 26 trials measuring the impact of 21 drugs on respiratory drive and OSAHS, including acetazolamide, medroxyprogesterone, aminophylline, theophylline, protriptyline and paroxetine, concluded that there was insufficient evidence to recommend drug therapy as a treatment for OSAHS [105]. Aminophylline increases minute ventilation, V_T, respiratory rate and parasternal intercostal muscle activity (electromyography) during hypoxia in humans; methylxanthines may also increase respiratory drive [106, 107].

In addition, in eight OHS patients, a high blood bicarbonate blood content was shown to blunt the ventilatory response to carbon dioxide and decrease occlusion pressure (measured 100 ms after initiation of tidal inspiration, an estimation of respiratory drive). Conversely, in these patients, acetazolamide reduced bicarbonate concentration and increased the ventilatory response to carbon dioxide [108]. The clinical relevance of these findings in the treatment of OHS remains undetermined and no medication can presently be considered as a surrogate for NIV in OHS.

Long-term oxygen therapy

Hypoxaemia results from two different physiological mechanisms in OHS, which may be combined: alveolar hypoventilation and ventilation (V')/perfusion (Q') mismatch. NIV and CPAP improve alveolar ventilation either by unloading the respiratory muscles and resetting the ventilatory response to carbon dioxide (NIV), or by decreasing UA resistance (related to OSAHS) and, thus, work of breathing (CPAP and NIV) [14, 15, 55, 57, 59]. Both approaches improve hypoxaemia and reduce V'/Q' mismatch [55]. Residual hypoxaemia under CPAP [109] or NIV is, however, well described [14, 74, 110, 111]: indeed, need for supplemental oxygen is an independent predictor of mortality in OHS patients treated by NIV [15, 53].

There is no clear rationale for long-term oxygen therapy (LTOT) without either CPAP or NIV in OHS, as LTOT does not decrease the work of breathing and, thus, will not improve alveolar ventilation, will have no effect on V'/Q' mismatch and alveolar recruitment, and may prolong obstructive hypopnoea or apnoea. Oxygen therapy may, in fact, have a deleterious impact in OHS [88, 89]. MASA *et al.* [58] studied 11 obese patients (42.9 ± 8 kg·m^{-2}) with nocturnal hypoventilation, treated sequentially by home nocturnal

Table 1. Treatments for obesity hypoventilation other than noninvasive positive pressure ventilation

Rehabilitation programmes are recommended for increasing exercise tolerance and daily activity, although RCTs are lacking
The initiation of nocturnal NIV could be the appropriate time to start a rehabilitation programme
Bariatric surgery induces more effective weight loss than medical and supportive management alone, improves sleep apnoea indices and hypoventilation in subjects with OHS and OSAHS
Respiratory stimulant drugs have a marginal impact in OHS and cannot be recommended
Long-term oxygen therapy must not be considered as an alternative to positive pressure therapy but may be indicated after optimal titration of NIV for "resistant hypoxaemia", although its long-term benefit has not been established

NIV: noninvasive ventilation; OHS: obesity hypoventilation syndrome; OSAHS: obstructive sleep apnoea–hypopnoea syndrome.

oxygen supplementation for 2 weeks followed by an equivalent period with nocturnal NIV. Oxygen tended to worsen nocturnal hypoventilation, aggravated morning headaches and morning obnubilation, and decreased sleep efficiency compared with room air or NIV. Thus, even in the absence of RCTs, available evidence shows that LTOT alone is inappropriate in OHS. Current evidence does not support the prescription of supplemental oxygen during adequately titrated nocturnal positive pressure therapy in patients with persistent desaturation who are not eligible for LTOT based on their daytime ABGs (PaO_2 <7.3 or <8 kPa with pulmonary hypertension, signs of cor pulmonale or right HF) (table 1).

References

1. Mokhlesi B. Obesity hypoventilation syndrome: a state-of-the-art review. *Respir Care* 2010; 55: 1347–1362.
2. Kessler R, Chaouat A, Schinkewitch P, *et al.* The obesity-hypoventilation syndrome revisited: a prospective study of 34 consecutive cases. *Chest* 2001; 120: 369–376.
3. Resta O, Foschino-Barbaro MP, Bonfitto P, *et al.* Prevalence and mechanisms of diurnal hypercapnia in a sample of morbidly obese subjects with obstructive sleep apnoea. *Respir Med* 2000; 94: 240–246.
4. Laaban JP, Chailleux E. Daytime hypercapnia in adult patients with obstructive sleep apnea syndrome in France, before initiating nocturnal nasal continuous positive airway pressure therapy. *Chest* 2005; 127: 710–715.
5. Manuel AR, Hart N, Stradling JR. Is a raised bicarbonate, without hypercapnia, part of the physiological spectrum of obesity-related hypoventilation? *Chest* 2014 [In press DOI: 10.1378/chest.14-1279].
6. Hart N, Mandal S, Manuel A, *et al.* Obesity hypoventilation syndrome: does the current definition need revisiting? *Thorax* 2014; 69: 83–84.
7. Tulaimat A, Littleton S. Defining obesity hypoventilation syndrome. *Thorax* 2014; 69: 491.
8. Berg G, Delaive K, Manfreda J, *et al.* The use of health-care resources in obesity-hypoventilation syndrome. *Chest* 2001; 120: 377–383.
9. Trakada GP, Steiropoulos P, Nena E, *et al.* Prevalence and clinical characteristics of obesity hypoventilation syndrome among individuals reporting sleep-related breathing symptoms in northern Greece. *Sleep Breath* 2010; 14: 381–386.
10. Berry RB, Budhiraja R, Gottlieb DJ, *et al.* Rules for scoring respiratory events in sleep: update of the 2007 AASM Manual for the Scoring of Sleep and Associated Events. Deliberations of the Sleep Apnea Definitions Task Force of the American Academy of Sleep Medicine. *J Clin Sleep Med* 2012; 8: 597–619.
11. Borel JC, Borel AL, Monneret D, *et al.* Obesity hypoventilation syndrome: from sleep disordered breathing to systemic comorbidities and the need to offer combined treatment strategies. *Respirology* 2012; 17: 601–610.
12. BaHammam A, Syed S, Al-Mughairy A. Sleep-related breathing disorders in obese patients presenting with acute respiratory failure. *Respir Med* 2005; 99: 718–725.
13. Borel J, Burel B, Tamisier R, *et al.* Comorbidities and mortality in hypercapnic obese under domiciliary noninvasive ventilation. *PLoS One* 2013; 8: e52006.
14. Perez de Llano LA, Golpe R, Ortiz Piquer M, *et al.* Short-term and long-term effects of nasal intermittent positive pressure ventilation in patients with obesity-hypoventilation syndrome. *Chest* 2005; 128: 587–594.
15. Priou P, Hamel JF, Person C, *et al.* Long-term outcome of noninvasive positive pressure ventilation for obesity hypoventilation syndrome. *Chest* 2010; 138: 84–90.
16. Carrillo A, Ferrer M, Gonzalez-Diaz G, *et al.* Noninvasive ventilation in acute hypercapnic respiratory failure caused by obesity hypoventilation syndrome and chronic obstructive pulmonary disease. *Am J Respir Crit Care Med* 2012; 186: 1279–1285.
17. Pepin JL, Borel JC, Janssens JP. Obesity hypoventilation syndrome: an underdiagnosed and undertreated condition. *Am J Respir Crit Care Med* 2012; 186: 1205–1207.
18. Mokhlesi B, Saager L, Kaw R. Q: Should we routinely screen for hypercapnia in sleep apnea patients before elective noncardiac surgery? *Cleve Clin J Med* 2010; 77: 60–61.
19. Akashiba T, Kawahara S, Kosaka N, *et al.* Determinants of chronic hypercapnia in Japanese men with obstructive sleep apnea syndrome. *Chest* 2002; 121: 415–421.
20. Golpe R, Jimenez A, Carpizo R. Diurnal hypercapnia in patients with obstructive sleep apnea syndrome. *Chest* 2002; 122: 1100–1101.
21. Leech JA, Onal E, Baer P, *et al.* Determinants of hypercapnia in occlusive sleep apnea syndrome. *Chest* 1987; 92: 807–813.
22. Nowbar S, Burkart KM, Gonzales R, *et al.* Obesity-associated hypoventilation in hospitalized patients: prevalence, effects, and outcome. *Am J Med* 2004; 116: 1–7.

23. Flegal KM, Carroll MD, Ogden CL, *et al.* Prevalence and trends in obesity among US adults, 1999–2008. *JAMA* 2010; 303: 235–241.

24. Sturm R. Increases in morbid obesity in the USA: 2000–2005. *Public Health* 2007; 121: 492–496.

25. Yanovski SZ, Yanovski JA. Obesity prevalence in the United States – up, down, or sideways? *N Engl J Med* 2011; 364: 987–989.

26. Jennum P, Kjellberg J. Health, social and economical consequences of sleep-disordered breathing: a controlled national study. *Thorax* 2011; 66: 560–566.

27. Akashiba T, Akahoshi T, Kawahara S, *et al.* Clinical characteristics of obesity-hypoventilation syndrome in Japan: a multi-center study. *Intern Med* 2006; 45: 1121–1125.

28. Mokhlesi B, Tulaimat A, Faibussowitsch I, *et al.* Obesity hypoventilation syndrome: prevalence and predictors in patients with obstructive sleep apnea. *Sleep Breath* 2007; 11: 117–124.

29. Behazin N, Jones SB, Cohen RI, *et al.* Respiratory restriction and elevated pleural and esophageal pressures in morbid obesity. *J Appl Physiol* 2010; 108: 212–218.

30. Lee MY, Lin CC, Shen SY, *et al.* Work of breathing in eucapnic and hypercapnic sleep apnea syndrome. *Respiration* 2009; 77: 146–153.

31. Lin CC, Wu KM, Chou CS, *et al.* Oral airway resistance during wakefulness in eucapnic and hypercapnic sleep apnea syndrome. *Respir Physiol Neurobiol* 2004; 139: 215–224.

32. Pankow W, Hijjeh N, Schuttler F, *et al.* Influence of noninvasive positive pressure ventilation on inspiratory muscle activity in obese subjects. *Eur Respir J* 1997; 10: 2847–2852.

33. Babb TG, Wyrick BL, DeLorey DS, *et al.* Fat distribution and end-expiratory lung volume in lean and obese men and women. *Chest* 2008; 134: 704–711.

34. Lazarus R, Sparrow D, Weiss ST. Effects of obesity and fat distribution on ventilatory function: the normative aging study. *Chest* 1997; 111: 891–898.

35. Lin WY, Yao CA, Wang HC, *et al.* Impaired lung function is associated with obesity and metabolic syndrome in adults. *Obesity (Silver Spring)* 2006; 14: 1654–1661.

36. Vassilakopoulos T, Hussain SN. Ventilatory muscle activation and inflammation: cytokines, reactive oxygen species, and nitric oxide. *J Appl Physiol* 2007; 102: 1687–1695.

37. Kelly TM, Jensen RL, Elliott CG, *et al.* Maximum respiratory pressures in morbidly obese subjects. *Respiration* 1988; 54: 73–77.

38. Weiner P, Waizman J, Weiner M, *et al.* Influence of excessive weight loss after gastroplasty for morbid obesity on respiratory muscle performance. *Thorax* 1998; 53: 39–42.

39. Sampson MG, Grassino K. Neuromechanical properties in obese patients during carbon dioxide rebreathing. *Am J Med* 1983; 75: 81–90.

40. Monneret D, Borel JC, Pepin JL, *et al.* Pleiotropic role of IGF-I in obesity hypoventilation syndrome. *Growth Horm IGF Res* 2010; 20: 127–133.

41. Rapoport DM. Obesity hypoventilation syndrome: more than just severe sleep apnea. *Sleep Med Rev* 2011; 15: 77–78.

42. Kaw R, Hernandez AV, Walker E, *et al.* Determinants of hypercapnia in obese patients with obstructive sleep apnea: a systematic review and metaanalysis of cohort studies. *Chest* 2009; 136: 787–796.

43. Ayappa I, Berger KI, Norman RG, *et al.* Hypercapnia and ventilatory periodicity in obstructive sleep apnea syndrome. *Am J Respir Crit Care Med* 2002; 166: 1112–1115.

44. Berger KI, Ayappa I, Sorkin IB, *et al.* Postevent ventilation as a function of CO_2 load during respiratory events in obstructive sleep apnea. *J Appl Physiol* 2002; 93: 917–924.

45. Becker HF, Piper AJ, Flynn WE, *et al.* Breathing during sleep in patients with nocturnal desaturation. *Am J Respir Crit Care Med* 1999; 159: 112–118.

46. Chouri-Pontarollo N, Borel JC, Tamisier R, *et al.* Impaired objective daytime vigilance in obesity-hypoventilation syndrome: impact of noninvasive ventilation. *Chest* 2007; 131: 148–155.

47. Norman RG, Goldring RM, Clain JM, *et al.* Transition from acute to chronic hypercapnia in patients with periodic breathing: predictions from a computer model. *J Appl Physiol* 2006; 100: 1733–1741.

48. O'Donnell C P, Schaub CD, Haines AS, *et al.* Leptin prevents respiratory depression in obesity. *Am J Respir Crit Care Med* 1999; 159: 1477–1484.

49. Montague CT, Farooqi IS, Whitehead JP, *et al.* Congenital leptin deficiency is associated with severe early-onset obesity in humans. *Nature* 1997; 387: 903–908.

50. Maffei M, Halaas J, Ravussin E, *et al.* Leptin levels in human and rodent: measurement of plasma leptin and ob RNA in obese and weight-reduced subjects. *Nat Med* 1995; 1: 1155–1161.

51. Caro JF, Kolaczynski JW, Nyce MR, *et al.* Decreased cerebrospinal-fluid/serum leptin ratio in obesity: a possible mechanism for leptin resistance. *Lancet* 1996; 348: 159–161.

52. Schwartz MW, Peskind E, Raskind M, *et al.* Cerebrospinal fluid leptin levels: relationship to plasma levels and to adiposity in humans. *Nat Med* 1996; 2: 589–593.

53. Budweiser S, Riedl SG, Jorres RA, *et al.* Mortality and prognostic factors in patients with obesity-hypoventilation syndrome undergoing noninvasive ventilation. *J Intern Med* 2007; 261: 375–383.

54. de Lucas-Ramos P, de Miguel-Diez J, Santacruz-Siminiani A, *et al.* Benefits at 1 year of nocturnal intermittent positive pressure ventilation in patients with obesity-hypoventilation syndrome. *Respir Med* 2004; 98: 961–967.

55. Heinemann F, Budweiser S, Dobroschke J, *et al.* Non-invasive positive pressure ventilation improves lung volumes in the obesity hypoventilation syndrome. *Respir Med* 2007; 101: 1229–1235.

56. Janssens JP, Derivaz S, Breitenstein E, *et al.* Changing patterns in long-term noninvasive ventilation: a 7-year prospective study in the Geneva Lake area. *Chest* 2003; 123: 67–79.

57. Masa JF, Celli BR, Riesco JA, *et al.* The obesity hypoventilation syndrome can be treated with noninvasive mechanical ventilation. *Chest* 2001; 119: 1102–1107.

58. Masa JF, Celli BR, Riesco JA, *et al.* Noninvasive positive pressure ventilation and not oxygen may prevent overt ventilatory failure in patients with chest wall diseases. *Chest* 1997; 112: 207–213.

59. Borel JC, Tamisier R, Gonzalez-Bermejo J, *et al.* Noninvasive ventilation in mild obesity hypoventilation syndrome: a randomized controlled trial. *Chest* 2012; 141: 692–702.

60. Mokhlesi B, Tulaimat A, Evans AT, *et al.* Impact of adherence with positive airway pressure therapy on hypercapnia in obstructive sleep apnea. *J Clin Sleep Med* 2006; 2: 57–62.

61. Murphy PB, Davidson C, Hind MD, *et al.* Volume targeted *versus* pressure support non-invasive ventilation in patients with super obesity and chronic respiratory failure: a randomised controlled trial. *Thorax* 2012; 67: 727–734.

62. Ojeda Castillejo E, de Lucas Ramos P, Lopez Martin S, *et al.* Ventilación mecánica no invasiva en pacientes con síndrome de obesidad-hipoventilación. Evolución a largo plazo y factores pronósticos. [Noninvasive mechanical ventilation in patients with obesity hypoventilation syndrome. Long-term outcome and prognostic factors.] *Arch Bronconeumol* 2014 [In press DOI: 10.1016/j.arbres.2014.02.015].

63. Castro-Anon O, Golpe R, Perez-de-Llano LA, *et al.* Haemodynamic effects of non-invasive ventilation in patients with obesity-hypoventilation syndrome. *Respirology* 2012; 17: 1269–1274.

64. Kauppert CA, Dvorak I, Kollert F, *et al.* Pulmonary hypertension in obesity-hypoventilation syndrome. *Respir Med* 2013; 107: 2061–2070.

65. Storre JH, Seuthe B, Fiechter R, *et al.* Average volume-assured pressure support in obesity hypoventilation: a randomized crossover trial. *Chest* 2006; 130: 815–821.

66. Rapoport DM, Sorkin B, Garay SM, *et al.* Reversal of the "Pickwickian syndrome" by long-term use of nocturnal nasal-airway pressure. *N Engl J Med* 1982; 307: 931–933.

67. Piper AJ, Sullivan CE. Effects of short-term NIPPV in the treatment of patients with severe obstructive sleep apnea and hypercapnia. *Chest* 1994; 105: 434–440.

68. Resta O, Guido P, Picca V, *et al.* Prescription of nCPAP and nBIPAP in obstructive sleep apnoea syndrome: Italian experience in 105 subjects. A prospective two centre study. *Respir Med* 1998; 92: 820–827.

69. Schafer H, Ewig S, Hasper E, *et al.* Failure of CPAP therapy in obstructive sleep apnoea syndrome: predictive factors and treatment with bilevel-positive airway pressure. *Respir Med* 1998; 92: 208–215.

70. Berger KI, Ayappa I, Chatr-Amontri B, *et al.* Obesity hypoventilation syndrome as a spectrum of respiratory disturbances during sleep. *Chest* 2001; 120: 1231–1238.

71. Piper AJ, Wang D, Yee BJ, *et al.* Randomised trial of CPAP *vs* bilevel support in the treatment of obesity hypoventilation syndrome without severe nocturnal desaturation. *Thorax* 2008; 63: 395–401.

72. Hida W, Okabe S, Tatsumi K, *et al.* Nasal continuous positive airway pressure improves quality of life in obesity hypoventilation syndrome. *Sleep Breath* 2003; 7: 3–12.

73. Kushida CA, Chediak A, Berry RB, *et al.* Clinical guidelines for the manual titration of positive airway pressure in patients with obstructive sleep apnea. *J Clin Sleep Med* 2008; 4: 157–171.

74. Banerjee D, Yee BJ, Piper AJ, *et al.* Obesity hypoventilation syndrome: hypoxemia during continuous positive airway pressure. *Chest* 2007; 131: 1678–1684.

75. Berry RB, Chediak A, Brown LK, *et al.* Best clinical practices for the sleep center adjustment of noninvasive positive pressure ventilation (NPPV) in stable chronic alveolar hypoventilation syndromes. *J Clin Sleep Med* 2010; 6: 491–509.

76. Janssens JP, Borel JC, Pepin JL. Nocturnal monitoring of home non-invasive ventilation: the contribution of simple tools such as pulse oximetry, capnography, built-in ventilator software and autonomic markers of sleep fragmentation. *Thorax* 2011; 66: 438–445.

77. Mokhlesi B, Tulaimat A. Recent advances in obesity hypoventilation syndrome. *Chest* 2007; 132: 1322–1336.

78. Piper AJ, Sullivan CE. Effects of long-term nocturnal nasal ventilation on spontaneous breathing during sleep in neuromuscular and chest wall disorders. *Eur Respir J* 1996; 9: 1515–1522.

79. Contal O, Adler D, Borel JC, *et al.* Impact of different back-up respiratory rates on the efficacy of non-invasive positive pressure ventilation in obesity hypoventilation syndrome: a randomized trial. *Chest* 2013; 143: 37–46.

80. Parreira VF, Delguste P, Jounieaux V, *et al.* Glottic aperture and effective minute ventilation during nasal two-level positive pressure ventilation in spontaneous mode. *Am J Respir Crit Care Med* 1996; 154: 1857–1863.

81. Battisti A, Tassaux D, Janssens JP, *et al.* Performance characteristics of 10 home mechanical ventilators in pressure-support mode: a comparative bench study. *Chest* 2005; 127: 1784–1792.

82. Guo YF, Sforza E, Janssens JP. Respiratory patterns during sleep in obesity-hypoventilation patients treated with nocturnal pressure support: a preliminary report. *Chest* 2007; 131: 1090–1099.

83. Meyer TJ, Pressman MR, Benditt J, *et al.* Air leaking through the mouth during nocturnal nasal ventilation: effect on sleep quality. *Sleep* 1997; 20: 561–569.

84. Gonzalez-Bermejo J, Perrin C, Janssens JP, *et al.* Proposal for a systematic analysis of polygraphy or polysomnography for identifying and scoring abnormal events occurring during non-invasive ventilation. *Thorax* 2012; 67: 546–552.

85. Janssens JP, Metzger M, Sforza E. Impact of volume targeting on efficacy of bi-level non-invasive ventilation and sleep in obesity-hypoventilation. *Respir Med* 2009; 103: 165–172.

86. Windisch W, Storre JH. Target volume settings for home mechanical ventilation: great progress or just a gadget? *Thorax* 2012; 67: 663–665.

87. BaHammam A. Acute ventilatory failure complicating obesity hypoventilation: update on a "critical care syndrome". *Curr Opin Pulm Med* 2010; 16: 543–551.

88. Wijesinghe M, Williams M, Perrin K, *et al.* The effect of supplemental oxygen on hypercapnia in subjects with obesity-associated hypoventilation: a randomized, crossover, clinical study. *Chest* 2011; 139: 1018–1024.

89. Hollier CA, Harmer AR, Maxwell LJ, *et al.* Moderate concentrations of supplemental oxygen worsen hypercapnia in obesity hypoventilation syndrome: a randomised crossover study. *Thorax* 2014; 69: 346–353.

90. Flum DR, Belle SH, King WC, *et al.* Perioperative safety in the longitudinal assessment of bariatric surgery. *N Engl J Med* 2009; 361: 445–454.

91. Sjostrom L, Narbro K, Sjostrom CD, *et al.* Effects of bariatric surgery on mortality in Swedish obese subjects. *N Engl J Med* 2007; 357: 741–752.

92. Sugerman HJ, Fairman RP, Sood RK, *et al.* Long-term effects of gastric surgery for treating respiratory insufficiency of obesity. *Am J Clin Nutr* 1992; 55: Suppl., 597S–601S.

93. Boone KA, Cullen JJ, Mason EE, *et al.* Impact of vertical banded gastroplasty on respiratory insufficiency of severe obesity. *Obes Surg* 1996; 6: 454–458.

94. Marti-Valeri C, Sabate A, Masdevall C, *et al.* Improvement of associated respiratory problems in morbidly obese patients after open Roux-en-Y gastric bypass. *Obes Surg* 2007; 17: 1102–1110.

95. De Cesare A, Cangemi B, Fiori E, *et al.* Early and long-term clinical outcomes of bilio-intestinal diversion in morbidly obese patients. *Surg Today* 2014; 44: 1424–1433.

96. Ashrafian H, le Roux CW, Rowland SP, *et al.* Metabolic surgery and obstructive sleep apnoea: the protective effects of bariatric procedures. *Thorax* 2012; 67: 442–449.

97. Budweiser S, Heidtkamp F, Jorres RA, *et al.* Predictive significance of the six-minute walk distance for long-term survival in chronic hypercapnic respiratory failure. *Respiration* 2008; 75: 418–426.

98. Gungor G, Karakurt Z, Adiguzel N, *et al.* The 6-minute walk test in chronic respiratory failure: does observed or predicted walk distance better reflect patient functional status? *Respir Care* 2013; 58: 850–857.

99. Jordan KE, Ali M, Shneerson JM. Attitudes of patients towards a hospital-based rehabilitation service for obesity hypoventilation syndrome. *Thorax* 2009; 64: 1007.

100. Holland AE, Wadell K, Spruit MA. How to adapt the pulmonary rehabilitation programme to patients with chronic respiratory disease other than COPD. *Eur Respir Rev* 2013; 22: 577–586.

101. Dreher M, Kabitz HJ, Burgardt V, *et al.* Proportional assist ventilation improves exercise capacity in patients with obesity. *Respiration* 2010; 80: 106–111.

102. Schonhofer B, Rosenbluh J, Voshaar T, *et al.* Die Ergometrie trennt das Schlafapnoesyndrom vom Obesitas-Hypoventilationssyndrom auch unter Therapie mit Positivdruckbeatmung [Ergometry separates sleep apnea syndrome from obesity-hypoventilation after therapy positive pressure ventilation therapy]. *Pneumologie* 1997; 51: 1115–1119.

103. Spruit MA, Singh SJ, Garvey C, *et al.* An official American Thoracic Society/European Respiratory Society statement: key concepts and advances in pulmonary rehabilitation. *Am J Respir Crit Care Med* 2013; 188: e13–e64.

104. Villiot-Danger JC, Villiot-Danger E, Borel JC, *et al.* Respiratory muscle endurance training in obese patients. *Int J Obes (Lond)* 2011; 35: 692–699.

105. Smith I, Lasserson TJ, Wright J. Drug therapy for obstructive sleep apnoea in adults. *Cochrane Database Syst Rev* 2006: CD003002.

106. Gorini M, Duranti R, Misuri G, *et al.* Aminophylline and respiratory muscle interaction in normal humans. *Am J Respir Crit Care Med* 1994; 149: 1227–1234.

107. Javaheri S, Guerra L. Lung function, hypoxic and hypercapnic ventilatory responses, and respiratory muscle strength in normal subjects taking oral theophylline. *Thorax* 1990; 45: 743–747.

108. Powers MA. Obesity hypoventilation syndrome: bicarbonate concentration and acetazolamide. *Respir Care* 2010; 55: 1504–1505.

109. Mokhlesi B. Positive airway pressure titration in obesity hypoventilation syndrome: continuous positive airway pressure or bilevel positive airway pressure. *Chest* 2007; 131: 1624–1626.
110. Cuvelier A, Muir JF. Acute and chronic respiratory failure in patients with obesity-hypoventilation syndrome: a new challenge for noninvasive ventilation. *Chest* 2005; 128: 483–485.
111. Mokhlesi B, Tulaimat A, Parthasarathy S. Oxygen for obesity hypoventilation syndrome: a double-edged sword? *Chest* 2011; 139: 975–977.

Disclosures: J.C. Borel is employed by AGIR à dom (a nonprofit homecare provider), and has received grants and personal fees from Philips Healthcare. J.L. Pépin reports receiving grants and personal fees from Vivatech, personal fees from Resmed, Perimetres, Philips, Fisher & Paykel, Astra Zeneca and HealthID, and other funding from AGIR à dom, Teva, ResMed, Philips, GSK, Fondation de le Recherche Médicale, Direction de la Recherche Clinique du CHU de Grenoble and Fonds de dotation "Agir pour les maladies chroniques".

Chapter 11

Specific diagnosis and clinical pathways in at-risk populations

Eusebi Chiner[1], José N. Sancho-Chust[1] and Ferran Barbé[2,3]

OSA is a highly prevalent disorder with limited diagnostic resources. Alternatives to "gold standard" in-laboratory PSG include clinical prediction models, single-channel devices, home respiratory polygraphy and home PSG. In addition, ambulatory strategies or integrated models (with ambulatory and hospital elements) can be used in the diagnostic approach. Patients with the following have a high risk of developing OSA: obesity, HF, atrial fibrillation, hypertension, type 2 diabetes mellitus, stroke, pulmonary hypertension and a history of bariatric surgery evaluation. Specific diagnostic considerations in these patients are reviewed in this chapter, including commentaries regarding the selection of the diagnostic devices or clinical pathways in these groups of patients.

OSA syndrome (respiratory disturbances during sleep and daytime symptoms) is a highly prevalent disorder in the general population, as demonstrated by many studies from different countries. The current prevalence estimates of moderate-to-severe sleep disordered breathing (AHI $\geqslant 15$ events·h^{-1}) are: 10% among 30–49-year-old men; 17% among 50–70-year-old men; 3% among 30–49-year-old women; and 9% among 50–70-year-old women. These estimated prevalence rates represent substantial increases over the last two decades (relative increases of between 14% and 55% depending on the subgroup). This level increases in a direct relationship with age [1, 2].

Diagnostic OSA procedures include a wide range of tests (table 1), including in-laboratory, fully attended, multichannel procedures, and home, unattended, single-channel devices [3].

Better recognition of OSA in recent years has meant that the number of patients referred with suspected OSAS has considerably increased. This can overload diagnostic and follow-up resources. To guarantee efficiency in the diagnostic management of patients with suspected OSA, alternatives to traditional methods need to be considered [4–6].

In addition, a comprehensive evaluation may be undertaken in some patients who are at high risk of OSA (table 2). High-risk patients include those with obesity, HF, atrial

[1]Pulmonology Section, University Hospital of Sant Joan d'Alacant, Alicante, Spain. [2]Respiratory Dept, Hospital Universitari Arnau de Vilanova and Santa Maria, IRB Lleida, Lleida, Spain. [3]Centro de Investigación Biomédica en Red de Enfermedades Respiratorias (CIBERES), Madrid, Spain.

Correspondence: Eusebi Chiner Vives, Secció de Pneumologia, Hospital Universitari Sant Joan d'Alacant, Ctra. Alacant-València s/n, CP: 03550, Sant Joan d'Alacant, Spain. E-mail: chiner_eus@gva.es

Table 1. Type of monitors for diagnosis of OSA according to the American Academy of Sleep Medicine

Type of monitor	Definition
Type 1	Full attended PSG (≥7 channels) in a laboratory setting
Type 2	Full unattended PSG (≥7 channels)
Type 3	Limited-channel devices (usually respiratory polygraphy using 4–7 channels)
Type 4	1–2 channels (usually oximetry or single devices)

fibrillation, hypertension, type 2 diabetes mellitus (T2DM), stroke, some group 3 patients within the World Health Organization clinical classification of pulmonary hypertension, and those being evaluated for bariatric surgery [7].

Laboratory diagnostic strategies

The current gold standard test in the diagnosis of OSA is hospital-based PSG. This method has been proven to be accurate with a low failure rate because it includes many channels and because it is attended by technical staff. PSG monitors many body functions including brain (electroencephalography), eye movements (electro-oculography), muscle activity or skeletal muscle activation (electromyography) and heart rhythm (ECG) during sleep. The frequency of obstructive events is reported as a RDI. OSA severity is defined (by consensus) as mild for RDI ≥5 and <15, moderate for RDI ≥15 and ≤30, and severe for RDI >30 events·h^{-1} [7, 8]. PSG provides far more information than just respiratory events, and it is the only accurate way to assess body position (rotational and vertical) and total sleep time (as opposed to total recording time). It also provides accurate assessment of sound measurement and, thereby, assessment of snoring in relation to sleep stage and body position.

However, PSG is considered relatively expensive and technically complex, and it is not always widely available. These reasons may lead to undesirable delays in diagnosis using only PSG [9].

Home-based strategies

There are many alternative diagnostic strategies with increasing technical complexity and different results in terms of diagnostic efficacy compared with in-laboratory PSG (table 3).

Table 2. Patients at high risk of OSA

Obesity
HF
Atrial fibrillation
Hypertension
Type 2 diabetes mellitus
Stroke
Pulmonary hypertension
Pre-operative for bariatric surgery

Table 3. Comparison of alternative diagnostic strategies in OSA

	Quality of evidence	Sensitivity %	Specificity %
Clinical prediction models	Low	36–97	18–89
Single-channel devices	Moderate	27–100	67–100
Home respiratory polygraphy	Moderate	83–97	48–100
Home PSG	Moderate	88–94	36–77

Clinical prediction models

A good history and examination does not replace a diagnostic test. Patients with OSA report snoring, witnessed apnoeas, waking up with a choking sensation and excessive sleepiness. Other common symptoms are nonrestorative sleep, difficulty initiating or maintaining sleep, fatigue or tiredness, and morning headache. Indicators include a family history of the disease or physical attributes suggestive of OSA, such as a small oropharyngeal airway or markers of obesity (e.g. large neck circumference) [10].

Several clinical screening questionnaires have been developed to help identify patients who are at high risk of OSA. The most studied is the Berlin questionnaire and the questionnaire with the highest methodological quality is the STOP-BANG (snoring, tiredness, observed sleep, BP, BMI, age, neck circumference and gender) [11, 12]. When questionnaires were compared, STOP-BANG had the highest sensitivity, odds ratio and area under the curve (AUC), but rather low specificity, and the Four-Variable Screening Tool had the highest specificity [13, 14]. A meta-analysis of clinical studies for the diagnosis of OSA revealed that clinical models have higher odds ratios for diagnosis and severity than questionnaire-based models (10.49 and 17.24 versus 5.02 and 10.12, respectively) [15].

Based on these clinical questionnaires, the clinical prediction models seek to establish a reliable diagnosis avoiding the need to perform objective sleep tests. These models are constructed from the analysis of the clinical characteristics of a sample of patients with suspected OSA, who then undergo an objective sleep test to establish the diagnosis and severity of disease. However, the results have not confirmed the utility of these tools and their potential use is limited to the prioritisation of an objective diagnostic test [16].

Single-channel devices

The most widely studied single-channel test is pulse oximetry. Respiratory events are identified indirectly via their impact on the nocturnal saturation curve. The total number of desaturations is divided by the number of hours in bed and an ODI per hour is obtained. The accuracy of pulse oximeters in measuring transient changes in arterial oxygen saturation (SaO_2) may be affected by the oximeter time response. The misestimation of SaO_2 induced by settings of oximeter averaging time that are within the range selectable in conventional oximeters may be of epidemiological significance when pulse oximetry is used as a complementary diagnostic tool to classify sleep events in sleep apnoea–hypopnoea syndrome (SAHS). The settings required (averaging time and sampling frequency), displays (maximum, mean and minimum SaO_2) and heart rate need to be checked for a correct interpretation. This technique can led false negatives, especially in young patients, as well as false positives in patients with comorbidities [7, 17]. The sensitivity of pulse oximetry at different cut-off points can range between 82% (using a cut-off of 5% desaturation) and 62% (15% desaturation), while specificity varies between 76% (5% desaturation) and 93% (15% desaturation) [4]. When the population studied has a high prevalence of SAHS or the severity is high, the sensitivity and specificity may improve because the accuracy lies in the detection of apnoeas, while hypopnoeas are underdiagnosed. A simplified two-stage model was validated for identifying OSA in primary care using a screening questionnaire followed by home sleep-monitoring oximetry. A 3% dip rate was highly predictive of OSA (receiver operating characteristic AUC 0.96, 95% CI 0.91–1.0; p<0.001). The two-stage diagnostic model showed a sensitivity of 0.97 (95% CI 0.81–1.00) and specificity of 0.87 (95% CI 0.74–0.95) in the development group, and a sensitivity of 0.88 (95% CI 0.60–0.98) and specificity of 0.82 (95% CI 0.70–0.90) in the validation group [18, 19].

Other single-channel devices are based on the log of the air flow, with special interest in the ambulatory setting. For example, the SleepStrip (Jant Pharmacal Corportation, Encino, CA, USA) is a small, lightweight device that consists of flow sensors (oral and nasal thermistors) and is worn underneath the nose and above the upper lip. Correlation between RDI in PSG and score based on the device is good, with a sensitivity and specificity varying depending on the RDI thresholds [20]. Another single-channel device is the MicroMESAM (ResMed, San Diego, CA, USA); it measures respiratory pressure *via* a nasal cannula, with high correlation with PSG. The sensitivity and specificity change at different RDI thresholds [21]. The ApneaLink (ResMed) device measures airflow through a nasal cannula connected to a pressure transducer. Compared with PSG, it has shown the best results at an RDI $\geqslant$15 events$\cdot$h^{-1} (sensitivity 91%, specificity 95%) [22].

Although the results using single-channel devices are promising, studies are relatively scarce. Single-channel devices are not recommended for diagnostic purposes and their usefulness may lie in rapid screening to prioritise more complete diagnostic tests [7].

Home respiratory polygraphy

Home respiratory polygraphy (HRP) records airflow, respiratory effort and oxygen saturation, identifying the respiratory events and episodes of desaturation necessary for diagnosis [3]. Several studies have evaluated the role of HRP in the diagnosis of OSA, but there is a great variability in terms of design, methodology, definitions of respiratory events, cut-off points for diagnosis and the types of device used. Moderate-quality evidence showed that HRP can predict RDI scores that are suggestive of OSA. The sensitivities and specificities showed a wide range between studies. Under economic evaluation, the HRP showed a cost approximately 50% less than that hospital-based PSG [23–35]. The utility of portable monitors for patients with serious comorbid conditions has not been adequately verified [36]. Based on this, HRP is recommended as a valid and efficient diagnostic test for the diagnosis of OSA in patients without serious comorbid conditions and when PSG is not available [36].

Home PSG

Some studies have used PSG in the patient's home to add to the information obtained by including neurological variables, while avoiding the first-night effect often experienced by patients when they attend sleep laboratories. Although most of the studies proved PSG to be less efficient at home, the differences were not significant. In contrast, there was an improvement in sleep quality and a reduction in costs (of nearly 75%) with high patient satisfaction. However, in clinical practice, patients get wired up in the laboratory then go home and set up the device at home, or a technician visits the home and sets up the patient. Importantly, signal drop out is high (estimates approaching 70%) and many patients do not wish to take responsibility for signal quality, so this can greatly affect the results. When one considers redo tests and staff time, home PSG can be more expensive that in-laboratory PSG. This diagnostic strategy may be more widely evaluated in subjects with high suspicion of OSA [37, 38].

Integrated models

The need for cost-efficiency in the diagnostic approach to OSA requires the development of alternatives to traditional hospital management. Some investigators have evaluated integrated models, including in-hospital and ambulatory elements. In addition, these integrated models attempt to address the follow-up of the disease. One of the main aspects to consider in the follow-up of OSA is treatment compliance, especially CPAP compliance because it is the first-line treatment in OSA and compliance problems have been shown since the first studies.

One study evaluated the results obtained using a HRP as an ambulatory diagnostic approach and a follow-up period, after starting CPAP therapy, assessed by a nurse rather than a sleep specialist. After 3 months of nursing follow-up subsequent to the home diagnosis, the results were comparable to those obtained in patients followed up by traditional methods. Although the results were very positive, the study did not have a control group, so more research is needed to evaluate this type of intervention [39].

Another study took home strategy one step further. They divided their patients into two groups: home diagnosis and nurse-based ambulatory follow-up *versus* in-laboratory diagnosis and follow-up. The strategies showed no differences in terms of efficacy and adherence to the treatment, but the former required fewer visits during the follow-up period. The final conclusion was that the nursing strategy is cheaper, without any effect on compliance. The cost differential is largely attributable to the type of diagnosis, as the first arm used oximetry and the second used PSG [40].

In another work, three different alternatives were simultaneously evaluated: one group with home diagnosis and follow-up, another with hospital diagnosis and follow-up, and a third group with home diagnosis and hospital follow-up. No differences in terms of efficacy or adherence to the treatment were found. A cost study showed significant differences in the home monitoring group and the group with HRP and hospital follow-up, compared with the group that was exclusively treated in the hospital. The final conclusion was that a strategy that was fully geared to a patient's home is cost-effective, without any disadvantage to the diagnosis and management of the patients [41].

Diagnosis in high-risk populations

An important issue is that patients sometimes seek medical attention because of excessive sleepiness associated with snoring, socially disturbing snoring or CVD (HF, atrial fibrillation, stroke, resistant systemic hypertension). At other times, medical attention can be sought due to high-risk surgical procedures (peri-operative assessment). The test required is very dependent upon the patient's circumstances and availability of investigative services.

Obesity

Obesity is a major risk factor for the development of OSA. Approximately 40% of obese individuals with no complaints of sleep disorders, 55% of all adolescents who undergo bariatric surgery and up to 71% of morbidly obese individuals develop OSA [42–44].

A patient's probability of having OSA can be estimated using the ESS and the adjusted neck circumference (ANC). If a patient has hypersomnolence (usually ESS ⩾10) or is at intermediate to high risk based on ANC, a sleep study is recommended in these obese patients [45, 46].

PSG is desirable when available, but specific validation of portable monitors has been specifically developed in obese patients, with similar results to PSG [47].

A proposed diagnostic approach in obese patients is shown in figure 1 [45].

Heart failure

Sleep apnoea is frequently observed in patients with HF. In general, sleep apnoea consists of two types: OSA and CSA. OSA results from UA collapse, whereas CSA arises from reductions in central respiratory drive. In patients with OSA, BP is frequently elevated as a result of sympathetic nervous system over-activation. The generation of exaggerated negative intrathoracic pressure during obstructive apnoeas further increases left ventricular afterload, reduces cardiac output, and may promote the progression of HF. IH and post-apnoeic reoxygenation cause vascular endothelial damage and possibly atherosclerosis, and consequently, coronary artery disease and ischaemic cardiomyopathy. CSA is also characterised by apnoea, hypoxia and increased sympathetic nervous activity, and when present in HF, is associated with an increased risk of death [48]. Studies of

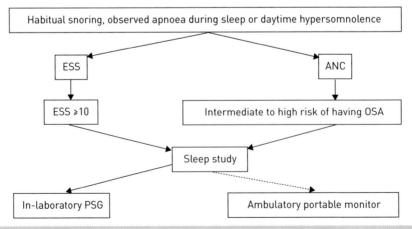

Figure 1. Proposed diagnostic algorithm of OSA in obese patients. ANC: adjusted neck circumference. Reproduced and modified from [45] with permission from the publisher.

consecutive patients with HF revealed that OSA is present in approximately one half of subjects [49].

The importance of the recognition of OSA in HF patients is that effective treatment with CPAP has shown improvement in left ventricular ejection fraction and sympathetic activity [50].

Keeping in mind that OSA is a highly prevalent condition with known negative impact, for which treatment is available and diagnosis is feasible, active screening may be recommended. Physicians caring for HF patients, especially cardiologists, may start with an active investigation into OSA symptoms. If OSA is clinically suspected, admission to sleep units is recommended [49, 50].

In-laboratory PSG is desirable in patients with HF, as ECG recording is included. However, specific validation of HRP in HF patients has shown excellent results. Thus, HF patients may be diagnosed using portable monitors in an ambulatory setting [51]. Thermistor measurements have traditionally been used to determine airflow during PSG. However, low accuracy in detecting hypopneas is a major drawback. The use of nasal prongs connected to a pressure transducer is a noninvasive, sensitive method to detect respiratory events with a good time response that allows the detection of several flow-related phenomena, in addition to apnoea and hypopnoea. The incorporation of nasal prongs in routine, full-night studies is an attainable technical option that provides adequate recordings adding relevant information not scored by thermistors is obtained for flow-related respiratory events, thus increasing diagnostic accuracy. Portable monitors should incorporate nasal prongs in patients with HF [52, 53]. Some authors have taken the findings a step further, validating the use of respiratory polygraphy during hospitalisation because of decompensated HF [54].

Demonstration of feasibility and reliability of in-patient testing for OSA should be followed in the future by the evaluation of the effect of in-patient treatment with CPAP in acute HF. Preliminary reports showed an improvement in 30-day hospital readmission among cardiac patients (HF and other cardiac conditions). If benefit is confirmed, systematic screening in patients with acute HF could be considered [55].

Atrial fibrillation

The prevalence of OSA among patients with atrial fibrillation is estimated to be approximately 32–49%. The association between OSA and atrial fibrillation is related to the extent of hypoxaemia and, therefore, the severity of sleep apnoea but also state change (REM *versus* non-REM), and intrathoracic pressure swings and autonomic activity [56, 57].

Patients with OSA have significantly greater atrial fibrillation recurrence rates after catheter ablation. In addition to other factors, a diagnosis of OSA merits special consideration when evaluating patients for AF ablation [58]. CPAP is an important therapy in the natural history of the disease, as adequate treatment with CPAP in coexisting OSA–atrial fibrillation patients reduces the risk of atrial fibrillation recurrence [59].

On the basis of these data, careful consideration for the presence of OSA has to be kept in mind in atrial fibrillation patients. If OSA is clinically suspected, evaluation in a sleep unit is recommended. An ambulatory diagnostic approach with home PSG has been used in atrial fibrillation patients with good results, with the advantage of including the ECG recording. The use of more simple portable monitors, such HRP, in an ambulatory setting should be investigated in this specific group of patients [60].

Hypertension

OSA increases the risk of daytime hypertension. There are several underlying mechanisms that include IH with release of cytokines, angiogenic inhibitors, free radicals and adhesion molecules. Although part of this association may be explained by co-existing risk factors (*e.g.* obesity), a large body of evidence supports an independent role of OSA in the pathogenesis of daytime hypertension. More than 60% of subjects with severe OSA were found to be hypertensive. Conversely, approximately 40% of hypertensive patients are diagnosed with OSA [61].

OSA is the most frequent cause of resistant hypertension. More than 70% of patients with resistant hypertension have OSA. In fact, international guidelines recommend the screening of OSA in resistant hypertension patients [62]. CPAP treatment has shown an effect in the reduction of BP in hypertensive patients, including those without daytime hypersomnolence or resistant hypertension [63, 64].

Specific recommendations have been made in hypertensive patients. A proposed diagnostic algorithm is shown in figure 2 [65].

Type 2 diabetes mellitus

The relative role of OSA in the pathogenesis of glucose alterations has been intensively studied in clinical and experimental models. Metabolic changes, haemodynamic alterations and systemic inflammation are involved. The identified mediators include leptin, angiotensinogen, resistin, C-reactive protein, TNF and plasminogen activator inhibitor [66].

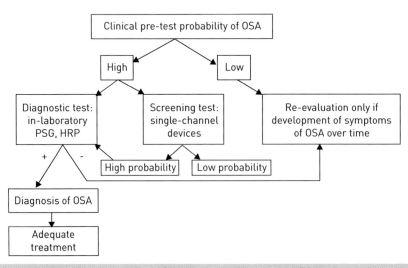

Figure 2. Proposed diagnostic algorithm of OSA in hypertensive patients. HRP: home respiratory polygraphy. Reproduced and modified from [65] with permission from the publisher.

T2DM prevalence increases with OSA severity, from 6% in subjects without OSA to 29% in those with severe OSA. Furthermore, diabetic subjects with more severe OSA have worse glycaemic control than those without OSA [67].

CPAP treatment is associated with improvement in insulin resistance, indicating treating OSA can positively impact the symptoms of T2DM [68]. Various diagnostic tests are used in screening for OSA among T2DM patients. In-laboratory PSG, HRP, home PSG and single-channel devices have been used with good results [69–72].

Specific recommendations to diabetes services have been proposed. The possibility of OSA should be considered in the assessment of all patients with T2DM and the metabolic syndrome, with a "low threshold" for referral to sleep clinics because of the established benefits of therapy [73].

A possible diagnostic approach in T2DM patients is shown in figure 3.

Stroke

After adjustment for confounding factors, OSA is associated with an increased risk of stroke. Prospective studies showed that severe OSA patients have an approximately three-fold increased risk of stroke. In addition, OSA is a negative predictor of all-cause mortality and recurrent vascular events in stroke patients [74, 75].

The relationship between OSA and stroke is complex, with shared risk factors, although an independent association is recognised for some factors. Postulated mechanisms of OSA as an independent risk factor for stroke include tachyarrhythmias, BP fluctuations or enhanced inflammation and oxidative stress associated with intermittent hypoxaemia [76].

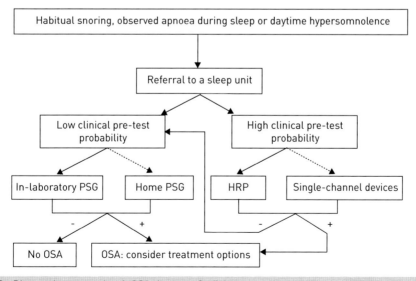

Figure 3. Diagnostic approach of OSA in type 2 diabetes mellitus patients. HRP: home respiratory polygraphy.

The effect of CPAP treatment has been related to benefits in acute and chronic outcomes in stroke patients. In the chronic phase, CPAP has positive effects on the incidence of cardiovascular events, mortality and outcomes of rehabilitation. In the acute phase, the early use of CPAP has been associated with acceleration of neurological recovery [77–82].

In-laboratory PSG is the gold standard test, but resources are limited. In addition, the transfer of patients with an acute stroke to sleep units is not desirable. The use of portable monitors allows patients to remain on the stroke units while undergoing a study with more rapid results at less cost. The use of respiratory polygraphy is feasible, cost-effective and has been widely validated in subacute inpatients with stroke [77–82].

Accepted recommendations in the management of subacute inpatients with stroke include the evaluation of the stroke aetiology (vascular diagnostic tests, cardiac monitoring or imaging tests) and the establishment of prevention efforts related to many recognised cardiovascular factors (hypertension, hyperlipidaemia, diabetes, cigarette smoking, alcohol consumption, atrial fibrillation or extracranial carotid disease). As evidence is accumulating that CPAP is among a handful of interventions demonstrated to improve functional outcome after stroke, clinical guidelines may include specific recommendations about OSA screening [83].

A possible diagnostic approach in stroke patients is shown in figure 4.

Pulmonary hypertension

OSA constitutes an independent risk factor for the development of pulmonary hypertension, which is ameliorated by CPAP treatment. At least 20% of patients with OSA exhibit day-time pulmonary hypertension, which can be reversed with CPAP treatment [84, 85].

Conversely, 16% of PH patients suffer from mild-to-moderate OSA. Acute increases in pulmonary artery pressure and alveolar hypoxia have been proposed as possible mechanisms. Male sex and obesity have been identified as risk factors for the diagnosis of OSA in PH patients [86].

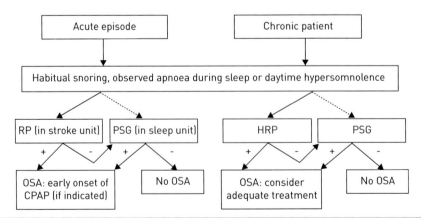

Figure 4. Diagnostic approach of OSA in stroke patients. HRP: home respiratory polygraphy; RP: unattended respiratory polygraphy.

HRP has been used for the recognition of OSA in class II–III pulmonary hypertension patients with good results. This diagnostic test should be used if there is clinical suspicion (particularly in male and obese patients) of OSA in pulmonary hypertension patients. If there is any doubt over the presence of CSA after HRP, full PSG can be performed.

Bariatric surgery candidates

The incidence of OSA has been underestimated in patients who present for evaluation for bariatric surgery. Several studies have shown an extremely high incidence of OSA in these patients (up to 94%) with a significant number of patients who are previously undiagnosed (up to 38%). OSA is associated with an increased risk of all-cause mortality and adverse outcomes in bariatric surgery patients, which can be neutralised by adequate CPAP therapy [87–89].

For all the above reasons, in patients presenting for bariatric surgery, screening for OSA is recommended. Pre-operative management with CPAP (if indicated) is also recommended. International guidelines reflect these recommendations [90].

The validation of HRP and single-channel devices has been performed with good results, and these could be the first option if PSG is not widely available [91, 92].

Conclusion

The need for cost-efficiency in the diagnostic approach to OSA requires the development of alternatives to "gold standard" in-laboratory PSG. Ambulatory strategies or integrated models (including hospital and ambulatory elements) are valid alternatives. Clinical prediction models and single-channel devices can be used to prioritise the use of resources. HRP is recommended as a valid and efficient diagnostic test for the diagnosis of OSA in patients without serious comorbid conditions and when PSG is not available.

High-risk patients include those with obesity, HF, atrial fibrillation, hypertension, T2DM, stroke or pulmonary hypertension, and those being evaluated for bariatric surgery. High clinical suspicion of OSA is needed in the evaluation of these patients. If OSA is suspected, some specific diagnostic considerations should be taken into account.

References

1. Greenstone M, Hack M. Obstructive sleep apnoea. *BMJ* 2014; 348: g3745.
2. Peppard PE, Young T, Barnet JH, *et al.* Increased prevalence of sleep-disordered breathing in adults. *Am J Epidemiol* 2013; 177: 1006–1114.
3. Collop NA, Anderson WM, Boehlecke B, *et al.* Clinical guidelines for the use of unattended portable monitors in the diagnosis of obstructive sleep apnea in adult patients. Portable Monitoring Task Force of the American Academy of Sleep Medicine. *J Clin Sleep Med* 2007; 3: 737–747.
4. Chiner E, Signes-Costa J, Arriero JM, *et al.* Nocturnal oximetry for the diagnosis of the sleep apnoea hypopnoea syndrome: a method to reduce the number of polysomnographies? *Thorax* 1999; 54: 968–971.
5. Lloberes P, Sampol G, Levy G, *et al.* Influence of setting on unattended respiratory monitoring in the sleep apnoea/hypopnoea syndrome. *Eur Respir J* 2001; 18: 530–534.
6. Flemons WW, Littner MR, Rowley JA, *et al.* Home diagnosis of sleep apnea: a systematic review of the literature. An evidence review cosponsored by the American Academy of Sleep Medicine, the American College of Chest Physicians, and the American Thoracic Society. *Chest* 2003; 124: 1543–1579.

7. Epstein LJ, Kristo D, Strollo PJ Jr, *et al.* Clinical guideline for the evaluation, management and long-term care of obstructive sleep apnea in adults. *J Clin Sleep Med* 2009; 5: 263–276.
8. Berry RB, Budhiraja R, Gottlieb DJ, *et al.* Rules for scoring respiratory events in sleep: update of the 2007 AASM Manual for the Scoring of Sleep and Associated Events. Deliberations of the Sleep Apnea Definitions Task Force of the American Academy of Sleep Medicine. *J Clin Sleep Med* 2012; 8: 597–619.
9. Masa Jimenez JF, Barbé Illa F, Capote Gil F, *et al.* Resources and delays in the diagnosis of sleep apnea-hypopnea syndrome. *Arch Bronconeumol* 2007; 43: 188–198.
10. Jordan AS, McSharry DG, Malhotra A. Adult obstructive sleep apnoea. *Lancet* 2014; 383: 736–747.
11. Netzer NC, Stoohs RA, Netzer CM, *et al.* Using the Berlin Questionnaire to identify patients at risk for the sleep apnea syndrome. *Ann Intern Med* 1999; 131: 485–491.
12. Chung F, Yegneswaran B, Liao P, *et al.* STOP questionnaire: a tool to screen patients for obstructive sleep apnea. *Anesthesiology* 2008; 108: 812–821.
13. Takegami M, Hashino Y, Chin K, *et al.* Simple four-variable screening tool for identification of patients with sleep-disordered breathing. *Sleep* 2009; 32: 939–948.
14. Pataka A, Daskalopoulou E, Kalamaras G, *et al.* Evaluation of five different questionnaires for assessing sleep apnea syndrome in a sleep clinic. *Sleep Med* 2014; 15: 776–781.
15. Ramachandran SK, Josephs LA. A meta-analysis of clinical screening tests for obstructive sleep apnea. *Anesthesiology* 2009; 110: 928–939.
16. Rowley JA, Aboussouan LS, Badr MS. The use of clinical prediction formulas in the evaluation of obstructive sleep apnea. *Sleep* 2000; 23: 929–938.
17. Zamarrón C, Gude F, Barcala J, *et al.* Utility of oxygen saturation and heart rate spectral analysis obtained from pulse oximetric recordings in the diagnosis of sleep apnea syndrome. *Chest* 2003; 123: 1567–1576.
18. Chiner E, Signes-Costa J, Arriero JM, *et al.* Nocturnal oximetry for the diagnosis of the sleep apnoea hypopnoea syndrome: a method to reduce the number of polysomnographies? *Thorax* 1999; 54: 968–971.
19. Chai-Coetzer CL, Antic NA, Rowland LS, *et al.* A simplified model of screening questionnaire and home monitoring for obstructive sleep apnoea in primary care. *Thorax* 2011; 66: 213–219.
20. Shochat T, Hadas N, Kerkhofs M, *et al.* The SleepStrip^{TM}: an apnoea screener for the early detection of sleep apnoea syndrome. *Eur Respir J* 2002; 19: 121–126.
21. Wang Y, Teschler T, Weinreich G, *et al.* Validation of microMESAM as screening device for sleep disordered breathing. *Pneumologie* 2003; 57: 734–740.
22. Erman MK, Stewart D, Einhorn D, *et al.* Validation of the ApneaLink™ for the screening of sleep apnea: a novel and simple single-channel recording device. *J Clin Sleep Med* 2007; 3: 387–392.
23. Dingli K, Coleman EL, Vennelle M, *et al.* Evaluation of a portable device for diagnosing the sleep apnoea/hypopnoea syndrome. *Eur Respir J* 2003; 21: 253–259.
24. Su S, Baroody FM, Kohrman M, *et al.* A comparison of polysomnography and a portable home sleep study in the diagnosis of obstructive sleep apnea syndrome. *Otolaryngol Head Neck Surg* 2004; 131: 844–850.
25. Yin M, Miyazaki S, Ishikawa K. Evaluation of type 3 portable monitoring in unattended home setting for suspected sleep apnea: factors that may affect its accuracy. *Otolaryngol Head Neck Surg* 2006; 134: 204–209.
26. García-Díaz E, Quintana-Gallego E, Ruiz A, *et al.* Respiratory polygraphy with actigraphy in the diagnosis of sleep apnea-hypopnea syndrome. *Chest* 2007; 131: 725–732.
27. Ayappa I, Norman RG, Seelall V, *et al.* Validation of a self-applied unattended monitor for sleep disordered breathing. *J Clin Sleep Med* 2008; 4: 26–37.
28. Alonso Alvarez ML, Terán Santos J, Cordero Guevara J, *et al.* Reliability of home respiratory polygraphy for the diagnosis of sleep apnea-hypopnea syndrome: analysis of costs. *Arch Bronconeumol* 2008; 44: 22–28.
29. Santos-Silva R, Sartori DE, Truksinas V, *et al.* Validation of a portable monitoring system for the diagnosis of obstructive sleep apnea syndrome. *Sleep* 2009; 32: 629–636.
30. Tonelli de Oliveira AC, Martinez D, Vasconcelos LF, *et al.* Diagnosis of obstructive sleep apnea syndrome and its outcomes with home portable monitoring. *Chest* 2009; 135: 330–336.
31. Ng SS, Chan TO, To KW, *et al.* Validation of Embletta portable diagnostic system for identifying patients with suspected obstructive sleep apnoea syndrome (OSAS). *Respirology* 2010; 15: 336–342.
32. Cheliout-Heraut F, Senny F, Djouadi F, *et al.* Obstructive sleep apnoea syndrome: comparison between polysomnography and portable sleep monitoring based on jaw recordings. *Neurophysiol Clin* 2011; 41: 191–198.
33. Driver HS, Pereira EJ, Bjerring K, *et al.* Validation of the MediByte® type 3 portable monitor compared with polysomnography for screening of obstructive sleep apnea. *Can Respir J* 2011; 18: 137–143.
34. Masa JF, Corral J, Pereira R, *et al.* Effectiveness of home respiratory polygraphy for the diagnosis of sleep apnoea and hypopnoea syndrome. *Thorax* 2011; 66: 567–573.
35. Masa JF, Corral J, Sanchez de Cos J, *et al.* Effectiveness of three sleep apnea management alternatives. *Sleep* 2013; 36: 1799–1807.
36. Qaseem A, Dallas P, Owens DK. Diagnosis of obstructive sleep apnea in adults: a clinical practice guideline from the American College of Physicians. *Ann Intern Med* 2014; 161: 210–220.

37. Bruyneel M, Sanida C, Art G, et al. Sleep efficiency during sleep studies: results of a prospective study comparing home-based and in-hospital polysomnography. *J Sleep Res* 2011; 20: 201–206.

38. Campbell AJ, Neill AM. Home set-up polysomnography in the assessment of suspected obstructive sleep apnea. *J Sleep Res* 2011; 20: 207–213.

39. Tomlinson M, Gibson M. Obstructive sleep apnoea syndrome: a nurse-led domiciliary service. *J Adv Nursing* 2006; 55: 391–397.

40. Antic NA, Buchan C, Esterman A, et al. A randomized controlled trial of nurse-led care for symptomatic moderate-severe obstructive sleep apnea. *Am J Respir Crit Care Med* 2009; 179: 501–508.

41. Andreu AL, Chiner E, Sancho-Chust JN, et al. Effect of an ambulatory diagnostic and treatment programme in patients with sleep apnoea. *Eur Respir J* 2012; 39: 305–312.

42. Vgontzas A, Tan TL, Bixler EO, et al. Sleep apnea and sleep disruption in obese patients. *Arch Intern Med* 1994; 154: 1705–1711.

43. Kalra M, Inge T, Garcia V, et al. Obstructive sleep apnea in extremely overweight adolescents undergoing bariatric surgery. *Obes Res* 2005; 13: 1175–1179.

44. Frey W, Pilcher J. Obstructive sleep-related breathing disorders in patients evaluated for bariatric surgery. *Obes Surg* 2003; 13: 676–683.

45. Flemons WW. Obstructive sleep apnea. *N Engl J Med* 2002; 347: 498–504.

46. De Sousa AG, Cercato C, Mancini MC, et al. Obesity and obstructive sleep apnea-hypopnea syndrome. *Obes Rev* 2008; 9: 340–354.

47. Fredheim JM, Røislien J, Hjelmesæth J. Validation of a portable monitor for the diagnosis of obstructive sleep apnea in morbidly obese patients. *J Clin Sleep Med* 2014; 10: 751–757.

48. Rosen D, Roux FJ, Shah N. Sleep and breathing in congestive heart failure. *Clin Chest Med* 2014; 35: 521–534.

49. Javaheri S, Caref EB, Chen E, et al. Sleep apnea testing and outcomes in a large cohort of medicare beneficiaries with newly diagnosed heart failure. *Am J Respir Crit Care Med* 2011; 183: 539–546.

50. Kaneko Y, Floras JS, Usui K, et al. Cardiovascular effects of continuous positive airway pressure in patients with heart failure and obstructive sleep apnea. *N Engl J Med* 2003; 348: 1233–1241.

51. Quintana-Gallego E, Villa-Gil M, Carmona-Bernal C, et al. Home respiratory polygraphy for diagnosis of sleep-disordered breathing in heart failure. *Eur Respir J* 2004; 24: 443–448.

52. Hernández L, Ballester E, Farré R, et al. Performance of nasal prongs in sleep studies: spectrum of flow-related events. *Chest* 2001; 119: 442–450.

53. BahHammam A. Comparison of nasal prong pressure and thermistor measurements for detecting respiratory events during sleep. *Respiration* 2004; 71: 385–390.

54. Khayat RN, Jarjoura D, Patt B, et al. In-hospital testing for sleep disordered breathing in hospitalized patients with decompensated heart failure – report of prevalence and patient characteristics. *J Card Fail* 2009; 15: 739–746.

55. Kauta SR, Keenan BT, Goldberg L, et al. Diagnosis and treatment of sleep disordered breathing in hospitalized cardiac patients: a reduction in 30-day hospital readmission rates. *J Clin Sleep Med* 2014; 10: 1051–1059.

56. Gami AS, Hodge DO, Herges RM, et al. Obstructive sleep apnea, obesity, and the risk of incident atrial fibrillation. *J Am Coll Cardiol* 2007; 49: 565–571.

57. Digby GC, Baranchuk A. Sleep apnea and atrial fibrillation; 2012 update. *Curr Cardiol Rev* 2012; 8: 265–272.

58. Ng CY, Liu T, Shehata M, et al. Meta-analysis of obstructive sleep apnea as predictor of atrial fibrillation recurrence after catheter ablation. *Am J Cardiol* 2011; 108: 47–51.

59. Fein AS, Shvilkin A, Shah D, et al. Treatment of obstructive sleep apnea reduces the risk of atrial fibrillation recurrence after catheter ablation. *J Am Coll Cardiol* 2013; 62: 300–305.

60. Stevenson IH, Teichtahl H, Cunnington D. Prevalence of sleep disordered breathing in paroxysmal and persistent atrial fibrillation patients with normal left ventricular function. *Eur Heart J* 2008; 29: 1662–1669.

61. Mohsenin V. Obstructive sleep apnea and hypertension: a critical review. *Curr Hypertens Rep* 2014; 16: 482–484.

62. Chobanian AV, Bakris GL, Black HR, et al. The seventh report of the joint national committee on prevention, detection, evaluation, and treatment of high blood pressure: the JNC 7 Report. *JAMA* 2003; 289: 2560–2572.

63. Barbe F, Duran-Cantolla J, Capote F, et al. Long-term effect of continuous positive airway pressure in hypertensive patients with sleep apnea. *Am J Respir Crit Care Med* 2010; 181: 718–726.

64. Martínez-García MA, Capote F, Campos-Rodríguez F, et al. Effect of CPAP on blood pressure in patients with obstructive sleep apnea and resistant hypertension: the HIPARCO randomized clinical trial. *JAMA* 2013; 310: 2407–2415.

65. Parati G, Lombardi C, Hedner J, et al. Recommendations for the management of patients with obstructive sleep apnoea and hypertension. *Eur Respir J* 2013; 41: 523–538.

66. Levy P, Bonsignore MR, Eckel J. Sleep, sleep-disordered breathing and metabolic consequences. *Eur Respir J* 2009; 34: 243–260.

67. Kent BD, Grote L, Ryan S, et al. Diabetes mellitus prevalence and control in sleep-disordered breathing: the European Sleep Apnea Cohort (ESADA) Study. *Chest* 2014; 146: 982–990.

68. Chen L, Pei JH, Chen HM. Effects of continuous positive airway pressure treatment on glycaemic control and insulin sensitivity in patients with obstructive sleep apnoea and type 2 diabetes: a meta-analysis. *Arch Med Sci* 2014; 10: 637–642.

69. Foster GD, Sanders MH, Millman R, *et al.* Obstructive sleep apnea among obese patients with type 2 diabetes. *Diabetes Care* 2009; 32: 1017–1019.

70. Laaban JP, Daenen S, Leger D, *et al.* Prevalence and predictive factors of sleep apnoea syndrome in type 2 diabetic patients. *Diabetes Metab* 2009; 35: 372–327.

71. Einhorn D, Stewart DA, Erman MK, *et al.* Prevalence of sleep apnea in a population of adults with type 2 diabetes mellitus. *Endocr Pract* 2007; 13: 355–362.

72. Rusu A, Todea D, Rosca L, *et al.* The development of a sleep apnea screening program in Romanian type 2 diabetic patients: a pilot study. *Acta Diabetol* 2012; 49: 105–109.

73. Shaw JE, Punjabi NM, Wilding JP, *et al.* Sleep-disordered breathing and type 2 diabetes: a report from the International Diabetes Federation Taskforce on Epidemiology and Prevention. *Diabetes Res Clin Pract* 2008; 81: 2–12.

74. Redline S, Yenokyan G, Gottlieb DJ, *et al.* Obstructive sleep apnea-hypopnea and incident stroke: the sleep heart health study. *Am J Respir Crit Care Med* 2010; 182: 269–277.

75. Birkbak J, Clark AJ, Rod NH. The effect of sleep disordered breathing on the outcome of stroke and transient ischemic attack: a systematic review. *J Clin Sleep Med* 2014; 10: 103–108.

76. Yaggi HK, Concato J, Kernan WN, *et al.* Obstructive sleep apnea as a risk factor for stroke and death. *N Engl J Med* 2005; 353: 2034–2041.

77. Martínez-García MA, Campos-Rodríguez F, Soler-Cataluña JJ, *et al.* Increased incidence of nonfatal cardiovascular events in stroke patients with sleep apnoea: effect of CPAP treatment. *Eur Respir J* 2012; 39: 906–912.

78. Parra O, Sánchez-Armengol Á, Capote F, *et al.* Efficacy of continuous positive airway pressure treatment on 5-year survival in patients with ischaemic stroke and obstructive sleep apnea: a randomized controlled trial. *J Sleep Res* 2015; 24: 47–53.

79. Ryan CM, Bayley M, Green R, *et al.* Influence of continuous positive airway pressure on outcomes of rehabilitation in stroke patients with obstructive sleep apnea. *Stroke* 2011; 42: 1062–1067.

80. Parra O, Sánchez-Armengol A, Bonnin M, *et al.* Early treatment of obstructive apnoea and stroke outcome: a randomised controlled trial. *Eur Respir J* 2011; 37: 1128–1136.

81. Väyrynen K, Kortelainen K, Numminen H. Screening sleep disordered breathing in stroke unit. *Sleep Disord* 2014; 317615.

82. Brown DL, Chervin RD, Hickenbottom SL, *et al.* Screening for obstructive sleep apnea in stroke patients: a cost-effectiveness analysis. *Stroke* 2005; 36: 1291–1293.

83. Davis AP, Billings ME, Longstreth WT Jr, *et al.* Early diagnosis and treatment of obstructive sleep apnea after stroke: Are we neglecting a modifiable stroke risk factor? *Neurol Clin Pract* 2013; 3: 192–201.

84. Alchanatis M, Tourkohoriti G, Kakouros S, *et al.* Daytime pulmonary hypertension in patients with obstructive sleep apnea: the effect of continuous positive airway pressure on pulmonary hemodynamics. *Respiration* 2001; 68: 566–572.

85. Arias MA, García-Río F, Alonso-Fernández A, *et al.* Pulmonary hypertension in obstructive sleep apnoea: effects of continuous positive airway pressure: a randomized, controlled cross-over study. *Eur Heart J* 2006; 27: 1106–1113.

86. Dumitrascu R, Tiede H, Eckermann J, *et al.* Sleep apnea in precapillary pulmonary hypertension. *Sleep Med* 2013; 14: 247–251.

87. Lopez PP, Stefan B, Schulman CI, *et al.* Prevalence of sleep apnea in morbidly obese patients who presented for weight loss surgery evaluation: more evidence for routine screening for obstructive sleep apnea before weight loss surgery. *Am Surg* 2008; 74: 834–838.

88. Nepomnayshy D, Hesham W, Erickson B, *et al.* Sleep apnea: is routine preoperative screening necessary? *Obes Surg* 2013; 23: 287–291.

89. Rasmussen JJ, Fuller WD, Ali MR. Sleep apnea syndrome is significantly underdiagnosed in bariatric surgical patients. *Surg Obes Relat Dis* 2012; 8: 569–573.

90. Mechanick JI, Youdim A, Jones DB, *et al.* Clinical practice guidelines for the perioperative, nutritional, metabolic, and nonsurgical support of the bariatric surgery patient – 2013 update: cosponsored by American Association of Clinical Endocrinologists, the Obesity Society, and American Society for Metabolic & Bariatric Surgery. *Endocr Pract* 2013; 19: 337–372.

91. Malbois M, Giusti V, Suter M. Oximetry alone *versus* portable polygraphy for sleep apnea screening before bariatric surgery. *Obes Surg* 2010; 20: 326–331.

92. Fredheim JM, Røislien J, Hjelmesæth J. Validation of a portable monitor for the diagnosis of obstructive sleep apnea in morbidly obese patients. *J Clin Sleep Med* 2014; 10: 751–757.

Disclosures: None declared.

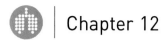
COPD and other pulmonary diseases

José M. Marin

Increased prevalence of OSA is not seen amongst those with chronic pulmonary diseases such as COPD, asthma, pulmonary fibrosis or pulmonary hypertension. However, prognosis does worsen when OSA and chronic pulmonary diseases overlap. Obesity is a key risk factor for OSA development, not only in the general population but also in patients with chronic respiratory diseases. Sleep in pulmonary patients with OSA overlap is characterised by higher sleep fragmentation and more severe hypoxaemia than in those with COPD or OSA alone. Untreated OSA is associated with increased mortality in the classic "overlap syndrome" (OSA plus COPD); noninvasive ventilation reduces such excessive risk. OSA is an independent risk factor for asthma exacerbations and worsened respiratory symptoms in patients with asthma and pulmonary fibrosis. CPAP is a very effective treatment for OSA. All patients with chronic pulmonary diseases should be carefully evaluated to rule out the coexistence of OSA.

In healthy subjects, sleep is accompanied by changes in the circulation and respiration that are not associated with significant adverse effects. However, in patients with chronic pulmonary diseases such as COPD, asthma and pulmonary fibrosis, sleep is associated with adaptive changes in the airway, lung and chest mechanics. The immediate consequences of these changes are the development of disproportionate hypoxaemia and hypercapnia, and bronchoconstriction in asthma. In the long-term, they can contribute to worsened prognosis for these diseases. This chapter reviews the overlap syndromes of OSA in patients with COPD, asthma, pulmonary fibrosis and pulmonary hypertension. Here, we understand the concept of "overlap syndromes" as the coexistence of one of these chronic respiratory conditions with OSA in the same patient.

COPD and OSA

Definitions and classifications

According to the most recent Global Initiative for Chronic Obstructive Lung Disease (GOLD) strategy document, COPD is a preventable and treatable disease, characterised by persistent airflow limitation that is usually progressive and associated with an enhanced

University of Zaragoza School of Medicine, and Respiratory Dept, Hospital Miguel Servet, Zaragoza, and CIBERES, Madrid, Spain.

Correspondence: José M. Marin, Respiratory Dept, Hospital Miguel Servet, 1–3, Avda Isabel la Católica, 50006-Zaragoza, Spain. E-mail: jmmarint@unizar.es

Copyright ©ERS 2015. Print ISBN: 978-1-84984-059-0. Online ISBN: 978-1-84984-060-6. Print ISSN: 2312-508X. Online ISSN: 2312-5098.

chronic inflammatory response in the airways and the lung to noxious particles or gases. The GOLD definition of COPD also emphasises that "exacerbations and comorbidities contribute to the overall severity in individual patients" [1]. Clearly, the coexistence of OSA is one of these comorbidities. A clinical diagnosis of COPD should be considered in any patient who has dyspnoea, chronic cough and/or sputum production, and a history of exposure to risk factors for the disease. Spirometry is required to make the diagnosis; a post-bronchodilator FEV_1/FVC <0.70 confirms the presence of persistent airflow limitation and thus COPD. Classification of airflow limitation severity in COPD is also based on spirometry results. The severity of COPD is classified using post-bronchodilator FEV_1: mild FEV_1 ⩾80% predicted; moderate FEV_1 50–<80% pred; severe FEV_1 30–<50% pred; or very severe FEV_1 <30% pred.

OSA is a sleep disorder characterised by increased UA resistance associated with an intermittent decrease or absence of inspiratory airflow, causing sympathetic activation, arousals during sleep and often accompanied by intermittent oxyhaemoglobin desaturation [2]. The diagnosis of OSA requires a PSG study. An AHI of ⩾5 events·h^{-1} is consistent with OSA [3]. The consensus definitions of severity in OSA used the following AHI cut-points. Mild sleep apnoea: ⩾5–<15 episodes·h^{-1}; moderate sleep apnoea: ⩾15–<30 episodes·h^{-1}; and severe sleep apnoea: ⩾30 episodes·h^{-1}. This consensus is in part based on published literature that has found an association between the severity of OSA and increased mortality [4–8].

David Flenley first described the coexistence of COPD and OSA as the "overlap syndrome" almost 30 years age [9]. In order to determine the presence of associated OSA, he suggested that a sleep study should be considered in obese COPD patients, in those who snore, and in those who complain of headache following nocturnal oxygen therapy. He questioned the administration of nocturnal oxygen in these patients and believed that in overlap patients, the clinical course and prognosis was worse than in patients suffering from COPD or OSA alone. This argument still holds true today.

Epidemiology

OSA, COPD and asthma are the most regularly seen chronic respiratory disorders in pulmonary clinics. Overall, it is estimated that a mean of 10% of the general population have moderate-to-severe COPD, defined as FEV_1/FVC <0.7 and FEV_1 <80% pred [10]. COPD prevalence increases with age and is directly related to tobacco smoking, but outdoor and indoor air pollution are also major COPD risk factors. The prevalence and burden of COPD are projected to increase in the coming decades due to continued exposure to COPD risk factors and the ageing of the world's population.

In the Wisconsin Sleep Cohort Study, 20% of men and 9% of women had an AHI of ⩾5 events·h^{-1} between the ages of 30 and 60 years [11]. This report was published 20 years ago. From the same ongoing cohort, the current prevalence estimates of moderate-to-severe sleep disordered breathing (AHI ⩾15 events·h^{-1}) showed a substantial increase over the last two decades, with relative increases of 14–55% depending on the age subgroup [12]. Although it is typically thought of as a condition affecting men, the OSA sex disparity ends around 55 years of age, with a sharp rise among post-menopausal women [12–14].

No study has directly assessed the prevalence of overlap. As COPD and OSA are increasing throughout the world and as the population age is rising, overlap syndrome is likely to become more prevalent. In a clinical series, it was noted that ~11% of patients with OSA syndrome have airflow limitation on spirometry [15]. In a European population study that predominantly included mild COPD patients, OSA syndrome occurred in 3% of the subjects [16]. The Sleep Heart Health Study (SHHS), a large community-based cohort study, included 5954 participants who underwent PSG and spirometry at baseline [17]. A total of 1132 participants (19%) had predominantly mild airway obstruction (FEV1/FVC <0.7) and 1644 (27.6%) had a RDI >10 events h^{-1}. No increase in OSA prevalence was seen in subjects with airway obstruction compared with the non-obstructed population. 254 participants (4.3%) had both characteristics (COPD and sleep apnoea).

The overall prevalence of COPD, OSA and overlap syndrome is presented in figure 1.

Sleep in patients with COPD and OSA

In the SHHS, subjects with mild airflow obstruction without OSA showed no change in sleep efficiency and no increase in sleepiness as measured by the ESS [18]. However, patients with airflow obstruction and OSA had a lower total sleep time, lower sleep efficiency and a higher ESS score. They were also more likely to have greater O_2 desaturation compared with those who only have either OSA or airway obstruction [17]. In a recent European survey, 78.1% of patients with COPD reported some degree of night-time symptoms. As the severity of airflow limitation increased, so did the prevalence of night-time symptoms [19]. Nocturnal COPD symptoms, such as dyspnoea, cough, sputum and wheezing, are associated with arousals and difficulty in maintenance of sleep, which are likely to contribute to the daytime hypersomnolence that many patients report.

More than 50% of COPD patients who have a daytime arterial oxygen saturation (S_aO_2) >90% and no experience of sleep apnoea experience significant desaturation during sleep [20]. Daytime gas exchange abnormalities, particularly a low arterial oxygen tension (P_aO_2), are predictive of sleep O_2 desaturation [21]. When compared with patients with either COPD or OSA alone, patients with overlap syndrome display more profound oxygen desaturations during sleep, as well as daytime hypoxaemia and hypercapnia [15].

Risk factor for overlap syndrome

In addition to the common risk factors for OSA in adults, such as obesity, UA abnormalities and family aggregation, among patients with COPD, active smoking,

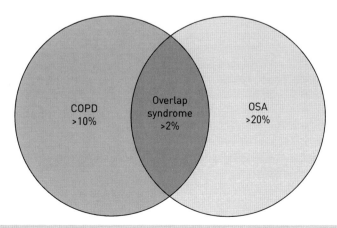

Figure 1. Overall prevalence of COPD, OSA and overlap syndrome.

peripheral oedema and oral corticosteroids increase the risk of obstructive apnoea events. When present among COPD patients, obesity is a key contributor to sleep disordered breathing, accelerated pulmonary hypertension and obesity hypoventilation syndrome, irrespective of airflow obstruction severity [22]. These patients particularly resemble the so-called "blue bloater" COPD phenotype. Smoking is associated with upper and lower airway inflammation, nasal airflow resistance and snoring [23]. In the Wisconsin Sleep Cohort, an AHI of >5 events·h^{-1} was three times more likely in current smokers than in never-smokers. In the study, heavy smokers (>40 cigarettes per day) had an odds ratio of 6.74 for an AHI of >5 events·h^{-1} [24]. Fluid accumulation around the pharynx increases pharyngeal resistance [25], meaning COPD patients treated with corticosteroids or with the coexistence of HF had an increased susceptibility to pharyngeal obstruction during sleep in response to rostral fluid redistribution. By contrast, some patients with advanced COPD can lose weight and consequently reduce the risk for UA obstruction (fig. 2).

Overlap syndrome pathophysiology

Respiratory mechanics during sleep have not been measured specifically in patients with overlap syndrome. Increased diaphragmatic and abdominal muscle effort is required during apnoeic episodes to overcome UA resistance and maintain adequate airflow to the lung. This can be particularly difficult for COPD patients who already have increased intrathoracic airway resistance and lung hyperinflation at baseline. In this scenario, the ribcage's contribution to breathing reduces, diaphragmatic efficiency decreases and the accessory muscles' contribution to breathing increases [26]. The result is a reduction in FRC, which may augment ventilation/perfusion mismatch. As obesity also reduces FRC during sleep, overweight/obese patients with overlap syndrome are particularly prone to reduced alveolar volume and increased gas exchange abnormalities during apnoea episodes (fig. 3). Respiratory control centre output is reduced during sleep, especially during REM sleep [27]. Moreover, patients with COPD also have blunted ventilatory responses and

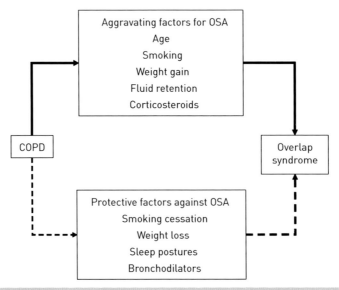

Figure 2. Interactions between COPD and OSA.

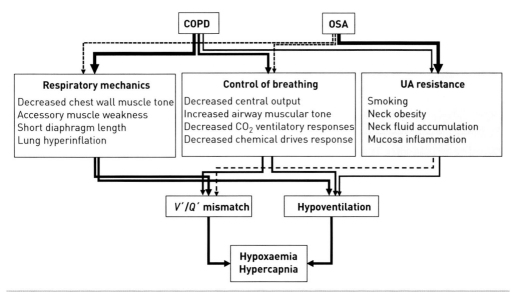

Figure 3. Pathways involved in nocturnal hypoxaemia and hypercapnia in overlap syndrome. V'/Q': ventilation/perfusion. Thick line: greater cause–effect relationship; thin line: lesser cause–effect relationship; interrupted line: a possible but unproven relationship.

mouth occlusion pressure responses to carbon dioxide and chemical drives [28]. When these patients develop apnoeic episodes, the compensatory response of the respiratory centre is slower, apnoeas are longer and changes in arterial oxygen tension (PaO$_2$) and carbon dioxide tension are more intense. Finally, because many COPD patients have awake hypoxaemia, those with overlap syndrome are particularly prone to nocturnal oxygen desaturation as they are on the steep portion of the oxyhaemoglobin dissociation curve.

Clinical features of the overlap syndrome

Compared with COPD or OSA populations, overlap patients with similar ages tend to be more obese and have more comorbid conditions [29]. They also report more daytime sleepiness [17] and worse quality of life [30]. Sleep recordings from overlap patients show a lower total sleep time, lower sleep efficiency and higher sleep fragmentation than those from COPD or OSA patients. More severe nocturnal oxygen desaturation is a characteristic feature in overlap patients. Subjects with OSA alone return to normal oxygen saturation baseline between obstructive events (IH); in COPD, due to hypoventilation and ventilation/perfusion mismatch, nocturnal oxygen saturation reduces more evenly throughout the night and at the end of an apnoea episode, SaO$_2$ does not tend to return to the initial baseline level (fig. 4). A typical patient with overlap syndrome has a reduced baseline SaO$_2$, lower mean SaO$_2$ and spends more time in hypoxaemia than patients with OSA or COPD.

The majority of patients with OSA do not develop significant night hypercapnia due to inter-apnoea hyperventilation. Nevertheless, if the patient also has COPD, the ventilatory response to apnoea episodes is reduced by the deficit of thoracic mechanics, and post-apnoea carbon dioxide levels may not return to baseline. Over time, a progressive desensitisation of the respiratory centre in response to hypoxic–hypercapnic episodes develops and then the patients can remain hypercapnic during sleep when blunting takes

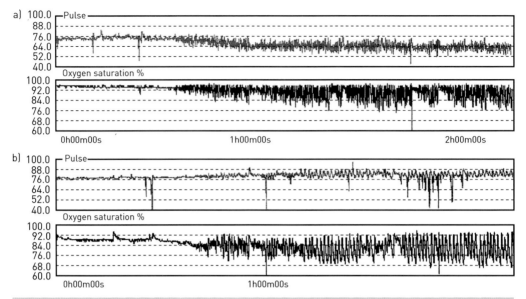

Figure 4. Sleep pattern of a patient with a) OSA alone and b) overlap syndrome. Reproduced from [31] with permission from the publisher.

place [32]. CPAP treatment can partially reverse this phenomenon [33]. Although daytime hypercapnia can develop in OSA alone, it is much more frequent in patients with overlap [34]. Both daytime hypoxaemia and hypercapnia have been found to be predictors of right-heart failure [35] and should therefore be considered markers of poor prognosis.

Overlap syndrome diagnosis

In the appropriate clinical context, PSG and a spirometry test should be performed to confirm the existence of the syndrome and to establish its severity. Routine PSG is not indicated in patients with COPD. There has been no progress on this issue since, in the second edition of his textbook, Neil Douglas recommended PSG in patients with COPD: "when OSA is suspected because of either symptoms or the development of hypoxemic complications – cor pulmonale and polycythaemia – with daytime PaO$_2$ greater than 60 mmHg" [36].

Major consequences of overlap syndrome

Daytime somnolence

Due to excessive sleepiness in patients with OSA, school and work performance are reduced [37]. There is also a strong association between sleep apnoea, as measured by AHI, and the risk of traffic accidents [38]. In patients with overlap syndrome, these "daytime consequences" of the disease have not been evaluated specifically, but they may reflect the sum of the severity of the sleep disorders of both entities, COPD and OSA separately.

Metabolic disorders

OSA is considered an independent risk factor for insulin resistance. In cohort studies controlling for multiple confounders, initial OSA severity predicted a subsequent risk of incident diabetes [39]. COPD has not been linked with the risk of metabolic disorders;

however, the so called "blue bloater" phenotype characterised by chronic bronchitis and high BMI may be particularly predisposed to develop OSA and metabolic diseases.

Cardiovascular disorders

Epidemiological data show a strong association between OSA and incident arterial hypertension, with prevalence rates of ~45% [40]. OSA is also common in refractory hypertension. In COPD, hypertension prevalence is similar to that of the general population and patients with overlap have the same rates as patients with OSA alone [29].

Almost all types of arrhythmia have been described during sleep in patients with OSA. Untreated OSA patients are particularly susceptible to the development of atrial fibrillation, as demonstrated in the Seep Heart Health Study [41]. Furthermore, patients with COPD also suffer a higher number of arrhythmias during sleep, which has been related to nocturnal desaturation [42] and is associated with an increased likelihood of atrial fibrillation/flutter [43]. It is therefore to be expected that patients with overlap suffer from an increased risk of arrhythmias. In fact, in a recent community-based retrospective cohort analysis, data collected from 2873 who were >65 years of age showed an increased risk of new-onset atrial fibrillation in overlap syndrome as compared with the presence of OSA or COPD alone [44].

Both OSA and COPD are medical conditions associated with an increased risk of cardiovascular morbidity and mortality. Epidemiological data indicate that the incidence of coronary artery disease, stroke and HF increase in OSA [4, 5, 45] and COPD [46]. There are no such studies in overlap syndrome but the coexistence of OSA and COPD in the same patient is likely to increase the risk of cardiovascular events if both diseases are not adequately treated. In support of this idea, the presence of several intermediate mechanisms that may accelerate the development of CVD in overlap syndrome has been documented. In addition to an increased risk of atrial fibrillation, CHAOUAT et al. [15] demonstrated that patients with overlap syndrome have increased daytime pulmonary vascular resistance compared with patients with OSA alone. SHARMA et al. [47] recently added important knowledge to this field when they demonstrated higher right ventricular mass and remodelling indices in overlap patients compared with COPD patients. Arterial stiffness, a surrogate marker of subclinical atherosclerosis, has been found to be significantly higher in subjects with overlap syndrome than in those with OSA alone [48]. Finally, oxidative stress occurs in COPD and OSA and there is evidence of increased circulating inflammatory cytokines and leukocytes in both disorders [49, 50]. These are key factors for endothelial dysfunction and atherosclerosis and ultimately CVDs (fig. 5). However, no study has been performed that determines whether overlap is a state of systemic hyper-inflammation with respect to its components and whether this syndrome may represent an extra risk of cardiovascular death in sufferers.

Mortality

Untreated OSA in patients with COPD is associated with increased mortality. In both conditions, the risk of mortality increases in accordance with the severity of the disorder. In OSA, a higher rate of mortality is seen in younger individuals [51]; in COPD, a higher rate of mortality is seen in older individuals [52]. In overlap patients, the evidence indicates that mortality is increased. A study of OSA patients attending sleep clinics found that the coexistence of COPD and OSA increased the risk of death [53]. We subsequently confirmed this data in a large cohort of patients with suspected sleep disordered breathing. All patients routinely underwent spirometry as well as a sleep study [29]. Patients had an average age of 57 years and the median follow-up time was >9 years. All-cause mortality was found to be

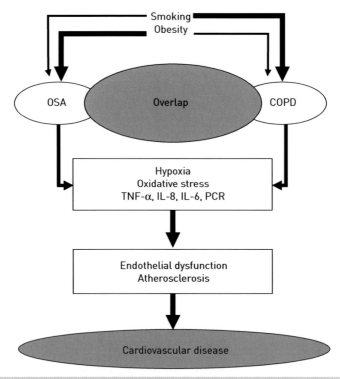

Figure 5. Pathways involved in accelerated CVD in COPD and OSA.

higher in the untreated overlap group (42.2%) than in the COPD-only group (24.2%) (fig. 6). In COPD patients, comorbid untreated OSA remained a risk factor for death after adjusting for FEV1 (% pred) as a surrogate of COPD severity. In this study there was a significantly higher number of cardiovascular deaths in patients with untreated overlap syndrome (14.6%) compared with overlap patients treated appropriately with CPAP (7.5%)

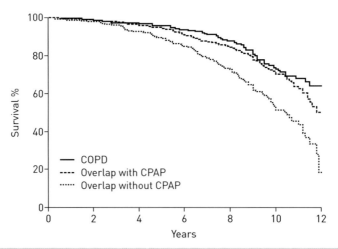

Figure 6. Kaplan–Meier survival curves in COPD patients without OSA, overlap syndrome patients not treated with CPAP, and overlap syndrome patients treated with CPAP. p<0.001. Reproduced and modified from [29] with permission from the publisher.

or COPD only (5.7%) [29]. Interestingly, in this non-aged population, the second most frequent cause of death was cancer, raising the question currently in debate about the excess risk of cancer in both OSA and COPD [54, 55].

Nocturnal death appears to increase in COPD during exacerbations [56]. Among >10 000 individuals referred for sleep study, nocturnal hypoxaemia, an important pathophysiological feature of OSA, strongly predicted sudden cardiac death especially at night, independently of well-established risk factors [57]. There are no data about this in overlap syndrome, although in the report by McNicholas and FitzGerald [56], nocturnal death was highest amongst "blue-bloater" patients with respiratory failure, a COPD phenotype commonly associated with OSA.

Overlap syndrome management

There are no specific guidelines for the treatment of overlap syndrome. The therapeutic management of these patients should be based on optimising treatment for both conditions (COPD and OSA) following the corresponding clinical recommendations [1, 37]. The goals of therapy are improvement in patient-related outcomes (such as sleep fragmentation, sleep quality and daytime sleepiness) and more objective data (such as daytime activity and COPD exacerbation). Correction of hypoxaemia and hypercapnia during sleep is particularly important for the reduction of cardiovascular complications and extension of survival.

Noninvasive ventilation

PAP is delivered nasally or through a face mask and is the most effective treatment for OSA. CPAP is the most commonly used PAP therapy for most patients with OSA. BPAP offers high-pressure delivery during inspiration and lower pressure during expiration; it is recommended for patients with severe OSA who require high levels of PAP as it is better tolerated than CPAP. BPAP is also preferred for patients with OSA and obesity hypoventilation syndrome because it provides a pressure gradient that increases alveolar ventilation.

In COPD, noninvasive ventilation (NIV) is highly effective in an acute setting. In COPD patients with chronic hypercapnia, the effects of NIV on quality of life, lung function, gas exchange and long-term survival are contradictory due to the absence of long-term studies with a large enough number of subjects [58]. Nevertheless, in the USA, Medicare and Medicaid have agreed to treat patients with severe COPD in the following situations: when OSA has been ruled out; when arterial carbon dioxide tension is $\geqslant$52 mmHg; when sleep oximetry shows a S_aO_2 $\leqslant$88% for $\geqslant$5 min while breathing oxygen at 2 L·min^{-1}; or when a patient is prescribed inspiratory oxygen fraction [59]. In a long-term cohort study, overlap patients who were not treated with CPAP demonstrated an increased risk of death from any cause and hospitalisation due to COPD exacerbations, compared with overlap patients who were treated with and adhered to CPAP [29]. In another observational study, the use of CPAP and long-term oxygen therapy improved survival among overlap patients with chronic respiratory failure [60]. Finally, in a retrospective analysis of 227 patients with overlap syndrome who were attending an outpatient clinic and were treated with CPAP, it was shown that more time on CPAP was associated with a reduced risk of death after controlling for common risk factors [61]. Taken together, the results of these studies seem to show that NIV is effective in patients with overlap syndrome.

The choice between CPAP and BPAP can be determined based on the pattern of sleep disordered breathing. In cases where OSA is the predominant condition, CPAP may be most appropriate; in cases where there is evidence of significant nocturnal hypoventilation with associated periods of sustained hypoxaemia, BPAP may be more appropriate. Newer modalities of pressure support, such as adaptive servoventilation, may be particularly suited to patients with the overlap syndrome. Supplemental oxygen should be added if CPAP or BPAP therapy alone fails to provide satisfactory oxygenation. The ideal place to adjust this treatment is the sleep laboratory and this should be conducted by well-trained technicians.

Additional medical treatment

In COPD alone, nocturnal hypoxaemia should be corrected with supplemental oxygen through a nasal cannula. Alveolar ventilation is dependent on the peripheral stimulant effect of hypoxaemia. Therefore, in order to minimise the tendency towards carbon dioxide retention, particularly during sleep hours, oxygen supplementation should be titrated carefully. Morning headache after oxygen initiation in patients with COPD is an indication that PSG should be performed in order to exclude the coexistence of OSA or to investigate the development of carbon dioxide retention.

In OSA alone, oxygen treatment can eliminate or reduce nocturnal hypoxaemia; however, AHI is not reduced, daytime hypersomnolence is not improved [62] and no change in nocturnal BP is seen [63]. The roll of oxygen supplementation as nocturnal therapy in overlap syndrome has not been explored and at present it should only be used to complement NIV.

There is currently no effective pharmacological treatment for OSA. Patients with COPD should receive the appropriate treatment according to current recommendations [1]. The most common drugs currently prescribed in stable COPD, such as long-acting anticholinergics (LAMA) and long-acting β-agonists (LABA), have been shown to improve nocturnal SaO_2 but without a clear improvement on the quality of sleep [64, 65]. Theophylline, which has been used as an oral bronchodilator for decades, has effects that may be useful in patients with COPD and sleep disordered breathing; it stimulates the respiratory centre and enhances the activity of the respiratory muscles [66]. However, there are conflicting results regarding its effect on the quality of sleep in these patients and its use should be determined on an individual basis and as a second-line treatment following LAMA and LABA. Inhaled corticosteroids are often used in patients with stable COPD and their use has not been linked with sleep disruption. No specific studies have been performed that evaluate the effects of these drugs in patients with overlap syndrome. Sleep aids, especially benzodiazepines, should be avoided in patients with COPD and OSA because they decrease arousal response to hypercapnia, induce hypoventilation and decrease muscular tone. Non-benzodiazepinic hypnotics, such as zolpidem, could be used for a limited time as there is evidence that this drug does not decrease respiratory drive and does not cause daytime drowsiness [67].

Surgical treatment

Patients with very severe COPD could be candidates for lung transplantation. They usually have nocturnal hypoxaemia but very rarely OSA as most of them are very thin. Other patients with COPD can present with severe emphysema and may be candidates for emphysema surgery. Ideally, all of these patients should undergo PSG and should be treated according to the findings arising from this. Thoracic surgery is not contraindicated in overlap syndrome but during post-operative care these patients must be closely monitored and NIV with oxygen supplementation should be added if there is coexistent diurnal and/or nocturnal hypoxaemia or hypercapnia.

There are no studies about the effect of UA surgery or the use of oral appliances in the treatment of OSA in overlap syndrome. In patients with this syndrome, surgery should be considered an adjunctive therapy and reserved for patients who have problems tolerating treatment with PAP due to nasal or pharyngeal obstruction.

Asthma and OSA

Definitions and classifications

According to the Global Strategy for Asthma Management and Prevention report, by the Global Initiative for Asthma (GINA), asthma is defined as a heterogeneous disease, usually characterised by chronic airway inflammation. It is defined by the history of respiratory symptoms, such as wheeze, shortness of breath, chest tightness and cough that vary over time and in intensity, together with variable expiratory airflow limitation [68]. Current asthma prevalence across all ages in the USA is 8.2% [69]. In adults, diseases with a known association with asthma include gastro-oesophageal reflux disease, rhinosinusitis, obesity, mental disorders and sleep apnoea. The GINA initiative recommended the investigation of the coexistence of OSA in all patients with asthma, especially in those with severe asthma, difficult-to-control asthma and asthma with associated obesity [68]. As asthma is more difficult to control in obese patients and obesity is the main risk factor for OSA, it is important that a sleep study is performed in obese asthmatics; if OSA is identified, it should be treated appropriately.

Epidemiology

There are no population-based studies that use PSG to identify the prevalence and severity of OSA in asthmatics. In a study using the Berlin Questionnaire, the prevalence of OSA symptoms was found to be higher in an asthmatic population (39.5%) than among primary care patients (27.2%; p=0.004) [70]. In a Canadian cohort of patients with asthma, OSA was defined using an AHI $\geqslant 15$ events·h^{-1} of sleep and was present in 88% patients with severe asthma, 58% of patients with moderate asthma and 31% of controls without asthma [71]. REDLINE et al. [72] performed an epidemiological study using home overnight multichannel monitoring in 399 children and adolescents of 2–18 years of age. They demonstrated that sinus problems and persistent wheeze each independently (of the other) predicted OSA independently of age, race and obesity. Overall, OSA appears to be approximately doubled in asthmatic populations compared with nonasthmatics.

Sleep in patients with asthma

Patients with nocturnal asthma complain of frequent arousals and poor sleep quality. The persistence of nocturnal symptoms like cough, wheeze or chest strain indicate poor control of asthma and the need to modify anti-asthmatic treatment. Indeed, reversal of nocturnal symptoms is an important goal of treatment in asthmatics [68]. Patients with nocturnal asthma attacks suffer from insomnia and daytime sleepiness. Sleep studies performed in a time in which the effective current asthma treatment was not available showed a lower sleep efficiency, more awakenings and less stage 3–4 sleep compared with normal subjects [73]. Cognitive performance as assessed using psychometric testing has also been found to be impaired in these patients [74]. Nevertheless, in a case–control study, a circadian peak expiratory flow variation of $\geqslant 20\%$ (a surrogate parameter of asthma instability) was associated with a poorer daytime cognitive performance when compared with healthy controls [75]. In the study, effective asthma treatment resulted in the recovery of cognitive impairment to a level of performance comparable to that of healthy control subjects, which was paralleled by a reduction of circadian peak expiratory flow variation of <10% and by the disappearance of nocturnal asthma symptoms.

Pathophysiology of nocturnal asthma

No isolated mechanism justifies nocturnal asthma in all cases. It is not the purpose of this chapter to provide an in-depth review of this topic; the interested reader is referred to [76]. Table 1 summarises a number of mechanisms implicated in the worsening of nocturnal asthma.

Risk factors for OSA in asthma

Weight gain
Obesity is a risk factor for both asthma and OSA. There is a dose–response effect of the increase in BMI over the increase in the risk of incident asthma, particularly in women [77]. In asthmatics, particularly those with exercise-induced asthma and nocturnal asthma, exercise restriction and daytime sleepiness contribute to weight gain and fat deposits in the pharynx. Therefore, as an asthmatic's weight increases, so the probability of having OSA increases (fig. 7).

Rhinitis, sinusitis, polyps
Many patients with nonatopic asthma and most atopic asthmatics suffer from nasal obstruction due to one or more of these comorbid conditions. Rhinitis and chronic sinusitis cause nasal congestion and airflow resistance. Nasopharyngeal polyps also reduce

Table 1. Mechanisms of nocturnal asthma

Mechanism	All types of asthma	Nocturnal asthma
Airway inflammation	The main underlying mechanism of bronchial hyperresponsiveness	Greater inflammatory markers in bronchoalveolar lavage at night compared with during the day.
Parasympathetic tone	Enhanced in some patients	Enhanced in all patients. Anticholinergics are effective.
Cold	Causes bronchoconstriction in most patients	Breathing warm and humidified air can prevent some nocturnal asthma attacks.
Allergens	Key issue for allergic asthma	Bedroom allergens can trigger nocturnal asthma attacks.
Gastro-oesophageal reflux	Present in ~50% of patients	Very common. Gastric acid suppressors are very effective for decreasing nocturnal symptoms.
Airway secretions	Increased in most patients	Sleep suppress cough reflex and impaired mucociliary clearance. Airway secretion is more pronounced at night compared with during the day.
OSA	More prevalent than in nonasthmatic population	Very common. OSA exacerbates asthma by neurally mediated reflex bronchoconstriction and inflammation of the UA.

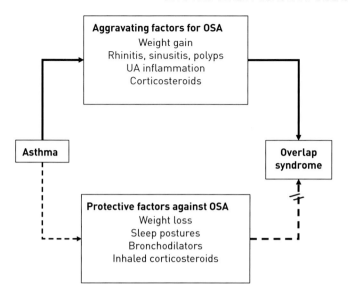

Figure 7. Interactions between asthma and OSA.

airway calibre. All of these, as well as increasing intrathoracic and pharyngeal negative pressure, promote UA collapse during inspiration, snoring and obstructive apnoea [78].

UA inflammation
In patients with long-term chronic asthma there is permanent airway mucosal inflammation. This process affects the UA by decreasing the cross-sectional area of the pharynx and promoting airway collapse [79].

Asthma medications
Inhaled corticosteroids are the most effective and most commonly used drugs in asthma. Their long-term effects on the collapsibility of the pharynx remain unknown. However, the effects of oral corticosteroids on the UA are well known and include myopathy of the muscles of the pharynx, fatty infiltration of the pharyngeal wall and accumulation of liquid in the neck. In a pulmonary outpatient clinic, asthmatics on oral corticosteroids or requiring frequent bursts of oral corticosteroids had a very high prevalence of OSA (>90%) [80].

Factors that may help reduce the risk of OSA in patients with asthma include those seen in COPD patients: weight loss, sleep in lateral decubitus and quitting smoking to reduce local inflammation. The effect of asthma medication in patients with concomitant OSA has not been studied. In nonasthmatic patients with OSA, there is molecular and clinical evidence regarding the ability of inhaled corticosteroids to reduce UA inflammation and improve AHI in a subgroup of patients with concomitant allergic rhinitis [81]. In clinical practice, nasal inhaled corticosteroids and oral anti-leukotrienes may be beneficial for reducing snoring and obstructive apnoeas in children with asthma and OSA, but their effect has not been proven in adults.

OSA worsens asthma

In contrast to overlap syndrome, no long-term cohort studies have been conducted that have evaluated asthma outcomes among patients with comorbid OSA. Nevertheless, CPAP treatment for comorbid OSA has been shown to improve asthma symptoms, reduce use of rescue medication and improve disease-specific quality of life [81–84].

The mechanisms by which OSA worsens asthma are multifactorial. Apnoeic episodes are associated with corresponding repeated arousals, heightened sympathetic activity and intermittent oxygen desaturation [37]. Sleep fragmentation has been associated with ventricular dysfunction and weight gain. Increased vagal tone during apnoea episodes can contribute to nocturnal asthma through muscarinic receptor stimulation of the central airway and UA. Negative intrathoracic pressure during obstructive events leads to intermittent loss of lower oesophageal sphincter tone. Gastro-oesophageal reflux disease is very common in OSA and is associated with arousal during sleep, UA oedema and bronchial micro-aspiration of gastric acid promoting nocturnal asthma. By stimulation of carotid body receptors, IH can enhance the bronchial responsiveness through vagal pathways [85]. Chronic IH in OSA induces a low-grade systemic inflammation characterised by the elevation of serum pro-inflammatory cytokines and chemokines. Local inflammatory changes of the UA similar to that noted in asthma are also prominent in OSA. All of these inflammatory changes reduce airway calibre, increase the underlying bronchial hyperresponsiveness and trigger asthma.

Treatment

There are no specific guidelines for the management of patients with OSA–asthma overlap. In a short-term randomised trial, CPAP decreased airway reactivity in asthmatics without OSA, probably through the reduction of bronchial inflammation [86]. Longer studies are needed to determine whether CPAP can also decrease asthma symptoms and/or medication use, and identify asthmatic subjects who can best be treated with CPAP. In OSA patients with comorbid asthma, CPAP has important collateral beneficial effects for asthmatics: it reduces gastro-oesophageal reflux, local and systemic inflammation, and airway smooth muscle contractility [87]. Therefore, CPAP can be an especially effective treatment for OSA–asthma overlap syndrome. Given the high prevalence of rhinitis, sinusitis and polyps, all patients with OSA and asthma should be carefully evaluated by an ear, nose and throat specialist and appropriately treated before starting treatment with CPAP.

Second-line treatments for OSA, such as MAD and UA surgery, have not been prospectively evaluated in patients with asthma overlap. Bariatric surgery for patients with OSA–asthma overlap and morbid obesity is especially effective not only for OSA resolution but also for asthma improvement [88]. There are no studies assessing asthma medication in OSA–asthma overlap. Therefore, asthma in patients with OSA should be treated according to current guidelines [68], in addition to optimising their OSA treatment.

Pulmonary fibrosis

Idiopathic pulmonary fibrosis (IPF) is the most common and severe form of interstitial lung disease. IPF is a fibrotic lung disease of unknown cause, characterised by progressive dyspnoea, hypoxaemia and restrictive-ventilatory limitation. IPF should be suspected in the appropriate clinical context when there is evidence of impairment of gas exchange or restrictive lung function deficit. Confirmation comes when there is a pattern of usual interstitial pneumonia on lung biopsy or on computed tomography scan [89]. The prevalence reported in Europe ranges 1.25–23.4 cases per 100 000 [90]. The incidence of

IPF appears to be increasing mainly because of improvements in the ability to diagnose the condition due to advances in chest imaging [91]. The natural history of IPF is unpredictable in the individual, with a median survival of 3–5 years from diagnosis [92].

Sleep is often disturbed among patients with IPF. Most patients report nocturnal cough as an important cause of nocturnal awakenings. Gastro-oesophageal reflux, which is also very prevalent in IPF and the pulmonary fibrotic process itself, are the main intermediate mechanisms that explain nocturnal cough. Hypoxaemia, particularly during exercise, is a characteristic feature of IPF. Oxygen desaturation during sleep is also very common and can contribute to pulmonary hypertension and poor outcomes [93]. OSA is very prevalent in IPF but clearly under-recognised. In a sample of 50 patients with stable IPF, OSA was confirmed using PSG in 88% [94]. Of those, 68% were moderate-to severe (AHI >15 events·h^{-1}). It appears that severity of OSA, as indicated by AHI, inversely correlates with total lung capacity and, interestingly, poorly correlates with BMI [95].

The mechanistic relationship between OSA and IPF and the impact of comorbid OSA on the natural history of ILD remains unknown. Nevertheless, clinicians should to evaluate the potential coexistence of sleep disordered breathing in patients with ILD as the appropriate treatment can improve the patient's quality of life and may improve survival.

References

1. Vestbo J, Hurd SS, Agusti AG, *et al.* Global strategy for the diagnosis, management, and prevention of chronic obstructive pulmonary disease. *Am J Respir Crit Care Med* 2013; 187: 347–365.
2. Strollo PJ Jr, Rogers RM. Obstructive sleep apnea. *N Engl J Med* 1996; 334: 99–104.
3. Sleep-related breathing disorders in adults: recommendations for syndrome definition and measurement techniques in clinical research. The Report of an American Academy of Sleep Medicine Task Force. *Sleep* 1999; 22: 667–689.
4. Marin JM, Carrizo SJ, Vicente E, *et al.* Long-term cardiovascular outcomes in men with obstructive sleep apnoea-hypopnoea with or without treatment with continuous positive airway pressure: an observational study. *Lancet* 2005; 365: 1046–1053.
5. Yaggi HK, Concato J, Kernan WN, *et al.* Obstructive sleep apnea as a risk factor for stroke and death. *N Engl J Med* 2005; 353: 2034–2041.
6. Young T, Finn L, Peppard PE, *et al.* Sleep disordered breathing and mortality: eighteen-year follow-up of the Wisconsin sleep cohort. *Sleep* 2008; 31: 1071–1078.
7. Marshall NS, Wong KK, Liu PY, *et al.* Sleep apnea as an independent risk factor for all-cause mortality: the Busselton Health Study. *Sleep* 2008; 31: 1079–1085.
8. Punjabi NM, Caffo BS, Goodwin JL, *et al.* Sleep-disordered breathing and mortality: a prospective cohort study. *PLoS Med* 2009; 6: e1000132.
9. Flenley DC. Sleep in chronic obstructive lung disease. *Clin Chest Med* 1985; 6: 651–661.
10. Buist AS, McBurnie MA, Vollmer WM, *et al.* International variation in the prevalence of COPD (the BOLD study): a population-based prevalence study. *Lancet* 2007; 370: 741–750.
11. Young T, Palta M, Dempsey J, *et al.* The occurrence of sleep-disordered breathing among middle-aged adults. *N Engl J Med* 1993; 328: 1230–1235.
12. Peppard PE, Young T, Barnet JH, *et al.* Increased prevalence of sleep-disordered breathing in adults. *Am J Epidemiol* 2013; 177: 1006–1014.
13. Bixler EO, Vgontzas AN, Lin HM, *et al.* Prevalence of sleep-disordered breathing in women: effects of gender. *Am J Respir Crit Care Med* 2001; 163: 608–613.
14. Dancey DR, Hanly PJ, Soong C, *et al.* Impact of menopause on the prevalence and severity of sleep apnea. *Chest* 2001; 120: 151–155.
15. Chaouat A, Weitzenblum E, Krieger J, *et al.* Association of chronic obstructive pulmonary disease and sleep apnea syndrome. *Am J Respir Crit Care Med* 1995; 151: 82–86.
16. Bednarek M, Plywaczewski R, Jonczak L, *et al.* There is no relationship between chronic obstructive pulmonary disease and obstructive sleep apnea syndrome: a population study. *Respiration* 2005; 72: 142–149.

17. Sanders MH, Newman AB, Haggerty CL, *et al.* Sleep Heart Health Study. Sleep and sleep-disordered breathing in adults with predominantly mild obstructive airway disease. *Am J Respir Crit Care Med* 2003; 167: 7–14.
18. Johns MW. A new method for measuring daytime sleepiness: the Epworth sleepiness scale. *Sleep* 1991; 14: 540–545.
19. Price D, Small M, Milligan G, *et al.* Impact of night-time symptoms in COPD: a real-world study in five European countries. *Int J Chron Obstruct Pulmon Dis* 2013; 8: 595–603.
20. Lewis CA, Fergusson W, Eaton T, *et al.* Isolated nocturnal desaturation in COPD: prevalence and impact on quality of life and sleep. *Thorax* 2009; 64: 133–138.
21. Mulloy E, McNicholas WT. Ventilation and gas exchange during sleep and exercise in severe COPD. *Chest* 1996; 109: 387–394.
22. Chaouat A, Bugnet AS, Kadaoui N, *et al.* Severe pulmonary hypertension and chronic obstructive pulmonary disease. *Am J Respir Crit Care Med* 2005; 172: 189–194.
23. Franklin KA, Gíslason T, Omenaas E, *et al.* The influence of active and passive smoking on habitual snoring. *Am J Respir Crit Care Med* 2004; 170: 799–803.
24. Wetter DW, Young TB, Bidwell TR, *et al.* Smoking as a risk factor for sleep-disordered breathing. *Arch Intern Med* 1994; 154: 2219–2224.
25. White LH, Motwani S, Kasai T, *et al.* Effect of rostral fluid shift on pharyngeal resistance in men with and without obstructive sleep apnea. *Respir Physiol Neurobiol* 2014; 192: 17–22.
26. Johnson MW, Remmers JE. Accessory muscle activity during sleep in chronic obstructive pulmonary disease. *J Appl Physiol* 1984; 57: 1011–1017.
27. Ballard RD, Clover CW, Suh BY. Influence of sleep on respiratory function in emphysema. *Am J Respir Crit Care Med* 1995; 151: 945–951.
28. Radwan L, Maszczyk Z, Koziorowski A, *et al.* Control of breathing in obstructive sleep apnoea and in patients with the overlap syndrome. *Eur Respir J* 1995; 8: 542–545.
29. Marin JM, Soriano JB, Carrizo SJ, *et al.* Outcomes in patients with chronic obstructive pulmonary disease and obstructive sleep apnea: the overlap syndrome. *Am J Respir Crit Care Med* 2010; 182: 325–331.
30. Mermigkis C, Kopanakis A, Fodvary-Schaefer N, *et al.* Health-related quality of life in patients with obstructive sleep apnea and chronic obstructive pulmonary disease (overlap syndrome). *Int J Clin Pract* 2007; 61: 207–211.
31. McNicholas WT, Verbraecken J, Marin JM. Sleep disorders in COPD: the forgotten dimension. *Eur Respir Rev* 2013; 22: 365–375.
32. Berger KI, Norman RG, Ayappa I, *et al.* Potential mechanism for transition between acute hypercapnia during sleep to chronic hypercapnia during wakefulness in obstructive sleep apnea. *Adv Exp Med Biol* 2008; 605: 431–436.
33. Verbraecken J, De Backer W, Willemen M, *et al.* Chronic CO_2 drive in patients with obstructive sleep apnea and effect of CPAP. *Respir Physiol* 1995; 101: 279–287.
34. Bradley TD, Rutherford A, Lue F, *et al.* Role of diffuse airway obstruction in the hypercapnia of obstructive apnea. *Am Rev Respir Dis* 1986; 134: 920–924.
35. Chaouat A, Weitzenblum E, Kessler R, *et al.* Sleep-related O_2 desaturation and daytime pulmonary haemodynamics in COPD patients with mild hypoxaemia. *Eur Respir J* 1997; 10: 1730–1735.
36. Douglas NJ. Breathing during sleep in patients with chronic obstructive pulmonary disease. *In*: Kryger MH, Roth T, Dement WC. *Principles and Practice of Sleep Medicine.* 2nd Edn. Philadelphia, WB Saunders Co., 1994; pp. 758–768.
37. Malhotra A, White DP. Obstructive sleep apnoea. *Lancet* 2002; 360: 237–245.
38. Teran J, Jiménez-Gómez A, Cordero-Guevara J. The association between sleep apnea and the risk of traffic accidents. Cooperative Group Burgos-Santander. *N Engl J Med* 1999; 340: 847–851.
39. Kendzerska T1, Gershon AS, Hawker G, *et al.* Obstructive sleep apnea and incident diabetes: a historical cohort study. *Am J Respir Crit Care Med* 2014; 190: 218–225.
40. Marin JM, Agusti A, Villar I, *et al.* Association between treated and untreated obstructive sleep apnea and risk of hypertension. *JAMA* 2012; 307: 2169–2176.
41. Mehra R, Benjamin EJ, Shahar E, *et al.* Sleep Heart Health Study. Association of nocturnal arrhythmias with sleep-disordered breathing: The Sleep Heart Health Study. *Am J Respir Crit Care Med* 2006; 173: 910–916.
42. Tirlapur VG, Mir MA. Nocturnal hypoxemia and associated electrocardiographic changes in patients with chronic obstructive airways disease. *N Engl J Med* 1982; 306: 125–130.
43. Konecny T, Park JY, Somers KR, *et al.* Relation of chronic obstructive pulmonary disease to atrial and ventricular arrhythmias. *Am J Cardiol* 2014; 114: 272–277.
44. Ganga HV, Nair SU, Puppala VK, *et al.* Risk of new-onset atrial fibrillation in elderly patients with the overlap syndrome: a retrospective cohort study. *J Geriatr Cardiol* 2013; 10: 129–134.
45. Gottlieb DJ1, Yenokyan G, Newman AB, *et al.* Prospective study of obstructive sleep apnea and incident coronary heart disease and heart failure: the sleep heart health study. *Circulation* 2010; 122: 352–360.
46. Müllerova H, Agusti A, Erqou S, *et al.* Cardiovascular comorbidity in COPD: systematic literature review. *Chest* 2013; 144: 1163–1178.

47. Sharma B, Neilan TG, Kwong RY, *et al.* Evaluation of right ventricular remodeling using cardiac magnetic resonance imaging in co-existent chronic obstructive pulmonary disease and obstructive sleep apnea. *COPD* 2013; 10: 4–10.

48. Shiina K, Tomiyama H, Takata Y, *et al.* Overlap syndrome: additive effects of COPD on the cardiovascular damages in patients with OSA. *Respir Med* 2012; 106: 1335–1341.

49. Gan WQ, Man SF, Senthilselvan A, *et al.* Association between chronic obstructive pulmonary disease and systemic inflammation: a systematic review and a metaanalysis. *Thorax* 2004; 59: 574–580.

50. Yokoe T, Minoguchi K, Matsuo H, *et al.* Elevated levels of C-reactive protein and interleukin-6 in patients with obstructive sleep apnea syndrome are decreased by nasal continuous positive airway pressure. *Circulation* 2003; 107: 1129–1134.

51. Lavie P1, Lavie L, Herer P. All-cause mortality in males with sleep apnoea syndrome: declining mortality rates with age. *Eur Respir J* 2005; 25: 514–520.

52. Thun MJ, Carter BD, Feskanich D, *et al.* 50-year trends in smoking-related mortality in the United States. *N Engl J Med* 2013; 368: 35–64.

53. Lavie P, Herer P, Peled R, *et al.* Mortality in sleep apnea patients: a multivariate analysis of risk factors. *Sleep* 1995; 18: 149–157.

54. Nieto FJ, Peppard PE, Young T, *et al.* Sleep-disordered breathing and cancer mortality: results from the Wisconsin Sleep Cohort Study. *Am J Respir Crit Care Med* 2012; 186: 190–194.

55. de Torres JP, Marín JM, Casanova C, *et al.* Lung cancer in patients with chronic obstructive pulmonary disease - incidence and predicting factors. *Am J Respir Crit Care Med* 2011; 184: 913–919.

56. McNicholas WT, FitzGerald MX. Nocturnal death among patients with chronic bronchitis and emphysema. *BMJ* 1984; 289: 878.

57. Gami AS, Olson EJ, Shen WK, *et al.* Obstructive sleep apnea and the risk of sudden cardiac death: a longitudinal study of 10,701 adults. *J Am Coll Cardiol* 2013; 62: 610–616.

58. Struik FM1, Lacasse Y, Goldstein R, *et al.* Nocturnal non-invasive positive pressure ventilation for stable chronic obstructive pulmonary disease. *Cochrane Database Syst Rev* 2013; 6: CD002878.

59. Centers for Medicare & Medicaid Services. Documentation checklist. https://www.cgsmedicare.com/jc/mr/PDF/MR_checklist_RAD_E0470.pdf Date last accessed: May 18, 2014. Date last updated: August 27, 2014.

60. Machado MC, Vollmer WM, *et al.* CPAP and survival in moderate-to-severe obstructive sleep apnoea syndrome and hypoxaemic COPD. *Eur Respir J* 2010; 35: 132–137.

61. Stanchina ML, Welicky LM, Donat W, *et al.* Impact of CPAP use and age on mortality in patients with combined COPD and obstructive sleep apnea: the overlap syndrome. *J Clin Sleep Med* 2013; 9: 767–772.

62. Phillips BA, Schmitt FA, Berry DTR, *et al.* Treatment of obstructive sleep apnea: a preliminary report comparing nasal CPAP to nasal oxygen in patients with mild OSA. *Chest* 1990; 98: 325–330.

63. Gottlieb DJ, Punjabi NM, Mehra R, *et al.* CPAP versus oxygen in obstructive sleep apnea. *N Engl J Med* 2014; 370: 2276–2285.

64. McNicholas WT, Calverley PMA, Lee A, *et al.* Long-acting inhaled anticholinergic therapy improves sleeping oxygen saturation in COPD. *Eur Respir J* 2004; 23: 825–831.

65. Ryan S, Doherty LS, Rock C, *et al.* Effects of salmeterol on sleeping oxygen saturation in chronic obstructive pulmonary disease. *Respiration* 2010; 79: 475–481.

66. Aubier M, De Troyer A, Sampson M, *et al.* Aminophylline improves diaphragmatic contractility. *N Engl J Med* 1981; 305: 249–252.

67. Cirignotta F, Mondini S, Zucconi M, *et al.* Zolpidem-polysomnographic study of the effect of a new hypnotic drug in sleep apnea syndrome. *Pharmacol Biochem Behav* 1988; 29: 807–809.

68. Global Initiative for Asthma. Global Strategy for Asthma Management and Prevention. http://www.ginasthma.org/local/uploads/files/GINA_Report_2014_Aug12.pdf Date last accessed: May 18, 2014.

69. Akinbami LJ, Moorman JE, Liu X. Asthma prevalence, health care use, and mortality: United States, 2005–2009. *Natl Health Stat Report* 2011; 32: 1–14.

70. Auckley D, Moallem M, Shaman Z, *et al.* Findings of a Berlin Questionnaire survey: comparison between patients seen in an asthma clinic versus internal medicine clinic. *Sleep Med* 2008; 9: 494–499.

71. Julien JY, Martin JG, Ernst P, *et al.* Prevalence of obstructive sleep apnea-hypopnea in severe *versus* moderate asthma. *J Allergy Clin Immunol* 2009; 124: 371–376.

72. Redline S, Tishler PV, Schluchter M, *et al.* Risk factors for sleep-disordered breathing in children. Associations with obesity, race, and respiratory problems. *Am J Respir Crit Care Med* 1999; 159: 1527–1532.

73. Montplaisir J, Walsh J, Malo JL. Nocturnal asthma: features of attacks, sleep and breathing patterns. *Am Rev Respir Dis* 1982; 125: 18–22.

74. Fitzpatrick MF, Engleman H, Whyte KF, *et al.* Morbidity in nocturnal asthma: sleep quality and daytime cognitive performance. *Thorax* 1991; 46: 569–573.

75. Weersink EJ, van Zomeren EH, Koëter GH, *et al.* Treatment of nocturnal airway obstruction improves daytime cognitive performance in asthmatics. *Am J Respir Crit Care Med* 1997; 156: 1144–1150.

76. Greenberg H, Cohen RI. Nocturnal asthma. *Curr Opin Pulm Med* 2012; 18: 57–62.

77.   Beuther DA, Sutherland ER. Overweight, obesity, and incident asthma: a meta-analysis of prospective epidemiologic studies. *Am J Respir Crit Care Med* 2007; 175: 661–666.

78.   Young T, Finn L, Kim H. Nasal obstruction as a risk factor for sleep disordered breathing. *J Allergy Clin Immunol* 1997; 99: S757–S762.

79.   Collett PW, Brancatisano AP, Engel LA. Upper airway dimensions and movements in bronchial asthma. *Am Rev Respir Dis* 1986; 133: 1143–1149.

80.   Yigla M, Tov N, Solomonov A, *et al.* Difficult-to-control asthma and obstructive sleep apnea. *J Asthma* 2003; 40: 865–871.

81.   Lavigne F, Petrof BJ, Johnson JR, *et al.* Effect of topical corticosteroids on allergic airway inflammation and disease severity in obstructive sleep apnoea. *Clin Exp Allergy* 2013; 43: 1124–1133.

82.   Chan CS, Woolcock AJ, Sullivan CE. Nocturnal asthma: role of snoring and obstructive sleep apnea. *Am Rev Respir Dis* 1988; 137: 1502–1504.

83.   Guilleminault C, Quera-Salva MA, Powell N, *et al.* Nocturnal asthma: snoring, small pharynx and nasal CPAP. *Eur Respir J* 1988; 1: 902–907.

84.   Lafond C, Séries F, Lemiere C. Impact of CPAP on asthmatic patients with obstructive sleep apnoea. *Eur Respir J* 2007; 29: 307–311.

85.   Denjean A, Canet E, Praud JP, *et al.* Hypoxia-induced bronchial responsiveness in awake sheep: role of carotid chemoreceptors. *Respir Physiol* 1991; 83: 201–210.

86.   Busk M, Busk N, Puntenney P, *et al.* Use of continuous positive airway pressure reduces airway reactivity in adults with asthma. *Eur Respir J* 2013; 41: 317–322.

87.   Yim S, Fredberg JJ, Malhotra A. Continuous positive airway pressure for asthma: not a big stretch? *Eur Respir J* 2007; 29: 226–228.

88.   Simard B, Turcotte H, Marceau P, *et al.* Asthma and sleep apnea in patients with morbid obesity: outcome after bariatric surgery. *Obes Surg* 2004; 14: 1381–1388.

89.   Raghu G, Collard HR, Egan JJ, *et al.* An official ATS/ERS/JRS/ALAT statement: idiopathic pulmonary fibrosis: evidence-based guidelines for diagnosis and management. *Am J Respir Crit Care Med* 2011; 183: 788–824.

90.   Fernandez Perez ER, Daniels CE, Schroeder DR, *et al.* Incidence, prevalence, and clinical course of idiopathic pulmonary fibrosis: a population-based study. *Chest* 2010; 137: 129–137.

91.   Olson AL, Swigris JJ, Lezotte DC, *et al.* Mortality from pulmonary fibrosis increased in the United States from 1992 to 2003. *Am J Respir Crit Care Med* 2007; 176: 277–284.

92.   Mannino DM, Etzel RA, Parrish RG. Pulmonary fibrosis deaths in the United States, 1979–1991. An analysis of multiple cause mortality data. *Am J Respir Crit Care Med* 1996; 153: 1548–1552.

93.   Rasche K, Orth M. Sleep and breathing in idiopathic pulmonary fibrosis. *J Physiol Pharmacol* 2009; 60: Suppl. 5, 13–14.

94.   Lancaster LH, Mason WR, Parnell JA, *et al.* Obstructive sleep apnea is common in idiopathic pulmonary fibrosis. *Chest* 2009; 136: 772–778.

95.   Mermigkis C, Stagaki E, Tryfon S, *et al.* How common is sleep disordered eating in patients with idiopathic pulmonary fibrosis. *Sleep Breath* 2010; 14: 387–390.

Disclosures: None declared.

Chapter 13

Traffic accident risk

Vinod Palissery[1], Akshay Dwarakanath[2] and Mark Elliott[1]

There is a strong association between OSA syndrome (OSAS) and road traffic accidents (RTAs). The reason for the high risk of RTAs in OSAS is probably related to excessive sleepiness and impaired cognitive function. The most important and effective method to reduce RTAs in OSAS is treatment with CPAP. The evidence for other treatments reducing RTAs is weak.

The assessment of driving risk in an individual patient with OSAS is challenging. The use of subjective and objective tests has limitations. Driving simulators are potentially an important tool for the assessment of driving risk, but at this stage can only be used for research and cannot yet be recommended for routine clinical practise. It is unlikely that a single test with a clear cut-off, pass or fail, will ever be able to accurately predict who is safe and not safe to drive. The clinician will continue to have a major role, weighing up a number of different factors that are likely to impact upon safe driving.

Worldwide, road traffic accidents (RTAs) are among the three leading causes of death in people aged between 5 and 44 years and are predicted to become the fifth leading cause for all age groups, resulting in an estimated 2.4 million deaths each year [1]. In 2011, more than 30000 people died on roads in the European Union, which is equivalent to the population of a medium-sized town. For every death on Europe's roads there are an estimated four permanently disabling injuries, such as damage to the brain or spinal cord, eight serious injuries and 50 minor injuries [2]. The economic consequences of RTAs have been estimated to be between 1% and 3% of the respective gross national product of all countries worldwide, reaching a total of over $500 billion. Reducing road casualties and fatalities would reduce suffering, unlock growth and free up resources for more productive use [1]. A United Nations General Assembly resolution (64/255) from March 2010 proclaimed 2011–2020 the "Decade of Action" for road safety [3], with a global goal of stabilising and reducing the forecasted level of global road fatalities by increasing activities conducted at national, regional and global levels.

There is convincing evidence that sleepiness, regardless of the cause, is a major risk factor for motor vehicle crashes [4–8]. It is difficult to estimate the exact number, but previous studies indicate sleepiness is a contributing factor in a significant proportion of road crashes (5–20%) [4–10]. Sagaspe et al. [6] carried out telephone interviews with 4774 French drivers and found that 11.8% of the sample had an ESS ⩾11; 28.6% reported experiencing sleepiness

[1]Dept of Respiratory Medicine, St James' University Hospital, Leeds, UK. [2]Dept of Respiratory Medicine, Mid Yorkshire Hospitals NHS Trust, Pinderfields Hospital, Wakefield, UK.

Correspondence: Mark Elliott, Dept of Respiratory Medicine, St James' University Hospital, Beckett Street, Leeds, LS9 7TF, UK. E-mail: mark.elliott2@nhs.net

at the wheel (severe enough to require stopping), 46.8% reported feeling sleepy during night-time driving and 39.4% during daytime driving. 10% of respondents had a near-miss accident during the previous year (of which 46% were reportedly sleep related) and 6% had a driving accident (of which 5.2% were sleep related) [6]. RTAs related to sleepiness are common if driving alone or for a long distance without a break in the 18–28-year age group, shift workers and those with untreated sleep disorders [11]. Two or more risk factors may synergistically increase the risk for drowsy driving and RTAs [12]. Professional drivers are at high risk of sleepiness due to a combination of factors, including shift work; sleepiness in professional drivers is particularly dangerous. In sleep questionnaire data obtained from 677 drivers (25 female) employed at bus depots within 30 miles of Edinburgh, UK, 20% reported an ESS >10. 8% of drivers reported falling asleep at the wheel at least once a month, 7% reported having had an accident and 18% reported having had a near-miss accident due to sleepiness while working [13]. A survey of 996 heavy goods vehicle drivers reported an average accident liability of 0.26 accidents in a 3-year recall period [14]. Accident liability increased with increasing ESS scores [14]. The morbidity and mortality associated with sleep-related RTAs are high, probably because of the greater speed on impact and lack of reaction of a sleepy driver to an impending crash [5, 11].

Poor sleep hygiene is the commonest cause of EDS. Long hours of work or social activities, circadian factors and sleep disorders increase the risk; OSA syndrome (OSAS) is the most common medical disorder causing EDS [15]. However, the relationship between sleepiness in general and RTAs is not consistent. TERAN-SANTOS et al. [16] did not find any relationship; however, a large study from China reported a higher chance of RTAs (OR 2.07) in people with chronic sleepiness when assessed by ESS (>10) [17].

OSAS and driving risk

OSAS is highly prevalent. Since the late 1980s several studies have been published in medical journals showing an association between OSAS and RTAs (table 1) [16, 20–28].

It is difficult to establish the exact incidence of RTAs in patients with OSAS. Studies have shown that patients are reluctant to report accidents and under report symptoms [29, 30]. Even data from police, licensing authorities and insurers may underestimate the problem because not all accidents are reported; in particular, near misses or episodes of falling asleep at the wheel that have not resulted in an accident. However, OSAS induced

Table 1. Studies showing association between OSA syndrome (OSAS) and road traffic accidents (RTAs)

First author [ref.]	Study subjects	Risk of RTAs in OSAS
FINDLEY [18]	Case: n=29; control: n=35	OR 7.0
HARALDSSON [19]	Case: n=140; control: n=142	OR 12.0
YOUNG [20]	General population: n=913	OR 3.4
GEORGE [21]	Case: n=460; control: n=581	OR 2.0
TERAN-SANTOS [16]	Case: n=102; control: n=152	OR 6.3 if AHI >10 events·h^{-1}
HORSTMANN [22]	Case: n=156; control: n=160	OR 12.0
MULGREW [23]	Case: n=783; control: n=783	Severe OSAS: RR 2.0

OR: odds ratio; RR: relative risk.

impairment in performance and EDS is associated with an increased risk of RTAs compared with the general population of drivers [15, 16, 19, 20, 22–25, 27, 28, 31, 32]. A meta-analysis comparing the risks of RTAs in all medical conditions showed that OSAS had the highest increased risk, with a relative risk of 3.71, second only to age and sex as a general risk factor for RTAs [33]. A systematic review and meta-analysis of OSA-related risk of RTAs in commercial motor vehicle drivers published in 2009 showed that the mean crash rate ratio associated with OSAS is likely to fall within the range of 1.21–4.89 [34]. Characteristics that may predict crashes in drivers with OSAS include BMI, AHI, oxygen saturation and, possibly, daytime sleepiness [34]. YOUNG et al. [20] showed that there are a large number of people with undiagnosed OSAS who are also at higher risk of RTAs. Based on their population-based study, men with an AHI >5 events·h^{-1} were significantly more likely to have had at least one accident in 5 years and men and women with an AHI >15 events·h^{-1} were significantly more likely to have multiple accidents in 5 years (OR 7.3).

Driving a motor vehicle is a complex activity, which requires alertness, vigilance, complex integrated higher cortical function and hand-eye coordination [35]. While EDS is generally considered the most obvious cause for impaired driving in patients with OSAS, the literature is less consistent on this point. Using neuroimaging techniques, significant changes to brain structure and metabolism have been observed in OSAS patients [36]. The effects of neural, cognitive and daytime functional impairments [36, 37], may be an important co-factor in the increased risk of RTAs in OSAS.

Assessing driving risk in patients with OSAS

Driving is an essential part of modern life and most patients with OSAS drive motor vehicles. Results from a survey conducted in 2013 by the British Lung Foundation showed that among 2671 OSAS patients attending sleep clinics in the UK, 82% of responders held a current driving licence, 62% drove a motor vehicle and 16% held a professional driving licence or drove for a living (22%) [38]. Therefore, doctors dealing with patients with OSAS will need to make an assessment of driving risk; this is one of the most important challenges facing the sleep medicine community. There are a number of different factors to take into consideration and several potential approaches.

Assessment of sleepiness

Subjective scoring
The ESS was initially validated in medical students in 1992 [39] and is the most commonly used scoring system to assess EDS. It is easy to administer and is useful in measuring changes in sleepiness over time. There are various limitations to the ESS. For example, one study in older adults concluded that the majority of older adults were not able to answer all of the ESS items and the ESS may underestimate sleepiness severity in older subjects [40]. Close relative-evaluated ESS performs as well as, if not better than, self-evaluated ESS and may be useful in some situations [41]. The key issue is whether patients experience sleepiness while driving. MASA et al. [32] suggested that asking about EDS while driving, rather than sleepiness in general, may better predict which subjects with OSAS are at risk of RTAs. All subjective measures of sleepiness rely on the insight and honesty of the patient (or their close relative) and this is a major limitation.

Objective tests of sleepiness

No test is considered as the gold standard. The Multiple Sleep Latency Test (MSLT) [42], the Maintenance of Wakefulness Test (MWT) [43] and the Oxford sleep resistance (OSLER) test [44] are all useful clinical tests for the evaluation of EDS. The MSLT assesses the patient's ability to fall asleep; however, patients do not try to fall asleep when driving and this test is not appropriate to assess fitness to drive [45]. YOUNG *et al.* [20] found no difference in MSLT test scores between subjects involved in a RTA and those who were not.

The MWT, or the behavioural alternative the OSLER test, is more logical. The MWT is a validated, objective measure of the ability of an individual to stay awake, and this is more reflective of what an individual does when driving, *i.e.* tries to maintain alertness. It appears to be useful in estimating the driving performance in sleepy patients [46–48], but its suitability to evaluating real world performances and/or risks has been questioned [49]. Pathological sleep latencies on the MWT predict simulator driving impairment in patients suffering from hypersomnias of central origin, as well as in OSAS patients [48]. In a small study comparing patients with untreated OSAS and controls, PHILIP *et al.* [47] showed that sleepy patients had more inappropriate line crossings than control drivers ($p<0.05$) and this correlated with MWT scores ($r^2=-0.339$; $p<0.05$). However, this is not sufficiently discriminating for everyday practise. Furthermore patients can reasonably question a decision to disallow driving based on an abnormal MWT, arguing that when driving they are stimulated and concentrating, which is not the case when performing the MWT (or OSLER test).

Driving simulators

Performing studies during real driving is not feasible for reasons of safety and practicality and, therefore, simulators have been developed with varying degrees of sophistication and realism [50, 51]. They provide a safe, controllable and low-cost environment in which to assess effects of sleepiness on driving. The important challenge is how to provide all the visual, vestibular and proprioceptive changes that occur during driving on the road.

Various studies have been performed reporting driving simulator performance in OSAS and controls. Using a personal computer programme simulating a monotonous motorway drive, FINDLEY *et al.* [18] showed that OSAS patients perform worse than controls "driving" for 30 min. OSAS patients had significantly more events than controls (44 ± 52 *versus* 9 ± 7, $p<0.05$). GEORGE *et al.* [52] developed a laboratory-based divided attention driving simulator (DADS) and studied performance in sober controls, controls under the influence of alcohol (mean blood alcohol level 95 ± 25 mg·dL^{-1}) and male OSAS patients. Simulator performance was worse in OSAS patient than controls in all measures, with the largest difference noted in tracking error. Half of the patients were worse than any control subject, with some showing performance worse than control subjects impaired by alcohol [52]. Using the Steer-Clear computer program BARBÉ *et al.* [53] investigated the association between OSAS, RTAs and simulator performance. OSAS patients reported more accidents than controls (OR 2.3, 95% CI 0.97–5.33) and were more likely to have had more than one accident (OR 5.2, 95% CI 1.07–25.29; $p<0.05$). They had a lower level of vigilance and poorer driving performance ($p<0.01$). However, there was no correlation between the degree of daytime sleepiness, severity of OSAS, level of vigilance, simulator performance and risk of RTAs [53]. In a case–control study using a computer-based driving simulator, RISSER *et al.* [54] recorded lane position variability, speed variability, steering rate variability and crash frequency. The frequency and duration of EEG-defined attention lapses were also measured. The authors showed that OSAS patients demonstrated greater variability in speed, lane position and steering rate, and had more crashes than controls. The poor performance appeared to be related to EEG-defined attention lapses. Lane position variability appeared to be the most sensitive measure for assessing and quantifying impairment. This study showed that poorer driving performance and crashes are not entirely due to EDS, but also inattention due to sleepiness [54]. JUNIPER et al. [55] developed a steering simulator with a realistic view of the road ahead that allowed separate assessment of two visual tasks required for steering a car: 1) immediate positioning on the road with reference to the road edges; and 2) assessment of the curve of the oncoming road. While steering, a subject is required to scan the four corners and identify a target digit each time it appears by pressing a button on either side of steering wheel. OSAS patients performed significantly worse on the three different drive fields as measured by steering error (p<0.001), time to detect the target number (p<0.03) and off-road events (p<0.03) [55]. TURKINGTON et al. [56] showed that there was a relationship with history of accidents in the previous year and performance on the DADS. In a study involving 129 OSAS patients and using both a Steer-Clear simulator and the divided attention steering simulator, PICHEL et al. [57] showed that alcohol and the Short-Form-36 questionnaire, a measure of self-reported health status, were associated with poor simulator outcome. PHILIP et al. [47] showed that the driving outcome in OSAS patients with a 90-min real-life driving session correlated with MWT and ESS.

One problem with simple simulators is that they lack credibility. In the study of TURKINGTON et al. [56] patients had multiple off-road events during the 20 min drive. In another study, also using the DADS during four 20-min drives, although compared to patients with OSAS controls performed significantly better, they still had ~40 off-road events during the 20 min drive [58]. A patient who is told that they cannot drive because of poor performance on such a test could reasonably question what relationship it had to real driving.

On road testing is not widely applicable and is ethically questionable in patients at high risk of having an accident. Fully immersive simulators provide all the visual, vestibular and proprioceptive changes that occur during on road driving, but are very expensive to build and impractical for routine clinical use. A more sophisticated computer-based simulator has been described, which incorporates the visual graphics from a fully immersive simulator [59]. In this study over 50% of patients with OSAS of sufficient severity to warrant a trial of CPAP were able to complete a 90 km stretch of motorway driving for ~50 min without crashing, veering out of the lane or colliding with another vehicle. Three groups of patients could be identified: 1) those who crash when they really should not; 2) those who do not crash at all; and 3) an intermediate group who crash in a situation in which even a reasonably alert driver might crash. In this study, 72 patients were included in the exploratory phase of the study and 133 patients in the validation phase. Prediction models could predict "fails" with a sensitivity of 82% and specificity of 96%. The models were subsequently confirmed in the validation phase. These were based on the standard deviation of lane position and the reaction time to an event [59]. Similar computer-based simulators have been used to investigate driving performance in patients with OSAS and have shown that patients are more vulnerable to the effects of alcohol and sleep restriction than normal subjects [60]. However, there are as yet insufficient data to recommend that these simulators can be used in routine clinical practise to advise individuals of whether they are safe to drive or not. They are, however, useful research tools for understanding factors that may affect driving safety in patients with OSAS.

How should fitness to drive be assessed?

Clinicians will have to continue to advise patients using their best judgement. In a recent survey from the British Thoracic Society, clinicians were asked to indicate whether they would allow driving in a number of patient vignettes. In the least contentious scenario, 94% of clinicians would allow driving; in the most contentious a patient had a 50% chance of being allowed to drive. Such variation shows that clinicians require more guidance in the assessment of driving in patients with OSAS [61]. There is a weak relationship between the severity of OSAS and the risk of RTAs [22, 25, 34] and patients should not be prevented from driving on the basis of the presence of OSAS alone. American Thoracic Society clinical practise guideline on OSAS, sleepiness and driving risk in non-commercial drivers considers patients with OSAS to be high-risk drivers if there is moderate-to-severe sleepiness plus previous RTAs (including near-miss events associated with driver behaviour that raise clinical alarm to an equivalent level) [62]. The clinician assessing patients with OSAS should ask specific questions regarding driving behaviour, previous accidents or near-miss events, *etc.* There is synergistic increase in risk when two or more risk factors occur in the same individual [12]. Therefore, the clinician should assess co-existing conditions that may increase the risk for drowsy driving, such as medication history (*e.g.* sedatives), substance use (*e.g.* alcohol), other sleep problems (*e.g.* sleep restriction) and medical comorbidities; all of which probably increase the driving risk by increasing sleepiness [62]. Despite their limitations, in the absence of better tests the objective tests described above may still have a role, but given the lack of evidence results must not be given undue weight.

Methods to reduce driving risk in OSAS

There are a number of reasons to treat OSAS, not least to improve the patient's daily quality of life. Treatment of OSAS with CPAP reduces accident risk in OSAS patients [30, 63–68] and improves driving simulator performance [69–74]. Two studies found that CPAP treatment of OSAS patients returned driving simulator performance to the level of healthy control subjects [69, 74], while another clinical observational study reported that CPAP therapy reduced motor vehicle accident rates to the background rate of the general population [65]. A meta-analysis found a significant reduction in the incidence of RTAs (OR 0.21, 95% CI 0.12–0.35), near-misses (OR 0.09, 95% CI 0.04–0.21) and RTA-related events in a driving simulator (standard mean difference 21.20 events, 95% CI 21.75–20.064 events) after the initiation CPAP treatment for OSAS [75]. Sassani *et al.* [76] assessed the impact of RTAs related to OSAS in the USA, and calculated that treating all drivers suffering from OSAS with CPAP would cost US$3.18 billion, but would save US $11.1 billion in collision costs and save 980 lives annually. The studies analysing the effect of CPAP on real life crashes and near miss accidents, or the effects of CPAP on driving simulator performance are shown in table 2.

Once a patient is established on CPAP their average risk of an RTA is reduced. However, what constitutes acceptable symptom control and compliance with CPAP has not been defined and is open to interpretation. In the British Thoracic Society survey, using vignettes of patients following treatment with CPAP, clinicians' interpretation of what constituted residual drowsiness was inconsistent. In each vignette the same clinician was more likely to say "yes" to "excessive" than to "irresistible" (71±12% *versus* 42±10%, p=0.0045). There was also a lack of consensus regarding "adequate CPAP compliance"; "yes" responses ranged

Table 2. Studies analysing the effect of CPAP on real life crashes, near miss accidents or driving simulator performance

First author [ref.]	Outcomes
Findley [18]	CPAP treatment improved driving simulator performance
Cassel [64]	Accident rate significantly reduced during an 80 min vigilance test following 12 months of CPAP treatment
Kreiger [77]	Reduction in accident and near miss events after CPAP treatment
Hack [70]	Improvement in simulator performance after 1 month of CPAP treatment
Yamamoto [67]	33% of OSA syndrome patients had accidents/near misses before treatment and no mishaps after CPAP treatment
Turkington [73]	Improvement in simulator performance after 7 days of CPAP treatment
Orth [72]	Improvement in simulator performance with reduced accident rate after CPAP treatment
Mazza [74]	CPAP treatment reduced the reaction time and number of accidents

from 13% to 64% [61]. Some patients remain sleepy despite using CPAP well. For these patients, modafinil has been shown be effective in treating EDS [78, 79] and armodafinil has been shown to improve driving simulator performance [80]. However, the European Medicines Agency has recommended a restriction in licencing to narcolepsy only. It is not recommended for shift work sleep disorders or for residual daytime sleepiness in patients with OSAS despite adequate CPAP use. This recommendation has, however, been disputed [81]. However, wake promoting or stimulant drugs should not be used just to allow a patient with OSAS to retain their driving licence.

One small study examined driving simulator performance between nine patients treated with a MAD and 10 patients treated with CPAP and found a similar result [71]. In a randomised crossover trial, Phillips et al. [82] compared the effects of 1 month each of CPAP and MAD treatment and showed that driving simulator performance improved equally between MAD and CPAP therapies in over 100 patients.

Effective control of OSAS, particularly a reduction in sleepiness, however achieved, is likely to reduce driving risk and this is accepted by licencing authorities. There is an issue of what to do when a patient is unable to tolerate treatment for OSAS and accepts that they are sleepy, but denies that there is a problem during driving. The same principles that apply at diagnosis are still relevant.

What should the clinician do if the driver considered to be at risk continues to drive?

In general, a clinician has a duty to the patient to take steps to reduce the foreseeable risk that the patient will harm themselves, including the task of operating a motor vehicle. This obligation would ordinarily include describing the risks of a medical impairment and warning the patient to take appropriate precautions. If a patient's disorder also poses a danger to other people, the clinician has a duty to these potential victims to take appropriate precautions to reduce the risks of harm to them [62]. It is the clinician's responsibility to inform an OSAS patient that they suffer from a disorder associated with an increased risk of traffic accidents, and to warn against the hazards of driving while untreated. The clinician should also inform the patient about the current regulations in their country, if relevant. In some countries it is also the clinician's duty to inform the licencing authorities. A meta-analysis of the literature from 1990–2011 indicates that trying to get people to take the issue of potentially unsafe driving seriously using threat appeal (*e.g.* graphical representations of the death and injury that may occur as a result of a RTA), generate/evoke fear, but do not translate into positive behavioural change resulting in less risky driving behaviour [83]. A recent Canadian study showed that clinicians' warnings to patients who are potentially unfit to drive may contribute to a decrease in subsequent trauma from road crashes, but they may also exacerbate mood disorders and compromise the doctor–patient relationship [84]. Some clinicians do not feel that making decisions about whether an individual is safe to drive is their responsibility. In particular, there is concern that they may be held accountable if they allow an individual to drive who is subsequently involved in an accident caused by driver sleepiness. The European Commission driving licence committee established a Working Group on OSAS in 2012. This group developed a report in 2013, with the aim of making it possible to introduce OSAS in Annex III of the European Directive in the near future [85]. A screening strategy has been devised (by the Working Group on OSAS) composed of simply available objective data, mainly anthrpometric, complemented by questions on the presence of RTAs, symptoms and complaints frequently associated with OSAS, and ESS. This provides a simple semi-quantitative analysis of the probability of the applicant being afflicted by OSAS, thus needing a complementary medical advice procedure before an unrestricted licence can be delivered [85]. Under measures currently being considered by the European Union [85, 86], drivers will be asked questions that raise the possibility of a diagnosis of OSAS as part of the application, and reapplication, process for a driving licence. If the answers to these questions suggest OSAS, patients will be given a restricted licence unless a clinician states otherwise. This will place responsibility very clearly with the clinician. Depriving an individual of their licence has major potential implications for them and society. This may well bring doctors into conflict with their patients. However, no one else is better placed than the clinician to make these difficult decisions.

Ultimately, the individual driver is responsible for their own actions and this should be reinforced to them. No one, whether they have a medical condition that causes sleepiness or not, should drive on any occasion when they feel tired and unable to guarantee the ability to maintain full concentration and vigilance. An individual with well-controlled OSAS may be safe to drive most of the time, but not on a long journey after little sleep. Another individual with no medical cause for sleepiness, but for instance working shifts [87, 88], may be a greater risk than a patient with OSAS. Public education about the dangers of driving when tired and encouraging safe practise are important [85, 89]. The 2013 report of the Working Group on OSA recommends police personnel involved in RTA reporting should receive information on sleepiness and falling asleep at the wheel as a potential cause of a RTA, and should be able to assess and inform on this possibility in the official forms to be completed in case the of a RTA [85].

Conclusion

Advising patients with sleep apnoea about whether they are safe to drive or not remains one of the major challenges for the sleep clinician. It is unlikely that a single test with a clear cut-off, pass or fail, will ever be able to accurately predict who is and who is not safe to drive. The clinician will continue to have a major role, weighing up a number of different factors that are likely to impact upon safe driving. Further research is needed to understand what aspects of OSAS increase driving risk and how this can best be assessed. In particular, objective tests that are a credible test of driving need to be developed and validated to the clinician in this difficult area. The patient should be advised of their personal responsibility and of the dangers, regardless of the cause, of driving when not able to guarantee to maintain full concentration and vigilance.

References

1. World Health Organisation. Global Plan for the Decade of Action for Road Safety 2011–2020. www.who.int/roadsafety/decade_of_action/plan/en. Date last accessed: August 30, 2014.
2. European Commission. Road Safety. Statistics – accidents data. http://ec.europa.eu/transport/road_safety/specialist/statistics/index_en.htm Date last updated: October 13, 2014. Date last accessed: August 29, 2014.
3. United Nations Resolution adopted by General Assembly May 10, 2010. www.who.int/violence_injury_prevention/publications/road_traffic/UN_GA_resolution-54-255-en.pdf
4. Horne JA, Reyner LA. Driver sleepiness. *J Sleep Res* 1995; 4: 23–29.
5. Horne JA, Reyner LA. Sleep related vehicle accidents. *BMJ* 1995; 310: 565–567.
6. Sagaspe P, Taillard J, Bayon V, *et al.* Sleepiness, near-misses and driving accidents among a representative population of French drivers. *J Sleep Res* 2010; 19: 578–584.
7. Garbarino S, Nobili L, Beelke M, *et al.* The contributing role of sleepiness in highway vehicle accidents. *Sleep* 2001; 24: 203–206.
8. Garbarino S, Repice AM, Traversa F, *et al.* [Commuting accidents: the influence of excessive daytime sleepiness. A review of an Italian Police officers population]. *G Ital Med Lav Ergon* 2007; 29: Suppl. 3, 324–326.
9. Garbarino S, Traversa F, Spigno F. [Sleepiness, safety on the road and management of risk]. *G Ital Med Lav Ergon* 2012; 34: Suppl. 3, 322–325.
10. Flatley D, Horne JA, Reyner LA. *Sleep-related crashes on sections of different road types in the UK (1995–2001).* London, Department of Transport, 2004.
11. Pack AI, Pack AM, Rodgman E, *et al.* Characteristics of crashes attributed to the driver having fallen asleep. *Accid Anal Prev* 1995; 27: 769–775.
12. Arnedt JT, Wilde GJ, Munt PW, *et al.* Simulated driving performance following prolonged wakefulness and alcohol consumption: separate and combined contributions to impairment. *J Sleep Res* 2000; 9: 233–241.
13. Vennelle M, Engleman HM, Douglas NJ. Sleepiness and sleep-related accidents in commercial bus drivers. *Sleep Breath* 2010; 14: 39–42.
14. Maycock G. Sleepiness and driving: the experience of heavy goods vehicle drivers in the UK. *J Sleep Res* 1997; 6: 238–244.
15. George CF. Sleep apnea, alertness, and motor vehicle crashes. *Am J Respir Crit Care Med* 2007; 176: 954–956.
16. Teran-Santos J, Jimenez-Gomez A, Cordero-Guevara J. The association between sleep apnea and the risk of traffic accidents. Cooperative Group Burgos-Santander. *N Engl J Med* 1999; 340: 847–851.
17. Liu GF, Han S, Liang DH, *et al.* Driver sleepiness and risk of car crashes in Shenyang, a Chinese northeastern city: population-based case-control study. *Biomed Environ Sci* 2003; 16: 219–226.
18. Findley LJ, Fabrizio MJ, Knight H, *et al.* Driving simulator performance in patients with sleep apnea. *Am Rev Respir Dis* 1989; 140: 529–530.
19. Haraldsson PO, Carenfelt C, Diderichsen F, *et al.* Clinical symptoms of sleep apnea syndrome and automobile accidents. *ORL J Otorhinolaryngol Relat Spec* 1990; 52: 57–62.
20. Young T, Blustein J, Finn L, *et al.* Sleep-disordered breathing and motor vehicle accidents in a population-based sample of employed adults. *Sleep* 1997; 20: 608–613.
21. George CF, Smiley A. Sleep apnea and automobile crashes. *Sleep* 1999; 22: 790–795.
22. Horstmann S, Hess CW, Bassetti C, *et al.* Sleepiness-related accidents in sleep apnea patients. *Sleep* 2000; 23: 383–389.
23. Mulgrew AT, Nasvadi G, Butt A, *et al.* Risk and severity of motor vehicle crashes in patients with obstructive sleep apnoea/hypopnoea. *Thorax* 2008; 63: 536–541.
24. Howard ME, Desai AV, Grunstein RR, *et al.* Sleepiness, sleep-disordered breathing, and accident risk factors in commercial vehicle drivers. *Am J Respir Crit Care Med* 2004; 170: 1014–1021.
25. Shiomi T, Arita AT, Sasanabe R, *et al.* Falling asleep while driving and automobile accidents among patients with obstructive sleep apnea-hypopnea syndrome. *Psychiatry Clin Neurosci* 2002; 56: 333–334.

26. Stoohs RA, Guilleminault C, Itoi A, et al. Traffic accidents in commercial long-haul truck drivers: the influence of sleep-disordered breathing and obesity. Sleep 1994; 17: 619–623.
27. George CF, Nickerson PW, Hanly PJ, et al. Sleep apnoea patients have more automobile accidents. Lancet 1987; 2: 447.
28. Aldrich MS. Automobile accidents in patients with sleep disorders. Sleep 1989; 12: 487–494.
29. Engleman HM, Hirst WS, Douglas NJ. Under reporting of sleepiness and driving impairment in patients with sleep apnoea/hypopnoea syndrome. J Sleep Res 1997; 6: 272–275.
30. Findley L, Smith C, Hooper J, et al. Treatment with nasal CPAP decreases automobile accidents in patients with sleep apnea. Am J Respir Crit Care Med 2000; 161: 857–859.
31. Wu H, Yan-Go F. Self-reported automobile accidents involving patients with obstructive sleep apnea. Neurology 1996; 46: 1254–1257.
32. Masa JF, Rubio M, Findley LJ. Habitually sleepy drivers have a high frequency of automobile crashes associated with respiratory disorders during sleep. Am J Respir Crit Care Med 2000; 162: 1407–1412.
33. Vaa T. Impairments, diseases, age and their relative risks of accident involvement: results from a metaanalysis. TØI report 690/2003. Oslo, Institute of Transport Economics, 2003.
34. Tregear S, Reston J, Schoelles K, et al. Obstructive sleep apnea and risk of motor vehicle crash: systematic review and meta-analysis. J Clin Sleep Med 2009; 5: 573–581.
35. Land M, Horwood J. Which parts of the road guide steering? Nature 1995; 377: 339–340.
36. Morrell MJ, Jackson ML, Twigg GL, et al. Changes in brain morphology in patients with obstructive sleep apnoea. Thorax 2010; 65: 908–914.
37. Jackson ML, Howard ME, Barnes M. Cognition and daytime functioning in sleep-related breathing disorders. Prog Brain Res 2011; 190: 53–68.
38. British Lung Foundation. OSA patient experience survey. www.blf.org.uk/Page/OSA-patient-experience-survey. Date last accessed: August 28, 2014.
39. Johns MW. Reliability and factor analysis of the Epworth Sleepiness Scale. Sleep 1992; 15: 376–381.
40. Onen F, Moreau T, Gooneratne NS, et al. Limits of the Epworth Sleepiness Scale in older adults. Sleep Breath 2013; 17: 343–350.
41. Li Y, Zhang J, Lei F, et al. Self-evaluated and close relative-evaluated Epworth Sleepiness Scale vs. multiple sleep latency test in patients with obstructive sleep apnea. J Clin Sleep Med 2014; 10: 171–176.
42. Carskadon MA, Dement WC, Mitler MM, et al. Guidelines for the multiple sleep latency test (MSLT): a standard measure of sleepiness. Sleep 1986; 9: 519–524.
43. Littner MR, Kushida C, Wise M, et al. Practice parameters for clinical use of the multiple sleep latency test and the maintenance of wakefulness test. Sleep 2005; 28: 113–121.
44. Bennett LS, Stradling JR, Davies RJ. A behavioural test to assess daytime sleepiness in obstructive sleep apnoea. J Sleep Res 1997; 6: 142–145.
45. Wise MS. Objective measures of sleepiness and wakefulness: application to the real world? J Clin Neurophysiol 2006; 23: 39–49.
46. Sagaspe P, Taillard J, Chaumet G, et al. Maintenance of wakefulness test as a predictor of driving performance in patients with untreated obstructive sleep apnea. Sleep 2007; 30: 327–330.
47. Philip P, Sagaspe P, Taillard J, et al. Maintenance of wakefulness test, obstructive sleep apnea syndrome, and driving risk. Ann Neurol 2008; 64: 410–416.
48. Philip P, Chaufton C, Taillard J, et al. Maintenance of wakefulness test scores and driving performance in sleep disorder patients and controls. Int J Psychophysiol 2013; 89: 195–202.
49. Bonnet MH. ACNS clinical controversy: MSLT and MWT have limited clinical utility. J Clin Neurophysiol 2006; 23: 50–58.
50. Philip P, Sagaspe P, Taillard J, et al. Fatigue, sleepiness, and performance in simulated versus real driving conditions. Sleep 2005; 28: 1511–1516.
51. Helland A, Jenssen GD, Lervåg LE, et al. Comparison of driving simulator performance with real driving after alcohol intake: a randomised, single blind, placebo-controlled, cross-over trial. Accid Anal Prev 2013; 53: 9–16.
52. George CF, Boudreau AC, Smiley A. Simulated driving performance in patients with obstructive sleep apnea. Am J Respir Crit Care Med 1996; 154: 175–181.
53. Barbé, Pericás J, Muñoz A, et al. Automobile accidents in patients with sleep apnea syndrome. An epidemiological and mechanistic study. Am J Respir Crit Care Med 1998; 158: 18–22.
54. Risser MR, Ware JC, Freeman FG. Driving simulation with EEG monitoring in normal and obstructive sleep apnea patients. Sleep 2000; 23: 393–398.
55. Juniper M, Hack MA, George CF, et al. Steering simulation performance in patients with obstructive sleep apnoea and matched control subjects. Eur Respir J 2000; 15: 590–595.
56. Turkington PM, Sircar M, Allgar V, et al. Relationship between obstructive sleep apnoea, driving simulator performance, and risk of road traffic accidents. Thorax 2001; 56: 800–805.
57. Pichel F, Zamarrón C, Magán F, et al. Sustained attention measurements in obstructive sleep apnea and risk of traffic accidents. Respir Med 2006; 100: 1020–1027.

58. Mazza S, Pepin JL, Naëgelé B, *et al.* Most obstructive sleep apnoea patients exhibit vigilance and attention deficits on an extended battery of tests. *Eur Respir J* 2005; 25: 75–80.

59. Ghosh D, Jamson SL, Baxter PD, *et al.* Continuous measures of driving performance on an advanced office-based driving simulator can be used to predict simulator task failure in patients with obstructive sleep apnoea syndrome. *Thorax* 2012; 67: 815–821.

60. Vakulin A, Baulk SD, Catcheside PG, *et al.* Effects of alcohol and sleep restriction on simulated driving performance in untreated patients with obstructive sleep apnea. *Ann Intern Med* 2009; 151: 447–455.

61. Dwarakanath A, Twiddy M, Ghosh D, *et al.* Variability in clinicians' opinions regarding fitness to drive in patients with obstructive sleep apnoea syndrome (OSAS). *Thorax* 2014 [in press DOI: 10.1136/thoraxjnl-2014-206180].

62. Strohl KP, Brown DB, Collop N, *et al.* An official American Thoracic Society Clinical Practice Guideline: sleep apnea, sleepiness, and driving risk in noncommercial drivers. An update of a 1994 Statement. *Am J Respir Crit Care Med* 2013; 187: 1259–1266.

63. Barbé F, Sunyer J, de la Peña A, *et al.* Effect of continuous positive airway pressure on the risk of road accidents in sleep apnea patients. *Respiration* 2007; 74: 44–49.

64. Cassel W, Ploch T, Becker C, *et al.* Risk of traffic accidents in patients with sleep-disordered breathing: reduction with nasal CPAP. *Eur Respir J* 1996; 9: 2606–2611.

65. George CF. Reduction in motor vehicle collisions following treatment of sleep apnoea with nasal CPAP. *Thorax* 2001; 56: 508–512.

66. Krieger J, Meslier N, Lebrun T, *et al.* Accidents in obstructive sleep apnea patients treated with nasal continuous positive airway pressure: a prospective study. The Working Group ANTADIR, Paris and CRESGE, Lille, France. Association Nationale de Traitement à Domicile des Insuffisants Respiratoires. *Chest* 1997; 112: 1561–1566.

67. Yamamoto H, Akashiba T, Kosaka N, *et al.* Long-term effects nasal continuous positive airway pressure on daytime sleepiness, mood and traffic accidents in patients with obstructive sleep apnoea. *Respir Med* 2000; 94: 87–90.

68. Tregear S, Reston J, Schoelles K, *et al.* Continuous positive airway pressure reduces risk of motor vehicle crash among drivers with obstructive sleep apnea: systematic review and meta-analysis. *Sleep* 2010; 33: 1373–1380.

69. George CF, Boudreau AC, Smiley A. Effects of nasal CPAP on simulated driving performance in patients with obstructive sleep apnoea. *Thorax* 1997; 52: 648–653.

70. Hack M, Davies RJ, Mullins R, *et al.* Randomised prospective parallel trial of therapeutic *versus* subtherapeutic nasal continuous positive airway pressure on simulated steering performance in patients with obstructive sleep apnoea. *Thorax* 2000; 55: 224–231.

71. Hoekema A, Stegenga B, Bakker M, *et al.* Simulated driving in obstructive sleep apnoea-hypopnoea; effects of oral appliances and continuous positive airway pressure. *Sleep Breath* 2007; 11: 129–138.

72. Orth M, Duchna HW, Leidag M, *et al.* Driving simulator and neuropsychological testing in OSAS before and under CPAP therapy. *Eur Respir J* 2005; 26: 898–903.

73. Turkington PM, Sircar M, Saralaya D, *et al.* Time course of changes in driving simulator performance with and without treatment in patients with sleep apnoea hypopnoea syndrome. *Thorax* 2004; 59: 56–59.

74. Mazza S, Pépin JL, Naëgelé B, *et al.* Driving ability in sleep apnea patients before and after CPAP treatment: evaluation on a road safety platform. *Eur Respir J* 2006; 28: 1020–1028.

75. Antonopoulos CN, Sergentanis TN, Daskalopoulou SS, *et al.* Nasal continuous positive airway pressure (nCPAP) treatment for obstructive sleep apnea, road traffic accidents and driving simulator performance: a meta-analysis. *Sleep Med Rev* 2011; 15: 301–310.

76. Sassani A, Findley LJ, Kryger M, *et al.* Reducing motor-vehicle collisions, costs, and fatalities by treating obstructive sleep apnea syndrome. *Sleep* 2004; 27: 453–458.

77. Krieger J, Meslier N, Lebrun T, *et al.* Accidents in obstructive sleep apnoea patients treated with nasal continuous positive airway pressure: a prospective study. *Chest* 1997; 112: 1561–1566.

78. Dinges DF, Weaver TE. Effects of modafinil on sustained attention performance and quality of life in OSA patients with residual sleepiness while being treated with nCPAP. *Sleep Med* 2003; 4: 393–402.

79. Black JE, Hirshkowitz M. Modafinil for treatment of residual excessive sleepiness in nasal continuous positive airway pressure-treated obstructive sleep apnea/hypopnea syndrome. *Sleep* 2005; 28: 464–471.

80. Kay GG, Feldman N. Effects of armodafinil on simulated driving and self-report measures in obstructive sleep apnea patients prior to treatment with continuous positive airway pressure. *J Clin Sleep Med* 2013; 9: 445–454.

81. British Sleep Society. The use of modafinil. Excessive daytime sleepiness. www.sleepsociety.org.uk/information/the-use-of-modafinil Date last accessed: October 10, 2014.

82. Phillips CL, Grunstein RR, Darendeliler MA, *et al.* Health outcomes of continuous positive airway pressure versus oral appliance treatment for obstructive sleep apnea: a randomized controlled trial. *Am J Respir Crit Care Med* 2013; 187: 879–887.

83. Carey RN, McDermott DT, Sarma KM. The impact of threat appeals on fear arousal and driver behavior: a meta-analysis of experimental research 1990–2011. *PLoS One* 2013; 8: e62821.

84. Redelmeier DA, Yarnell CJ, Thiruchelvam D, *et al.* Physicians' warnings for unfit drivers and the risk of trauma from road crashes. *N Engl J Med* 2012; 367: 1228–1236.

85. European Commission. Road Safety. Fitness to drive. http://ec.europa.eu/transport/road_safety/topics/behaviour/fitness_to_drive/index_en.htm Date last updated: October 24, 2014. Date last accessed: November 25, 2014.

86. Rodenstein D. Driving in Europe: the need of a common policy for drivers with obstructive sleep apnoea syndrome. *J Sleep Res* 2008; 17: 281–284.

87. Ftouni S, Sletten TL, Howard M, *et al.* Objective and subjective measures of sleepiness, and their associations with on-road driving events in shift workers. *J Sleep Res* 2013; 22: 58–69.

88. Barger LK, Cade BE, Ayas NT, *et al.* Extended work shifts and the risk of motor vehicle crashes among interns. *N Engl J Med* 2005; 352: 125–134.

89. Department for Transport. Think! Fatigue. Don't drive tired. http://think.direct.gov.uk/fatigue.html Date last accessed: October 16, 2014.

Disclosures: M. Elliott reports honoraria, travel expenses and fees for speaking and attendance at advisory boards from Resmed. He has also received travel expenses and fees for speaking from Phillips Respironics and Curative Medical, as well as stock options for an advisory role from Curative Medical.

Chapter 14

Resistant hypertension

Miguel Ángel Martinez-García[1,2], Francisco Campos-Rodríguez[3],
María José Selma Ferrer[1] and Cristina Navarro Soriano[1]

Resistant hypertension (RH) is defined as BP that stays above the goal despite the concurrent use of three anti-hypertensive agents at optimal doses. The prevalence of RH could be higher than 20% in hypertensive individuals, representing an additional cardiovascular risk in these patients.

OSA is present in more than 70–80% of RH patients. Several pathophysiological mechanisms have been invoked to explain this relationship including an increased sympathetic tone and hyperaldosteronism. Obesity is the major confounder since it is highly prevalent in both OSA and RH.

Some clinical trials have found that CPAP treatment has a beneficial effect on BP in patients with RH, with effects greater than those seen in well-controlled hypertensive patients.

Current scientific evidence indicates that every patient with chronic snoring and RH (especially those with obesity), independent of the presence or absence of daytime hypersomnolence, should undergo a sleep study. This is due to the high prevalence of OSA with this high-risk cardiovascular profile and the potential beneficial effect of CPAP treatment.

Arterial hypertension (AHT) affects 25% of the general population worldwide and becomes more prevalent with age [1]. Both OSA and AHT are significant cardiovascular risk factors, particularly AHT, which is responsible for over 60% of cerebrovascular events, 50% of cases of ischaemic heart disease and the death of more than 7 million people every year [2].

OSA has been associated with an increase in cardiovascular morbidity and mortality [3–6]. Of all the cardiovascular risk factors associated with OSA, the relationship between OSA and AHT has possibly been the most thoroughly investigated. Various studies have established that OSA is associated with an increase in the prevalence [7, 8] and incidence of AHT [9, 10]. This relationship seems to be more pronounced in cases of more severe OSA or uncontrolled BP [11–13]. Consequently, several international guidelines on the diagnosis and management of AHT recognise OSA as one of the most important treatable causes of AHT [1, 14].

Several meta-analyses have confirmed that treatment with CPAP, not only in normotensive patients but also in hypertensive patients, can produce a modest reduction in BP (between

[1]Pneumology Service, Hospital Universitario y Politécnico La Fe, Valencia, Spain. [2]CIBER de enfermedades respiratorias, Bunyoles, Spain. [3]Sleep-Disordered Breathing Unit, Respiratory Dept, Hospital Universitario de Valme, Seville, Spain

Correspondence: Miguel Ángel Martinez-García, Pneumology Service, Hospital Universitario y Politécnico La Fe, Avenida Fernando Abril Martorell, no. 106, 46026-Valencia, Spain. E-mail: mianmartinezgarcia@gmail.com

1.5 and 2.5 mmHg). This reduction seems to be more marked in those patients with more severe OSA and poorer hypertension control and in nocturnal BP readings [15–18].

Of all the types of AHT, those with an incomplete or negative response to anti-hypertensive treatment are particularly important. It has been established that over half of all hypertensive patients remain uncontrolled and that up to 30% require a combined treatment to stabilise their BP [1, 14], although the cause of this poor control is often unknown. The close relationship between OSA and uncontrolled BP, and the capacity of CPAP treatment to improve this control has been the subject of several studies in recent years, especially in those patients who are more resistant or refractory to medical treatment and, therefore, present a greater cardiovascular risk.

Resistant hypertension

The American Hypertension Association (AHA) defined resistant hypertension (RH) as BP that stays above the goal despite the concurrent use of three anti-hypertensive agents of different classes, with one of them being a diuretic. All these agents should be prescribed at their optimal doses. This definition of RH also embraces patients whose BP is controlled with more than three medications [19], but the first criterion is more widely used in clinical studies. The diagnosis of RH should be made on the basis of 24-h ambulatory BP monitoring (ABPM) as stated in the European Society of Hypertension practice guidelines [1]. There are no conclusive data on the real epidemiology of RH. Approximately 20–30% of hypertensive patients need at least three drugs to stabilise their BP readings. The prevalence of RH has been calculated as around 12–30% of hypertensive patients, depending on the definition of RH used, the population of the study in question and the inclusion (or otherwise) of patients with white-coat hypertension or poor compliance with anti-hypertensive treatments [20–23]. DAUGHERTY et al. [21] observed that patients with RH have a 50% greater probability of a cardiovascular event than other hypertensive patients after 4 years of follow-up. The high prevalence of AHT in the general population, and its diagnosis and management, particularly in those patients with RH, pose a challenge that has inspired various studies to seek new treatments for these patients. The AHA guidelines [19] recognise OSA as one of most frequent (if not the most frequent) causes of RH (table 1).

Pathophysiological links between OSA and RH

Some pathophysiological mechanisms and confounders have been described to explain the relationship between OSA and arterial hypertension, including: age, obesity, metabolic disturbances, sympathetic activation, inflammation, haemodynamic response to stress, oxidative stress, endothelial dysfunction, hyperaldosteronism status, sleep inefficiency,

Table 1. Secondary causes of resistant hypertension

Common	Uncommon
OSA	Pheochromocytoma
Renal parenchymal disease	Hyperparathyroidism
Primary aldosteronism	Cushing's disease
Renal artery stenosis	Aortic coarctation
	Intracranial tumour

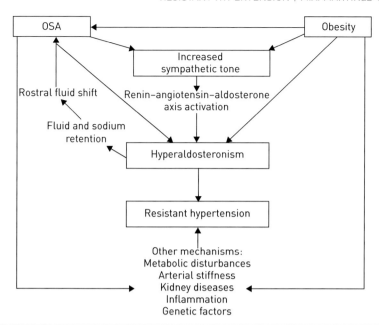

Figure 1. Pathophysiological scheme of the relationship between OSA, obesity, sympathetic activation, hyperaldosteronism, rostral fluid shift and resistant hypertension.

endothelin-mediated vasoconstriction, intermittent hypoxaemia, genetic factors and fluid shifts [24–26]. However, not all the above mechanisms have been studied in the context of the relationship between OSA and RH. The effect of sleep disordered breathing on the sympathetic system and the renin–angiotensin–aldosterone axis seems to be particularly important, as is the role played by obesity (fig. 1) [27–30]. Endothelial dysfunction [31], arterial stiffness [32] and rostral fluid shift [33, 34] have also been investigated.

Renin–angiotensin–aldosterone system activation

Various studies have observed that up to 20% of patients with RH present with a primary hyperaldosteronism [35, 36]. Since the prevalence of OSA in RH patients is extremely high [37–41], and since obesity is found in a high percentage of both OSA and RH patients [42, 43] and has also been associated with an increase in the prevalence of hyperaldosteronism [44], some authors have suggested that OSA may play a role in the emergence of hyperaldosteronism as an intermediate factor to explain the uncontrolled BP observed in RH patients (fig. 1). Pratt-Ubunama et al. [45] observed a correlation between the AHI as a marker of the severity of OSA and plasma levels of aldosterone in RH patients, although this was not the case in a control group with the same AHI but no RH. Other studies have replicated these results with varying degrees of success, either via patients with RH and primary hyperaldosteronism who presented with a greater severity of OSA or via OSA patients who presented with higher levels of aldosterone [46–49]. Although we have not yet been able to establish any causal relationship, the results of these studies give rise to two hypotheses that are not mutually exclusive. On the one hand, it is possible that the presence of hyperaldosteronism explains the uncontrolled BP in OSA patients with RH, while on the other hand, the presence of hyperaldosteronism in patients with RH could cause OSA, or exacerbate pre-existing OSA.

Increased sympathetic tone

The most widely accepted explanation of the relationship between OSA and AHT is probably activation of the nocturnal sympathetic system during apnoeic events, which can continue during the daytime. BP normally goes down in the transition between wakefulness and non-REM sleep, due to an increase in parasympathetic activity and a decrease in sympathetic activity. In OSA, however, these mechanisms are counteracted by apnoea-related stimuli for sympathetic activation and parasympathetic withdrawal during sleep. The mechanisms that translate these recurrent nocturnal increases in BP into sustained daytime hypertension may be mediated by central or peripheral upward resetting of sympathetic vasoconstriction tone, increased circulatory activity of vasoactive hormones or abnormalities in the vascular endothelial function [50–53]. This pathophysiological route has barely been investigated in the subgroup of patients with RH, but its importance can be hypothesised for various reasons. First, sympathetic renal stimulation is capable of activating the renin–angiotensin–aldosterone axis and thereby exacerbating uncontrolled hypertension [54]. Secondly, some studies have shown that renal denervation is particularly useful in reducing the BP of patients with RH [55–57]. Finally, LOGAN et al. [58] observed that treatment with CPAP for a single night was capable of modulating the baroreflex response mediated by the sympathetic system in patients with RH and OSA.

Rostral fluid shift

Some authors have observed that the pathophysiological relationship between OSA and RH could be two-way, i.e. RH could also exacerbate pre-existing OSA. The mechanism that is possibly responsible for this effect is known as rostral fluid shift. Hyperaldosteronism associated with RH induces the retention of water and sodium and, therefore, the presence of oedemas in the lower body (normally the legs). In a supine position, liquid would move from the legs to the neck during sleep, thereby reducing the diameter of the UA due to oedema in the pharyngeal musculature, consequently making the UA more likely to collapse [33, 34]. In this respect, FRIEDMAN et al. [33] concluded that rostral fluid displacement in RH patients is closely associated with OSA severity, and is approximately twice that observed in well-controlled hypertensive patients (346 versus 176 mL; p=0.01). This hypothesis was further endorsed by a study by GADDAM et al. [59], in which 8 weeks of treatment with aldosterone inhibitors (spironolactone 25–50 mg·day^{-1}) reduced the AHI in patients with RH. This phenomenon could explain, at least in part, the high prevalence of OSA found in patients with RH.

Epidemiological association between OSA and RH

Approximately 50% of patients with OSA present with AHT [7, 60], while 30–50% of patients with AHT present with OSA [61]. These figures are even higher in patients with more severe OSA or uncontrolled hypertension [11–13].

The prevalence of OSA is particularly high in hypertensive patients with poorly controlled BP or a poor response to treatment [37–41, 45, 46]. Table 2 shows some of the most relevant studies that have established the prevalence of OSA in patients with RH, along with their main characteristics. Depending on the AHI cut-off point selected and the chosen definition of RH, the prevalence of OSA in the majority of studies ranges from 85% to 90% in patients with an AHI ⩾5 events·h^{-1}; from 70% to 85% with an AHI ⩾10 events·h^{-1}; and from 40% to 70%

Table 2. Prevalence of OSA in patients with resistant hypertension and characteristics of the patients included in the studies

First author [ref.]	Patients n	Age years	Males	BMI kg·m^{-2}	ESS	SBP mmHg	DBP mmHg	Non-dipper	AHI events·h^{-1}	OSA	Anti-AHT drugs %
LOGAN [41]	41	57.2±1.6$^{#}$	58.5	34±0.9$^{#}$		149±2.6$^{#}$ men; 151±3.7$^{#}$ women	86±2$^{#}$ men; 84±1.9$^{#}$ women	64.1	24.7±3.2$^{#}$	AHI ≥10: 83	3.6±0.1$^{#}$
MARTINEZ-GARCÍA [38]	49	68.1±9.1	62	34.5±5.3	6.3±4.1	152±13	89±8.5	89	26.2±19.5	AHI ≥10: 81.4 AHI ≥30: 40.8	3.5±0.9
GONÇALVES [40]	63	59±7	33	30±3		141±17	84±12		21±17.6	AHI ≥10: 71	3.4±0.6
PRATT-UBUNAMA [45]	71	56±9.8		34.1±7.8		156±27	83±15		24.1±24.7	AHI ≥10: 85	≥3
LLOBERES [37]	62	59±10	67.3	31.1±0.6	6.4±0.4	D: 143±1.2 N: 131±2.3	D: 84±1.4 N: 76±1.5	46.8 Sd; 30.6 Dd	47.8±23.4	AHI ≥5: 90 AHI ≥30: 71	3.5±0.1
PEDROSA [39]	125	52±10	43	31.5±6.2	8 (5–13)	D: 146±21 N: 135±21	D: 89±16 N: 78±15	61 Sd; 39 Dd	18 (10–40)	AHI ≥15: 64	5 (4–6)
FLORCZAK [46]	204	48.4±10.6	60.3	30.1±4.7		N: 132±19	D: 90±13 N: 79±12			AHI ≥5: 72.1 AHI ≥30: 26.5	4 (4–5)

Data are presented as mean±SD, % or median (interquartile range), unless otherwise stated. AHT: arterial hypertension; D: diurnal; N: nocturnal; Sd: systolic non-dippers; Dd: diastolic non-dippers. #: data are presented as mean±SEM.

with an AHI $\geqslant$30 events$\cdot$h^{-1}. As can be seen in table 2, most studies investigated patients aged 50–70 years with obesity (BMI $\geqslant$30 kg$\cdot$m^{-2}) and a mean AHI of 18–48 events$\cdot$h^{-1} (moderate-severe OSA). GONÇALVES et al. [40] observed, in a case–control study of 63 patients with RH compared with the same number of patients with well-controlled AHT, that the presence of OSA (AHI $\geqslant$10 events$\cdot$h^{-1}) was 4.8 times higher in RH patients, and that the more severe the OSA the higher the prevalence of RH. Similarly, MARTINEZ-GARCÍA et al. [38] found a correlation between the AHI and the 24-h SBP and 24-h DBP figures (both daytime and night-time), along with a higher intake of anti-hypertensive drugs in patients with OSA. It is particularly striking that these patients present few OSA-related symptoms. Accordingly, those studies that have analysed the ESS have found values that lie between 6 and 8 points, which is in the normal range. MARTINEZ-GARCÍA et al. [38] found that only 70% of patients with OSA and RH were snorers and that very few presented having witnessed apnoeas. Furthermore, PEDROSA et al. [39] found, in 125 patients with RH, that the most commonly associated disorder was OSA. The predictors of OSA were neck circumference, the presence of snoring and age >50 years, but not the ESS, obesity or BP readings. These results confirm the fact that questionnaires on OSA symptoms (such as the Berlin questionnaire) are not valid when they are used to screen for OSA in patients with RH, or to make an assessment of which patients would benefit from treatment with CPAP [62]. This means that every patient with chronic snoring and RH (especially those with obesity), independent of the presence or absence of daytime hypersomnolence, should undergo a sleep study, due to his/her high risk of OSA with a high-risk cardiovascular profile and the potential beneficial effect of CPAP treatment [63].

Another notable finding is that all the analysed studies show a mean BMI of up to 30 kg$\cdot$m^{-2}, rising to 35 kg$\cdot$m^{-2} in those studies with a higher prevalence of OSA. This is probably due to both RH and OSA patients presenting with a high prevalence of obesity. Obesity, therefore, emerges as a crucial confounder when it comes to explaining the epidemiological relationship between OSA and RH. There have been no studies of the relationship between OSA and RH in non-obese patients, although some of the data could indicate that OSA and obesity could play an additive role in RH. MARTINEZ-GARCÍA et al. [38] observed that the presence of obesity and the AHI value were two independent risk factors for uncontrolled BP in patients with RH. Another hypothesis is that part of the observed relationship between obesity and a higher prevalence of RH can be explained by the presence of OSA as an intermediate variable. GONÇALVES et al. [40], for example, observed in a case–control study that the presence of OSA, but not BMI, was a strong independent predictor of RH in patients with AHT. Finally, as mentioned earlier, some authors have also hypothesised that this high prevalence of OSA observed in patients with RH is partly due to rostral fluid displacement [33, 34].

Treatment of OSA and RH

Lifestyle changes

Being overweight or obese is common in patients who present with OSA and RH. Weight reduction has been shown to improve both OSA and BP in RH [64], although no study in the literature has produced any specific data on the effect of weight reduction on BP readings in patients with OSA and RH.

The presence of RH can exacerbate pre-existing OSA as a result of rostral fluid shift during sleep, particularly in the supine position [33, 34]. It is, therefore, advisable for patients to sleep with the top end of their bed raised, to avoid the effect of gravity on the displacement of liquid accumulated in the lower limbs to the neck.

Sodium restriction

Excessive sodium intake in the diet makes a significant contribution to the development of RH [65]. PIMENTA et al. [66] concluded, in a study of 97 patients with RH with a 77% prevalence of OSA and a 29% prevalence of hyperaldosteronism, that the urinary sodium level was an independent predictor of severity of OSA only in patients with hyperaldosteronism, and that dietary salt is related to the severity of OSA in patients with RH and hyperaldosteronism. These results support dietary salt restriction as a treatment strategy for the reduction of OSA severity in these patients.

Renal denervation

Therapeutic renal sympathetic denervation, through the application of discreet, low-dose radio frequency energy to the endothelial surface of the renal artery *via* a percutaneous catheter-based procedure, has been reported to reduce BP by selectively reducing renal sympathetic efferent and afferent signalling [55–57]. Furthermore, some authors have found, in the majority of their patients, unexpected improvements in glycaemic control and reduced OSA severity after renal denervation, probably as a result of reduced displacement of fluid from the legs to the neck during sleep [67].

Diuretics

As one of the most important mechanisms in the genesis of RH is hyperaldosteronism, it can be assumed that anti-aldosterone drugs would be effective. CHAPMAN et al. [68] observed that treatment with spironolactone effectively lowers BP in patients with RH. As OSA is also associated with hyperaldosteronism, and as the latter could be an intermediary mechanism in the relationship between OSA and RH (which in turn could increase the severity of OSA by means of rostral fluid shift), it is logical to think that spironolactone could have a positive effect on the severity of OSA. GADDAM et al. [59] concluded that treatment with a mineralocorticoid receptor antagonist substantially reduced the severity of OSA: the mean±SD AHI dropped from 39.8±19.5 to 22±6.8 events·h^{-1} (p<0.05). Finally, KASAI et al. [69] observed that intensified diuretic therapy (doubling the doses of metolazone and spironolactone over 1 week) significantly reduced the AHI, the overnight change in leg fluid volume and overnight change in neck circumference. There was an inverse correlation between change in leg fluid volume and AHI, suggesting that the effect may be secondary to decreases in pharyngeal oedema and consequent reductions in UA resistance, although RCTs are needed to confirm this finding.

CPAP treatment

There have been seven studies to date that have tried to evaluate the effect of CPAP on BP in patients with RH [58, 70–75]. Of these, three used an observational methodology [73–75] and four were RCTs [72–75]. Table 3 shows the general characteristics of the most significant studies published to date.

Observational studies

LOGAN et al. [58] evaluated the effect of CPAP over 2 months on 11 patients with OSA (AHI ≥15 events·h^{-1}) and RH, with a mean±SEM drop of 10.5±4.2 mmHg of SBP and 5.7±2.5 mmHg of DBP in both the daytime and at night-time. MARTINEZ-GARCÍA et al. [70] carried out a study on 33 patients, of whom 23 presented good tolerance of CPAP over 3 months, with a significant

Table 3. Studies that evaluate the effect of treatment with CPAP on BP readings in patients with resistant hypertension (RH)

First author [ref.]	Study type	Subjects	Age years	Males %	BMI kg·m⁻²	CPAP duration months	24-h initial SBP mmHg	24-h initial DBP mmHg	ESS	BP measure	AHI events·h⁻¹	CPAP compliance h·day⁻¹	Anti-AHT drugs
Logan [58]	Obs	11	57±2#	91	34.4±2.4#	2	147.2±3.3#	88.3±2.2#		ABPM	36.6±6.6#	4.2±0.4#	>3
Martinez-Garcia [70]	Obs	33 by ITT 23 by PP	70.2±7.5	52	34.2±5	3	154.8±14	90±8.8	6.3±4.5	ABPM	37.7±18.2	5.9±2.7	3.6±0.7
Dernaika [71]	Obs Retr	42 RH versus 56 well-controlled AHT	61.8±8.9	97.5	38.5±10.2	12	146±8.4	84.8±7.2		Office	60.1±36.2	6.5±1.2	3.4±0.8
Lozano [72]	RCT (PP)	64 [29 CPAP and 35 control], 41 true RH¶ [20 CPAP and 21 control]	59.2±9.9	68.8	30.8±5	3	129.9±13.7	76±10	6.1±3.3	ABPM	52.7±21.5	5.6±1.5	3.5±0.57
Pedrosa [73]	RCT (ITT)	40 random 37 analysed 19 CPAP 16 control	56±1#	77	32 [28-39]	6	Diurnal (control versus CPAP) 145.8±4 versus 148.4±2.5#; nocturnal 136.6±4.4 versus 136.2±3.0#	Diurnal (control versus CPAP) 88.4±3.4 versus 85.4±2.3#; nocturnal 78.4±3.4 versus 80.3±2.7#	10±1#	ABPM	29 [24-48]	6.01±0.2#	4 (4-5)
Martinez-Garcia [74]	RCT (ITT)	98 CPAP 96 control	56±9.5	68.6	34.1±5.4	3	144.2±12.5	83±10.5	9.1±3.7	ABPM	40.4±18.9	5±1.9	3.8±0.9
De Oliveira [75]	RCT (ITT)	47 [24 CPAP and 23 sham-CPAP]	59.4±7.7	57	29.8±4.4	2	148±17	88±13	10 [6-15]	ABPM	20 [18-31]		4±1

Data are presented as n, mean±SD, or median (interquartile range), unless otherwise stated. AHT: arterial hypertension; Obs: observational; ABPM: ambulatory BP monitoring; ITT: intention-to-treat; PP: per protocol; Retr: retrospective. #: data are presented as mean±SEM; ¶: true RH indicates RH confirmed by 24-h ABPM.

improvement in the 24-h SBP readings (of −5.2 mmHg), especially at night (−6.1 mmHg), without any variations in the DBP. DERNAIKA *et al.* [71] observed, in a retrospective study on 42 patients with RH, that treatment with CPAP progressively reduced BP (−5.6 mmHg on 24-h mean BP) over a year with the beneficial effects beginning after 6 months of treatment.

RCTs

The general characteristics of the patients included in the four published RCTs are shown in table 3 [72–75]. They were aged 56–60 years (57–77% men), with a BMI of 30–34 kg·m^{-2} and an EES of 9–10 points. BP was measured in every case using ABPM, with baseline 24-h SBP readings of 130–148 mmHg and 24-h DBP readings of 76–88 mmHg. The mean AHI was 20–52.7 events·h^{-1}. CPAP treatment was used for 2–6 months, depending on the study, with a mean compliance of 5–6 h per night. Practically all the studies ruled out any secondary forms of RH and those caused by poor compliance with the treatment or by white-coat hypertension. Most of the studies also monitored BMI and compliance with anti-hypertensive drugs and CPAP during follow-up. The CPAP was usually titrated *via* autoCPAP, with subsequent treatment at fixed pressure. The most frequent main outcome for those studies with a calculated sample size was change in 24-h SBP. The basic differences between the studies were, above all, the definition of RH (which ranged between 125 and 140 mmHg for SBP and between 80 and 90 mmHg for DBP measured by 24-h ABPM), followed by the AHI cut-off point for randomisation (from 5 to 15 events·h^{-1}, although most of the studies chose an AHI of 15 events·h^{-1}), the diagnostic method used (respiratory polygraphy *versus* full PSG) and the use of sham CPAP (only used in one study) [75]. Figure 2 shows the effect of CPAP treatment on both daytime and night-time systolic and diastolic readings in the RCTs undertaken to date. Only a few of the studies analysed the effect of CPAP on nocturnal BP patterns [70, 73, 75], observing a drop in the percentage of patients with nocturnal riser patterns and an increase in patients who recovered a dipper pattern.

A recent meta-analysis [76] that included two of the observational studies and three of the clinical studies described above found a drop of −4.6 mmHg (−6.4−−3 mmHg) in 24-h

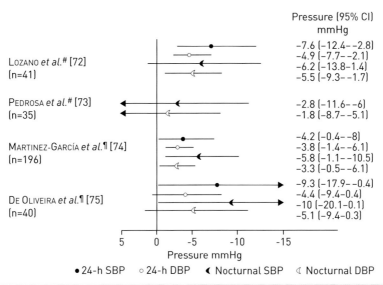

Figure 2. Role of CPAP on BP in patients with resistant hypertension. Data from RCTs are expressed as the change in mean BP (95% CI). #: effect of CPAP on BP in the CPAP arm; ¶: effect of CPAP on BP as a difference between CPAP and control arms.

SBP (−3.96 mmHg when only the RCTs were considered) and of −2.93 mmHg (−4.49–1.38 mmHg) in 24-h DBP (−3.49 mmHg in the RCTs alone). These drops were significantly larger than those observed in OSA patients with nonresistant AHT or those without AHT who were being treated with CPAP. This meta-analysis does not include the very recent study by DE OLIVEIRA *et al.* [75], which used sham CPAP in 23 patients and active CPAP in 24, with a significant drop of 9.3 mmHg in 24-h SBP and of 4.4 mmHg in 24-h DBP, particularly in the nocturnal readings.

Uvulopalatopharyngoplasty

Only one study has evaluated the effectiveness of surgical treatment with uvulopalato-pharyngoplasty in patients with RH and OSA. ZHENG *et al.* [77] performed uvulopalatopha-ryngoplasty on 36 patients with moderate-severe OSA and RH and obtained after 6 months a reduction in the AHI from 37.5 to 9.5 events·h^{-1}, and a drop in 24-h BP of 18.3 mmHg for SBP and of 19 mmHg for DBP. They also observed a close correlation between the drop in AHI and the drop in BP, as well as a reduction in the need for anti-hypertensive treatment, which fell from 3.6 to 2.9 drugs per day.

Mechanisms of action of CPAP treatment

CPAP treatment has proved beneficial in attenuating practically all the intermediate pathophysiological mechanisms that explain the relationship between OSA and AHT [22]. Focusing specifically on patients with RH, LOGAN *et al.* [58] observed that CPAP treatment in RH patients is capable of significantly reducing BP in a single night (by 12.3 mmHg in SBP and 4.8 mmHg in DBP) (fig. 3) and decreasing heart rate. This effect is achieved by acting on the attenuation of the baroreflex that is dependent on the activation of the sympathetic system, which means that the effect of CPAP can be attributed, at least in part, to a normalisation of sympathetic activity that could also continue during the daytime.

Furthermore, three studies have also analysed the effect of CPAP on the concentration of aldosterone in patients with OSA and RH. ZHANG *et al.* [78] observed in 13 patients that after 3 months of treatment with CPAP the plasma concentration of aldosterone dropped significantly, unlike the plasma renin activity, which was unchanged. These results contrast with other studies that did not find any changes in the concentration of aldosterone after

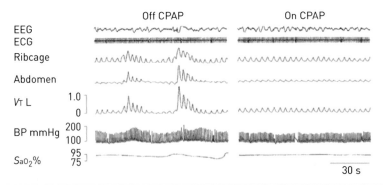

Figure 3. Stabilisation of BP in a patient with resistant hypertension and OSA during treatment with CPAP. EEG: electroencephalogram; V_T: tidal volume; Sa_{O_2}: arterial oxygen saturation. Reproduced from [58] with permission from the publisher.

treatment with CPAP [48, 72], although LLOBERES *et al.* [49] did find a significant correlation with nocturnal desaturation in patients with RH.

Compliance with CPAP

Compliance with CPAP treatment was acceptable, even in those patients with only mild symptoms of OSA. Some of these studies established CPAP use for at least 4 h per night as acceptable [70, 73, 75], and 70–95% of patients satisfied this criterion (4.2–6.5 h·night^{-1}). Some authors failed to observe any greater effect of CPAP with greater compliance or any evidence that the variable "number of hours" was an independent factor in the drop in BP [73]. However, the HIPARCO study [74], the largest RCT on this subject to date, did find a correlation between the number of hours of CPAP use and reduced BP.

Future challenges

There is still a great deal of important information that has yet to be uncovered about the relationship between OSA, greater resistance to anti-hypertensive treatment and the possible effect of OSA treatment on improved control of BP in patients with RH. In this unknown territory, the most important information may require the exploration of new pathophysiological routes, as well as the role of obesity in this process (studies of non-obese patients with RH and OSA would be very illuminating in this respect). As for CPAP treatment, some important questions remain unanswered. For example, CPAP is not usually an anti-hypertensive treatment (*i.e.* one that normalises BP), which usually means that patients have to continue with anti-hypertensive pills to some extent. There is, therefore, a need to clarify the position of CPAP in the therapeutic algorithm of RH, what it would offer in combination with other treatments, which other treatments would be optimal as combinations with CPAP, and what changes these treatments would require when combined with CPAP. Moreover, the longest study with CPAP lasted 12 months [71] and was retrospective. Major long-term studies are, therefore, needed to establish the role of CPAP, find out whether drops in BP change over time and investigate the impact on cardiovascular morbidity and mortality, although this type of study could give rise to ethical issues. Finally, further clinical, biological and genetic studies are required to reliably determine which RH patients have a greater probability of suffering from OSA and, above all, which patients are suitable for treatment with CPAP and would have a good adherence/response to this treatment.

Conclusion

The prevalence of OSA in patients with RH is extremely high. It has been postulated that the main pathophysiological mechanisms determining this relationship could be the activation of the sympathetic system and the hyperaldosteronism present in a high proportion of patients with OSA and RH, as well as in obese patients. Even when they experience OSA, RH patients present barely any associated sleep-related symptoms, which makes a sleep study indispensable in every case because of the additional cardiovascular risk involved. Moreover, the information currently available from four RCTs demonstrates that treatment with CPAP is capable of reducing BP more substantially in RH patients than in those with nonresistant hypertension (around 4–5 mmHg drop in SBP and DBP), as well as improving the nocturnal BP patterns. Given the importance of OSA, RH and obesity, in epidemiological, prognostic and therapeutic terms, further studies are required to conclusively establish the optimal treatment for these patients.

References

1. Parati G, Stergiou G, O'Brien E, et al. European Society of Hypertension practice guidelines for ambulatory blood pressure monitoring. J Hypertens 2014; 32: 1359–1366.
2. World Health Organization. The World Health Report 2002: Reducing Risks, Promoting Healthy Life. Geneva, World Health Organization, 2002.
3. Barbé F, Durán-Cantolla J, Sánchez de la Torre M, et al. Effect of continuous positive airway pressure on the incidence of hypertension and cardiovascular events in nonsleepy patients with obstructive sleep apnea: a randomized-controlled trial. JAMA 2012; 307: 2161–2168.
4. Campos-Rodriguez F, Martinez-Garcia MA, de la Cruz-Moron I, et al. Cardiovascular mortality in women with obstructive sleep apnea with or without continuous positive airway pressure treatment: a cohort study. Ann Intern Med 2012; 156: 115–122.
5. Martinez-García MA, Campos-Rodríguez F, Catalán-Serra P, et al. Cardiovascular mortality in obstructive sleep apnea in the elderly: role of long-term continuous positive airway pressure treatment: a prospective observational study. Am J Respir Crit Care Med 2012; 186: 909–916.
6. Marin JM, Carrizo SJ, Vicente E, et al. Long-term cardiovascular outcomes in men with obstructive sleep apnoea-hypopnea syndrome with or without treatment with continuous positive airway pressure: an observational study. Lancet 2005; 365: 1046–1053.
7. Lavie P, Herer P, Hoffstein V. Obstructive sleep apnea syndrome as a risk factor for hypertension: population study. BMJ 2000; 320: 479–482.
8. Young T, Peppard P, Palta M, et al. Population-based study of sleep-disordered breathing as a risk factor for hypertension. Arch Intern Med 1997; 157: 1746–1752.
9. Peppard PE, Young T, Palta M, et al. Prospective study of the association between sleep-disordered breathing and hypertension. N Engl J Med 2000; 342: 1378–1384.
10. Marin JM, Agustí A, Villar I, et al. Association between treated and untreated obstructive sleep apnea and risk of hypertension. JAMA 2012; 307: 2169–2176.
11. Grote L, Hedner J, Peter JH. Sleep-related breathing disorder is an independent risk factor for uncontrolled hypertension. J Hypertens 2000; 18: 679–685.
12. Lavie P, Hoffstein V. Sleep apnea syndrome: a possible contributing factor to resistant hypertension. Sleep 2011; 24: 721–725.
13. Logan AG, Perlikowski SM, Mente A, et al. High prevalence of unrecognized sleep apnoea in drug-resistant hypertension. J Hypertens 2001; 19: 2271–2277.
14. Chobanian AV, Bakris GL, Black HR, et al. Seventh report of the Joint National Committee on prevention, detection, evaluation, and treatment of high blood pressure. Hypertension 2003; 42: 1206–1252.
15. Bazzano LA, Khan Z, Reynolds K, et al. Effect of nocturnal nasal continuous positive airway pressure on blood pressure in obstructive sleep apnea. Hypertension 2007; 50: 417–423.
16. Alajmi M, Mulgrew AT, Fox J, et al. Impact of continuous positive airway pressure therapy on blood pressure in patients with obstructive sleep apnea hypopnea: a meta-analysis of randomized controlled trials. Lung 2007; 185: 67–72.
17. Haentjens P, Van Meerhaeghe A, Moscariello A, et al. The impact of continuous positive airway pressure on blood pressure in patients with obstructive sleep apnea syndrome: evidence from a meta-analysis of placebo-controlled randomized trials. Arch Intern Med 2007; 167: 757–764.
18. Fava C, Dorigoni S, Dalle Vedove F, et al. Effect of CPAP on blood pressure in patients with OSA/hypopnea a systematic review and meta-analysis. Chest 2014; 145: 762–771.
19. Calhoun DA, Jones D, Textor S, et al. Resistant hypertension: diagnosis, evaluation, and treatment. A scientific statement from the American Heart Association Professional Education Committee of the Council for High Blood Pressure Research. Hypertension 2008; 51: 1403–1419.
20. Egan BM, Zhao Y, Axon RN. US trends in prevalence, awareness, treatment, and control of hypertension, 1998–2008. JAMA 2010; 303: 2043–2050.
21. Daugherty SL, Powers JD, Magid DJ, et al. Incidence and prognosis of resistant hypertension in hypertensive patients. Circulation 2012; 125: 1635–1642.
22. Egan BM, Zhao Y, Axon RN, et al. Uncontrolled and apparent treatment resistant hypertension in the United States, 1988 to 2008. Circulation 2011; 124: 1046–1058.
23. De la Sierra A, Segura J, Banegas JR, et al. Clinical features of 8295 patients with resistant hypertension classified on the basis of ambulatory blood pressure monitoring. Hypertension 2011; 57: 898–902.
24. Shamsuzzaman AS, Gersh BJ, Somers VK. Obstructive sleep apnea: implications for cardiac and vascular disease. JAMA 2003; 290: 1906–1914.
25. Prabhakar NR, Kumar GK, Peng YJ. Sympatho-adrenal activation by chronic intermittent hypoxia. J Appl Physiol 2012; 113: 1304–1310.

26. Ip MS, Tse HF, Lam B, *et al.* Endothelial function in obstructive sleep apnea and response to treatment. *Am J Respir Crit Care Med* 2004; 169: 348–353.

27. Pimenta E, Calhoun DA, Oparil S. Sleep apnea, aldosterone, and resistant hypertension. *Prog Cardiovasc Dis* 2009; 51: 371–380.

28. Goodfriend TL, Calhoun DA. Resistant hypertension, obesity, sleep apnea, and aldosterone: theory and therapy. *Hypertension* 2004; 43: 518–524.

29. Dudenbostel T, Calhoun DA. Resistant hypertension, obstructive sleep apnoea and aldosterone. *J Hum Hypertens* 2012; 26: 281–287.

30. Parati G, Ochoa JE, Bilo G, *et al.* Obstructive sleep apnea syndrome as a cause of resistant hypertension. *Hypertens Res* 2014; 37: 601–613.

31. Kato M, Roberts-Thompson P, Phillips BG, *et al.* Impairment of endothelium-dependent vasodilation of resistance vessels in patients with obstructive sleep apnea. *Circulation* 2000; 102: 2607–2610.

32. Doonan RJ, Scheffler P, Lalli M, *et al.* Increased arterial stiffness in obstructive sleep apnea: a systematic review. *Hypertens Res* 2011; 34: 23–32.

33. Friedman O, Bradley TD, Chan CT, *et al.* Relationship between overnight rostral fluid shift and obstructive sleep apnea in drug-resistant hypertension. *Hypertension* 2010; 56: 1077–1082.

34. Egan BM. Overnight rostral fluid shift and obstructive sleep apnea in treatment resistant hypertension: connecting the dots clarifies the picture. *Hypertension* 2010; 56: 1040–1041.

35. Gallay BJ, Ahmad S, Xu L, *et al.* Screening for primary aldosteronism without discontinuing hypertensive medications: plasma aldosterone-renin ratio. *Am J Kidney Dis* 2001; 37: 699–705.

36. Eide IK, Torjesen PA, Drolsum A, *et al.* Low-renin status in therapy-resistant hypertension: a clue to efficient treatment. *J Hypertens* 2004; 22: 2217–2226.

37. Lloberes P, Lozano L, Sampol G, *et al.* Obstructive sleep apnoea and 24-h blood pressure in patients with resistant hypertension. *J Sleep Res* 2010; 19: 597–602.

38. Martinez-García MA, Gomez R, Gil T, *et al.* Trastornos respiratorios durante el sueño en pacientes con hipertensión arterial de dificil control [Sleep-disordered breathing in patients with difficult-to-control hypertension]. *Arch Bronconeumol* 2006; 42: 14–20.

39. Pedrosa RP, Drager LF, Gonzaga CC, *et al.* Obstructive sleep apnea: the most common secondary cause of hypertension associated with resistant hypertension. *Hypertension* 2011; 58: 811–817.

40. Gonçalves SC, Martinez D, Gus M, *et al.* Obstructive sleep apnea and resistant hypertension: a case-control study. *Chest* 2007; 132: 1858–1862.

41. Logan AG, Perlikowski SM, Mente A, *et al.* High prevalence of unrecognized sleep apnoea in drug-resistant hypertension. *J Hypertens* 2001; 19: 2271–2277.

42. Wolk R, Shamsuzzaman AS, Somers VK. Obesity, sleep apnea, and hypertension. *Hypertension* 2003; 42: 1067–1074.

43. Bramlage P, Pittrow D, Wittchen HU, *et al.* Hypertension in overweight and obese primary care patients is highly prevalent and poorly controlled. *Am J Hypertens* 2004; 17: 904–910.

44. Goodfriend TL, Egan BM, Kelley DE. Aldosterone in obesity. *Endocr Res* 1998; 24: 789–796.

45. Pratt-Ubunama MN, Nishizaka MK, Boedefeld RL, *et al.* Plasma aldosterone is related to severity of obstructive sleep apnea in subjects with resistant hypertension. *Chest* 2007; 131: 453–459.

46. Florczak E, Prejbisz A, Szwench-Pietrasz E, *et al.* Clinical characteristics of patients with resistant hypertension: the RESIST-POL study. *J Hum Hypertens* 2013; 27: 678–685.

47. Gonzaga CC, Calhoun DA. Resistant hypertension and hyperaldosteronism. *Curr Hypertens Rep* 2008; 10: 496–503.

48. Calhoun DA, Nishizaka MK, Zaman MA, *et al.* Aldosterone excretion among subjects with resistant hypertension and symptoms of sleep apnea. *Chest* 2004; 125: 112–117.

49. Lloberes P, Sampol G, Espinel E, *et al.* A randomized controlled study of CPAP effect on plasma aldosterone concentration in patients with resistant hypertension and obstructive sleep apnea. *J Hypertens* 2014; 32: 1650–1657.

50. Fletcher EC. The relationship between systemic hypertension and obstructive sleep apnea: facts and theory. *Am J Med* 1995; 98: 118–128.

51. Carlson JT, Rångemark C, Hedner JA. Attenuated endothelium-dependent vascular relaxation in patients with sleep apnoea. *J Hypertens* 1996; 14: 577–584.

52. Marrone O, Riccobono L, Salvaggio A, *et al.* Catecholamines and blood pressure in obstructive sleep apnea syndrome. *Chest* 1993; 103: 722–727.

53. Solin P, Kaye DM, Little PJ, *et al.* Impact of sleep apnea on sympathetic nervous system activity in heart failure. *Chest* 2003; 123: 1119–1126.

54. Tsioufis C, Kordalis A, Flessas D, *et al.* Pathophysiology of resistant hypertension: the role of sympathetic nervous system. *Int J Hypertens* 2011; 2011: 642416.

55. Krum H, Schlaich M, Whitbourn R, *et al.* Catheter-based renal sympathetic denervation for resistant hypertension: a multicentre safety and proof-of-principle cohort study. *Lancet* 2009; 373: 1275–1281.

56. Esler MD, Krum H, Sobotka PA, et al. Renal sympathetic denervation in patients with treatment-resistant hypertension (the Symplicity HTN-2 Trial): a randomised controlled trial. Lancet 2010; 376: 1903–1909.
57. Egan BM. Renal sympathetic denervation: a novel intervention for resistant hypertension, insulin resistance, and sleep apnea. Hypertension 2011; 58: 542–543.
58. Logan AG, Tkacova R, Perlikowski SM, et al. Refractory hypertension and sleep apnoea: effect of CPAP on blood pressure and baroreflex. Eur Respir J 2003; 21: 241–247.
59. Gaddam K, Pimenta E, Thomas SJ, et al. Spironolactone reduces severity of obstructive sleep apnoea in patients with resistant hypertension: a preliminary report. J Hum Hypertens 2010; 24: 532–537.
60. Nieto FJ, Young TB, Lind BK, et al. Association of sleep-disordered breathing, sleep apnea, and hypertension in a large community-based study. Sleep Heart Health Study. JAMA 2000; 283: 1829–1836.
61. Sjöström C, Lindberg E, Elmasry A, et al. Prevalence of sleep apnoea and snoring in hypertensive men: a population based study. Thorax 2002; 57: 602–607.
62. Margallo VS, Muxfeldt ES, Guimarães GM, et al. Diagnostic accuracy of the Berlin questionnaire in detecting obstructive sleep apnea in patients with resistant hypertension. J Hypertens 2014; 32: 2030–2036.
63. Lloberes P, Durán-Cantolla J, Martinez-García MÁ, et al. Diagnosis and treatment of sleep apnea-hypopnea syndrome. Spanish Society of Pulmonology and Thoracic Surgery. Arch Bronconeumol 2011; 47: 143–156.
64. Buchwald H, Avidor Y, Braunwald E, et al. Bariatric surgery: a systematic review and meta-analysis. JAMA 2004; 292: 1724–1737.
65. Pimenta E, Gaddam KK, Oparil S, et al. Effects of dietary sodium reduction on blood pressure in subjects with resistant hypertension: results from a randomized trial. Hypertension 2009; 54: 475–481.
66. Pimenta E, Stowasser M, Gordon RD, et al. Increased dietary sodium is related to severity of obstructive sleep apnea in patients with resistant hypertension and hyperaldosteronism. Chest 2013; 143: 978–983.
67. Witkowski A, Kadziela J. Obstructive sleep apnoea, resistant hypertension and renal denervation. EuroIntervention 2013; 9: Suppl R, R105–R109.
68. Chapman N, Dobson J, Wilson S, et al. Effect of spironolactone on blood pressure in subjects with resistant hypertension. Hypertension 2007; 49: 839–845.
69. Kasai T, Bradley TD, Friedman O, et al. Effect of intensified diuretic therapy on overnight rostral fluid shift and obstructive sleep apnoea in patients with uncontrolled hypertension. J Hypertens 2014; 32: 673–680.
70. Martinez-García MA, Gómez R, Soler-Cataluña JJ, et al. Positive effect of CPAP treatment on the control of difficult-to-treat hypertension. Eur Respir J 2007; 29: 951–957.
71. Dernaika TA, Kinasewitz GT, Tawk MM. Effects of nocturnal continuous positive airway pressure therapy in patients with resistant hypertension and obstructive sleep apnea. J Clin Sleep Med 2009; 15: 103–107.
72. Lozano L, Tovar JL, Sampol G, et al. Continuous positive airway pressure treatment in sleep apnea patients with resistant hypertension: a randomized, controlled trial. J Hypertens 2010; 28: 2161–2168.
73. Pedrosa RP, Drager LF, de Paula LKG, et al. Effects of OSA treatment on BP in patients with resistant hypertension: a randomized trial. Chest 2013; 144: 1487–1494.
74. Martinez-García MA, Capote F, Campos-Rodríguez F, et al. Effect of CPAP on blood pressure in patients with obstructive sleep apnea and resistant hypertension: the HIPARCO randomized clinical trial. JAMA 2013; 310: 2407–2415.
75. De Oliveira AC, Martinez D, Massierer D, et al. The antihypertensive effect of positive airway pressure on resistant hypertension of patients with obstructive sleep apnea: a randomized, double-blind, clinical trial. Am Respir J Crit Care Med 2014; 190: 345–347.
76. Varounis C, Katsi V, Kallikazaros IE, et al. Effect of CPAP on blood pressure in patients with obstructive sleep apnea and resistant hypertension: a systematic review and meta-analysis. Int J Cardiol 2014; 175: 195–198.
77. Zheng T, Zhang L, Tian GY, et al. [Effect of uvulopalatopharyngoplasty on obstructive sleep apnea hypopnea syndrome in patients with resistant hypertension]. Zhonghua Er Bi Yan Hou Tou Jing Wai Ke Za Zhi 2012; 47: 383–387.
78. Zhang XL, Li YQ. [Efficacy of continuous positive airway pressure therapy upon resistant hypertension in patients with obstructive sleep apnea hypopnea syndrome]. Zhonghua Yi Xue Za Zhi 2009; 89: 1811–1814.

Disclosures: **None declared.**

Chapter 15

Cancer: an epidemiological perspective

F. Javier Nieto

Emerging epidemiological research linking OSA with cancer outcomes is based on strong evidence from laboratory and animal experiments, which show that intermittent hypoxaemia can enhance cancer growth and/or metastasis by promoting angiogenesis, changes on immune function, or inflammatory changes and oxidative stress. In this chapter the epidemiological evidence linking OSA and cancer incidence or cancer mortality is critically analysed.

Using Hill's causality analysis framework, this review found moderately strong evidence that OSA might promote cancer growth and decrease cancer survival. Evidence in support of a role of OSA as a risk factor for cancer incidence is substantially weaker but this hypothesis cannot be ruled out at this time.

In addition to mechanistic studies, future research should include studies in different population settings and further clarification as to whether OSA increases cancer incidence, mortality or both. An additional critical area for further research is whether cancer patients with OSA would benefit from OSA treatment.

As evidenced by the large body of literature reviewed in this *Monograph* and elsewhere, the immediate and measurable consequences of OSA, intermittent hypoxaemia and sleep fragmentation may have serious pathophysiological consequences on a variety of metabolic, endocrine, neurological, sympathetic and homeostatic systems [1–3]. Unsurprisingly, OSA has been in turn associated with a growing number of health outcomes, including psychopathological disorders (depression, reduced quality of life), increased risk of occupational and motor vehicle injuries, CVD, hypertension and metabolic syndrome [4–7].

As discussed by Almendros *et al.* [8] in this *Monograph*, growing evidence from laboratory studies suggests that IH and sleep fragmentation might play a role at different stages of carcinogenesis, either as cancer initiators or by facilitating cancer progression. As Abrams pointed out in his brief 2007 commentary [9], emerging evidence from laboratory studies in support of this hypothesis contrasts with the lack of published

Dept of Population Health Sciences, School of Medicine and Public Health, University of Wisconsin, Madison, WI, USA.

Correspondence: F. Javier Nieto, Dept of Population Health Sciences, School of Medicine and Public Health, University of Wisconsin, 610 Walnut Street, WARF Building 707C, Madison, WI 53726, USA. E-mail: fjnieto@wisc.edu

reports documenting an association between sleep apnoea and cancer in humans. A critical tipping point was the publication of a series of landmark experimental studies from a Spanish research group led by Ramon Farré. In these studies, a melanoma mouse model that was subjected to an intermittent hypoxaemia regimen closely mimicking that occurring in humans with OSA, resulted in a marked acceleration of tumour growth and metastasis [10–12]. These experiments inspired a 20-year follow-up analysis of existing data from the Wisconsin Sleep Cohort, which demonstrated a strikingly strong association between baseline OSA and cancer mortality [13]. Additional reports exploring the association between different surrogate measures of OSA and a variety of cancer outcomes (incidence or mortality; site-specific or all cancers) have been published in the last couple of years. Due to its emerging nature, however, this body of literature still raises more questions than it answers [14–17].

This chapter reviews the existing epidemiological evidence and uses a classic causal analysis framework to discuss the strength of the evidence in support of the hypothesis that OSA might be causally involved in either carcinogenesis or cancer progression. The chapter concludes with a review of some of the remaining knowledge gaps and suggests further areas of research in this area.

Epidemiological studies in human populations

Following the evidence stemming from laboratory and animal experiments, a number of recently published studies have considered whether OSA is associated with increased cancer incidence or mortality in human populations. These studies are reviewed in this section.

One common characteristic of these studies is that they were all secondary or *ad hoc* analyses of existing cohorts or clinical databases. Indeed, because of the novel nature of this hypothesis, none of the studies published thus far has been specifically designed to address this hypothesis. This is one reason why the existing evidence needs to be interpreted critically, as discussed in the following section.

OSA and cancer mortality

The first epidemiological study on this topic was an extension of a previously published follow-up analysis of mortality associated with OSA in participants in the Wisconsin Sleep Cohort study [18]. Established in 1989, the Wisconsin Sleep Cohort is the longest ongoing cohort study of sleep apnoea and other sleep disorders in a population-based sample [19, 20]. It is defined as "population-based" as its sample frame is the general population rather than patients attending healthcare facilities. Study participants were recruited from rosters of Wisconsin state government employees, ranging from those in administrative and clerical roles, to educators and managerial professionals. A total of 2940 people were invited and 1546 participated in at least one baseline examination, which included a full 18-channel PSG and extensive evaluation of the participants' sociodemographic characteristics, health history, behaviours, psychosocial status, cognitive status, a physical exam (including BP and anthropometric measurements) and the collection of biological specimens, including urine and blood. Follow-up was both passive (linkage with vital statistics to assess mortality) and active (repeated contact that for most participants included additional exams (with repeated PSG)).

A Wisconsin Sleep Cohort study published in 2008 documented a strong association between sleep apnoea and both total and cardiovascular mortality over a follow-up period of ≤18 years [18]. Relative to those with no OSA, and after controlling for possible confounding variables (age, sex and BMI), the adjusted hazard ratios of total and cardiovascular mortality associated with severe OSA were 3.0 (95% CI 1.4–6.3) and 2.9 (95% CI 0.8–10.0), respectively.

In view of the emerging evidence of a putative OSA–carcinogenesis connection, an updated analysis focusing exclusively on cancer mortality was published in 2012 [13]. For this analysis, ≤22 years of follow-up were available, during which 50 cancer deaths were identified. Categories of OSA severity were defined based on widely used criteria [21] as follows: absent (AHI of <5 events·h^{-1}), mild (AHI of ≥5–<15 events·h^{-1}), moderate (AHI of ≥15–<30 events·h^{-1}) and severe (AHI ≥30 events·h^{-1}). The corresponding rates of cancer mortality (per 1000 person-years) for these categories were 1.5, 1.9, 3.6 and 7.3, respectively. Figure 1 demonstrates how the survival over time progressively decreased with increasing levels of OSA severity. Other features and some of the main results from this study are summarised in table 1. The main multivariate analyses (controlling for age, sex, BMI and smoking) revealed that, compared to subjects without OSA, the adjusted hazard ratios of cancer mortality were 1.1 (95% CI 0.5–2.7) for mild OSA, 2.0 (95% CI 0.7–5.5) for moderate OSA, and 4.8 (95% CI 1.7–13.2) for severe OSA (trend test, p=0.0052). These hazard ratios remained virtually unchanged after further adjustment for other possible confounders (physical activity, alcohol use, education, diabetes, waist circumference and sleep duration).

When the hypoxaemia index (HI) (% sleep time with oxygen saturation <90%) was used to characterise OSA instead of the AHI, the association was even stronger. In the absence of a predetermined set of criteria, the cut-off points used to define the HI categories for this analysis were based on the same quantile distribution as the AHI cut-points for mild,

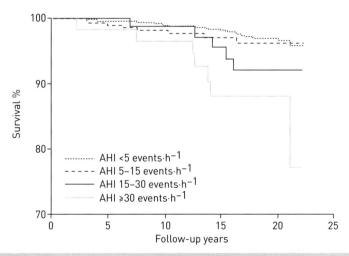

Figure 1. Survival free of cancer mortality according to categories of sleep disordered breathing, Wisconsin Sleep Cohort, 1989–2011; Kaplan-Meier estimates. Reproduced and modified from [13] with permission from the publisher.

Table 1. Summary of published epidemiological cohort studies on the association between OSA and cancer mortality

First author [ref.]	Location	Study type	Participants	Follow-up	OSA assessment	Cancer[#] deaths n	Main results	Potential confounders	Stratified analyses
NIETO [13]	WI, USA	Population-based	1522 state employees	18 years	Full PSG	50	AHI (ref.: <5 events·h⁻¹) 5–14.9 events·h⁻¹: HR 1.1 15–29.9 events·h⁻¹: HR 2.0 ≥30 events·h⁻¹: HR 4.8¶ HI (ref.: <0.8%) 0.8–3.5%: HR 1.6 3.6–11.2%: HR 2.9 >11.2%: HR 8.6¶	Age, sex, BMI, smoking, physical activity, alcohol use, education, diabetes, waist circumference and sleep duration	Association present in both sexes and within categories defined according to age, obesity (slightly stronger among the non-obese) and sleepiness status
MARTINEZ-GARCIA [22]	Multicenter, Spain	Clinic-based	5427 patients referred to sleep clinics (3958 <65 years of age)	4.5 years	Respiratory polygraphy (68%) Full PSG (32%)	90 (26 in patients <65 years of age)	AHI tertiles (ref.: <19.1 events·h⁻¹) 19.1–44.5 events·h⁻¹: HR 0.8 >44.5 events·h⁻¹: HR 1.0 HI tertiles (ref.: <1.2%) 1.2–13%: HR 1.6 >13%: HR 2.1¶	Age, sex, BMI, smoking, alcohol intake, type of sleep study, enrolment hospital	In age-stratified analyses association limited to patients <65 years of age, HR for same categories in previous cell: AHI tertiles: 1.0; 2.7¶; 4.0¶ HI tertiles: 1.0; 7.6¶; 14.4¶
MARSHALL [23]	Busselton, Australia	Population-based	389 town residents without cancer history	20 years	MESAM 4 home sleep monitor (no EEG)	39	RDI (ref.: <5) 5–14.9: HR 0.8 ≥15: HR 3.9¶	Age, sex, BMI, smoking, waist circumference	

HR: hazard ratio (comparing each category to the reference); HI: hypoxaemia index; EEG: electroencephalogram. #: all cancers. ¶: 95% CI for the HR do not include 1.0.

moderate and severe OSA. As seen in table 1, the hazard ratios showed a clearly graded dose–response relationship that was highly statistically significant (trend test, p=0.0008); those with severe OSA (HI ⩾11.2%) were over eight times more likely to die of cancer than those without OSA (HI <0.8%).

In the study, stratified analysis revealed that the association between OSA and cancer mortality was present across groups defined by sex, age and the presence of sleepiness. When stratified according to obesity status, the association was slightly stronger among the non-obese. Given the small number of events, the study was not able to analyse mortality from specific cancers [13].

Two other studies have further explored the association between OSA and cancer mortality (table 1). Martinez-García et al. [22] analysed data from a retrospective multicentre cohort study of adult patients referred to sleep laboratories in Spanish hospitals due to suspicion of OSA. The study included a total sample of ~5400 patients who were followed for a median of 4.5 years; 90 deaths were observed. OSA status was determined using respiratory polygraphy in about two-thirds of the patients; the rest received a full PSG. In this study, OSA was not associated with cancer mortality when defined according to the AHI; however, a significant dose–response association was observed between increasing mortality and increasing levels of HI, up to a 2.1-fold hazard ratio of cancer mortality comparing the top to the bottom tertile of HI (95% CI 1.7–4.6), an association that was slightly stronger among the 3219 study participants who did not receive OSA treatment. The association was present in both women and men but was strongly modified by age: it was practically absent among participants ⩾65 years of age but very strong (even stronger than in the Wisconsin Sleep Cohort results described above) among the 3958 participants <65 years of age (the same age range as the original Wisconsin Sleep Cohort); the hazard ratios of cancer mortality comparing top to bottom tertiles were 4.0 (95% CI 1.1–3.6) for AHI and 14.4 (95% CI 1.9–111.6) for HI.

The recent retrospective cohort study from Busselton in Western Australia provides additional support to the OSA–cancer mortality hypothesis [23]. Among ~400 Busselton residents who received a home MESAM 4 polygraphy study at baseline, 39 cancer deaths were observed over a 20-year follow-up period. After controlling for demographic variables, smoking, BMI and waist circumference, a RDI of ⩾15 was associated with a 3.4-fold increase in cancer mortality (95% CI 1.1–10.2) when compared with a RDI of <5.

In summary, even though only three studies have been published so far, these studies strongly suggest an association between OSA and mortality in humans. However, because data on cancer diagnosis in these analyses were not available or considered, the studies were unable to discern whether the observed association was attributable to an increased incidence of cancer (fig. 2, option 1) or to an accelerated progression (decreased survival) after cancer initiation (fig. 2, option 2). As these hypotheses may involve different pathophysiologic mechanisms, existing evidence in support of each of them is examined separately in the following sections, even though a third hypothesis (that OSA affects both cancer initiation and cancer progression (fig. 2, option 3)) cannot be ruled out at this time (discussed further later).

OSA and cancer survival after diagnosis

Unfortunately, only one study published to date has directly examined option 2 in figure 2. In the study by Martinez-García et al. [22], a subset survival analysis of the 263

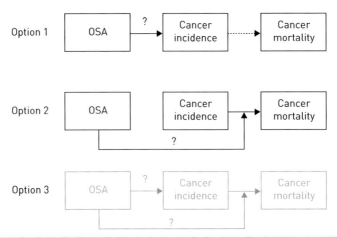

Figure 2. Possible ways to explain an association between OSA and increased cancer mortality. Option 1: OSA is carcinogenetic (cancer initiation) and results in an increased number of cases (incidence), which in turns results in a higher mortality. Option 2: OSA affects tumour growth and metastasis (cancer progression) and affects prognosis (increases mortality). Option 3: OSA affects both cancer initiation and cancer progression.

participants who were <65 years of age and who were diagnosed with cancer (62 deaths) showed that, compared with the bottom tertile of HI, the hazard ratio of cancer fatality were 8.6 (95% CI 1.1–68.8) for the second tertile and 12.8 (95% CI 1.1–10.2) for the highest tertile. Additional support for the hypothesis that intermittent hypoxaemia might play a role in cancer progression comes from a clinical study showing that melanoma tumour aggressiveness (as measured by mitotic rate, Breslow index and other markers) was significantly correlated with the degree of nocturnal ODI (a direct measure of intermittent hypoxaemia) among 56 melanoma patients [24].

Studies that have explored option 1 in figure 2 are discussed in the following section.

OSA and cancer incidence

The first published study to examine OSA and cancer incidence was from the same Spanish multicentre clinic-based cohort described above [25]. As seen for the mortality results, there was no association between AHI and cancer incidence (table 2). However, when HI was used to define OSA, a statistically significant dose–response increase in cancer incidence with rising OSA severity (tertiles of HI) was found (table 2, fig. 3); the adjusted hazard ratio of cancer incidence associated with a 10-unit increase in the HI was 1.1 (95% CI 1.0–1.1). In stratified analyses, the hazard ratios were only significantly higher among younger (<65 years of age) subjects and among male patients.

In another population-based study conducted in Denmark, 8783 participants in the third wave of the Copenhagen City Heart Study were followed for an average of 13 years to assess the relationship between OSA symptoms at baseline and the incidence of cancer, overall and by cancer subtype [26]. The main independent variables in this study were participant self-reported snoring and breathing cessation. Daytime sleepiness data (assessed using the ESS [30]) was available for 5894 participants in one of the follow-up visits. The study found no relationship between OSA symptoms and cancer incidence (table 2). However, in

Table 2. Summary of published epidemiologic cohort studies on the association between OSA and cancer incidence

First author [ref.]	Location	Study type	Participants	Follow-up	OSA assessment	Cases n	Main results	Potential confounders included in model	Stratified analyses
Campos Rodriguez [25]	Spain	Multicentre, clinic-based	4910 patients referred to sleep clinics [3958 <65 years]	4.5 years	Respiratory polygraphy [68%], full PSG [32%]	261	AHI tertiles [ref: <18.7] 18.7–43: HR 1.1 >43: HR 1.2 HI tertiles [ref: <1.2%] 1.2–12%: HR 1.6[#] >12%: HR 2.3[#]	Age, sex, BMI, smoking, alcohol intake, type of sleep study, enrolment hospital	Younger [<65 years of age]: $HR_{HI>12\%}$ 2.9[#] Older [≥65 years of age]: $HR_{HI>12\%}$ 1.6 Females: $HR_{HI>12\%}$ 1.8 Males: $HR_{HI>12\%}$ 2.6[#]
Christensen [26]	Copenhagen, Denmark	Population-based	8783 random population sample [5894 for sleepiness analysis]	13 years	Snoring, breathing pauses; self-reported	1985 [1097 for sleepiness analysis]	Snoring [ref: no snoring] Sometimes: HR 1.0 Often: HR 1.0 Don't know: HR 1.0 Number of sleep symptoms [ref: 0] 1: HR 1.2 2–3: HR 1.2	Age, sex, BMI, marital status, education, physical activity, alcohol and smoking	For sleepiness: Alcohol-related cancers [HR 4.9] Virus-related cancers [HR 2.7] For 2–3 OSA symptoms: Smoking-related cancers [HR 1.7]
Kendzerska [27]	Toronto, Canada	Clinic-based [electronic health records]	9629 clinical records	7.8 years	Full PSG	627	AHI [ref: <5] 5–14.9: HR 1.0 15–29.9: HR 1.0 >30: HR 1.0 HI >12 versus <1.2: HR 1.1	Age, sex, BMI, smoking	
Chen [28]	Taiwan	Clinic-based [medical	92 220 claim records	10 years	Full PSG	38 [central nervous	AHI [ref: <5] ≥5: HR 1.5[#]	Age, sex, comorbidities	Stronger HR if OSA was associated with

Continued

211

Table 2. Continued

First author [ref.]	Location	Study type	Participants	Follow-up	OSA assessment	Cases n	Main results	Potential confounders included in model	Stratified analyses
		claims database]				system cancers]		[cardiovascular, hypertension, diabetes, chronic kidney, liver, Alzheimer's disease (no adjustment for BMI or smoking)]	insomnia (HR 2.2#)
CHANG [29]	Taiwan	Clinic-based (National Health insurance database)	846 OSA patients (PSG-verified) and 4230 non-OSA controls	5 years	Breast cancer		Adjusted HR 2.1#	Age, income, urbanisation level, geographic region, comorbidities (hypertension, hyperlipidemia, diabetes), alcohol intake, obesity	
MARSHALL [23]	Busselton, Australia	Population-based	389 Busselton residents without cancer history	20 years	MESAM 4 home sleep monitor (no EEG)	125	RDI (ref: <5) 5–14.9: HR 0.7 ≥15 HR 2.5#	Age, sex, BMI, smoking, waist circumference	

HI: hypoxaemia index; HR: hazard ratio comparing each category to the reference; $HR_{HI>12\%}$: HR associated with an HI >12%; EEG: electroencephalogram. #: 95% CI for the HR do not include 1.0.

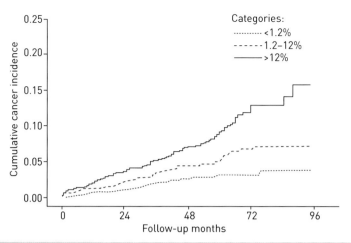

Figure 3. Kaplan–Meier curves showing cumulative cancer incidence according to percentage of night-time with <90% oxygen saturation categories (tertiles) in the Spanish multicentre cohort study. Log-rank test p < 0.0005. Reproduced and modified from [25] with permission from the publisher.

subset analyses, a strong association was found between sleepiness and cancer incidence among younger participants (<50 years of age), although this observation was based on just five cases in the top category of sleepiness (ESS score of >15). The study also reported "significant" associations between OSA symptoms and smoking-related cancers, and between sleepiness and both alcohol- and virus-related cancers. These results should be interpreted with caution, however, because of the potential multiple comparisons problem. An important limitation of this study is the exclusive characterisation of OSA based on self-reported symptoms, which may have biased the results towards null [16].

Three studies using healthcare records or claims databases have recently been reported (table 2) [27–29]. A study using electronic health records from 9600 patients who received PSG in a Toronto hospital and were followed for ~8 years, found no association between either AHI or HI and cancer incidence once BMI and smoking were controlled for in the analysis [27]. In an analyses from a large medical claims database in Taiwan (which included >92 000 records) that specifically looked at central nervous system cancers (38 cases), the hazard ratio comparing those with at least mild OSA (AHI of $\geqslant 5$ events·h^{-1}) to those without was 1.5 (95% CI 1.0–2.4) [28]. A nested case–control study based on a large national insurance longitudinal database in Taiwan, which compared patients with a sleep apnoea diagnosis to controls, resulted in an estimated 2.1-fold adjusted hazard ratio (95% CI 1.1–4.1) of breast cancer incidence over a 5-year follow-up period [29].

Finally, in the 20-year follow-up analyses of the Busselton cohort described above [23], moderate-to-severe OSA (RDI $\geqslant 15$ events·h^{-1}) was associated with a 2.5-fold increase in cancer incidence (95% CI 1.2–5.0) (table 2).

OSA and cancer: association or causation?

The epidemiological research presented in the previous section reveals that OSA is associated with cancer mortality (and possibly cancer incidence). A further question is whether or not these associations imply causality, i.e. whether or not OSA may act as a contributing factor in the initiation or clinical progression of cancer. There are two distinct phases in the natural history of cancer, *i.e.* factors that influence cancer inception (carcinogenesis) might be completely different to factors that affect cancer progression (cancer growth or metastasis). Therefore, the evidence in support of one or the other (fig. 2, Options 1 and 2) needs to be independently evaluated.

This section critically reviews the existing evidence in support of the hypothesis that OSA is causally linked with cancer incidence (*e.g.* involved in carcinogenesis) or with increased cancer mortality (*e.g.* a rise in case-fatality rate or poor prognosis after cancer diagnosis). Hill's classic causality criteria have been used as a guideline [31–33]; the findings of these criteria are briefly described in the following sections and are summarised in table 3.

Biological plausibility

Unlike many other situations, in which findings from epidemiological studies have led to further investigation of the biological mechanisms that might explain such observations, in this instance biology and pathophysiological discovery came first [9, 17], inspiring the interrogation of the epidemiological databases described in the preceding section. Until now, the strongest evidence has supported the role of OSA (particularly intermittent hypoxaemia) in cancer growth and poor cancer prognosis (fig. 2, option 2). There is substantial evidence that hypoxia increases the transcription of the hypoxia-inducible factor (HIF), thereby increasing both resistance to hypoxia and the expression of vascular endothelial growth factor (VEGF), as well as the formation of new capillaries that facilitate blood supply to the tumour and thus enhance its growth and metastatic potential [34–36]. Chronic hypoxia, a common feature in solid tumour tissue, has been associated with therapeutic resistance, tumour progression and metastasis [37–39]. *In vitro* studies have further demonstrated that cultured lung cancer cells subjected to IH are more resistant to radiation and apoptosis, and are more prone to metastasize [40]. Furthermore, both *in vivo* and *in vitro* studies have demonstrated that low-frequency IH (*e.g.* 4–2-min hypoxic periods) could also promote tumour development, and enhance tumour growth and

Table 3. The strength of the epidemiological evidence for each of Hill's guidelines [31–33] in the evaluation of causality in the association between OSA and either cancer incidence or cancer progression/mortality

Criterion	Cancer incidence (carcinogenesis)	Cancer fatality/mortality (cancer progression)
Biological plausibility	+	+++
Experimental evidence in animal models	−	+++
Temporal relationship	+++	+++
Strength of the association	+	+++
Dose–response relationship	+	+++
Consideration of alternative explanations	+	++
Replication of findings	+/−	+
Cessation of exposure	−	−

The criteria are described in the main text. −, +, ++, +++: strength of evidence for each criterion, ranked from no evidence (−) to significant evidence (+++).

angiogenesis [41–43]. Recent studies have also suggested that IH might enhance cancer growth and aggressiveness through changes in the immune system, particularly through the activation of tumour-associated macrophages [44, 45].

Possible biological mechanisms that could explain a carcinogenic role for hypoxia (promoting cancer incidence (fig. 2, option 1)) are currently more speculative. For example, studies have shown that hypoxia might induce oxidative stress [46, 47] and DNA oxidation [48, 49]. It is conceivable that increased oxidative stress and DNA oxidation could in turn result in mutations leading to cell malignisation, particularly in the context of the inflammatory background of patients with OSA [2, 50–52].

A third possibility that cannot currently be dismissed is that hypoxia increases both cancer incidence and cancer progression (fig. 2, option 3). Even though it is well known that the three stages of carcinogenesis (initiation, promotion and progression) might be affected by different factors [53], it is possible that hypoxia might promote both initiation and progression through combination of some of the previously described mechanisms.

Finally, and in addition to hypoxia, a role for OSA-induced sleep fragmentation in carcinogenesis has been suggested by some studies, including a recent animal model (see below) [54] and indirectly by the results of epidemiological studies which demonstrated that other non-OSA sleep disorders (short sleep duration, shift work, insomnia) might increase cancer risk [55–59].

Experimental evidence from animal models

Animal experiments do not currently provide any evidence in support of a carcinogenic (cancer initiation) role for OSA. In contrast, there is strong experimental evidence from animal models that supports a possible role of OSA (particularly intermittent hypoxaemia) and cancer growth and cancer prognosis. In an experimental model designed to simulate the level and frequency of IH occurring in human OSA, melanoma cancer cells were subcutaneously injected into the flank of identical young male mice distributed into two groups. The control group remained breathing room air. The animals in the other group were subjected to a pattern of IH by breathing air of varying oxygen concentrations: periodic cycles of 20 s of 5% oxygen followed by 40 s of room air (21% oxygen), ~60 apnoeic events·h^{-1}, for ~6 h per day during the light cycle. The growth of the melanoma tumour over a 2-week period was twice as great in the IH as it was in the control group [10]. Histological examination of the excised tumour revealed that the tumour was more necrotic in the animals under IH than in the controls; the increased tumour growth appeared to be associated with an increased expression of VEGF [11].

In subsequent experiments, the same mouse model was used to demonstrate that IH increases the rate of lung metastasis, both originating as spontaneous metastasis from the subcutaneously injected melanoma tumour, and when the melanoma cells were injected intravenously reaching the lung directly through the systemic circulation [12].

Two recent animal experiments provide further evidence of the effects of OSA on cancer risk [44, 54]. Lung epithelial TC1 cell tumours were 84% larger in mice subjected to IH for 28 days than in normoxic mice [44]. Interestingly, this effect appeared to be mediated by changes in the immune system, specifically by activation of tumour-associated macrophages.

In another recent study, experimentally induced sleep fragmentation (without hypoxaemia) in a murine model involving lung epithelial tumours was associated with a two-fold increase in tumour growth and an increased frequency of invasive features in surrounding tissues [54].

Temporal relationship

The epidemiological studies reviewed in the preceding section (and tables 1 and 2) were all cohort studies (even though they were retrospective analyses of existing cohorts, also known as "historical cohort studies"). Thus, the existing evidence meets the temporal criterion, which requires that the suspected risk factor (OSA) was measured before the presumed outcome (cancer incidence or mortality).

Strength of the association

The association between OSA and cancer mortality was found to be strong or very strong in all of the epidemiological studies published to date (table 1), with an eight to 14-fold increased mortality associated with moderate or severe OSA when characterised using the HI, even after possible confounding factors were taken into consideration [13, 22]. Even in the Busselton cohort, with its surrogate measure of OSA which tended to result in dilution bias, a strong four-fold adjusted relative risk was found. In contrast, OSA–cancer incidence found either no association [26, 27] or an association no stronger than two or 2.5-fold hazard ratio [23, 25, 28, 39].

Dose–response relationship

As with the previous criterion, studies using cancer incidence as an outcome have failed to show a clear dose–response relationship, whereas those for mortality have demonstrated increasing relative hazard with increasing levels of OSA severity in a clearly linear dose–response fashion (table 1, figs 1 and 3).

Consideration of alternative explanations

This criterion calls for the consideration of confounding factors as potential reasons for the observed association. All studies reviewed above adjusted for age and sex. Smoking is unlikely to be a strong confounder given its relatively weak association with OSA and the fact that virtually all studies controlled for smoking. The other major candidate for confounding is obesity, as it has been described as a risk factor for cancer [60] and is strongly associated with OSA [4]. However, most studies have controlled for BMI and other measures of adiposity (e.g. waist/hip ratio), and a strong association (especially for mortality) still persist. Furthermore, in stratified analyses in the Wisconsin Sleep Cohort study the association was stronger in non-obese than in obese participants, an observation that is consistent with the experimental results showing that intermittent hypoxaemia increases melanoma progression in lean but not in obese mice [11]. Overall, there is little evidence that obesity is a strong confounder in the adjusted analyses described previously. Furthermore, in addition to a confounding model (fig. 4a), an alternative causal model that

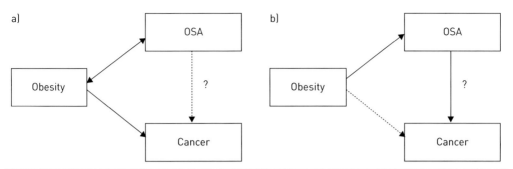

Figure 4. Two different models for understanding the relationship between obesity, OSA and cancer. a) Obesity is a confounding variable because it is associated with both OSA and cancer. b) OSA is one of the mechanisms whereby obesity causes cancer, in addition to other potential direct metabolic or pro-inflammatory effects.

could be postulated is one in which OSA constitutes one of the mechanisms whereby obesity is a risk factor for cancer, in addition to other direct metabolic or pro-inflammatory effects (fig. 4b).

Replication of findings

Only a relatively small number of studies have been published so far for both incidence and mortality. Therefore, this criterion is still not entirely fulfilled. Clearly there is an urgent need for additional studies in diverse populations and patient settings to replicate these findings.

Cessation of exposure

This criterion refers to evidence that the risk of an outcome diminishes or reverts when exposure is removed. In this case, it would be, for example, whether cancer patients with OSA who receive treatment (*e.g.* CPAP) have a better prognosis than their untreated counterparts. There is currently almost no evidence meeting this criterion, with the exception of the indirect observation in the studies described above, which found that the association between OSA and cancer mortality was slightly stronger when participants who were treated with CPAP during follow-up were excluded [13, 22]. Consequently, this is an area in urgent need of further research.

Conclusions and future directions

There is considerable but rapidly growing evidence from laboratory, experimental and epidemiological studies that supports the hypothesis that OSA might play a role in carcinogenesis or cancer progression. The evidence is particularly strong for the argument that OSA promotes cancer progression, resulting in a decrease in survival after cancer initiation or cancer diagnosis. It seems that this relationship can be explained by the effect of intermittent hypoxaemia on increasing activation of HIF-1 pathways, which in turn promotes angiogenesis and tumour growth, and increases rates of metastasis. Studies from a variety of laboratory settings and animal experiments all point in that direction. Remarkably, the epidemiological data also supports this hypothesis [17], namely through the consistent finding that the association between OSA and a variety of cancer outcomes in humans tends to be stronger when OSA is characterised using the HI than when using the AHI [13, 22, 25].

As critically reviewed in the previous section, the existing evidence of this hypothesis fits some of the key classic causality criteria [31], although the evidence in support of the carcinogenesis (cancer incidence) hypothesis is currently significantly weaker. However, there are important areas of weakness that require further research, including the need for additional studies replicating the findings described above in different populations and settings. Furthermore, studies that explore whether OSA treatment results in a decrease in cancer mortality are urgently needed, not only to reinforce the causal inference (the cessation of exposure criterion) but also because of the important implications that findings from this research might have for the clinical management of cancer patients with OSA.

Further exploration of whether OSA cancer-promotion effects are generic or cancer-specific is also required. Supporting laboratory evidence has been obtained in a variety of cell lines but most of the animal experiments were conducted using a melanoma model (largely for reasons of convenience). Most of the epidemiological studies used "total" cancer incidence and mortality, an approach often frowned upon by researchers concerned about the specificity of the biological mechanisms of different types of cancer. However, it is important to point out that as discussed elsewhere [13], this limitation is an unlikely explanation for the strong associations between OSA and cancer mortality in the studies described above. If associations are specific for distinct cancer sites but not others, combining all cancer mortality will result in the dilution of effects and thus tend to bias the results towards the null. Furthermore, the hypothesised pathophysiological mechanisms in this case (hypoxia leading to HIF-1 activation that results in increased angiogenesis and/or immune changes that in turn promote tumour growth and metastasis) may be so fundamental that they might actually be generic in nature, or at least applicable to many solid cancers.

Finally, there is clearly a need for additional research on the specific biological mechanisms involved, which are likely to be complex, perhaps complementary and synergistic, and might involve not only activation of angiogenesis but of oxidative stress, and inflammatory and immunologic changes [8].

If verified in future studies, the implication of the evidence presented here is profound. OSA might be one of the mechanisms in which obesity is a detrimental factor in cancer aetiology and natural history. From a clinical standpoint, assessing the presence of OSA (particularly in overweight or obese patients) and treating it if present might have to become a routine part of the clinical management of cancer patients.

References

1. Eckert DJ, Malhotra A. Pathophysiology of adult obstructive sleep apnea. *Proc Am Thoracic Soc* 2008; 5: 144–153.
2. Arnardottir ES, Mackiewicz M, Gislason T, *et al.* Molecular signatures of obstructive sleep apnea in adults: a review and perspective. *Sleep* 2009; 32: 447–470.
3. Punjabi NM, Ahmed MM, Polotsky VY, *et al.* Sleep-disordered breathing, glucose intolerance, and insulin resistance. *Respir Physiol Neurobiol* 2003; 136: 167–178.
4. Young T, Peppard PE, Gottlieb DJ. Epidemiology of obstructive sleep apnea: a population health perspective. *Am J Respir Crit Care Med* 2002; 165: 1217–1239.
5. Dempsey JA, Veasey SC, Morgan BJ, *et al.* Pathophysiology of sleep apnea. *Physiol Rev* 2010; 90: 47–112.
6. Institute of Medicine. IOM Committee on Sleep Medicine and Research BoHSP. Sleep Disorders and Sleep Deprivation: an Unmet Public Health Problem. Washington, Institutes of Medicine, 2006.

7. Punjabi NM. The epidemiology of adult obstructive sleep apnea. *Proc Am Thoracic Soc* 2008; 5: 136–143.

8. Almendros I, Gozal D, Farré R. Cancer: insights into biological plausibility. *In*: Barbé F, Pépin J-L, eds. Obstructive Sleep Apnoea. *ERS Monogr* 2015; 67: 24–36.

9. Abrams B. Cancer and sleep apnea – the hypoxia connection. *Med Hypotheses* 2007; 68: 232.

10. Almendros I, Montserrat JM, Ramirez J, *et al.* Intermittent hypoxia enhances cancer progression in a mouse model of sleep apnoea. *Eur Respir J* 2012; 39: 215–217.

11. Almendros I, Montserrat JM, Torres M, *et al.* Obesity and intermittent hypoxia increase tumor growth in a mouse model of sleep apnea. *Sleep Med* 2012; 13: 1254–1260.

12. Almendros I, Montserrat JM, Torres M, *et al.* Intermittent hypoxia increases melanoma metastasis to the lung in a mouse model of sleep apnea. *Respir Physiol Neurobiol* 2013; 186: 303–307.

13. Nieto FJ, Peppard PE, Young T, *et al.* Sleep-disordered breathing and cancer mortality: results from the Wisconsin Sleep Cohort Study. *Am J Respir Crit Care Med* 2012; 186: 190–194.

14. Redline S, Quan SF. Sleep apnea: a common mechanism for the deadly triad – cardiovascular disease, diabetes, and cancer? *Am J Respir Crit Care Med* 2012; 186: 123–124.

15. Martinez-Garcia MA, Campos-Rodriguez F, Farré R. Sleep apnoea and cancer: current insights and future perspectives. *Eur Respir J* 2012; 40: 1315–1317.

16. Peppard PE, Nieto FJ. Here come the sleep apnea-cancer studies. *Sleep* 2013; 36: 1409–1411.

17. Nieto FJ, Farré R. Association of sleep apnea and cancer: from animal studies to human epidemiologic data. *In*: Berger N, Redline S, eds. Impact of Sleep and Sleep Disturbances on Obesity and Cancer. New York, Springer, 2014; pp. 121–136.

18. Young T, Finn L, Peppard PE, *et al.* Sleep disordered breathing and mortality: eighteen-year follow-up of the Wisconsin sleep cohort. *Sleep* 2008; 31: 1071–1078.

19. Young T, Palta M, Dempsey J, *et al.* The occurrence of sleep-disordered breathing among middle-aged adults. *N Engl J Med* 1993; 328: 1230–1235.

20. Young T. Rationale, design and findings from the Wisconsin Sleep Cohort Study: toward understanding the total societal burden of sleep disordered breathing. *Sleep Med Clin* 2009; 4: 37–46.

21. American Academy of Sleep Medicine Task Force. Sleep-related breathing disorders in adults: recommendations for syndrome definition and measurement techniques in clinical research. *Sleep* 1999; 22: 667–689.

22. Martinez-García MA, Campos-Rodriguez F, Duran-Cantolla J, *et al.* Obstructive sleep apnea is associated with cancer mortality in younger patients. *Sleep Med* 2014; 15: 742–748.

23. Marshall NS, Wong KK, Cullen SR, *et al.* Sleep apnea and 20-year follow-up for all-cause mortality, stroke, and cancer incidence and mortality in the busselton health study cohort. *J Clin Sleep Med* 2014; 10: 355–362.

24. Martinez-García MA, Martorell-Calatayud A, Nagore E, *et al.* Association between sleep disordered breathing and aggressiveness markers of malignant cutaneous melanoma. *Eur Respir J* 2014; 43: 1661–1668.

25. Campos-Rodriguez F, Martinez-Garcia MA, Martinez M, *et al.* Association between obstructive sleep apnea and cancer incidence in a large multicenter Spanish cohort. *Am J Respir Crit Care Med* 2013; 187: 99–105.

26. Christensen AS, Clark A, Salo P, *et al.* Symptoms of sleep disordered breathing and risk of cancer: a prospective cohort study. *Sleep* 2013; 36: 1429–1435.

27. Kendzerska T, Leung RS, Hawker G, *et al.* Obstructive sleep apnea and the prevalence and incidence of cancer. *Can Med Assoc J* 2014; 186: 985–992.

28. Chen JC, Hwang JH. Sleep apnea increased incidence of primary central nervous system cancers: a nationwide cohort study. *Sleep Med* 2014; 15: 749–754.

29. Chang WP, Liu ME, Chang WC, *et al.* Sleep apnea and the subsequent risk of breast cancer in women: a nationwide population-based cohort study. *Sleep Med* 2014; 15: 1016–1020.

30. Johns MW. A new method for measuring daytime sleepiness: the Epworth sleepiness scale. *Sleep* 1991; 14: 540–545.

31. Hill AB. The environment and disease: association or causation? *Proc Royal Soc Med* 1965; 58: 295–300.

32. Gordis L. Epidemiology. Philadelphia, Elsevier Saunders, 2004.

33. Szklo M, Nieto FJ. Epidemiology: Beyond the Basics. 3rd Edn. Burlington, Jones & Bartlett Learning, 2013.

34. Harris AL. Hypoxia – a key regulatory factor in tumour growth. *Nature Rev Cancer* 2002; 2: 38–47.

35. Rankin EB, Giaccia AJ. The role of hypoxia-inducible factors in tumorigenesis. *Cell Death Differentiation* 2008; 15: 678–685.

36. Semenza GL. Oxygen sensing, homeostasis, and disease. *N Engl J Med* 2011; 365: 537–547.

37. Raghunand N, Gatenby RA, Gillies RJ. Microenvironmental and cellular consequences of altered blood flow in tumours. *Br J Radiol* 2003; 76: S11–S22.

38. Ahn GO, Brown M. Targeting tumors with hypoxia-activated cytotoxins. *Front Biosci* 2007; 12: 3483–3501.

39. Wouters A, Pauwels B, Lardon F, *et al.* Review: implications of *in vitro* research on the effect of radiotherapy and chemotherapy under hypoxic conditions. *Oncologist* 2007; 12: 690–712.

40. Liu Y, Song X, Wang X, *et al.* Effect of chronic intermittent hypoxia on biological behavior and hypoxia-associated gene expression in lung cancer cells. *J Cell Biochem* 2010; 111: 554–563.

41. Toffoli S, Michiels C. Intermittent hypoxia is a key regulator of cancer cell and endothelial cell interplay in tumours. *FEBS J* 2008; 275: 2991–3002.
42. Rofstad EK, Gaustad JV, Egeland TA, *et al.* Tumors exposed to acute cyclic hypoxic stress show enhanced angiogenesis, perfusion and metastatic dissemination. *Int J Cancer* 2010; 127: 1535–1546.
43. Karoor V, Le M, Merrick D, *et al.* Alveolar hypoxia promotes murine lung tumor growth through a VEGFR-2/ EGFR-dependent mechanism. *Cancer Prev Res* 2012; 5: 1061–1071.
44. Almendros I, Wang Y, Becker L, *et al.* Intermittent hypoxia-induced changes in tumor-associated macrophages and tumor malignancy in a mouse model of sleep apnea. *Am J Respir Crit Care Med* 2014; 189: 593–601.
45. Gozal D, Almendros I, Hakim F. Sleep apnea awakens cancer: a unifying immunological hypothesis. *Oncoimmunology* 2014; 3: e28326.
46. Federico A, Morgillo F, Tuccillo C, *et al.* Chronic inflammation and oxidative stress in human carcinogenesis. *Int J Cancer* 2007; 121: 2381–2386.
47. Weinberg F, Chandel NS. Reactive oxygen species-dependent signaling regulates cancer. *Cellular Mol Life Sci* 2009; 66: 3663–3673.
48. Yamauchi M, Nakano H, Maekawa J, *et al.* Oxidative stress in obstructive sleep apnea. *Chest* 2005; 127: 1674–1679.
49. Kontogianni K, Messini-Nikolaki N, Christou K, *et al.* DNA damage and repair capacity in lymphocytes from obstructive sleep apnea patients. *Environ Mol Mutagen* 2007; 48: 722–727.
50. Porta C, Larghi P, Rimoldi M, *et al.* Cellular and molecular pathways linking inflammation and cancer. *Immunobiology* 2009; 214: 761–777.
51. Wu Y, Zhou BP. Inflammation: a driving force speeds cancer metastasis. *Cell Cycle* 2009; 8: 3267–3273.
52. Li S, X. Qian XH, Zhou W, *et al.* Time-dependent inflammatory factor production and NFkappaB activation in a rodent model of intermittent hypoxia. *Swiss Med Weekly* 2011; 141: w13309.
53. Pitot HC, Dragan YP. Facts and theories concerning the mechanisms of carcinogenesis. *FASEB J* 1991; 5: 2280–2286.
54. Hakim F, Wang Y, Zhang SX, *et al.* Fragmented sleep accelerates tumor growth and progression through recruitment of tumor-associated macrophages and TLR4 signaling. *Cancer Res* 2014; 74: 1329–1337.
55. Qin Y, Zhou Y, Zhang X, *et al.* Sleep duration and breast cancer risk: a meta-analysis of observational studies. *Int J Cancer* 2014; 134: 1166–1173.
56. Jia Y, Lu Y, Wu K, *et al.* Does night work increase the risk of breast cancer? A systematic review and meta-analysis of epidemiological studies. *Cancer Epidemiol* 2013; 37: 197–206.
57. Kakizaki M, Kuriyama S, Sone T, *et al.* Sleep duration and the risk of breast cancer: the Ohsaki Cohort Study. *Br J Cancer* 2008; 99: 1502–1505.
58. McElroy JA, Newcomb PA, Titus-Ernstoff L, *et al.* Duration of sleep and breast cancer risk in a large population-based case-control study. *J Sleep Res* 2006; 15: 241–249.
59. Luo J, Sands M, Wactawski-Wende J, *et al.* Sleep disturbance and incidence of thyroid cancer in postmenopausal women the Women's Health Initiative. *Am J Epidemiol* 2013; 177: 42–49.
60. Renehan AG, Tyson M, Egger M, *et al.* Body-mass index and incidence of cancer: a systematic review and meta-analysis of prospective observational studies. *Lancet* 2008; 371: 569–578.

Support statement: F.J. Nieto is supported in part by a National Institutes of Health grant (R01HL062252-11) and by the University of Wisconsin Helfaer Endowed Chair of Public Health.

Disclosures: None declared.

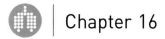
Metabolic syndrome

Maria R. Bonsignore[1,2] and Paschalis Steiropoulos[3]

OSA is a common disorder with major cardiovascular and metabolic consequences. OSA is often associated with metabolic syndrome, a cluster of cardiometabolic risk factors, and prevalence of metabolic syndrome is particularly high in OSA patients. The role of obesity as a risk factor for OSA has been shown in population and clinical studies, and increased adipose tissue volume and neck circumference are closely linked with OSA, even though major sex-related differences exist. Besides OSA treatment, cardiometabolic risk factors should be assessed and possibly corrected in all OSA patients in order to reduce adverse events. Occurrence of metabolic syndrome should be investigated, and modifiable risk factors aggressively treated especially in obese patients. Improvement of the metabolic state after OSA treatment with CPAP has been reported by some but not all studies, suggesting the need to treat additional cardiometabolic disorders and adopt strategies aimed at reducing body weight in OSA patients.

The metabolic syndrome is a cluster of risk factors including abdominal obesity, hypertension and dyslipidaemia associated with insulin resistance. Although there are several definitions of the metabolic syndrome, summarised in table 1 [1–4], the updated National Cholesterol Education Program – Adult Treatment Panel III (NCEP-ATP III) definition is the most widely used [2]. Such a definition has been criticised [5], but its simple criteria are easy to use in clinical practice, are highly popular among general practitioners, and can be considered a powerful screening tool for cardiometabolic risk in the general population [6].

Epidemiology of the metabolic syndrome in OSA patients

Metabolic syndrome is a common finding in patients with OSA, but prevalence rates are highly variable among studies (fig. 1). In elderly subjects with OSA, a very low prevalence of metabolic syndrome has been reported [7], but such findings should be interpreted cautiously since data were obtained in a general population sample, not in a clinical OSA sample as in most other studies. The highest prevalence rates were found in patients from the UK [9] and in cohorts of morbidly obese patients undergoing bariatric surgery [12, 13]. Prevalence in different countries ranged between 23% and 80% [8, 10, 11, 14–23]. Very high prevalence rates (between 65% and 80%) were found among Indian OSA patients

[1]Biomedical Dept of Internal and Specialist Medicine (DiBiMIS), Cardio-Respiratory Section, University of Palermo, Palermo, Italy. [2]Institute of Biomedicine and Molecular Immunology (IBIM), National Research Council (CNR), Palermo, Italy. [3]Dept of Pneumonology, Medical School, Democritus University of Thrace and University Hospital of Alexandroupolis, Alexandroupolis, Greece.

Correspondence: Maria R. Bonsignore, DiBiMIS, University of Palermo, Via Trabucco 180, 90146 Palermo, Italy.
E-mail: marisa@ibim.cnr.it

Table 1. Summary of the commonly used definitions of the metabolic syndrome

National Cholesterol Education Program – Adult Treatment Panel III (NCEP-ATP III), updated 2005 [1] and 2009 [2]	Presence of any three of the five following parameters: Elevated waist circumference (population- and country-specific definitions) Elevated triglycerides ≥150 mg·dL^{-1} (1.7 mmol·L^{-1}) or drug treatment for elevated triglycerides Reduced HDL-C <40 mg·dL^{-1} (1.0 mmol·L^{-1}) in males, <50 mg·dL^{-1} (1.3 mmol·L^{-1}) in females, or drug treatment for reduced HDL-C Elevated SBP (≥130 mmHg) and/or DBP (≥85 mmHg) or drug treatment for hypertension Elevated fasting glucose ≥100 mg·dL^{-1} (5.6 mmol·L^{-1}) or drug treatment for elevated blood glucose
International Diabetes Federation (IDF), 2006 [3]	Central obesity (elevated waist circumference with ethnicity-specific values) AND two of the following criteria: Raised triglycerides ≥150 mg·dL^{-1} (1.7 mmol·L^{-1}) or drug treatment for elevated triglycerides Reduced HDL-C <40 mg·dL^{-1} (1.03 mmol·L^{-1}) in males, <50 mg·dL^{-1} (1.29 mmol·L^{-1}) in females, or drug treatment for reduced HDL-C Raised BP (SBP ≥130 and/or DBP ≥85 mmHg), or treatment of previously diagnosed hypertension Raised fasting plasma glucose ≥100 mg·dL^{-1} (5.6 mmol·L^{-1}) or previously diagnosed type 2 diabetes
World Health Organization (WHO), 1999 [4]	Any one of diabetes mellitus, impaired glucose tolerance, impaired fasting glucose or insulin resistance, AND two of the following: BP ≥140/90 mmHg Central obesity: waist/hip ratio >0.90 (male), >0.85 (female), or BMI >30 kg·m^{-2} Dyslipidaemia: triglycerides ≥150 mg·dL^{-1} (1.7 mmol·L^{-1}) or HDL-C <35 mg·dL^{-1} (0.9 mmol·L^{-1}) [male], <39 mg·dL^{-1} (1.0 mmol·L^{-1}) [female] Microalbuminuria: urinary albumin excretion rate ≥20 µg·min^{-1} or albumin/creatinine ratio ≥30 mg·g^{-1}

HDL-C: high-density lipoprotein cholesterol.

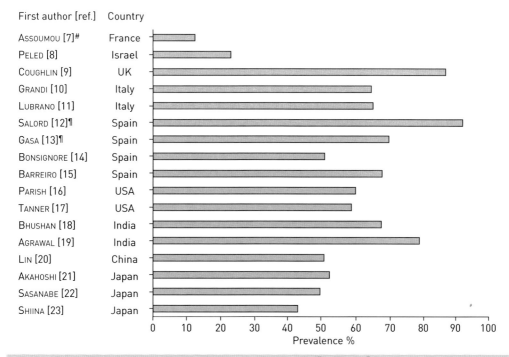

Figure 1. Prevalence rates of metabolic syndrome in OSA patients. #: elderly; ¶: morbidly obese.

[18, 19]. All studies agree on the finding that metabolic abnormalities worsen with increasing OSA severity. Therefore, the association of metabolic syndrome and OSA is very common in clinical practice, suggesting the opportunity to investigate and possibly correct metabolic abnormalities, which may contribute to the high cardiovascular risk in OSA patients.

Abdominal obesity and enlarged neck: markers of OSA with major sex differences

The role of obesity as a risk factor for OSA has been shown by several studies in both the general population and clinical cohorts [24, 25]. Due to the evolving obesity epidemics and the increase in obesity-related problems in clinical practice, the relationship between obesity and OSA is currently investigated with great attention [26]. Metabolic syndrome is defined by the presence of insulin resistance [27–31]; a direct relationship between insulin resistance and number of metabolic syndrome components, i.e. the metabolic index, has been shown in patients with OSA [14]. Moreover, the metabolic index increases with OSA severity [8, 14]. Conversely, the recently proposed visceral adiposity index did not correlate with OSA severity, possibly because systemic arterial BP is not included in its calculation [32]. Therefore, occurrence of metabolic syndrome should always be assessed in OSA patients, although it is still unclear whether the association is simply secondary to visceral obesity or whether OSA plays any independent role. Morbidly obese patients with OSA show a worse metabolic profile compared with non-OSA patients with a similar degree of obesity [13]. OSA could therefore play a pathogenic role in metabolic abnormalities. Alternatively, both metabolic syndrome and OSA could be markers of severe metabolic abnormalities associated with visceral obesity.

Neck circumference is a marker of visceral obesity and insulin resistance [33, 34] and of OSA risk [35, 36]. Recent reports from the Framingham Heart Study proposed increased neck circumference as an additional cardiovascular risk factor [28, 29], but concomitant occurrence of OSA was not investigated. Neck circumference normalised by height (neck/height ratio) strongly predicted OSA, but the slope of the relationship between AHI and neck/height ratio was higher in men than in women [37]. In a population study, neck circumference was increased in patients with metabolic syndrome, even after adjustment for all metabolic syndrome components, and predicted OSA only in male subjects [38].

Sex-related differences in the clinical characteristics of OSA are well known [39]. The amount and distribution of body fat differ physiologically between sexes: men tend to accumulate adipose tissue in the visceral compartment, whereas fat deposition in women preferentially occurs in the subcutaneous compartment, with a "peripheral" pattern of obesity compared with the "central" pattern typical of men [40]. Sex dimorphism in fat distribution depends on hormonal influences and may contribute, together with other factors, to the milder OSA severity found in middle-aged women compared with men with a similar BMI [41]. Recent studies have investigated sex-related differences in fat compartments [32, 42–46], with some variability in protocols but a quite uniform emerging picture (table 2). Men usually show an association of OSA with markers of central obesity (waist circumference, waist/hip ratio, neck circumference). Conversely, OSA in women is associated with markers of general obesity (BMI, increased subcutaneous fat, hip circumference) and often with increased neck circumference. In patients with OSA and metabolic syndrome, however, waist circumference, which is the most important marker of visceral obesity, was the only variable associated with AHI irrespective of sex [32]. Therefore, sex-related features of obesity should be considered in the diagnostic work-up of patients with suspected OSA. Different fat distribution patterns might be associated with variable cardiometabolic risk, although this issue has been little explored in OSA patients.

Mechanisms of metabolic dysregulation in OSA

The potential role of IH as a cause of metabolic abnormalities has been explored by several experimental studies in rodents and humans. IH caused insulin resistance in lean mice [47, 48], and exacerbated glucose intolerance, inflammation, oxidative stress and non-alcoholic fatty liver disease (NAFLD) in mice with diet-induced obesity [48].

The association of OSA with dyslipidaemia or NAFLD might be mediated by the effects of IH on adipose tissue. In vitro exposure of adipocytes to IH caused inflammatory activation [49], consistent with the possibility that OSA may exert a direct detrimental role on adipose tissue in obese subjects. Furthermore, recent studies in mice documented visceral fat remodelling after exposure to IH for 6 weeks, and lipectomy before IH exposure reduced the severity of vascular lesions, suggesting that adipose tissue dysfunction may accelerate cardiovascular alterations in OSA [50].

Besides the interaction of IH at the adipose tissue level, sympathetic activation may contribute to hyperglycaemia and suppression of insulin secretion, as recently suggested by a study on the effects of adrenal medullectomy in mice [51]. However, other studies found no evidence of sympathetically mediated metabolic changes in the model of acute IH in lean mice [47]. Given the complex interaction between IH, obesity and adipose and vascular tissues, the reader is referred to a recent review article on this topic [52].

Table 2. Summary of recent studies on sex-related differences in OSA: anthropometrics and metabolic abnormalities

First author [ref.]	Subjects	Methodology	Results
MARTINEZ-RIVERA [42]	152 men and 40 women with suspected OSA	PSG, truncal obesity measurements	BMI similar in snorers and OSA; waist/hip ratio predictive of OSA for values >1 in men and >0.85 in women; male sex and age >52 years also predictive of OSA
SIMPSON [43]	60 men and 36 women with suspected OSA	PSG, anthropometric measurements, body composition by DXA	AHI variance explained in men by % of fat in the neck and waist/hip ratio (R^2=0.37), in women by % of fat in the neck and BMI (R^2=0.33)
BOULOUKAKI [44]	2061 men and 629 women with suspected OSA	PSG, anthropometric measurements	AHI correlated with BMI in men, and with neck circumference, hip circumference and BMI in women; best model (R^2=0.27): neck circumference, BMI, EDS and sex
BEZERRA [45]	96 women undergoing PSG for suspected OSA, pre-bariatric surgery evaluation, snoring or insomnia	PSG, anthropometric measurements, body composition by DXA	BMI not predictive of OSA in women; for each 1% increase in total body fat, OSA risk increased by 12.8%; leptin higher in women with OSA
KRITIKOU [46]	Middle-aged patients with OSA (22 men and 20 post-menopausal women); age-matched controls (19 men and 20 women)	PSG, anthropometric measurements, CT scan assessment of abdominal VAT and SAT	Compared with controls, men with OSA showed increased VAT and high VAT/SAT ratio, but no increase in total fat; women with OSA showed increased VAT, SAT and total adipose tissue, with VAT/SAT ratio similar to controls; no effect of CPAP for 2 months on the amount/type of abdominal fat
MAZZUCA [32]	423 men and 105 women with suspected OSA	PSG, anthropometric measurements, assessment of the metabolic syndrome (NCEP-ATP III)	In men, BMI, waist circumference and metabolic syndrome diagnosis were associated with OSA severity (R^2=0.308); in women, hip circumference and neck circumference normalised by height were associated with OSA severity (R^2=0.339); similar results in subjects without metabolic syndrome; in subjects with OSA and metabolic syndrome, only waist circumference was associated with AHI independent of sex

DXA: dual-energy absorptiometry; CT: computed tomography; VAT: visceral adipose tissue; SAT: subcutaneous adipose tissue; NCEP-ATP III: National Cholesterol Education Program – Adult Treatment Panel III.

Relevance for cardiovascular risk

The association of OSA and metabolic syndrome has been extensively explored with regard to the potential detrimental effects of both conditions on cardiovascular risk. According to some investigators, OSA could actually be considered to be a component of the metabolic syndrome, both conditions being associated with visceral obesity [53]. Conversely, several clinical studies have shown that in patients with metabolic syndrome, occurrence of OSA is associated with a worse metabolic [54–56], inflammatory [57] and cardiovascular risk profile [58, 59]. Vascular function markers (intima media thickness, carotid diameter, pulse wave velocity) were more impaired in patients with metabolic syndrome and OSA than in patients with metabolic syndrome without OSA [60]. Compared with patients with metabolic syndrome without OSA or control subjects, patients with metabolic syndrome and OSA showed a profound autonomic dysfunction [61]. Overall, the available data suggest that, at least in obese patients, occurrence of OSA is associated with a worse metabolic profile. However, the role of OSA in increasing cardiovascular risk independent of obesity remains unproven.

Clinical assessment of the metabolic syndrome in OSA patients

It has been postulated that OSA is more than an epiphenomenon in the metabolic syndrome and represents an additional burden that actually increases the cardiovascular risk of metabolic syndrome [26]. Undiagnosed OSA may be a contributing factor to the observed metabolic dysregulation in patients with metabolic syndrome, and an effective OSA treatment could ameliorate at least a part of this metabolic derangement.

It is of clinical significance for OSA diagnosis that many patients with metabolic syndrome or diabetes and OSA may not present with EDS, which is a cardinal daytime symptom of OSA [57, 62]. Increased serum glucose levels [54, 56] and glycosylated haemoglobin [54] in subjects with metabolic syndrome may indicate the presence of OSA and the opportunity of further diagnostic procedures. AGRAWAL et al. [63] found that EDS was among the factors associated with OSA and metabolic syndrome, while two case–control studies in OSA patients without comorbidities reported that EDS predicted insulin resistance independent of obesity [64, 65]. Conversely, in a large "real-life" sample of OSA patients, metabolic syndrome occurred in about half of OSA patients irrespective of EDS [14]. In the European Sleep Apnea Database (ESADA) cohort, the presence and severity of OSA predicted poor glycaemic control [66, 67], independent of sleepiness. Therefore, the association of daytime sleepiness and metabolic disturbances remains controversial.

Clinicians should meticulously examine the possibility of occurrence of metabolic syndrome in OSA patients, given that metabolic syndrome is associated with increased risk for type 2 diabetes [68] and increased overall and cardiovascular mortality [69]. Since metabolic parameters probably contribute to the development of CVD in OSA, they should be monitored [70].

Among the metabolic syndrome components, BP showed the strongest relationship with OSA severity after correction for confounders [14]. Ambulatory BP monitoring (ABPM) should be considered in all OSA patients [71], since "masked hypertension" is common in OSA and many patients are not aware of their abnormal BP values, especially at night [72, 73]. Arterial hypertension, and the sympathetic hyperactivity associated with OSA, might be a major factor in increased cardiovascular risk [71].

It is important to emphasise that this complex picture needs assessment in OSA patients beyond the diagnostic procedures for sleep disordered breathing [74]. At present, some simple measurements (ABPM, fasting glucose levels, glycosylated haemoglobin, lipidaemic profile, *etc.*) should be obtained in OSA patients at diagnosis to investigate the occurrence of metabolic syndrome. Since obesity is usually associated with metabolic disturbances, these measurements should be obtained early during the diagnostic work-up of OSA as proposed in figure 2. Besides the obvious approach in patients who are overweight or obese, the need for metabolic assessment in normal-weight patients deserves some comment. At least two studies have reported glycaemic dysregulation in non-obese OSA patients, correlated with sleep fragmentation [75] or severity of nocturnal hypoxaemia [76], suggesting that metabolic status could be disrupted in OSA even in the absence of obesity.

In summary, screening in OSA patients for concurrent metabolic syndrome or some of its components is highly advisable, because both conditions are common and may synergistically contribute to cardiovascular morbidity.

Effects of CPAP treatment on metabolic syndrome

Summarising the results of cross-sectional studies on the association of OSA and metabolic syndrome [77], an improvement in cardiometabolic abnormalities could be expected after

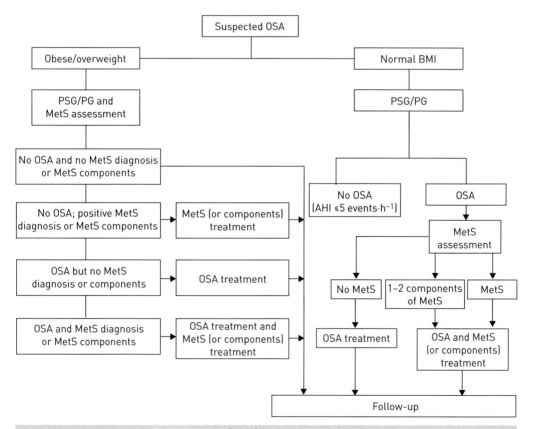

Figure 2. Assessment of metabolic syndrome (MetS) in OSA patients. PG: polygraphy.

CPAP treatment, but this is not strongly supported by hitherto conducted RCTs examining the effect of CPAP on metabolic parameters. Few studies specifically addressed the effects of CPAP treatment in OSA patients with concurrent metabolic syndrome. Additionally, there are no studies on the effect of CPAP on "hard" end-points, such as nonfatal and fatal cardiovascular events in patients with OSA according to the presence/absence of metabolic syndrome.

Studies have not yet reached a definitive conclusion regarding the impact of CPAP treatment on metabolic syndrome as an entity, or on its separate components. Several factors contribute to the observed discrepancies, notably the small sample size and the variability in characteristics of included populations, patients' adherence to therapy, variable duration of treatment, presence of comorbidities and the effect of physical exercise [78, 79].

Effect of CPAP on prevalence of metabolic syndrome

In a randomised, placebo-controlled, blinded, cross-over trial, COUGHLIN et al. [80] demonstrated that prevalence of metabolic syndrome, diagnosed with NCEP-ATP III criteria, changed neither in patients receiving effective CPAP treatment (even in the subgroup with adequate adherence) nor in those receiving sham therapy, despite effectiveness of CPAP treatment in decreasing BP levels and daytime sleepiness. Conversely, auto-adjusting positive airway pressure (APAP) therapy significantly reduced the prevalence of metabolic syndrome (diagnosed with NCEP-ATP III criteria) from 63.5% to 47.3% [81]. The reduction was more prevalent in patients who were adherent to APAP use and in patients with less severe OSA [81].

In a retrospective analysis [82] of data from a previously published RCT [83], 12 weeks of CPAP treatment had no effect on the prevalence of metabolic syndrome diagnosed according to the International Diabetes Federation (IDF) criteria. Reversal of metabolic syndrome occurred in 17% of the effective treatment receivers and in 7% of sham therapy receivers, while development of metabolic syndrome occurred in 14% of the effective treatment receivers and in 18% of the sham therapy receivers (p=0.28). Further analysis of the same data according to NCEP-ATP III criteria did not alter the findings.

In a nonrandomised trial, metabolic syndrome prevalence decreased by 45% after 1 year of CPAP treatment in 20 OSA patients and a significant difference was observed in waist circumference, high-density lipoprotein cholesterol levels and BMI after treatment [84]. In a nonrandomised study in patients with OSA and metabolic syndrome, diagnosed according to IDF criteria, DORKOVA et al. [85] reported a significant reduction of several components of metabolic syndrome including BP, triglycerides and glucose levels, among patients with good adherence ($\geqslant$4 h·night^{-1}) to 8 weeks of CPAP therapy.

Body fat distribution has been shown to be unaffected by OSA treatment for 8 weeks [86], and unchanged abdominal obesity after CPAP treatment was also reported by other studies [46, 83, 87]. Patients on CPAP tended to gain rather than lose weight in the first months of treatment [88]. Therefore, any potentially positive effect of CPAP on metabolism could be offset by increased/unchanged body weight in OSA patients, suggesting the opportunity to implement lifestyle intervention programmes together with OSA treatment [89].

Effect of CPAP on components of the metabolic syndrome

The majority of studies looking at the impact of CPAP on individual components of the metabolic syndrome did not come to a definite conclusion, due to a number of limitations, as already mentioned. In a double-blind RCT of therapeutic and placebo CPAP for 3 months in 42 men with type 2 diabetes and OSA, WEST et al. [90] did not show any significant improvement in glycosylated haemoglobin or insulin resistance measured by euglycaemic clamp and homeostasis model assessment, despite the observed improvement in sleepiness and quality of life. WEINSTOCK et al. [91] conducted oral glucose tolerance tests in order to measure insulin sensitivity in 50 moderate-to-severe patients with glucose intolerance before and after 2 months of CPAP treatment in a cross-over design with control treatment by sham CPAP. CPAP treatment did not reverse glucose intolerance or improve insulin sensitivity, except in patients with severe OSA (AHI >30 events·h^{-1}). Finally, HOYOS et al. [83] assessed insulin sensitivity in 65 male, moderate-to-severe OSA patients without diabetes. They were randomised to receive either real (n=34) or sham (n=31) CPAP for 12 weeks. At 12 weeks, all subjects received real CPAP for an additional 12 weeks. Improvement in insulin sensitivity was only observed after 24 weeks of CPAP use.

Table 3 summarises the published meta-analyses on the effect of CPAP on the metabolic parameters (insulin resistance, BP, lipids) included in the different metabolic syndrome definitions [92–103] and on glycosylated haemoglobin [104], as its measurement has recently been approved as a stand-alone diagnostic test for type 2 diabetes mellitus by the American Diabetes Association [105]. In general, these meta-analyses examined both RCTs and uncontrolled trials and documented only limited positive effects of CPAP on insulin resistance in severe OSA patients without diabetes, while RCTs found no improvement in glycaemic control after CPAP in diabetic OSA patients [92–96]. The impact of CPAP treatment on lipid profile [103] or glycosylated haemoglobin [104] is also a topic of considerable debate and no consistent results have been reported so far. Regarding BP, all but one of the meta-analyses [96–102] reported a favourable effect of CPAP treatment, which was more profound in specific subgroups of patients. In general, reductions of BP were statistically significant but small, raising the question of their clinical significance [106].

A significant limitation of the available studies is that none of them was fully controlled for physical activity and dietary habits of OSA patients. Hence, well-designed RCTs with larger populations and longer duration of treatment, well-accepted cut-off points for diagnosis and better patient compliance to CPAP treatment are necessary to define the impact of OSA treatment on metabolic and cardiovascular outcomes in patients with OSA and metabolic syndrome.

Lifestyle interventions and weight loss

Until recently, weight loss in patients with OSA was considered difficult to achieve in clinical practice. The high cardiovascular risk found in untreated patients with severe OSA and the positive effects of CPAP treatment [107] urged physicians to concentrate their efforts on optimising compliance to CPAP rather than actively promoting control of body weight. In the last decade, this attitude has slowly changed towards a comprehensive patient-centred treatment including weight loss [108]. Obesity has become a major problem in industrialised countries, causing increasing public health costs and reducing survival and quality of life [109]. Comprehensive programmes to obtain weight loss by medical therapy

Table 3. Summary of the meta-analyses on the effect of CPAP on components of metabolic syndrome

First author [ref.]	Studies n	Patients n	Main finding
Insulin resistance			
Hecht [92]	6	296	CPAP had no effect on insulin levels or HOMA index; one study reported increase of insulin sensitivity index
Yang [93]	9	185	CPAP use ≥4 h for 8–24 weeks improved HOMA-IR in nondiabetic patients with moderate-to-severe OSA (average reduction −0.75, p<0.001)
Yang [94]	15	367	CPAP for 8–24 weeks resulted in an average reduction of HOMA-IR of 0.55 (p=0.002)
Iftikhar [95]	5	244	CPAP had a favourable effect on HOMA-IR levels versus sham therapy in OSA patients without diabetes (pooled estimate of difference in means −0.44, p=0.02)
Arterial hypertension			
Giles [96]	36	1718	CPAP (short-term) resulted in lower 24-h SBP and DBP compared with controls
Alajmi [97]	10	587	CPAP caused no significant change in SBP (p=0.23) or in DBP (p=0.06); a trend for BP reduction was revealed in separate subgroups
Haentjens [98]	12#	572	CPAP resulted in a net decrease of 24-h mean BP by 1.69 mmHg; meta-regression analysis showed that for every 1 h of increase in CPAP use, a decrease of mean 24-h BP by 1.39 mmHg was observed
Bazzano [99]	16	818	CPAP resulted in a mean net reduction of SBP/DBP of −2.46/−1.83 mmHg, and mean net reduction of mean BP was −2.22 mmHg after 2–24 weeks of CPAP; only two studies included exclusively hypertensive patients; significant reductions were observed in patients with BP >130/80 mmHg
Montesi [100]	28	1948 diurnal BP analysis	CPAP resulted in a mean difference of −2.58/−2.01 mmHg in diurnal SBP/DBP
	10	661 nocturnal BP analysis	CPAP resulted in a mean difference of −4.09/−1.85 mmHg in nocturnal SBP/DBP
Fava [101]	29	1820	CPAP had a favourable effect; mean±SEM net difference in SBP and DBP were 2.6±0.6 mmHg and 2.0±0.4 mmHg, respectively; a sub-analysis of studies with 24-h ABPM revealed a significant reduction in both daytime and night-time measurements
Schein [102]	16	1166	CPAP resulted in small but significant BP reductions, but no change in daytime SBP and DBP was observed
Hyperlipidaemia			
Xu [103]	6	741¶	CPAP decreased levels of total cholesterol (p=0.01); this decrease was more profound in younger, more obese OSA patients who used CPAP for a period >12 weeks; CPAP did not alter levels of triglycerides, LDL cholesterol or HDL cholesterol
Glycosylated haemoglobin			
Iftikhar [104]	9	151	CPAP did not reduce levels of glycosylated haemoglobin; the mean net change was −0.06% (95% CI −0.24–0.12; p=0.5)

HOMA: homeostasis model assessment; HOMA-IR: HOMA-insulin resistance; ABPM: ambulatory BP monitoring; LDL: low-density lipoprotein; HDL: high-density lipoprotein. #: included only studies with ABPM; ¶: for total cholesterol levels (n=658 for triglyceride levels, n=550 for LDL cholesterol levels, n=525 for HDL cholesterol levels).

and/or surgical procedures have been developed and applied to obese patients, including those with OSA.

The effects of weight loss on OSA severity have been the major focus of studies addressing the effects of bariatric surgery or lifestyle interventions, such as diet, exercise programmes or both [110, 111]. Since bariatric surgery causes a greater weight loss compared with diet or exercise, it is not suprising that most patients undergoing bariatric surgery showed improved OSA after weight loss [112–115], although complete resolution of OSA occurred in only 25% of the cases [116]. Surgical weight loss was associated with better maintenance of weight and lower AHI in the long term, compared with conventional measures [117]. Larger metabolic improvements occurred after bariatric surgery compared with lifestyle interventions [118]. However, it is hard to dissect the probably small, independent effects of OSA on metabolism in the context of large reductions in body weight. Recent data from the Swedish Obese Subjects (SOS) study underlined that patients with residual AHI >20 events·h^{-1} after weight loss showed a worse metabolic, cardiovascular and inflammatory profile compared with patients with post-surgical AHI <20 events·h^{-1}, suggesting a detrimental effect of residual OSA on cardiometabolic risk [119].

Recent meta-analyses reported positive effects of diet and exercise training in OSA patients [120–122]. Intensive lifestyle interventions represent an interesting alternative to bariatric surgery and may in the long-term achieve similar results [123]. The improvement in AHI after intensive diet programmes was associated with a prevalent reduction of visceral fat [124, 125], and weight reduction was effective as a first-line treatment for mild OSA, not only for respiratory events during sleep but also for metabolic improvement [124]. Other studies reported favourable effects of exercise training in sedentary patients with severe OSA [126–128]. Therefore, although diet and exercise cause relatively small BMI changes, they might exert very positive effects on both OSA and the metabolic profile. It is still uncertain which type of intervention should be preferred, and positive small effects have also been reported following adoption of the Mediterranean diet for 6 months [129].

Pharmacological treatment could also help in achieving weight loss in obese patients. Unfortunately, appetite-suppressant drugs have major side-effects. Both rimonabant and sibutramine, two recently developed drugs for the treatment of obesity, had to be withdrawn from the market after initial enthusiasm because of psychiatric and cardiovascular side-effects [52, 108]. To date, metformin remains the most widely used drug for improving insulin sensitivity in obese patients, since it does not cause further weight gain. The combination of phentermine and topiramate has been successfully used in OSA patients [130], and other drugs are currently under study.

Unfortunately, a progressive regain in weight can occur after lifestyle interventions in the long term, confirming the difficulty in maintaining a healthy lifestyle in obese patients. In this regard, positive results came from the Sleep AHEAD (Action for Health in Diabetes) study in diabetic patients with OSA, showing persistent decrease in AHI after the intensive lifestyle intervention, despite partial weight gain over 4 years [131].

Although data on metabolism in OSA patients after weight loss are scarce, one study reported that an intensive lifestyle intervention programme for 1 year in men with visceral obesity was less successful in those who also had OSA compared with patients without OSA [132]. These results point to a relative "resistance" of OSA patients to lose weight. Treatment with CPAP is not associated with weight loss [133] or increased physical activity

[134]. A recent experimental study has shown that IH causes dysfunction of brown adipose tissue, with decreased expression of uncoupling protein-1 and failure to increase the metabolic rate [135]. Whether OSA patients are more resistant to weight loss, and the mechanism responsible for the negative effects of IH, require further study.

Future research

Future research should focus on specific areas, such as RCTs to identify the best approach to achieve weight loss in OSA patients, and the effects of weight loss and OSA treatment on clinical outcomes, *e.g.* incidence of cardiovascular or metabolic diseases. In addition, future studies on the effects of intensive lifestyle changes should include more studies in women, since sex has a major role in type/distribution of adipose tissue and women are usually less represented than men in clinical studies. Finally, treatment strategies combining CPAP with lifestyle interventions and/or drug treatment for obesity in OSA patients are still under study. A very recent RCT testing the effects of CPAP, weight loss or both in obese OSA patients reported positive effects of weight loss alone or combined with CPAP treatment, but not of CPAP alone, on metabolic and inflammatory variables after 24 weeks of treatment [136]. These results suggest that obesity rather than OSA is the main cause of metabolic abnormalities, but at present a possible synergistic role of OSA cannot be excluded.

In conclusion, the role of OSA and IH in metabolic disturbances is under intense investigation. Recent evidence suggests that weight loss exerts larger positive effects on metabolism compared with CPAP, but definitive proof is lacking. Clinicians should actively promote both CPAP treatment and a healthier lifestyle in OSA patients, in order to optimise treatment of respiratory events during sleep, hypertension and metabolic abnormalities, consequently reducing overall cardiovascular risk.

References

1. Grundy SM, Cleeman JI, Daniels SR, *et al.* Diagnosis and management of the metabolic syndrome: an American Heart Association/National Heart, Lung, and Blood Institute Scientific Statement. *Circulation* 2005; 112: 2735–2752.
2. Alberti KG, Eckel RH, Grundy SM, *et al.* Harmonizing the metabolic syndrome: a joint interim statement of the International Diabetes Federation Task Force on Epidemiology and Prevention; National Heart, Lung, and Blood Institute; American Heart Association; World Heart Federation; International Atherosclerosis Society; and International Association for the Study of Obesity. *Circulation* 2009; 120: 1640–1645.
3. International Diabetes Federation. The IDF consensus worldwide definition of the metabolic syndrome. 2006. www.idf.org/webdata/docs/MetS_def_update2006.pdf Date last accessed: August 25, 2014.
4. World Health Organization. Definition, Diagnosis and Classification of Diabetes Mellitus and its Complications. Report of a WHO Consultation. Geneva, World Health Organization, 1999.
5. Kahn R, Buse J, Ferrannini E, *et al.* The metabolic syndrome: time for a critical appraisal: joint statement from the American Diabetes Association and the European Association for the Study of Diabetes. *Diabetes Care* 2005; 28: 2289–2304.
6. Simmons RK, Alberti KG, Gale EA, *et al.* The metabolic syndrome: useful concept or clinical tool? Report of a WHO Expert Consultation. *Diabetologia* 2010; 53: 600–605.
7. Assoumou HG, Gaspoz JM, Sforza E, *et al.* Obstructive sleep apnea and the metabolic syndrome in an elderly healthy population: the SYNAPSE cohort. *Sleep Breath* 2012; 16: 895–902.
8. Peled N, Kassirer M, Shitrit D, *et al.* The association of OSA with insulin resistance, inflammation and metabolic syndrome. *Respir Med* 2007; 101: 1696–1701.
9. Coughlin SR, Mawdsley L, Mugarza JA, *et al.* Obstructive sleep apnoea is independently associated with an increased prevalence of metabolic syndrome. *Eur Heart J* 2004; 25: 735–741.

10. Grandi AM, Laurita E, Marchesi C, *et al.* OSA, metabolic syndrome and CPAP: effect on cardiac remodeling in subjects with abdominal obesity. *Respir Med* 2012; 106: 145–152.

11. Lubrano C, Saponara M, Barbaro G, *et al.* Relationships between body fat distribution, epicardial fat and obstructive sleep apnea in obese patients with and without metabolic syndrome. *PLoS One* 2012; 7: e47059.

12. Salord N, Mayos M, Miralda R, *et al.* Respiratory sleep disturbances in patients undergoing gastric bypass surgery and their relation to metabolic syndrome. *Obes Surg* 2009; 19: 74–79.

13. Gasa M, Salord N, Fortuna AM, *et al.* Obstructive sleep apnoea and metabolic impairment in severe obesity. *Eur Respir J* 2011; 38: 1089–1097.

14. Bonsignore MR, Esquinas C, Barceló A, *et al.* Metabolic syndrome, insulin resistance and sleepiness in real-life obstructive sleep apnoea. *Eur Respir J* 2012; 39: 1136–1143.

15. Barreiro B, Garcia L, Lozano L, *et al.* Obstructive sleep apnea and metabolic syndrome in Spanish population. *Open Respir Med J* 2013; 7: 71–76.

16. Parish JM, Adam T, Facchiano L. Relationship of metabolic syndrome and obstructive sleep apnea. *J Clin Sleep Med* 2007; 3: 467–472.

17. Tanner JM, Chang TI, Harada ND, *et al.* Prevalence of comorbid obstructive sleep apnea and metabolic syndrome: syndrome Z and maxillofacial surgery implications. *J Oral Maxillofac Surg* 2012; 70: 179–187.

18. Bhushan B, Misra A, Guleria R. Obstructive sleep apnea is independently associated with the metabolic syndrome in obese Asian Indians in northern India. *Metab Syndr Relat Disord* 2010; 8: 431–435.

19. Agrawal S, Sharma SK, Sreenivas V, *et al.* Prevalence of metabolic syndrome in a north Indian hospital-based population with obstructive sleep apnoea. *Indian J Med Res* 2011; 134: 639–644.

20. Lin QC, Chen LD, Yu YH, *et al.* Obstructive sleep apnea syndrome is associated with metabolic syndrome and inflammation. *Eur Arch Otorhinolaryngol* 2014; 271: 825–831.

21. Akahoshi T, Uematsu A, Akashiba T, *et al.* Obstructive sleep apnoea is associated with risk factors comprising the metabolic syndrome. *Respirology* 2010; 15: 1122–1126.

22. Sasanabe R, Banno K, Otake K, *et al.* Metabolic syndrome in Japanese patients with obstructive sleep apnea syndrome. *Hypertens Res* 2006; 29: 315–322.

23. Shiina K, Tomiyama H, Takata Y, *et al.* Concurrent presence of metabolic syndrome in obstructive sleep apnea syndrome exacerbates the cardiovascular risk: a sleep clinic cohort study. *Hypertens Res* 2006; 29: 433–441.

24. Stradling JR. Sleep-related breathing disorders. 1. Obstructive sleep apnoea: definitions, epidemiology, and natural history. *Thorax* 1995; 50: 683–689.

25. Young T, Peppard PE, Taheri S. Excess weight and sleep-disordered breathing. *J Appl Physiol* 2005; 99: 1592–1599.

26. Drager LF, Togeiro SM, Polotsky VY, *et al.* Obstructive sleep apnea: a cardiometabolic risk in obesity and the metabolic syndrome. *J Am Coll Cardiol* 2013; 62: 569–576.

27. Roberts CK, Hevener AL, Barnard RJ. Metabolic syndrome and insulin resistance: underlying causes and modification by exercise training. *Compr Physiol* 2013; 3: 1–58.

28. Preis SR, Massaro JM, Hoffmann U, *et al.* Neck circumference as a novel measure of cardiometabolic risk: the Framingham Heart study. *J Clin Endocrinol Metab* 2010; 95: 3701–3710.

29. Preis SR, Pencina MJ, D'Agostino RB Sr, *et al.* Neck circumference and the development of cardiovascular disease risk factors in the Framingham Heart Study. *Diabetes Care* 2013; 36: e3.

30. Preis SR, Massaro JM, Robins SJ, *et al.* Abdominal subcutaneous and visceral adipose tissue and insulin resistance in the Framingham heart study. *Obesity* 2010; 18: 2191–2198.

31. Preis SR, Hwang SJ, Coady S, *et al.* Trends in all-cause and cardiovascular disease mortality among women and men with and without diabetes mellitus in the Framingham Heart Study, 1950 to 2005. *Circulation* 2009; 119: 1728–1735.

32. Mazzuca E, Battaglia S, Marrone O, *et al.* Gender-specific anthropometric markers of adiposity, metabolic syndrome and visceral adiposity index (VAI) in patients with obstructive sleep apnea. *J Sleep Res* 2014; 23: 13–21.

33. Laakso M, Matilainen V, Keinanen-Kiukaanniemi S. Association of neck circumference with insulin resistance-related factors. *Int J Obes Relat Metab Disord* 2002; 26: 873–875.

34. Yang L, Samarasinghe YP, Kane P, *et al.* Visceral adiposity is closely correlated with neck circumference and represents a significant indicator of insulin resistance in WHO grade III obesity. *Clin Endocrinol* 2010; 73: 197–200.

35. Davies RJ, Ali NJ, Stradling JR. Neck circumference and other clinical features in the diagnosis of the obstructive sleep apnoea syndrome. *Thorax* 1992; 47: 101–105.

36. Kawaguchi Y, Fukumoto S, Inaba M, *et al.* Different impacts of neck circumference and visceral obesity on the severity of obstructive sleep apnea syndrome. *Obesity* 2011; 19: 276–282.

37. Dancey DR, Hanly PJ, Soong C, *et al.* Gender differences in sleep apnea: the role of neck circumference. *Chest* 2003; 123: 1544–1550.

38. Onat A, Hergenc G, Yuksel H, et al. Neck circumference as a measure of central obesity: associations with metabolic syndrome and obstructive sleep apnea syndrome beyond waist circumference. *Clin Nutr* 2009; 28: 46–51.

39. Yukawa K, Inoue Y, Yagyu H, et al. Gender differences in the clinical characteristics among Japanese patients with obstructive sleep apnea syndrome. *Chest* 2009; 135: 337–343.

40. White UA, Tchoukalova YD. Sex dimorphism and depot differences in adipose tissue function. *Biochim Biophys Acta* 2014; 1842: 377–392.

41. Lin CM, Davidson TM, Ancoli-Israel S. Gender differences in obstructive sleep apnea and treatment implications. *Sleep Med Rev* 2008; 12: 481–496.

42. Martinez-Rivera C, Abad J, Fiz JA, et al. Usefulness of truncal obesity indices as predictive factors for obstructive sleep apnea syndrome. *Obesity* 2008; 16: 113–118.

43. Simpson L, Mukherjee S, Cooper MN, et al. Sex differences in the association of regional fat distribution with the severity of obstructive sleep apnea. *Sleep* 2010; 33: 467–474.

44. Bouloukaki I, Kapsimalis F, Mermigkis C, et al. Prediction of obstructive sleep apnea syndrome in a large Greek population. *Sleep Breath* 2011; 15: 657–664.

45. Bezerra PC, do Prado M, Gaio E, et al. The use of dual-energy X-ray absorptiometry in the evaluation of obesity in women with obstructive sleep apnea-hypopnea syndrome. *Eur Arch Otorhinolaryngol* 2013; 270: 1539–1545.

46. Kritikou I, Basta M, Tappouni R, et al. Sleep apnoea and visceral adiposity in middle-aged male and female subjects. *Eur Respir J* 2013; 41: 601–609.

47. Iiyori N, Alonso LC, Li J, et al. Intermittent hypoxia causes insulin resistance in lean mice independent of autonomic activity. *Am J Respir Crit Care Med* 2007; 175: 851–857.

48. Drager LF, Li J, Reinke C, et al. Intermittent hypoxia exacerbates metabolic effects of diet-induced obesity. *Obesity* 2011; 19: 2167–2174.

49. Taylor CT, Kent BD, Crinion SJ, et al. Human adipocytes are highly sensitive to intermittent hypoxia induced NF-κB activity and subsequent inflammatory gene expression. *Biochem Biophys Res Commun* 2014; 447: 660–665.

50. Poulain L, Thomas A, Rieusset J, et al. Visceral white fat remodelling contributes to intermittent hypoxia-induced atherogenesis. *Eur Respir J* 2014; 43: 513–522.

51. Shin MK, Han W, Bevans-Fonti S, et al. The effect of adrenal medullectomy on metabolic responses to chronic intermittent hypoxia. *Respir Physiol Neurobiol* 2014; 203: 60–67.

52. Bonsignore MR, McNicholas WT, Montserrat JM, et al. Adipose tissue in obesity and obstructive sleep apnoea. *Eur Respir J* 2012; 39: 746–767.

53. Vgontzas AN, Bixler EO, Chrousos GP. Sleep apnea is a manifestation of the metabolic syndrome. *Sleep Med Rev* 2005; 9: 211–224.

54. Drager LF, Queiroz EL, Lopes HF, et al. Obstructive sleep apnea is highly prevalent and correlates with impaired glycemic control in consecutive patients with the metabolic syndrome. *J Cardiometab Syndr* 2009; 4: 89–95.

55. Angelico F, del Ben M, Augelletti T, et al. Obstructive sleep apnoea syndrome and the metabolic syndrome in an internal medicine setting. *Eur J Intern Med* 2010; 21: 191–195.

56. Papanas N, Steiropoulos P, Nena E, et al. Predictors of ostructive sleep apnea in males with metabolic syndrome. *Vasc Health Risk Manag* 2010; 6: 281–286.

57. Drager LF, Lopes HF, Maki-Nunes C, et al. The impact of obstructive sleep apnea on metabolic and inflammatory markers in consecutive patients with metabolic syndrome. *PLoS One* 2010; 5: e12065.

58. Trombetta IC, Maki-Nunes C, Toschi-Dias E, et al. Obstructive sleep apnea is associated with increased chemoreflex sensitivity in patients with metabolic syndrome. *Sleep* 2013; 36: 41–49.

59. Trombetta IC, Somers VK, Maki-Nunes C, et al. Consequences of comorbid sleep apnea in the metabolic syndrome – implications for cardiovascular risk. *Sleep* 2010; 33: 1193–1199.

60. Drager LF, Bortolotto LA, Maki-Nunes C, et al. The incremental role of obstructive sleep apnoea on markers of atherosclerosis in patients with metabolic syndrome. *Atherosclerosis* 2010; 208: 490–495.

61. Toschi-Dias E, Trombetta IC, Dias da Silva VJ, et al. Time delay of baroreflex control and oscillatory pattern of sympathetic activity in patients with metabolic syndrome and obstructive sleep apnea. *Am J Physiol Heart Circ Physiol* 2013; 304: H1038–H1044.

62. Schober AK, Neurath MF, Harsch IA. Prevalence of sleep apnoea in diabetic patients. *Clin Respir J* 2011; 5: 165–172.

63. Agrawal S, Sharma SK, Sreenivas V, et al. Stepped approach for prediction of syndrome Z in patients attending sleep clinic: a north Indian hospital-based study. *Sleep Breath* 2012; 16: 621–627.

64. Barceló A, Barbé F, de la Peña M, et al. Insulin resistance and daytime sleepiness in patients with sleep apnoea. *Thorax* 2008; 63: 946–950.

65. Nena E, Steiropoulos P, Papanas N, et al. Sleepiness as a marker of glucose deregulation in obstructive sleep apnea. *Sleep Breath* 2012; 16: 181–186.

66. Kent BD, Grote L, Bonsignore MR, et al. Sleep apnoea severity independently predicts glycaemic health in nondiabetic subjects: the ESADA study. *Eur Respir J* 2014; 44: 130–139.

67. Kent BD, Grote L, Ryan S, et al. Diabetes mellitus prevalence and control in sleep-disordered breathing: the European Sleep Apnea Cohort (ESADA) study. Chest 2014; 146: 982–990.

68. Lorenzo C, Williams K, Hunt KJ, et al. The National Cholesterol Education Program – Adult Treatment Panel III, International Diabetes Federation, and World Health Organization definitions of the metabolic syndrome as predictors of incident cardiovascular disease and diabetes. Diabetes Care 2007; 30: 8–13.

69. Ho JS, Cannaday JJ, Barlow CE, et al. Relation of the number of metabolic syndrome risk factors with all-cause and cardiovascular mortality. Am J Cardiol 2008; 102: 689–692.

70. Kostapanos MS, Mikhailidis DP, Elisaf MS, et al. Obstructive sleep apnoea syndrome and cardiovascular risk. Arch Med Sci 2012; 8: 1115–1116.

71. Parati G, Lombardi C, Hedner J, et al. Recommendations for the management of patients with obstructive sleep apnoea and hypertension. Eur Respir J 2013; 41: 523–538.

72. Baguet JP, Lévy P, Barone-Rochette G, et al. Masked hypertension in obstructive sleep apnea syndrome. J Hypertens 2008; 26: 885–892.

73. Baguet JP, Boutin I, Barone-Rochette G, et al. Hypertension diagnosis in obstructive sleep apnea: self or 24-hour ambulatory blood pressure monitoring? Int J Cardiol 2013; 167: 2346–2347.

74. Heatley EM, Harris M, Battersby M, et al. Obstructive sleep apnoea in adults: a common chronic condition in need of a comprehensive chronic condition management approach. Sleep Med Rev 2013; 17: 349–355.

75. Pamidi S, Wroblewski K, Broussard J, et al. Obstructive sleep apnea in young lean men: impact on insulin sensitivity and secretion. Diabetes Care 2012; 35: 2384–2389.

76. Borel AL, Monneret D, Tamisier R, et al. The severity of nocturnal hypoxia but not abdominal adiposity is associated with insulin resistance in non-obese men with sleep apnea. PLoS One 2013; 8: e71000.

77. Lam JC, Mak JC, Ip MS. Obesity, obstructive sleep apnoea and metabolic syndrome. Respirology 2012; 17: 223–236.

78. Pépin JL, Tamisier R, Lévy P. Obstructive sleep apnoea and metabolic syndrome: put CPAP efficacy in a more realistic perspective. Thorax 2012; 67: 1025–1027.

79. Steiropoulos P, Papanas N, Maltezos E, et al. Is there a metabolic effect of continuous positive airway pressure in sleep apnoea? Adherence should not be underestimated. Eur Respir J 2009; 34: 1209–1210.

80. Coughlin SR, Mawdsley L, Mugarza JA, et al. Cardiovascular and metabolic effects of CPAP in obese males with OSA. Eur Respir J 2007; 29: 720–727.

81. Mota PC, Drummond M, Winck JC, et al. APAP impact on metabolic syndrome in obstructive sleep apnea patients. Sleep Breath 2011; 15: 665–672.

82. Hoyos CM, Sullivan DR, Liu PY. Effect of CPAP on the metabolic syndrome: a randomised sham-controlled study. Thorax 2013; 68: 588–589.

83. Hoyos CM, Killick R, Yee BJ, et al. Cardiometabolic changes after continuous positive airway pressure for obstructive sleep apnoea: a randomised sham-controlled study. Thorax 2012; 67: 1081–1089.

84. Oktay B, Akbal E, Firat H, et al. CPAP treatment in the coexistence of obstructive sleep apnea syndrome and metabolic syndrome, results of one year follow up. Acta Clin Belg 2009; 64: 329–334.

85. Dorkova Z, Petrasova D, Molcanyiova A, et al. Effects of continuous positive airway pressure on cardiovascular risk profile in patients with severe obstructive sleep apnea and metabolic syndrome. Chest 2008; 134: 686–692.

86. Sivam S, Phillips CL, Trenell MI, et al. Effects of 8 weeks of continuous positive airway pressure on abdominal adiposity in obstructive sleep apnoea. Eur Respir J 2012; 40: 913–918.

87. Münzer T, Hegglin A, Stannek T, et al. Effects of long-term continuous positive airway pressure on body composition and IGF1. Eur J Endocrinol 2010; 162: 695–704.

88. Quan SF, Budhiraja R, Clarke DP, et al. Impact of treatment with continuous positive airway pressure (CPAP) on weight in obstructive sleep apnea. J Clin Sleep Med 2013; 9: 989–993.

89. Hoyos CM, Phillips CL, Grunstein RR. From couch potato to gym junkie – CPAP may not be the answer. J Clin Sleep Med 2014; 10: 473–474.

90. West SD, Nicoll DJ, Wallace TM, et al. Effect of CPAP on insulin resistance and HbA1c in men with obstructive sleep apnoea and type 2 diabetes. Thorax 2007; 62: 969–974.

91. Weinstock TG, Wang X, Rueschman M, et al. A controlled trial of CPAP therapy on metabolic control in individuals with impaired glucose tolerance and sleep apnea. Sleep 2012; 35: 617–625.

92. Hecht L, Möhler R, Meyer G. Effects of CPAP-respiration on markers of glucose metabolism in patients with obstructive sleep apnoea syndrome: a systematic review and meta-analysis. Ger Med Sci 2011; 9: Doc20.

93. Yang D, Liu Z, Yang H. The impact of effective continuous positive airway pressure on homeostasis model assessment insulin resistance in non-diabetic patients with moderate to severe obstructive sleep apnea. Diabetes Metab Res Rev 2012; 28: 499–504.

94. Yang D, Liu Z, Yang H, et al. Effects of continuous positive airway pressure on glycemic control and insulin resistance in patients with obstructive sleep apnea: a meta-analysis. Sleep Breath 2013; 17: 33–38.

95. Iftikhar IH, Khan MF, Das A, et al. Meta-analysis: continuous positive airway pressure improves insulin resistance in patients with sleep apnea without diabetes. Ann Am Thorac Soc 2013; 10: 115–120.

96.   Giles TL, Lasserson TJ, Smith BH, *et al.* Continuous positive airways pressure for obstructive sleep apnoea in adults. *Cochrane Database Syst Rev* 2006; 3: CD001106.
97.   Alajmi M, Mulgrew AT, Fox J, *et al.* Impact of continuous positive airway pressure therapy on blood pressure in patients with obstructive sleep apnea hypopnea: a meta-analysis of randomized controlled trials. *Lung* 2007; 185: 67–72.
98.   Haentjens P, Van Meerhaeghe A, Moscariello A, *et al.* The impact of continuous positive airway pressure on blood pressure in patients with obstructive sleep apnea syndrome: evidence from a meta-analysis of placebo-controlled randomized trials. *Arch Intern Med* 2007; 167: 757–764.
99.   Bazzano LA, Khan Z, Reynolds K, *et al.* Effect of nocturnal nasal continuous positive airway pressure on blood pressure in obstructive sleep apnea. *Hypertension* 2007; 50: 417–423.
100. Montesi SB, Edwards BA, Malhotra A, *et al.* The effect of continuous positive airway pressure treatment on blood pressure: a systematic review and meta-analysis of randomized controlled trials. *J Clin Sleep Med* 2012; 8: 587–596.
101. Fava C, Dorigoni S, Dalle Vedove F, *et al.* Effect of CPAP on blood pressure in patients with OSA/hypopnea: a systematic review and meta-analysis. *Chest* 2014; 145: 762–771.
102. Schein AS, Kerkhoff AC, Coronel CC, *et al.* Continuous positive airway pressure reduces blood pressure in patients with obstructive sleep apnea; a systematic review and meta-analysis with 1000 patients. *J Hypertens* 2014; 32: 1762–1773.
103. Xu H, Yi H, Guan J, *et al.* Effect of continuous positive airway pressure on lipid profile in patients with obstructive sleep apnea syndrome: a meta-analysis of randomized controlled trials. *Atherosclerosis* 2014; 234: 446–453.
104. Iftikhar IH, Blankfield RP. Effect of continuous positive airway pressure on hemoglobin A$_{1c}$ in patients with obstructive sleep apnea: a systematic review and meta-analysis. *Lung* 2012; 190: 605–611.
105. American Diabetes Association. Diagnosis and classification of diabetes mellitus. *Diabetes Care* 2011; 34: Suppl. 1, S62–S69.
106. Floras JS, Bradley TD. Treating obstructive sleep apnea: is there more to the story than 2 millimeters of mercury? *Hypertension* 2007; 50: 289–291.
107. Marin JM, Carrizo SJ, Vicente E, *et al.* Long-term cardiovascular outcomes in men with obstructive sleep apnoea-hypopnoea with or without treatment with continuous positive airway pressure: an observational study. *Lancet* 2005; 365: 1046–1053.
108. Bonsignore MR, Borel AL, Machan E, *et al.* Sleep apnoea and metabolic dysfunction. *Eur Respir Rev* 2013; 22: 353–364.
109. Dee A, Kearns K, O'Neill C, *et al.* The direct and indirect costs of both overweight and obesity: a systematic review. *BMC Res Notes* 2014; 7: 242.
110. Ashrafian H, le Roux CW, Rowland SP, *et al.* Metabolic surgery and obstructive sleep apnoea: the protective effects of bariatric procedures. *Thorax* 2012; 67: 442–449.
111. Tuomilehto H, Seppä J, Uusitupa M. Obesity and obstructive sleep apnea – clinical significance of weight loss. *Sleep Med Rev* 2013; 17: 321–329.
112. Buchwald H, Avidor Y, Braunwald E, *et al.* Bariatric surgery: a systematic review and meta-analysis. *JAMA* 2004; 292: 1724–1737.
113. Greenburg DL, Lettieri CJ, Eliasson AH. Effects of surgical weight loss on measures of obstructive sleep apnea: a meta-analysis. *Am J Med* 2009; 122: 535–542.
114. Bae EK, Lee YJ, Yun CH, *et al.* Effects of surgical weight loss for treating obstructive sleep apnea. *Sleep Breath* 2014; 18: 901–905.
115. Fredheim JM, Rollheim J, Sandbu R, *et al.* Obstructive sleep apnea after weight loss: a clinical trial comparing gastric bypass and intensive lifestyle intervention. *J Clin Sleep Med* 2013; 9: 427–432.
116. Noria SF, Grantcharov T. Biological effects of bariatric surgery on obesity-related comorbidities. *Can J Surg* 2013; 56: 47–57.
117. Dixon JB, Schachter LM, O'Brien PE, *et al.* Surgical *vs* conventional therapy for weight loss treatment of obstructive sleep apnea: a randomized controlled trial. *JAMA* 2012; 308: 1142–1149.
118. Gloy VL, Briel M, Bhatt DL, *et al.* Bariatric surgery *versus* non-surgical treatment for obesity: a systematic review and meta-analysis of randomised controlled trials. *BMJ* 2013; 347: f5934.
119. Kardassis D, Grote L, Sjöström L, *et al.* Sleep apnea modifies the long-term impact of surgically induced weight loss on cardiac function and inflammation. *Obesity* 2013; 21: 698–704.
120. Araghi MH, Chen YF, Jagielski A, *et al.* Effectiveness of lifestyle interventions on obstructive sleep apnea (OSA): systematic review and meta-analysis. *Sleep* 2013; 36: 1553–1562.
121. Thomasouli MA, Brady EM, Davies MJ, *et al.* The impact of diet and lifestyle management strategies for obstructive sleep apnoea in adults: a systematic review and meta-analysis of randomised controlled trials. *Sleep Breath* 2013; 17: 925–935.
122. Mitchell LJ, Davidson ZE, Bonham M, *et al.* Weight loss from lifestyle interventions and severity of sleep apnea: a systematic review and meta-analysis. *Sleep Med* 2014; 15: 1173–1183.

123. Miras AD, le Roux CW. Can medical therapy mimic the clinical efficacy or physiological effects of bariatric surgery? *Int J Obes* 2014; 38: 325–333.

124. Tuomilehto HP, Seppä JM, Partinen MM, *et al.* Lifestyle intervention with weight reduction: first-line treatment in mild obstructive sleep apnea. *Am J Respir Crit Care Med* 2009; 179: 320–327.

125. Johansson K, Neovius M, Lagerros YT, *et al.* Effect of a very low energy diet on moderate and severe obstructive sleep apnoea in obese men: a randomised controlled trial. *BMJ* 2009; 339: b4609.

126. Sengul YS, Ozalevli S, Oztura I, *et al.* The effect of exercise on obstructive sleep apnea: a randomized and controlled trial. *Sleep Breath* 2011; 15: 49–56.

127. Kline CE, Crowley EP, Ewing GB, *et al.* The effect of exercise training on obstructive sleep apnea and sleep quality: a randomized controlled trial. *Sleep* 2011; 34: 1631–1640.

128. Desplan M, Mercier J, Sabaté M, *et al.* A comprehensive rehabilitation program improves disease severity in patients with obstructive sleep apnea syndrome: a pilot randomized controlled study. *Sleep Med* 2014; 15: 906–912.

129. Papandreou C, Schiza SE, Bouloukaki I, *et al.* Effect of Mediterranean diet *versus* prudent diet combined with physical activity on OSAS: a randomised trial. *Eur Respir J* 2012; 39: 1398–1404.

130. Winslow DH, Bowden CH, DiDonato KP, *et al.* A randomized, double-blind, placebo-controlled study of an oral, extended-release formulation of phentermine/topiramate for the treatment of obstructive sleep apnea in obese adults. *Sleep* 2012; 35: 1529–1539.

131. Kuna ST, Reboussin DM, Borradaile KE, *et al.* Long-term effect of weight loss on obstructive sleep apnea severity in obese patients with type 2 diabetes. *Sleep* 2013; 36: 641–649.

132. Borel AL, Leblanc X, Alméras N, *et al.* Sleep apnoea attenuates the effects of a lifestyle intervention programme in men with visceral obesity. *Thorax* 2012; 67: 735–741.

133. Garcia JM, Sharafkhaneh H, Hirshkowitz M, *et al.* Weight and metabolic effects of CPAP in obstructive sleep apnea patients with obesity. *Respir Res* 2011; 12: 80.

134. Batool-Anwar S, Goodwin JL, Drescher AA, *et al.* Impact of CPAP on activity patterns and diet in patients with obstructive sleep apnea (OSA). *J Clin Sleep Med* 2014; 10: 465–472.

135. Fiori CZ, Martinez D, Baronio D, *et al.* Downregulation of uncoupling protein-1 mRNA expression and hypoadiponectemia in a mouse model of sleep apnea. *Sleep Breath* 2014; 18: 541–548.

136. Chirinos JA, Gurubhagavatula I, Teff K, *et al.* CPAP, weight loss, or both for obstructive sleep apnea. *N Engl J Med* 2014; 370: 2265–2275.

Disclosures: **None declared.**

Chapter 17

Lifestyle intervention and pharmaceutical therapies of sleep apnoea

Ding Zou and Jan Hedner

Excess body weight and lack of exercise are associated with increased risk of OSA. RCTs have shown that weight loss and physical activity improve sleep-disordered breathing in OSA patients. Moreover, long-term follow-up studies on the effect of an intensive lifestyle weight-management programme have yielded promising results. The therapeutic effect of weight-reduction drugs on OSA has not been systematically explored. Few drugs have been approved for pharmacological management of overweight and obesity in Europe despite an increasing obesity epidemic. Currently, there is no effective drug for OSA treatment in clinical practice. The fact that multiple pathophysiological mechanisms contribute to this complex disease highlights the importance of better patient phenotyping for tailored therapy. Recent advances in the field certainly bring hope for such a development.

In contrast with the high prevalence of OSA, available treatments aiming to eliminate apnoeic events and improve long-term outcome in OSA are relatively limited and primarily focused on mechanical PAP. However, the overall beneficial effect of PAP therapy is often compromised by incomplete compliance to treatment. In the light of this limitation, there is a need for alternative treatment options in OSA patients.

OSA is often associated with unhealthy lifestyle (*e.g.* low physical activity, excessive food intake). While PAP reduces daytime excessive sleepiness and cardiovascular morbidity in OSA patients, there is no change in physical activity and dietary habits [1]. In fact, there is evidence that associates PAP treatment with modest weight gain [2] which has been attributed to reduced energy expenditure during sleep with PAP [3]. It therefore appears important to consider lifestyle intervention as both a stand-alone and an added treatment option in OSA patients, especially those who are overweight. Such attention will also benefit the patients with respect to other comorbid conditions (*e.g.* cardiovascular, metabolic) associated with OSA.

Current research has recognised that OSA is a heterogeneous disorder caused by different pathophysiological mechanisms all predisposing to airway collapse during sleep. While some patients may have a reduced compensatory neuromuscular control of the UA, others

Sleep Disorders Center, Department of Pulmonary Medicine and Allergology, Sahlgrenska University Hospital, Gothenburg, Sweden.

Correspondence: Jan Hedner, Sleep Disorders Center, Department of Pulmonary Medicine and Allergology, Sahlgrenska University Hospital, 41345 Gothenburg, Sweden. E-mail: jan.hedner@lungall.gu.se

may suffer from an unstable central neurochemical ventilatory control during sleep [4]. This heterogeneity not only suggests that tailored therapies should be developed in OSA. It also illustrates the potential difficulty residing in the identification of a novel target for drug development in OSA. Although several attempts have been undertaken over the years, there is no drug currently available for OSA treatment.

In this chapter, we will briefly review current evidence from RCTs suggesting that physical exercise and weight loss may be effective in OSA treatment. In addition, potential targets for future drug development in OSA will be discussed.

Exercise

A physically active lifestyle is associated with numerous health benefits extending from reduced cardiovascular morbidity to reduction of all-cause mortality. Several studies have demonstrated that exercise training improves sleep quality both in healthy subjects and patients with insomnia [5–7]. In OSA patients, lack of exercise has been associated with increased severity of OSA independent of body habitus [8]. A modulation of chemoreflex sensitivity and breathing efficiency to exercise test has been reported in young sleep apnoea patients [9]. It has been suggested that physical exercise acts to enhance chemoreceptor sensitivity and increase respiratory drive in OSA patients. Moreover, regular physical exercise increases overall tone of skeletal muscles including the pharyngeal muscles [10]. KLINE et al. [11] randomised 43 sedentary and overweight/obese patients with moderate-to-severe sleep apnoea to a 12-week intense exercise training or a low-intensity stretching programme. Compared with stretching, exercise reduced AHI (exercise: 32.2±5.6 to 24.6±4.4, stretching: 24.4±5.6 to 28.9±6.4; p<0.01) as well as the ODI (p=0.03) but body weight was maintained. Non-REM (stage N3) and actigraphy-recorded sleep as well as subjective sleep quality also improved in the exercise group. In another RCT, SENGUL et al. [12] randomised 20 mild-to-moderate OSA patients to an exercise (breathing and aerobic exercise three-times per week) or a control group. After 12 weeks, AHI in the exercise group decreased from 15.2±5.4 to 11.0±5 (p=0.02) but this change was not significantly different from the control group (p=0.11). Body weight, respiratory muscle strength and other sleep measures were unchanged. Although data from RCT studies suggest a positive effect of exercise on OSA severity, the treatment effect is generally quite modest and the exact mechanisms are not fully understood. In a recent meta-analysis [13], it was estimated that exercise training in OSA patients was associated with a 6.3 events·h^{-1} reduction in AHI, a 5.8% increase of sleep efficiency, a 3.3-unit drop of ESS score, but no change of BMI. Hence, although potentially effective, physical activity cannot be recommended as a stand-alone therapy in OSA.

Exercise may be particularly beneficial in subgroup of OSA patients with cardiovascular comorbidities; for instance, congestive HF. In a prospective study by UENO et al. [14], 25 HF patients were recruited in a 4-month exercise training protocol consisting of 60 mins of exercise three times per week. Compared with baseline, exercise reduced muscle sympathetic nerve activity, increased limb blood-flow and improved endothelial function in all patients. Interestingly, exercise training improved AHI, minimum oxygen saturation and increased the proportion of slow wave sleep in patients with predominant OSA. In a subsequent RCT, 50 patients with chronic HF and sleep apnoea (proportion central apnoea unknown) were randomised to aerobic training, aerobic with strength training and a control group [15]. After three supervised exercise sessions, training groups underwent 3 months of home-based exercise sessions (three sessions per week at month 1 and 2, four sessions per week at month

3, on non-consecutive days). As expected, outcomes from the cardiopulmonary exercise test and isokinetic strength and endurance tests improved in both training groups compared with controls. In addition, AHI in the aerobic training and the aerobic with strength training groups decreased from 25.2 ± 24.7 to 16.7 ± 18.6 events·h^{-1} and from 26.4 ± 17.6 to 16.4 ± 11.1 events·h^{-1}, respectively, compared with baseline (all p⩽0.001). Sleep efficiency during the PSG night also improved in both exercise groups. Although small, these studies underline that exercise training may be beneficial for sleep apnoea patients with comorbid HF. The conditions chronic HF and sleep apnoea have both associated with increased sympathetic nerve activity. The reduction in sympathetic outflow and improved endothelial function following exercise training might help to normalise chemoreflex sensitivity and cardiac afterload. In addition, exercise-induced improvement of cardiac function may stabilise breathing *via* a shorter circulation time, reduced pulmonary vascular pressure and less overnight fluid shift to the neck. Hence, the possibility that exercise improved sleep-disordered breathing in patients with HF suggests that synergistic effects may be achieved with PAP treatment and this area certainly deserves further studies [16].

Weight management

Excess body weight is the dominant modifiable risk factor in OSA, and almost 70% of OSA patients are overweight or obese. Several mechanisms are believed to contribute to the obesity-related pathogenesis of OSA. First, increased parapharyngeal and tongue fat deposition narrows the UA diameter and increases the risk of UA collapsibility. Second, abdominal visceral adiposity may restrict diaphragmatic and ribcage movements, reduce chest wall compliance and lung volume, impair respiratory stability and increase OSA susceptibility. Finally, an obesity-related neurohormonal change (*e.g.* modified leptin secretion) may be involved in the chemoreflex regulation in OSA. In the Wisconsin Sleep Cohort, subjects with stable weight and those with a weight gain/loss over a 4-year period were compared [17]. A 10% weight gain predicted a 32% increase in AHI whereas a 10% weight loss was associated with a 26% reduction of AHI. Obesity is also likely to worsen the magnitude of IH associated with apnoeic events [18] and this may influence the likelihood of developing of cardiovascular comorbidity (*e.g.* hypertension) in OSA [19]. In addition, the metabolic derangement (*e.g.* leptin resistance) associated with OSA may further contribute to weight gain or resistance to weight loss [20].

Several different strategies for obesity management (table 1) including intensive diet and behavioural programmes, bariatric surgery and pharmacological intervention have been explored in OSA. All these methods may result in a body weight reduction and an associated reduction of sleep apnoea.

Diet and lifestyle intervention

The overall aim of dietary intervention in weight loss is to reduce caloric intake below the level used for energy expenditure. A very low calorie diet (VLCD), defined as a diet of 800 kcal·day^{-1} or less, is often used to obtain rapid weight loss in obese patients. Patients receive formulated liquid meals that contain the recommended daily requirements *e.g.* vitamins, minerals and protein. The programme may include intensified supervision or integration with other interventions (*e.g.* lifestyle, PAP). The effectiveness of weight loss on

Table 1. Recommendations for overweight and obesity management in adults from the 2013 American Heart Association/American College of Cardiology/The Obesity Society guideline

Identifying patients who need to lose weight	1) Cutpoints for overweight (BMI 25.0–29.9 kg·m^{-2}) and obesity (BMI $\geqslant$30 kg·m^{-2}) 2) Advise overweight and obese adults that the greater the BMI, the greater the risk of CVD, type 2 diabetes and all-cause mortality 3) Measure waist circumference in overweight and obese adults
Matching treatment benefits with risk profiles	Counsel overweight and obese adults: 1) Sustained weight loss of 3–5% is likely to result in clinically meaningful reductions in triglycerides, blood glucose, haemoglobin A1c, and the risk of developing type 2 diabetes 2) Greater amounts of weight loss will reduce BP, improve low-density lipoprotein cholesterol and high-density lipoprotein cholesterol, and reduce the need for medications to control BP, blood glucose, and lipids as well as further reduce triglycerides and blood glucose
Diets for weight loss	Prescribe a diet to achieve reduced calorie intake for obese or overweight individuals as part of a comprehensive lifestyle intervention (one of following methods) 1) Prescribe 1200–1500 kcal·day^{-1} for women and 1500–1800 kcal·day^{-1} for men (kilocalorie levels are usually adjusted for the individual's body weight) 2) Prescribe a 500–750 kcal·day^{-1} energy deficit 3) Prescribe one of the evidence-based diets that restricts certain food types (such as high-carbohydrate foods, low-fibre foods or high-fat foods) in order to create an energy deficit by reduced food intake
Lifestyle intervention and counselling	1) Advise overweight and obese adults to participate in a comprehensive lifestyle programme ($\geqslant$6 months) that assists participants in adhering to a lower-calorie diet and in increasing physical activity through the use of behavioural strategies 2) Prescribe on-site, high-intensity (*i.e.* $\geqslant$14 sessions in 6 months) comprehensive weight loss interventions provided in individual or group sessions by a trained health professional 3) Use a very-low-calorie diet (defined as <800 kcal·day^{-1}) only in limited circumstances and only when provided by trained practitioners in a medical care setting where medical monitoring and high-intensity lifestyle intervention can be provided; medical supervision is required because of the rapid rate of weight loss and potential for health complications 4) Advise overweight and obese individuals who have lost weight to participate long term ($\geqslant$1 year) in a comprehensive weight loss maintenance programme
Bariatric surgical treatment for obesity	Patient selection: a BMI $\geqslant$40 kg·m^{-2}, or BMI $\geqslant$35 kg·m^{-2} with obesity-related comorbid conditions who are motivated to lose weight and who have not responded to behavioural treatment with or without pharmacotherapy with sufficient weight loss to achieve targeted health outcome goals

Reproduced and modified from [21] with permission from the publisher.

OSA severity was shown a long time ago, but it was not until recently that RCTs were introduced in this area.

TUOMILEHTO et al. [22] performed the first prospective randomised controlled parallel-group study on weight reduction in overweight/obese patients with mild OSA. 72 subjects were randomised to routine, single-session lifestyle counselling or a 12-week VLCD programme (600–800 kcal·day^{-1}) and supervised lifestyle intervention for 1 year. At 12 months, the intervention group had lost more weight than the control group (−10.7 versus −2.4 kg; p<0.001) and there was a greater reduction in waist circumference and BMI (−11.6 versus −3.0 cm and −3.5 versus −0.8 kg·m^{-2}, respectively; p<0.001). AHI determined by cardiorespiratory polygraphy, decreased 4 events·h^{-1} in the intervention group whereas there was no change in the controls (p=0.017). The overnight oxygen saturation (e.g. mean oxygen saturation, percentage of time with oxygen saturation <90%) was improved in the intervention group. Changes in AHI were strongly associated with changes in weight and waist circumference. In addition, the intervention group showed a significant reduction of insulin and triglyceride levels, and better hypertension and diabetes control. Subjects were followed up for 1 year [23] and 4 years [24] after the intervention protocol, patients from intervention group sustained weight loss compared with controls: −4.5 (p=0.09) and −6.1 kg (p=0.025), respectively. The changes in AHI in the intervention group compared with the control group were −4.1 events·h^{-1} (p=0.049) and −5.8 events·h^{-1} (p=0.041), respectively. Importantly, the progression of OSA in the intervention group had decreased 61% compared with controls (p=0.04). Hence, despite slight increase of body weight after the intense dietary programme, the reduction of body weight and improvement of OSA was sustained up to 4 years after intervention. This series of studies provide strong evidence that a combination of dietary and lifestyle intervention may be very useful in the management of mild OSA in overweight/obese patients.

JOHANSSON et al. [25] conducted a RCT using VLCD alone for treatment of moderate and severe OSA in obese patients. 63 patients (aged 49±7 years, AHI 37±15 events h^{-1}, weight 112.5±14.2 kg, waist circumference 120±9 cm) were randomised to a 7-week standard 2.3 MJ·day^{-1} liquid energy diet programme followed by a 2-week normal food to reach 6.3 MJ·day^{-1}, or a usual diet. Supervision and group support were provided at 2-week intervals. At week 9, mean body weight and BMI change were −18.7±4.1 kg and −5.7±1.1 kg·m^{-2} in the intervention group and 1.1±1.9 kg and 0.3±0.6 kg·m^{-2} in the control group, respectively (all p<0.001 between groups). Waist circumference, neck circumference and percentage body fat decreased 17.7 cm, 4.2 cm and 8.5%, respectively, in the intervention group compared with controls. Group differences in AHI quantified by an ambulatory WatchPAT device (type IV of AASM) (Itamar Medical, Caesarea, Israel) [26] favoured intervention with a reduction of −23 (95% CI −30 to −15) events·h^{-1} (p<0.001). Overnight oxygenation and subjective daytime sleepiness assessed by ESS were concurrently improved. VLCD patients were subsequently followed up in a weight-loss maintenance programme from 9 to 52 weeks [27]. The programme included a 3-hour monthly group session headed by a nurse and dietitian. In case of weight regain, partial meal replacement or weight-reduction mediation was prescribed. After 1 year, the improvement of adiposity and OSA were largely maintained with a −12.1±9.0 kg body weight loss (BMI −3.7±2.7 kg·m^{-2}) and a −17 (95% CI −21 to −13) events·h^{-1} AHI reduction. There was a dose–response association between weight loss and AHI reduction and a 10 kg weight loss at the 1-year follow-up was associated with a 5 events·h^{-1} decrease in AHI. Patients with severe OSA had a greater improvement than those with moderate disease.

Promising data were also reported from the Sleep AHEAD (Action for Health in Diabetes) Study, a prospective multi-centre RCT, investigating weight loss on sleep apnoea improvement in overweight and obese OSA patients with type 2 diabetes [28, 29]. 264 patients (sex balanced, aged 61.2±6.5 years, weight 102.4±18.3 kg, BMI 36.7±5.7 kg·m^{-2}, AHI 23.2±16.5 events·h^{-1}) were randomised to an intensive life intervention (ILI) (protein-controlled diets for first 4 months and reduced use from months 5–12 plus moderate-intensity physical activity) or diabetes support and education programme and followed up for 4 years. Supervision was provided between years 2 and 4 including at least one on-site visit per month in the ILI group and three group sessions annually in the control group. Ambulatory PSG recording was used for assessment of sleep-related disordered breathing. 82, 79 and 66% from ILI group and 83, 80 and 60% from the control group completed the assessment at the 1, 2 and 4 years follow-up, respectively. Compared with baseline, weight, AHI and neck and waist circumference decreased significantly in the ILI group while, in the control group, there was no change in body composition, and AHI was modestly increased. The between-group differences on body weight were −10.8, −6.7 and −4.4 kg at 1, 2 and 4 years, respectively (all p<0.001). Despite weight regain at the 2- and 4-year follow-ups, the AHI improvement in the ILI group remained stable was −9.7, −8.0 and −7.7 events·h^{-1} compared with the control group at 1, 2 and 4 years, respectively (all p⩽0.001). 20.7% of patients in the ILI group and 3.6% from the control group had remission of OSA (AHI <5 events·h^{-1}) at 4 years. As expected, the greater changes in AHI occurred in patients with high AHI at baseline. Interestingly, ILI intervention was associated with AHI reduction over time, independent of body weight change, suggesting other components in the lifestyle intervention programme (e.g. physical activity) may also contribute to the change of AHI in the study. Although lifestyle intervention improves apnoea severity, the sleep architecture assessed by PSG did not differ compared with the control group after 1-, 2- and 4-year follow-up in these overweight/obese OSA patients with type 2 diabetes [30].

The effect of PAP treatment on body weight in OSA patients has remained an issue of debate. A modest reduction of body weight after 10 weeks of CPAP treatment was found in Asian patients with mild-to-moderate OSA [31]. Another randomised sham-CPAP-controlled study found no change of body weight after 24 weeks with CPAP in 65 male patients with moderate-to-severe OSA [32]. Alternatively, with sufficient sample size, large long-term follow-up RCTs have demonstrated that PAP treatment appears to induce modest increase in body weight compared with control or sham-CPAP [2]. Moreover, this effect was more pronounced in patients compliant with PAP therapy. Several mechanisms, including a reduction of energy expenditure with CPAP and leptin resistance in OSA, may contribute to a weight increase after PAP treatment in OSA. Hence, in overweight and obese patients, physical activity and dietary intervention needs to be incorporated in the treatment strategy in addition to PAP. It is worth noting that adding PAP in the weight-reduction programme may not change the effectiveness of weight loss [33]. In a recent randomised parallel-group 24-week study [34] of 181 obese moderate-to-severe OSA patients, combined CPAP and a dietary, physical activity and cognitive behavioural weight loss programme was found to reduce body weight and to improve insulin sensitivity and serum triglycerides better than CPAP alone (p<0.001, 0.01 and 0.046, respectively). In patients adherent with the study protocol, the combined interventions resulted in a larger SBP reduction than CPAP or weight loss alone (p<0.001 and 0.02, respectively). The reduction of C-reactive protein was greater in the weight-loss group compared with the CPAP group.

It may be concluded that weight loss achieved by lifestyle intervention reduces sleep apnoea severity in overweight and obese OSA patients. However, in the RCTs, patients typically received intense support in order to provide maximum adherence to the programme and this may be difficult to repeat in the clinical setting.

Surgical intervention

Bariatric surgery is an effective method to obtain long-term weight loss. Several different surgical procedures, including laparoscopic adjustable gastric banding (purely restrictive) and Roux-en-Y gastric bypass (restrictive with a malabsorptive component), have been used in treatment of morbid obesity (BMI >40 kg·m^{-2}) or obesity with cardiovascular/metabolic comorbidities (BMI >35 kg·m^{-2}). It was early determined that sham-controlled studies of bariatric surgery were not feasible due to ethical reasons. Uncontrolled studies and case series were used to assess the clinical effectiveness of bariatric surgery on weight loss in OSA. A recent systematic review including 13 900 patients from 69 studies found that OSA was reduced in more than 75% of patients after bariatric surgery [35]. The effectiveness appears to apply for all types of surgical procedures and it is suggested that weight loss, improvement of the metabolic condition and the inflammation status jointly contribute to the improvement of OSA. GREENBURG et al. [36] performed a meta-analysis on 342 patients undergoing bariatric surgery and found that the 32% BMI reduction (from 55.3 (95% CI 53.5–57.1) to 37.7 (36.6–38.9) kg·m^{-2}) was associated with an AHI reduction of 71% (from 55 (49–60) to 16 (13–19) events·h^{-1}).

FREDHEIM et al. [37] performed a non-randomised controlled study comparing effect of gastric bypass surgery and a 1-year ILI programme on OSA in 133 morbid obese patients (BMI 45.1±5.7 kg·m^{-2}, AHI 17.1±21.4 events·h^{-1}). The ILI programme aimed at inducing ⩾10% weight loss and included 4 intermittent in-hospital stays (7 weeks in total) with physical activity, dietary consultation and group sessions. Patients were contacted every 2 weeks at home to ensure motivation. Sleep apnoea was assessed by a cardiorespiratory polygraphy recording at baseline and at 1 year. Both the ILI and the surgery groups reduced body weight significantly (9.5 and 29.7%, respectively; between group difference p<0.001). AHI decreased 40 and 74% in the ILI and the surgery groups, respectively (between group difference p=0.003). The gastric bypass surgery was more effective in improving 3% ODI and mean arterial oxygen saturation measured by pulse oximetry than ILI. 66% of the surgery patients and 40% ILI patients had remission of OSA at 1 year of follow-up (p=0.028). However, a multivariate analysis showed that the effect on OSA was mediated by the weight loss rather than the type of treatment.

Drug-induced weight loss

In the light of the potential peri-operative morbidity and mortality risk associated with bariatric surgery, pharmacological management has been considered as an adjunct therapy to lifestyle intervention in obese patients. However, several recently developed drugs with weight reduction properties were found to have long-term psychiatric and cardiovascular side-effects which resulted in a withdrawal from the market (e.g. rimonabant, sibutramine). Currently, there are four anti-obesity drugs approved by the US Food and Drug Administration (FDA) for long-term use on the US market (orlistat, phentermine/ topiramate extended-release combination, lorcaserin and a naltrexone SR/bupropion SR combination). In Europe, there is only one approved drug (orlistat).

The gastric and pancreatic lipase inhibitor orlistat prevents dietary fat absorption (reduction ~25%). It is recommended for use in combination with a diet where 30% of calories come from fat. In a recent meta-analysis of RCTs, orlistat combined with lifestyle intervention resulted in a 1.80 (95% CI −2.54 to −1.06) kg weight reduction compared with placebo at 1 year [38]. The weight-loss effect was more pronounced among patients with orlistat 120 mg three times per day than 30/60 mg three times per day (−2.34 kg (−3.03 to −1.65) *versus* −0.70 kg (−1.92 to 0.52); p=0.02). Side effects included gastrointestinal events and a decrease in fat-soluble vitamin absorption. Despite this well-established, although moderate, weight-loss effect of orlistat, the compound has not been evaluated in studies of overweight and obese OSA patients. This is surprising considering that OSA severity may be expected to improve in parallel with a reduction of body weight.

Phentermine, a synthetic sympathomimetic amine, has been approved by the FDA for short-term (3 months) monotherapy in obesity. The compound has an appetite-suppressing effect and increases the resting energy expenditure *via* an augmentation of adrenergic signalling in the sympathetic nervous system. Consequently, heart rate and blood pressure may increase during treatment. Topiramate is an antiepileptic drug which also has been used for migraine management. Topiramate is known to suppress the appetite and to induce satiety. Several randomised controlled studies have confirmed the body weight-reducing effect of topiramate in obese patients [39–41] and a low-dose, controlled-release combination of phentermine and topiramate has been developed for long-term management of obesity [42, 43]. In a large randomised placebo-controlled trial [42], including 2487 overweight and obese patients, the change in body weight at 56 weeks was −1.4 (−1.8 to −0.7) kg, −8.1 kg (−8.5 to −7.1) −10.2 kg (−10.4 to −9.3) in patients receiving placebo, phentermine 7.5 mg plus topiramate 46 mg, and phentermine 15.0 mg plus topiramate 92 mg (all p<0.0001 *versus* placebo). The most common side-effects included dry-mouth, paresthesia, constipation, insomnia and dysgeusia. In the 2-year extension phase of the study, controlled-release phentermine/topiramate was associated with significant, sustained weight loss (−1.8, −9.3 and −10.5% for placebo, low and high dose treatment, respectively) [44]. The rate of adverse events was also reduced compared with the first year.

Extended-release phentermine/topiramate was also tested for treatment of OSA in obese patients. Winslow *et al.* [45] randomised 45 patients with moderate-to-severe OSA to receive placebo or phentermine 15 mg plus extended-release topiramate 92 mg daily for 28 weeks [45]. Both groups received lifestyle modification counselling. At week 28, AHI in phentermine/topiramate group decreased from 44 to 14 events·h^{-1} and in the placebo group from 45 to 27 events·h^{-1} (p=0.0084 between group) (fig. 1). A 10.2% weight reduction was achieved in phentermine/topiramate group compared with a 4.3% weight loss in patients receiving placebo (p=0.0006). The change of AHI was positively correlated with weight change in all the patients (p=0.0003). Overnight oxygen saturation and subjective sleep quality improved in phentermine/topiramate group whereas ESS score did not differ between the two groups. Phentermine/topiramate significantly decreased SBP (−15.0 mmHg *versus* −7.3 mmHg; p=0.0431) but tended to increase heart rate (7.7 bpm *versus* 1.7 bpm; p=0.0708) compared with placebo at 28 weeks. Hence, combination of lifestyle intervention and drug-induced weight loss seems to provide an effective treatment alternative in obese OSA patients not compliant to PAP therapy. Long-term follow-up study is needed to further elucidate the cardiovascular/cognitive side effect of the medication.

Lorcaserin was approved by the FDA as an adjunct to diet and exercise for chronic weight management in 2012. Lorcaserin is a selective agonist on the serotonin receptor 2C

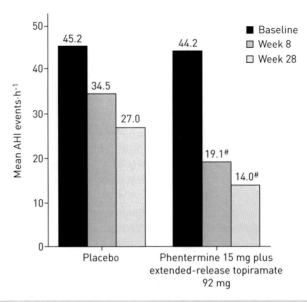

Figure 1. The effect of phentermine 15 mg plus extended-release topiramate 92 mg and placebo on AHI. Both groups received lifestyle modification counselling. #: p<0.01 *versus* placebo. Data from [45].

(5-HT2C), a receptor associated with increased hypothalamic pro-opiomelanocortin production which promotes satiety. Large phase III RCTs have shown that, in conjunction with lifestyle intervention, lorcaserin reduces body weight in a dose-dependent manner and maintains weight loss compared with placebo in overweight and obese patients [46, 47]. 22.6 and 17.4% of patients receiving lorcaserin 10 mg once or twice daily achieved a 10% weight loss compared with 9.7% in the placebo group (all p<0.001 *versus* lorcaserin 10 mg once/twice daily) at 1 year [47]. Lorcaserin was also associated with weight loss and improvement in glycemic control in patients with type 2 diabetes [48]. The side-effects of lorcaserin (*e.g.* headache, dizziness and nausea) are usually mild and well-tolerated. One of the concerns with serotonin agonist usage is increased risk of valvulopathy mainly due to activation of the 5-HT2b receptor. However, a recent analysis on lorcaserin based on 5249 patients from three prospective placebo-controlled trials did not suggest a significant increase of valvulopathy risk (risk ratio 1.16 (95% CI 0.81–1.67)) compared with placebo [49]. Whether the numerical risk increase is associated with greater body weight loss in lorcaserin group or the drug itself is still clear. Follow-up studies are needed to finally determine the risk of long-term usage associated with lorcaserin (*e.g.* tumour, psychiatric disorder and valvulopathy). To our knowledge, there is currently no study addressing the effect of lorcaserin in overweight/obese sleep apnoea patients.

A naltrexone and bupropion combination for sustained-release was recently approved by the FDA for chronic weight management in addition to a reduced-calorie diet and physical activity. Naltrexone is an opioid-receptor antagonist that has been explored in the treatment of alcohol and opioid dependence. Bupropion is a dopamine and norepinephrine reuptake inhibitor that is approved for treatment of depression, seasonal affective disorder as well as for smoking cessation. The combination stimulates hypothalamic pro-opiomelanocortin neurons (bupropion component) and blocks opioid-mediated pro-opiomelanocortin autoinhibition (naltrexone component) which increases energy expenditure and reduces appetite. In addition, this combination modulates the dopamine reward system which may provide a synergistic effect due to a reduction of food intake. Four phase III RCTs were performed to investigate the safety and efficacy of naltrexone plus bupropion in overweight and obese patients. In the Contrave Obesity Research (COR) Behavior Modification trial [50], a combination of naltrexone (32 mg·day^{-1}) and bupropion (360 mg·day^{-1}) was compared with placebo as an adjunct therapy to behavioural modification in 793 patients. At week 56, there was a 9.3±0.4% weight loss in the drug arm compared with a 5.1±0.6% reduction in the placebo group (p<0.001). However, SBP and DBP increased slightly compared with placebo despite an improvement of metabolic parameters. In the COR-I trial (n=1742) [51], two dosage levels of naltrexone (16 and 32 mg·day^{-1}) plus bupropion (360 mg·day^{-1}) were compared with placebo in addition to diet and exercise intervention. At 56 weeks the mean weight change was −6.1, −5.0 and −1.3% in the naltrexone 32 mg plus bupropion, naltrexone 16 mg plus bupropion and placebo group, respectively; 48, 39 and 16% of the participants lost at least 5% of their weight in the three groups, respectively. The combination treatment was not associated with depression or suicidality, but a small increase of blood pressure and heart rate was documented. The most common side-effects included nausea, headache and constipation. A similar weight-loss effect with improvement of metabolic risk markers was demonstrated in obese patients (COR-II study) and in overweight and obese patients with type 2 diabetes (COR-Diabetes study) [52, 53]. However, the change of blood pressure and heart rate in the naltrexone/bupropion combination group has sparked a concern and a RCT addressing long-term cardiovascular safety of the drug is now ongoing (the Light study; ClinicalTrials.gov number: NCT01601704). The effect of a naltrexone/bupropion combination on sleep disordered breathing has not been investigated.

Hence, it is evident that pharmacological therapy can effectively reduce body weight and consequently improve OSA in overweight and obese patients. The pharmacological properties of some of the investigated compounds (*e.g.* carbonic anhydrase inhibitory effect of topiramate [54]) may result in direct effects on respiration which provide an additive influence on the treatment effect. Moreover, these agents may be particularly useful in obese OSA patients with comorbid type II diabetes or hyperlipidaemia since glucose control and lipid metabolism appear to improve in addition to drug-induced weight reduction. Adverse cardiovascular effects (*e.g.* increase heart rate, valvulopathy), potential risk of psychiatric disorders (*e.g.* depression) and tumour development may limit the long-term usage of this type of treatment. Future prospective long-term follow-up studies are needed to examine the benefit and risk of the treatment in overweight and obese patients.

Drug treatment of OSA

Finding a novel drug candidate for OSA treatment has been the aim of various animal/ clinical studies since OSA was first described. Although modest-to-moderate therapeutic effects have been reported in several drug trials, it is generally accepted that there is currently no drug that could be uniformly recommended for treatment of OSA [55, 56]. While most studies focused on increase UA dilatory muscular tone and respiratory drive during sleep, there have been data suggesting that reduction of UA surface tension and overnight rostral-fluid shift also may improve sleep disordered breathing in a selected group of OSA patients. A more detailed overview of pharmacological management explored in OSA is provided in table 2 and in some previous reviews of the topic [77, 78].

Unlike PAP, which directly reverses UA collapse irrespective the pathogenesis of OSA, an effective drug therapy is likely to use a defined target for action. This means that systematic

Table 2. Some potential targets explored for pharmacological treatment of sleep apnoea

Physiological/ pharmacological target	Potential effect on sleep disordered breathing	Drug studied	Clinical relevance
Central nervous serotoninergic mechanisms	Elevation of UA dilator muscular tone during sleep	Paroxetine [57] Fluoxetine [58] Mirtazapine [59, 60]	Modest AHI reduction in non-REM sleep AHI reduction in REM sleep No significant change on AHI; induction of weight gain
Inhibition of carbonic anhydrase	Elevation of ventilatory drive by induction of metabolic acidosis	Acetazolamide [61–65]	Reduced AHI in OSA patients; improved oxygenation and reduction of a breathing disturbance at high altitude; reduced CSA and Cheyne–Stokes breathing in patients with HF Reduced AHI and oxygenation; reduction of body weight
Inhibition of acetylcholinesterase	Elevation of cholinergic activity with enhanced neuromuscular transmission, modified hypoglossal- to-phrenic nerve firing interval, increased saliva production and reduced surface tension	Zonisamide [66] Physostigmine [67] Donepezil [68, 69]	Modest reduction of AHI mainly in REM sleep, reduced total sleep time Modest reduction of AHI, improved oxygenation and daytime sleepiness, decreased sleep efficiency
Renal and systemic volume regulation	Reduction and redistribution of extracellular fluid accumulation/oedema, and increased pharyngeal calibre	Furosemide and spironolactone [70] Spironolactone [71] Metolazone and spironolactone [72] Topical lubricant [73]	Reduction of AHI in severe OSA with diastolic HF Improved AHI and time spent under 90% oxygen saturation in OSA patients with resistant hypertension Modest reduction of AHI in OSA patients with uncontrolled hypertension Modest reduction of AHI both supine and non-supine position
UA surface tension and nasal airway resistance	Reduced surface tension and increase UA compliance Reduction of nasal airflow resistance	Fluticasone [74] Xylometazoline [75] Tramazoline and dexamethasone [76]	Modest AHI reduction in OSA No change in AHI in OSA with chronic nasal congestion Improved nasal breathing and AHI (~20%) in OSA patients with normal nasal resistance at wakefulness

drug development in OSA needs to be based on a phenotypic subselection of patients responsive to a given therapy. In fact, there had been few rational and systematic drug developments originating from a molecular and animal experimental level in the early studies. Most attempts are based on clinical experimental protocols applying existing drugs, with already established toxicity/tolerability, that are used in other medical conditions [79]. It is also important to note a successful pharmacological management in OSA requests good tolerability and low adverse event rate for long-term usage. Drug candidates that potentially worsen the sleep structure and shorten sleep time may not provide a useful solution for long-term treatment of OSA. It is likely that the heterogeneity of the clinical presentation in OSA will provide a limiting factor as proper patient selection in studies need to be based on more detailed phenotypic characterisation of patients. Several recent studies have tried to address this issue using either pathophysiological traits [80] or clinical symptom and comorbidity [81] to phenotype OSA patients and specific drug interventions targeting these phenotypes have shown promising results [82–85].

Conclusion

In conclusion, abundant literature shows that body weight gain worsens OSA and conversely weight loss reduces OSA severity. There is also evidence suggesting that exercise independently of body habitus is associated with a reduced risk of OSA. Hence, lifestyle intervention (*e.g.* dietary, physical activity) is useful in the management of OSA. It is plausible that these interventions are more effective in overweight and obese OSA patients and in those with metabolic comorbidities. In fact, comorbid sleep apnoea attenuated the effect of a lifestyle intervention programme on body weight [86]. When considering the substantial benefits of weight control and physical activity for general health, lifestyle intervention should be recommended to OSA patients as a standard long-term treatment strategy. It appears rational to apply intensive life style intervention in mild-to-moderate OSA patients either alone or in combination with established therapies, such as PAP or oral devices. Different weight loss therapies (*e.g.* behavioural, surgical, and pharmacological) all reduce AHI in OSA patients. Several targets for pharmacological treatment have been studied in OSA. Although some promising concepts have emerged, there is yet no single effective drug for use in clinical practise. Identification of new outcome measures in OSA (*e.g.* hypoxic burden, hypercapnic load, biomarkers of inflammation or vascular dysfunction) may help us to identify patients at particular risk. Future drug development in OSA needs to follow such a "patient-centered" approach. It also needs to be based on vulnerability to various pathophysiological traits, clinical symptomatology and co-morbidity. The time has certainly come for a more diverse approach in the management of OSA.

References

1. West SD, Kohler M, Nicoll DJ, *et al.* The effect of continuous positive airway pressure treatment on physical activity in patients with obstructive sleep apnoea: a randomised controlled trial. *Sleep Med* 2009; 10: 1056–1058.
2. Quan SF, Budhiraja R, Clarke DP, *et al.* Impact of treatment with continuous positive airway pressure (CPAP) on weight in obstructive sleep apnea. *J Clin Sleep Med* 2013; 9: 989–993.
3. Stenlof K, Grunstein R, Hedner J, *et al.* Energy expenditure in obstructive sleep apnea: effects of treatment with continuous positive airway pressure. *Am J Physiol* 1996; 271: E1036–E1043.
4. Dempsey JA, Veasey SC, Morgan BJ, *et al.* Pathophysiology of sleep apnea. *Physiol Rev* 2010; 90: 47–112.
5. King AC, Oman RF, Brassington GS, *et al.* Moderate-intensity exercise and self-rated quality of sleep in older adults. A randomized controlled trial. *JAMA* 1997; 277: 32–37.

6. Tworoger SS, Yasui Y, Vitiello MV, et al. Effects of a yearlong moderate-intensity exercise and a stretching intervention on sleep quality in postmenopausal women. Sleep 2003; 26: 830–836.
7. Passos GS, Poyares D, Santana MG, et al. Effects of moderate aerobic exercise training on chronic primary insomnia. Sleep Med 2011; 12: 1018–1027.
8. Peppard PE, Young T. Exercise and sleep-disordered breathing: an association independent of body habitus. Sleep 2004; 27: 480–484.
9. Hargens TA, Guill SG, Aron A, et al. Altered ventilatory responses to exercise testing in young adult men with obstructive sleep apnea. Respir Med 2009; 103: 1063–1069.
10. Giebelhaus V, Strohl KP, Lormes W, et al. Physical exercise as an adjunct therapy in sleep apnea – an open trial. Sleep Breath 2000; 4: 173–176.
11. Kline CE, Crowley EP, Ewing GB, et al. The effect of exercise training on obstructive sleep apnea and sleep quality: a randomized controlled trial. Sleep 2011; 34: 1631–1640.
12. Sengul YS, Ozalevli S, Oztura I, et al. The effect of exercise on obstructive sleep apnea: a randomized and controlled trial. Sleep Breath 2011; 15: 49–56.
13. Iftikhar IH, Kline CE, Youngstedt SD. Effects of exercise training on sleep apnea: a meta-analysis. Lung 2014; 192: 175–184.
14. Ueno LM, Drager LF, Rodrigues AC, et al. Effects of exercise training in patients with chronic heart failure and sleep apnea. Sleep 2009; 32: 637–647.
15. Servantes DM, Pelcerman A, Salvetti XM, et al. Effects of home-based exercise training for patients with chronic heart failure and sleep apnoea: a randomized comparison of two different programmes. Clin Rehabil 2012; 26: 45–57.
16. Morgan BJ. Exercise: alternative therapy for heart failure-associated sleep apnea? Sleep 2009; 32: 585–586.
17. Peppard PE, Young T, Palta M, et al. Longitudinal study of moderate weight change and sleep-disordered breathing. JAMA 2000; 284: 3015–3021.
18. Peppard PE, Ward NR, Morrell MJ. The impact of obesity on oxygen desaturation during sleep-disordered breathing. Am J Respir Crit Care Med 2009; 180: 788–793.
19. Tkacova R, McNicholas WT, Javorsky M, et al. Nocturnal intermittent hypoxia predicts prevalent hypertension in the European Sleep Apnoea Database cohort study. Eur Respir J 2014; 44: 931–941.
20. Phillips BG, Kato M, Narkiewicz K, et al. Increases in leptin levels, sympathetic drive, and weight gain in obstructive sleep apnea. Am J Physiol Heart Circ Physiol 2000; 279: H234–H237.
21. Jensen MD, Ryan DH, Apovian CM, et al. 2013 AHA/ACC/TOS guideline for the management of overweight and obesity in adults: a report of the American College of Cardiology/American Heart Association Task Force on Practice Guidelines and The Obesity Society. J Am Coll Cardiol 2014; 63: 2985–3023.
22. Tuomilehto HP, Seppa JM, Partinen MM, et al. Lifestyle intervention with weight reduction: first-line treatment in mild obstructive sleep apnea. Am J Respir Crit Care Med 2009; 179: 320–327.
23. Tuomilehto H, Gylling H, Peltonen M, et al. Sustained improvement in mild obstructive sleep apnea after a diet- and physical activity-based lifestyle intervention: postinterventional follow-up. Am J Clin Nutr 2010; 92: 688–696.
24. Tuomilehto H, Seppa J, Uusitupa M, et al. Weight reduction and increased physical activity to prevent the progression of obstructive sleep apnea: A 4-year observational postintervention follow-up of a randomized clinical trial. JAMA Intern Med 2013; 173: 929–930.
25. Johansson K, Neovius M, Lagerros YT, et al. Effect of a very low energy diet on moderate and severe obstructive sleep apnoea in obese men: a randomised controlled trial. BMJ 2009; 339: b4609.
26. Zou D, Grote L, Peker Y, et al. Validation a portable monitoring device for sleep apnea diagnosis in a population based cohort using synchronized home polysomnography. Sleep 2006; 29: 367–374.
27. Johansson K, Hemmingsson E, Harlid R, et al. Longer term effects of very low energy diet on obstructive sleep apnoea in cohort derived from randomised controlled trial: prospective observational follow-up study. BMJ 2011; 342: d3017.
28. Foster GD, Borradaile KE, Sanders MH, et al. A randomized study on the effect of weight loss on obstructive sleep apnea among obese patients with type 2 diabetes: the Sleep AHEAD study. Arch Intern Med 2009; 169: 1619–1626.
29. Kuna ST, Reboussin DM, Borradaile KE, et al. Long-term effect of weight loss on obstructive sleep apnea severity in obese patients with type 2 diabetes. Sleep 2013; 36: 641A–649A.
30. Shechter A, St-Onge MP, Kuna ST, et al. Sleep architecture following a weight loss intervention in overweight and obese patients with obstructive sleep apnea and type 2 diabetes: relationship to apnea-hypopnea index. J Clin Sleep Med 2014; 10: 1205-11.
31. Lam B, Sam K, Mok WY, et al. Randomised study of three non-surgical treatments in mild to moderate obstructive sleep apnoea. Thorax 2007; 62: 354–359.
32. Hoyos CM, Killick R, Yee BJ, et al. Cardiometabolic changes after continuous positive airway pressure for obstructive sleep apnoea: a randomised sham-controlled study. Thorax 2012; 67: 1081–1089.
33. Kajaste S, Brander PE, Telakivi T, et al. A cognitive-behavioral weight reduction program in the treatment of obstructive sleep apnea syndrome with or without initial nasal CPAP: a randomized study. Sleep Med 2004; 5: 125–131.
34. Chirinos JA, Gurubhagavatula I, Teff K, et al. CPAP, weight loss, or both for obstructive sleep apnea. N Engl J Med 2014; 370: 2265–2275.

35. Sarkhosh K, Switzer NJ, El-Hadi M, *et al.* The impact of bariatric surgery on obstructive sleep apnea: a systematic review. *Obes Surg* 2013; 23: 414–423.

36. Greenburg DL, Lettieri CJ, Eliasson AH. Effects of surgical weight loss on measures of obstructive sleep apnea: a meta-analysis. *Am J Med* 2009; 122: 535–542.

37. Fredheim JM, Rollheim J, Sandbu R, *et al.* Obstructive sleep apnea after weight loss: a clinical trial comparing gastric bypass and intensive lifestyle intervention. *J Clin Sleep Med* 2013; 9: 427–432.

38. Dombrowski SU, Knittle K, Avenell A, *et al.* Long term maintenance of weight loss with non-surgical interventions in obese adults: systematic review and meta-analyses of randomised controlled trials. *BMJ* 2014; 348: g2646.

39. Bray GA, Hollander P, Klein S, *et al.* A 6-month randomized, placebo-controlled, dose-ranging trial of topiramate for weight loss in obesity. *Obes Res* 2003; 11: 722–733.

40. Wilding J, Van Gaal L, Rissanen A, *et al.* A randomized double-blind placebo-controlled study of the long-term efficacy and safety of topiramate in the treatment of obese subjects. *Int J Obes Relat Metab Disord* 2004; 28: 1399–1410.

41. Eliasson B, Gudbjörnsdottir S, Cederholm J, *et al.* Weight loss and metabolic effects of topiramate in overweight and obese type 2 diabetic patients: randomized double-blind placebo-controlled trial. *Int J Obes* 2007; 31: 1140–1147.

42. Gadde KM, Allison DB, Ryan DH, *et al.* Effects of low-dose, controlled-release, phentermine plus topiramate combination on weight and associated comorbidities in overweight and obese adults (CONQUER): a randomised, placebo-controlled, phase 3 trial. *Lancet* 2011; 377: 1341–1352.

43. Allison DB, Gadde KM, Garvey WT, *et al.* Controlled-release phentermine/topiramate in severely obese adults: a randomized controlled trial (EQUIP). *Obesity* 2012; 20: 330–342.

44. Garvey WT, Ryan DH, Look M, *et al.* Two-year sustained weight loss and metabolic benefits with controlled-release phentermine/topiramate in obese and overweight adults (SEQUEL): a randomized, placebo-controlled, phase 3 extension study. *Am J Clin Nutr* 2012; 95: 297–308.

45. Winslow DH, Bowden CH, DiDonato KP, *et al.* A randomized, double-blind, placebo-controlled study of an oral, extended-release formulation of phentermine/topiramate for the treatment of obstructive sleep apnea in obese adults. *Sleep* 2012; 35: 1529–1539.

46. Smith SR, Weissman NJ, Anderson CM, *et al.* Multicenter, placebo-controlled trial of lorcaserin for weight management. *N Engl J Med* 2010; 363: 245–256.

47. Fidler MC, Sanchez M, Raether B, *et al.* A one-year randomized trial of lorcaserin for weight loss in obese and overweight adults: the BLOSSOM trial. *J Clin Endocrinol Metab* 2011; 96: 3067–3077.

48. O'Neil PM, Smith SR, Weissman NJ, *et al.* Randomized placebo-controlled clinical trial of lorcaserin for weight loss in type 2 diabetes mellitus: the BLOOM-DM study. *Obesity* 2012; 20: 1426–1436.

49. Weissman NJ, Sanchez M, Koch GG, *et al.* Echocardiographic assessment of cardiac valvular regurgitation with lorcaserin from analysis of 3 phase 3 clinical trials. *Circ Cardiovasc Imaging* 2013; 6: 560–567.

50. Wadden TA, Foreyt JP, Foster GD, *et al.* Weight loss with naltrexone SR/bupropion SR combination therapy as an adjunct to behavior modification: the COR-BMOD trial. *Obesity* 2011; 19: 110–120.

51. Greenway FL, Fujioka K, Plodkowski RA, *et al.* Effect of naltrexone plus bupropion on weight loss in overweight and obese adults (COR-I): a multicentre, randomised, double-blind, placebo-controlled, phase 3 trial. *Lancet* 2010; 376: 595–605.

52. Apovian CM, Aronne L, Rubino D, *et al.* A randomized, phase 3 trial of naltrexone SR/bupropion SR on weight and obesity-related risk factors (COR-II). *Obesity* 2013; 21: 935–943.

53. Hollander P, Gupta AK, Plodkowski R, *et al.* Effects of naltrexone sustained-release/bupropion sustained-release combination therapy on body weight and glycemic parameters in overweight and obese patients with type 2 diabetes. *Diabetes Care* 2013; 36: 4022–4029.

54. Westwood AJ, Vendrame M, Montouris G, *et al.* Pearls & oy-sters: treatment of central sleep apnea with topiramate. *Neurology* 2012; 78: e97–e99.

55. Veasey SC, Guilleminault C, Strohl KP, *et al.* Medical therapy for obstructive sleep apnea: a review by the Medical Therapy for Obstructive Sleep Apnea Task Force of the Standards of Practice Committee of the American Academy of Sleep Medicine. *Sleep* 2006; 29: 1036–1044.

56. Randerath WJ, Verbraecken J, Andreas S, *et al.* Non-CPAP therapies in obstructive sleep apnoea. *Eur Respir J* 2011; 37: 1000–1028.

57. Kraiczi H, Hedner J, Dahlof P, *et al.* Effect of serotonin uptake inhibition on breathing during sleep and daytime symptoms in obstructive sleep apnea. *Sleep* 1999; 22: 61–67.

58. Prasad B, Radulovacki M, Olopade C, *et al.* Prospective trial of efficacy and safety of ondansetron and fluoxetine in patients with obstructive sleep apnea syndrome. *Sleep* 2010; 33: 982–989.

59. Carley DW, Olopade C, Ruigt GS, *et al.* Efficacy of mirtazapine in obstructive sleep apnea syndrome. *Sleep* 2007; 30: 35–41.

60. Marshall NS, Yee BJ, Desai AV, *et al.* Two randomized placebo-controlled trials to evaluate the efficacy and tolerability of mirtazapine for the treatment of obstructive sleep apnea. *Sleep* 2008; 31: 824–831.

61. Whyte KF, Gould GA, Airlie MA, *et al.* Role of protriptyline and acetazolamide in the sleep apnea/hypopnea syndrome. *Sleep* 1988; 11: 463–472.
62. Javaheri S. Acetazolamide improves central sleep apnea in heart failure: a double-blind, prospective study. *Am J Respir Crit Care Med* 2006; 173: 234–237.
63. Nussbaumer-Ochsner Y, Latshang TD, Ulrich S, *et al.* Patients with obstructive sleep apnea syndrome benefit from acetazolamide during an altitude sojourn: a randomized, placebo-controlled, double-blind trial. *Chest* 2012; 141: 131–138.
64. Latshang TD, Nussbaumer-Ochsner Y, Henn RM, *et al.* Effect of acetazolamide and autoCPAP therapy on breathing disturbances among patients with obstructive sleep apnea syndrome who travel to altitude: a randomized controlled trial. *JAMA* 2012; 308: 2390–2398.
65. Javaheri S, Sands SA, Edwards BA. Acetazolamide attenuates Hunter-Cheyne-Stokes breathing but augments the hypercapnic ventilatory response in patients with heart failure. *Ann Am Thorac Soc* 2014; 11: 80–86.
66. Eskandari D, Zou D, Karimi M, *et al.* Zonisamide reduces obstructive sleep apnoea: a randomised placebo-controlled study. *Eur Respir J* 2014; 44: 140–149.
67. Hedner J, Kraiczi H, Peker Y, *et al.* Reduction of sleep-disordered breathing after physostigmine. *Am J Respir Crit Care Med* 2003; 168: 1246–1251.
68. Moraes W, Poyares D, Sukys-Claudino L, *et al.* Donepezil improves obstructive sleep apnea in Alzheimer disease: a double-blind, placebo-controlled study. *Chest* 2008; 133: 677–683.
69. Sukys-Claudino L, Moraes W, Guilleminault C, *et al.* Beneficial effect of donepezil on obstructive sleep apnea: a double-blind, placebo-controlled clinical trial. *Sleep Med* 2012; 13: 290–296.
70. Bucca CB, Brussino L, Battisti A, *et al.* Diuretics in obstructive sleep apnea with diastolic heart failure. *Chest* 2007; 132: 440–446.
71. Gaddam K, Pimenta E, Thomas SJ, *et al.* Spironolactone reduces severity of obstructive sleep apnoea in patients with resistant hypertension: a preliminary report. *J Hum Hypertens* 2010; 24: 532–537.
72. Kasai T, Bradley TD, Friedman O, *et al.* Effect of intensified diuretic therapy on overnight rostral fluid shift and obstructive sleep apnoea in patients with uncontrolled hypertension. *J Hypertens* 2014; 32: 673–680.
73. Jokic R, Klimaszewski A, Mink J, *et al.* Surface tension forces in sleep apnea: the role of a soft tissue lubricant: a randomized double-blind, placebo-controlled trial. *Am J Respir Crit Care Med* 1998; 157: 1522–1525.
74. Kiely JL, Nolan P, McNicholas WT. Intranasal corticosteroid therapy for obstructive sleep apnoea in patients with co-existing rhinitis. *Thorax* 2004; 59: 50–55.
75. Clarenbach CF, Kohler M, Senn O, *et al.* Does nasal decongestion improve obstructive sleep apnea? *J Sleep Res* 2008; 17: 444–449.
76. Koutsourelakis I, Minaritzoglou A, Zakynthinos G, *et al.* The effect of nasal tramazoline with dexamethasone in obstructive sleep apnoea patients. *Eur Respir J* 2013; 42: 1055–1063.
77. Hedner J, Zou D. Pharmacological management of sleep-disordered breathing. *In:* McNicholas WT, Bonsignore MR, eds. Sleep Apnoea. *Eur Respir Monogr* 2010; 50: pp. 321–339.
78. Mason M, Welsh EJ, Smith I. Drug therapy for obstructive sleep apnoea in adults. *Cochrane Database Syst Rev* 2013; 5: CD003002.
79. Hedner J, Grote L, Zou D. Pharmacological treatment of sleep apnea: current situation and future strategies. *Sleep Med Rev* 2008; 12: 33–47.
80. Eckert DJ, White DP, Jordan AS, *et al.* Defining phenotypic causes of obstructive sleep apnea. Identification of novel therapeutic targets. *Am J Respir Crit Care Med* 2013; 188: 996–1004.
81. Ye L, Pien GW, Ratcliffe SJ, *et al.* The different clinical faces of obstructive sleep apnoea: a cluster analysis. *Eur Respir J* 2014; 44: 1600–1607.
82. Eckert DJ, Owens RL, Kehlmann GB, *et al.* Eszopiclone increases the respiratory arousal threshold and lowers the apnoea/hypopnoea index in obstructive sleep apnoea patients with a low arousal threshold. *Clin Sci* 2011; 120: 505–514.
83. Edwards BA, Sands SA, Eckert DJ, *et al.* Acetazolamide improves loop gain but not the other physiological traits causing obstructive sleep apnoea. *J Physiol* 2012; 590: 1199–1211.
84. Grace KP, Hughes SW, Horner RL. Identification of a pharmacological target for genioglossus reactivation throughout sleep. *Sleep* 2014; 37: 41–50.
85. Chapman JL, Kempler L, Chang CL, *et al.* Modafinil improves daytime sleepiness in patients with mild to moderate obstructive sleep apnoea not using standard treatments: a randomised placebo-controlled crossover trial. *Thorax* 2014; 69: 274–279.
86. Borel AL, Leblanc X, Almeras N, *et al.* Sleep apnea attenuates the effects of a lifestyle intervention programme in men with visceral obesity. *Thorax* 2012; 67: 735–741.

Disclosures: **None declared.**

Chapter 18

Mandibular advancement devices

Fernanda R. de Almeida[1,7], Peter Cistulli[2,3,7], Bernard Fleury[4,7] and Frederic Gagnadoux[5,6,7]

Nasal CPAP is the primary treatment of OSA, but many patients are unable or unwilling to comply with this treatment. MADs have emerged as the main non-CPAP therapeutic option for OSA. Despite its lower efficacy to reduce sleep disordered breathing, most trials comparing MADs and CPAP reported similar health outcomes. The greater efficacy of CPAP may be offset by a lower compliance relative to MADs. Individual titration of mandibular advancement is of primary importance to achieve successful MAD therapy. Younger, thinner patients with positional OSA and lower AHI appear to be most successful with MAD therapy. However, there is no reliable method to individually predict treatment response. The dentist plays a key role in determining whether the patient is a good dental candidate for MAD therapy, selecting the appropriate device and detecting side-effects during long-term MAD therapy.

We will review the evidence in favour of MAD therapy and discuss the main challenges to the success of MADs in treating OSA.

MADs are thought to primarily act through anterior movement of the tongue, and consequently increase the anteroposterior dimensions of the oropharynx. However, using a range of imaging modalities, many studies suggest that MADs increase the cross-sectional area of the velopharynx, in both the lateral and anteroposterior dimensions, and increase the lateral dimension of the oropharynx [1–3]. These changes are thought to be mediated through the palatoglossal and palatopharyngeal arches, which link the muscles of the tongue, soft palate, lateral pharyngeal walls and the mandibular attachments. Inter-individual variability in airway changes induced by mandibular advancement may reflect variations in anatomy and function, and this is likely to have major relevance to the variable clinical response associated with this treatment modality.

Patient selection

The American Academy of Sleep Medicine practice parameters on MADs, last published in 2006 but currently under review, advocate the use of MADs in patients with mild-to-moderate OSA who prefer this form of treatment over CPAP, or who do not respond

[1]Dept of Oral Health Sciences, University of British Columbia, Vancouver, BC, Canada. [2]Dept of Respiratory Medicine, Royal North Shore Hospital, Sydney, Australia. [3]University of Sydney, Sydney, Australia. [4]Sleep Unit, Saint-Hospital, Paris VI University, Paris, France. [5]Dept of Respiratory Diseases, University Hospital of Angers, Angers, France. [6]INSERM Unit 1063, Angers, France. [7]Authors contributed equally to this publication.

Correspondence: Frédéric Gagnadoux, Dépt de Pneumologie, CHU Angers, 4 rue Larrey, 49033 Angers, France.
E-mail: frgagnadoux@chu-angers.fr

to or are unable to tolerate CPAP [4]. Since then the evidence base supporting the use of MADs has grown considerably, thereby potentially expanding the scope for MAD therapy as a first-line therapy. Selection of appropriate patients for MAD therapy, based on the likelihood of successful treatment, remains a somewhat elusive goal at present. While considerable research using a variety of techniques has attempted to identify the factors that predict a good response, the clinical utility of such approaches remains to be proven. In the absence of clear selection criteria, patient selection largely relies on clinical judgment and patient preference.

Not all patients are medically suitable candidates for the use of MADs. A major clinical limitation of MAD therapy is that it generally takes some time (weeks) to attain optimal therapy, and hence caution is warranted in considering MAD therapy in circumstances where there is an urgent need to commence treatment quickly (*e.g.* concern about driving risk and co-existent unstable medical comorbidities). Moreover, this treatment modality has no known role in treating CSA or hypoventilation disorders. Given that in some patients' OSA is worsened by MADs [5, 6], and the known placebo effect [7, 8], there is a need for objective verification of treatment outcome using in-laboratory or home sleep testing.

The dentist plays a key role in determining whether or not the patient is a good dental candidate for MAD therapy. The patient should have the ability to protrude the mandible forward in order to achieve a therapeutic result, although it is unclear whether a minimum degree of protrusion is required. Caution is warranted in patients with temporomandibular joint problems. The presence of periodontal disease may promote excessive tooth movement under MADs. All these factors tend to limit the scope of this form of therapy, and one European study has suggested that up to one-third of patients are excluded on the basis of such factors [9]. Beyond appropriate patient selection, the dentist's role is also to select an appropriate device design for each patient, taking into account specific clinical features.

Predictors of treatment response

An important issue limiting the role of MADs for the treatment of OSA is the inability to reliably predict treatment response. Research has focussed on patient factors, including anthropomorphic and polysomnographic factors. Clinical characteristics reported to be associated with a better outcome include younger age, lower BMI, supine-dependent OSA, a smaller oropharynx, smaller overjet, shorter soft palate and smaller neck circumference [10]. In general, it is considered that a good response is more likely to be reported in lower degrees of OSA severity (mild-to-moderate), although benefit in severe OSA has been reported [11, 12]. Cephalometric variables, such as a shorter soft palate, longer maxilla, decreased distance between mandibular plane and hyoid bone, alone or in combination with other anthropomorphic and polysomnographic variables, are thought to be somewhat predictive [7, 13].

Physiological studies in the sleeping state indicate that primary retroglossal, rather than velopharyngeal, collapse is highly predictive of success [14]. A range of physiological measurements during wakefulness, including nasal resistance and flow–volume loops, have been reported to differ between responders and nonresponders. UA imaging during wakefulness may also assist in predicting treatment response. UA magnetic resonance imaging (MRI) studies suggest that baseline airway and soft tissue anatomical characteristics do not differ significantly between responders and nonresponders [2]. However, the changes resulting in mandibular advancement do differ such that an increase in airway volume is reasonably predictive of a favourable outcome. Application of computational modelling techniques to imaging studies appears to enhance prediction [15]. Whilst such sophisticated imaging studies are helpful in understanding fundamental mechanisms, the clinical utility of such approaches is limited due to cost and accessibility. A more clinically accessible imaging modality is nasendoscopy. Studies during wakefulness [3] and drug-induced sleep [16] have reported predictive potential. Lateral widening of the velopharynx during awake endoscopy in the supine position is associated with a higher likelihood of success [3]. Drug-induced sleep endoscopy without and with a mandibular advancement simulation bite has been used to visualise the magnitude and patterns of pharyngeal collapse [16]. Patients with a greater improvement in pharyngeal patency under mandibular advancement conditions were more likely to respond to treatment.

MAD titration

In anesthetised OSA patients [17], mandibular advancement produces a dose-dependent closing pressure reduction of all pharyngeal segments. In the same patients during normal sleep, repetitive overnight oximetry with and without MADs showed that each 2-mm mandibular advancement coincided with ~20% improvement in number and severity of nocturnal desaturations. These results established that MADs open the passive pharynx in a dose-dependent fashion. According to the pharyngeal anatomy, temporomandibular joint characteristics, elasticity of the soft tissues and mandibular advancement achieving maximal therapeutic effect is different among subjects and has to be individually determined. As for CPAP, an individual titration process is necessary.

At present, many MAD titration protocols have been proposed [18], but there is no emerging consensual gold standard procedure.

Remotely controlled mandibular protrusion during sleep

Four studies experimentally simulated the mechanical action of a MAD by progressively protruding the mandible during sleep under polysomnographic examination. The aim of this method was to recognise MAD responders in 1 night and determine the effective mandibular advancement. In the first study [19], a temporary MAD connected to a hydraulic system, which was progressively adjusted during the night, allowed the authors to determine an effective mandibular advancement decreasing the AHI to <10 events·h^{-1} in 42.9% of patients on follow-up PSG. In three other studies [20–22], a trial MAD was connected to a stepping motor. The rotation of the motor extended the lower tray of the MAD. The positive and negative predictive values of mandibular advancement titration for subsequent treatment success were high, and in two studies remotely controlled mandibular positioner titration predicted a reliable estimate of the therapeutic mandibular advancement [21, 22]. This elegant approach has the great advantage of quickly defining the effective mandibular advancement, but requires in-laboratory sleep recording and has a particular hardware.

Combined analysis of symptomatic benefit and sleep recordings

A combined analysis of repeated clinical evaluations (snoring and diurnal vigilance) and oximetric recordings was used in severe OSA patients who failed to continue CPAP therapy [23]. The mandible was advanced 1 mm every week until symptoms resolved and the ODI was reduced to <10, or a maximal comfortable limit of mandibular advancement was reached. A complete response (AHI <10 events·h^{-1}) was obtained in 63% of patients. Of note, 25% of mandibular advancement increases were motivated by an abnormal ODI, despite subjective resolution of the symptoms.

The course of snoring index and AHI has been studied during progressive mandibular advancement with a custom MAD using sequential limited sleep recordings [24]. Mandibular advancement was increased until either reduction of AHI to <10 events·h^{-1} or attainment of the maximal limit of comfort. On average, MADs improved AHI by 70% and snoring index by 60% at the final mandibular advancement. In 54% of complete responders and 29% of partial responders, AHI decreased by 83% and 71%, respectively, at the end of the titration procedure. Comparatively, a previous review pooling data from 74 studies including 2816 patients showed a mean reduction in AHI of only 55% on MADs [25], but in most included studies the degree of mandibular advancement had been arbitrarily set without any individual titration.

Several studies have combined self-adjustment of mandibular advancement by the patient followed by a polysomnographic evaluation to potentially decide further advancement. Two groups of mild-to-moderate OSA patients had a MAD set at 70% of the maximal protrusion and were randomly allocated to subjective self-adjustment for 6 weeks, or fixed 70% mandibular advancement for 3 weeks and then self-adjustment for 3 weeks after objective control using PSG [26]. The overall improvement obtained with the two methods was similar but the amount of further forward titration performed by the two groups of patients was very small. Of note, a majority of the patients (91%) in the objective group reported using the MADs every night compared to 69% in the subjective group.

In two studies [27, 28], self-adjustment of mandibular advancement to the point of good symptomatic control was followed by a titration PSG with the opportunity to further increase mandibular advancement during the night. In the two studies, 65–69% of the patients were efficiently treated after the self-adjustment period with AHI <10 events·h^{-1} and reduction of AHI by at least 50%. The incomplete responders had their MADs further titrated during titration PSG and this increased treatment success by about 30%.

Therapeutic effects of MADs

Sleep disordered breathing

RCTs comparing the effects of active *versus* inactive oral appliances in patients with mild-to-severe OSA have demonstrated that MADs reduce the number of respiratory disturbances during sleep and their immediate consequences on oxygen saturation, sleep structure and fragmentation [7, 29–34]. However, MADs are clearly less effective than CPAP in reducing sleep disordered breathing. Table 1 presents a summary of 11 RCTs (eight crossover and three parallel-group studies) comparing MADs with CPAP in OSA patients [5, 11, 12, 33, 35–41]. Most included patients had moderate OSA (mean AHI 26.4) and were mildly sleepy (mean ESS 11.4). On average, AHI was reduced by 61% for MADs *versus* 84% for CPAP. CPAP performed significantly better than MADs in terms of reduction of AHI in nine out of 11 studies. A complete treatment response, defined by an AHI <5 events·h^{-1}, was achieved in 19–43% of patients with MADs *versus* 34–75% with CPAP [11, 12, 36]. A recent meta-analysis confirmed the superiority of CPAP in reducing AHI [42].

Table 1. Summary of RCT comparing MADs and CPAP therapy in OSA

First author [ref.]	Study design	Sample size n	Baseline patient characteristics			AHI treatment		ESS treatment		CPAP versus MAD
			BMI kg m^{-2}	AHI	ESS	CPAP	MAD	CPAP	MAD	
FERGUSON [5]	Crossover, 2×16 weeks	25	30.4±4.8	24.5±8.8		3.6±1.7	9.7±7.3¶			Equivalent
FERGUSON [35]	Crossover, 2×16 weeks	20	32.0±8.2	25.3±15.0	10.6±3.4	4.0±2.0	14.2±14.7¶	5.1±3.3	4.7±2.6	Equivalent
ENGLEMAN [36]	Crossover, 2×8 weeks	48		31±26	14±4	8±6	15±16¶	8±5	12±5¶	Equivalent
RANDERATH [37]	Crossover, 2×6 weeks	20	31.2±6.4	17.5±7.7		3.2±2.9	10.5±7.5¶			MAD>CPAP
TAN [38]	Crossover, 2×8 weeks	24	31.9±6.8	22.2±9.6	13.4±4.6	3.1±2.8	8.0±10.9	8.1±4.1	9.0±5.1	MAD>CPAP
BARNES [39]	Crossover, 3×12 weeks	104	Mean±SEM: 31.0±0.6	Mean±SEM: 21.5±1.6	Mean±SEM: 10.2±0.5	Mean±SEM: 4.8±0.5	Mean±SEM: 14.0±1.1*	Mean±SEM: 9.2±0.4	Mean±SEM: 9.2±0.4	MAD>CPAP
LAM [40]	Parallel, 10 weeks#	109	Mean±SEM: 27.4± 0.6	CPAP: 23.8±1.9 MAD: 20.9±1.7	CPAP: 12±1 MAD: 12±1	Mean±SEM: 2.8±1.1	Mean±SEM: 10.6±1.7*	Mean±SEM: 7±1	Mean±SEM: 9±1¶	MAD>CPAP
HOEKEMA [41]	Parallel, 8–12 weeks	103		CPAP: 40.3±27.6 MAD: 39.4±30.8	CPAP:14.2±5.6 MAD: 12.9±5.6	2.4±4.2	7.8±14.4¶	5.9±4.8	6.9±5.5	Equivalent
GAGNADOUX [11]	Crossover, 2×8 weeks	56	26.7±3.5	34.2±13.0	10.6±4.5	6.9±5.7	2.7±3.5¶	8.2±3.9	7.7±4.0	MAD>CPAP
AARAB [33]	Parallel, 24 weeks#	57	28.9±3.4	CPAP: 20.9±9.8 MAD: 22.1±10.8	CPAP:10.2±4.7 MAD: 11.8±5.8	Δvalue 19.5±8.7	Δvalue 16.3±10.3			Equivalent
PHILLIPS [12]	Crossover, 2×4 weeks	108	29.5±5.5	26.6±12.3	9.1±4.2	4.5±6.6	11.1±12.1¶	Mean±SEM: 7.5±0.4	Mean±SEM: 7.2±0.4	MAD>CPAP
Mean			29.9	26.4	11.4	4.2	10.2	7.6	8.4	

Data are presented as mean±SD, unless otherwise stated. #: including placebo group; ¶: CPAP performed better than MAD.

Alertness, cognition and health-related quality of life

OSA is associated with impairment of daytime alertness, cognition, emotional state and health-related quality of life (HRQoL). Treatment with MADs more markedly improved daytime alertness, neurobehavioral functioning and HRQoL than inactive oral devices [8, 30–32]. Among nine RCTs with available data for ESS [11, 12, 33, 35, 36, 38–41], seven concluded on a similar improvement of daytime sleepiness with MADs and CPAP in mildly sleepy patients (mean baseline ESS 10.8) [11, 12, 33, 35, 38, 39, 41], and two studies including patients with more severe daytime sleepiness (mean baseline ESS 13) found a more marked reduction of ESS with CPAP [36, 40]. A similar impact of MADs and CPAP on ESS was found in a recent meta-analysis [42]. Three RCTs that included objective assessment of daytime alertness, either by the maintenance of wakefulness test [36, 39] or the Oxford Sleep Resistance Test [11], showed no difference between MADs and CPAP. No differences between the two treatments were observed in three RCTs reporting the outcome of cognitive performance tests [11, 12, 36] and in two studies evaluating driving simulator performances, which were improved to the same extent by both MADs and CPAP [12, 43]. Discordant findings were obtained in terms of HRQoL outcome with MADs *versus* CPAP [11, 12, 33, 36, 39, 41]. Out of six RCTs reporting the outcome of the Short Form-36 health survey (SF-36) [12, 33, 36, 39, 40, 43], two studies found that changes in SF-36 score were not different between the two treatments [33, 41], two concluded on a more marked improvement in several domains of the HRQoL with CPAP including "bodily pain", "physical functioning" [40], "health transition" and "mental component" [36], one found that only CPAP was more effective than placebo [39], and one recent crossover trial concluded that MADs performed better than CPAP by improving four out of eight SF-36 domains and the overall mental component score [12]. In another crossover trial reporting the outcome of the Nottingham Heath Profile general HRQoL questionnaire, MAD therapy was associated with a significant improvement in four out of six domains, whereas only two domains where improved with CPAP [11].

Blood pressure

A dose–response relationship between OSA severity and hypertension has clearly been documented by cross-sectional and longitudinal studies in both community- and clinic-based populations [44–48]. The most recent meta-analysis (based on 28 RCTs including 1948 patients with OSA) demonstrated a modest but significant reduction in SBP (≈-2.6 mmHg) and DBP (≈-2.0 mmHg) with CPAP therapy [49]. In a crossover trial comparing the outcome of 24-h ambulatory BP monitoring after 4 weeks of MAD therapy and 4 weeks of inactive oral appliance in 61 OSA patients, MAD therapy resulted in a significant reduction in 24-h DBP (mean±SD 1.8±0.5 mmHg), awake SBP (3.3±1.1 mmHg) and awake DBP (3.4±0.9 mmHg). A recent meta-analysis of seven studies enrolling 399 participants concluded on a favourable effect of MADs on SBP, DBP and mean arterial BP [50], but most of the included studies were observational. Only two RCTs compared the outcome of ambulatory BP monitoring in patients treated with MADs and CPAP [12, 39]. In a parallel-group study including a placebo arm, BARNES *et al.* [39] found that MAD therapy was associated with an improvement in night time DBP, but reported no other significant changes with either MADs or CPAP. In a recent crossover trial [12], neither treatment lowered BP from baseline in the entire group but similar 24-h BP improvements of between 2 and 4 mmHg were observed for all indexes with MADs and CPAP in the subgroup of patients with comorbid hypertension at diagnosis.

Cardiovascular outcomes

OSA is associated with an increased risk of CVDs including stroke, coronary heart disease and HF [51–54]. Regular CPAP therapy for moderate-to-severe OSA is associated with a decreased incidence of cardiovascular events compared to untreated OSA patients or subjects with poor CPAP compliance (<4 $h \cdot night^{-1}$) [54, 55]. A recent non-concurrent observational cohort study monitored cardiovascular mortality in 208 control subjects and 461 severe OSA patients (177 CPAP treated, 72 MAD treated and 212 untreated) for a median of 6.6 years. The cardiovascular mortality rate was significantly higher in the untreated OSA group than in either treatment group, with no difference between CPAP and MADs, despite a higher treatment AHI in MAD-treated patients [56]. Endothelial dysfunction has been recognised as a key early event that precedes or accelerates the development of atherosclerosis [57] and may be predictive of future cardiovascular events in at-risk patients [58]. A small randomised crossover trial involving 12 severe OSA patients has demonstrated a similar improvement in endothelial function as assessed by acetylcholine-induced vasodilation after 2 months of MADs and CPAP [59].

Treatment adherence

Treatment adherence can be affected by numerous factors and although major focus has been given to the type of therapy, such as oral appliance design or CPAP characteristics, there are also contributing factors such as patient preference, social and economic status, healthcare system/team, characteristics of the disease and other patient-related factors. The consequences of a non-tailored treatment with poor patient adherence are related to poor health outcomes and increased healthcare costs.

Current literature in the field of MADs has shown that treatment adherence to MADs differs depending on the type of appliance, disease severity and patient supervision [60, 61]. For example, adherence rates are greater with custom MADs than tongue retaining or non-custom MADs [62, 63]. QUINNELL et al. [64] described the nightly use of non-custom MADs to be significantly less compared to custom MADs (4.4 versus 5.7 $h \cdot night^{-1}$), and the discontinuation rate to be higher in non-custom MADs (17% versus 8%). Self-reported use of MADs has been reported as high, with 96% of patients using it most of the night (>75% of the night per week) and 80% of patients using their device for >75% of their sleep period [65]. In a large retrospective study including 630 patients using MAD therapy, MARKLUND et al. [66] described adherence rates of 75% of patients who remained adherent after 12 months of treatment. After a period of 2–5 years of follow-up, studies have revealed adherence rates of 48% up to 90% where 60% and 48% of patients reported continued regular use of their appliances at 1 and 2 years, respectively [24, 67, 68].

Previous experience with nasal CPAP suggests that self-reported treatment adherence tends to over estimation of actual use. As a recent development, three microsensors are currently available that can be integrated into MADs: TheraMon (Hargelsberg, Austria), Air Aid Sleep (AIR AID GmbH, Frankfurt, Germany) and DentiTrac (Braebon Medical Corporation, Kanata, Canada). All three microsensors are safe, comfortable and provide reliable and accurate wear-time once incorporated into custom MADs [69]. DIELTJENS et al. [70] evaluated 1-year objectively measured adherence during MAD therapy and compared it to self-reported use. The discontinuation rate was 9.8% at 1 year; the remaining patients used their MADs for an average of 6.1 h·night^{-1} for 83% of nights. Interestingly, the patient's self-reported compliance showed a mean 30-min overestimation when compared to objective compliance.

Overall therapeutic effectiveness

Despite the superior efficacy of CPAP to reduce AHI, most RCTs comparing MADs and CPAP in patients with moderate-to-severe OSA and mild-to-moderate daytime sleepiness reported similar health outcomes in terms of sleepiness, neurobehavioral functioning, quality of life and BP [11, 12, 33, 38, 39, 43]. Recent findings also suggest similar cardiovascular outcomes with MADs and CPAP [56, 59]. These finding can probably be explained by the fact that the superior efficacy of CPAP is offset by the poorer compliance relative to MADs, resulting in a similar overall therapeutic effectiveness [71]. A recent study defined mean disease alleviation as the product of objective MAD compliance measured by an embedded microsensor thermometer, adjusted by sleep duration and therapeutic efficacy [69]. MDA was used as a measure of overall therapeutic effectiveness. Figure 1 shows that MADs and CPAP and have similar overall therapeutic effectiveness, with mean disease alleviation values of 51.1% and 55.8%, respectively [12, 69].

Side-effects of MAD therapy

Although initial side-effects related to the use of MADs are usually classified as mild and transient, these side-effects, along with insufficient reduction of snoring, are the main reasons for discontinuing treatment [72]. Initial side-effects are excessive salivation, although dry mouth is also a complaint, mouth or teeth discomfort, morning-after occlusal changes and discomfort in the gums, muscle tenderness and jaw stiffness. Custom MADs can be adjusted to reduce pressure on the teeth and gums, and a decrease in the mandibular

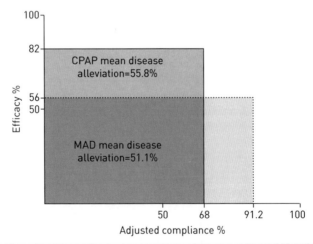

Figure 1. Overall therapeutic effectiveness of CPAP and MAD, measured as mean disease alleviation. Mean disease alleviation is equal to the area of the rectangle for which the length is given by the adjusted compliance (objective daily use/sleep duration), and the height is given by the therapeutic efficacy (baseline AHI–treatment AHI). Reproduced and modified from [69] with permission from the publisher.

advancement can also improve muscle tenderness. In the majority of the cases these side-effects resolve with time.

The impact of these side-effects on patient's comfort has been evaluated and compared to CPAP. Using the same visual analogue scale, GAGNADOUX et al. [11] found the impact of these side-effects to be small and presented similar scores between MADs and CPAP. Similar results have been found in other RCTs and, therefore, short-term side-effects to MADs are considered mild and acceptable.

The temporomandibular joint is often a concern for patients and professionals involved in MAD therapy. DE ALMEIDA et al. [73] assessed the temporomandibular joint of seven patients over a mean period of 11 months with MRI and found the MAD to move the temporomandibular joint within the normal limits and to be innocuous to the temporomandibular joint in OSA patients. Over a period of 2 years, DOFF et al. [74] evaluated the occurrence of temporomandibular disorders related to MADs and CPAP treatment. They found a limited long-term risk of developing pain or function impairment of the temporomandibular complex with either treatment. The occurrence of (pain-related) tempromandibular joint disorders increased in the initial period of MAD therapy, but tended to return to baseline values during a 2-year follow-up.

Craniofacial changes related to long-term use of MADs has been widely studied. Bite changes are commonly reported by patients after a period of 1 to 2 years of continuing MAD use [74–79]. Using a titratable MAD, ALMEIDA and co-workers [75, 76] demonstrated that using MADs for a mean period of 7.3 years has a significant impact on occlusal and dental structures. Changes observed in craniofacial structures were mainly related to significant tooth movements. PLISKA et al. [80] evaluated dental changes after an average observation period of 11 years. Clinically significant changes in occlusion were observed and were progressive, with a reduction in overbite (mean±SD 2.3±1.6 mm), overjet (1.9±1.9 mm) and mandibular crowding (1.3±1.8 mm). Dental side-effects, such as overjet, mandibular intercanine distance and lower arch crowding, all continuously decreased at a constant rate over time. Interestingly, by evaluating various studies on different appliance designs, such as herbst [77], mobloc [79], klearway [75], somnomed [78] and Thornton Adjustable Positioner (Airway Management Inc., Dallas, TX, USA) [81], it has been shown that the amount of change was related to the duration of therapy and not the type of appliance used. When comparing side-effects of MADs and CPAP over a 2-year period, DOFF et al. [81], found a significantly greater change in overbite and overjet with MADs compared to CPAP. Craniofacial changes related to MADs do occur and are mainly related to dental movements. It is important to notice that patient's perceptions do not typically correlate with objective measurements and occlusal changes often go unnoticed [82]. This may be explained by the development of new occlusal contacts resulting from new occlusal equilibrium over time [83]. Patient's perception of side-effects and the benefits of MADs have to be assessed in a patient-specific evaluation and despite the presence of irreversible long-term occlusal changes, oral appliance therapy should be considered as a lifelong treatment for patients with OSA.

Conclusion

There is increasing evidence that MADs constitute an effective therapeutic option for OSA with a higher compliance relative to CPAP that may compensate the lower efficacy of this treatment modality in reducing sleep disordered breathing. The recent development of embedded microsensors allowing objective measurement of MAD compliance offers the opportunity to validate this hypothesis and to perform long-term research on the comparative effectiveness of MADs and CPAP for the management of OSA. Additional studies are also required to improve our ability to predict treatment response and side-effects of long-term MADs. Efforts should also be made to standardise the procedure for optimal mandibular advancement titration that has to be implemented for every OSA patient for whom MAD therapy is considered.

References

1. Gale DJ, Sawyer RH, Woodcock A, et al. Do oral appliances enlarge the airway in patients with obstructive sleep apnoea? A prospective computerized tomographic study. Eur J Orthod 2000; 22: 159–168.
2. Chan AS, Sutherland K, Schwab RJ, et al. The effect of mandibular advancement on upper airway structure in obstructive sleep apnoea. Thorax 2010; 65: 726–732.
3. Chan AS, Lee RW, Srinivasan VK, et al. Nasopharyngoscopic evaluation of oral appliance therapy for obstructive sleep apnoea. Eur Respir J 2010; 35: 836–842.
4. Kushida CA, Morgenthaler TI, Littner MR, et al. Practice parameters for the treatment of snoring and obstructive sleep apnea with oral appliances: an update for 2005. Sleep 2006; 29: 240–243.
5. Ferguson KA, Ono T, Lowe AA, et al. A randomized crossover study of an oral appliance vs nasal-continuous positive airway pressure in the treatment of mild-moderate obstructive sleep apnea. Chest 1996; 109: 1269–1275.
6. Henke KG, Frantz DE, Kuna ST. An oral elastic mandibular advancement device for obstructive sleep apnea. Am J Respir Crit Care Med 2000; 161: 420–425.
7. Mehta A, Qian J, Petocz P, et al. A randomized, controlled study of a mandibular advancement splint for obstructive sleep apnea. Am J Respir Crit Care Med 2001; 163: 1457–1461.
8. Gotsopoulos H, Chen C, Qian J, et al. Oral appliance therapy improves symptoms in obstructive sleep apnea: a randomized, controlled trial. Am J Respir Crit Care Med 2002; 166: 743–748.
9. Petit FX, Pepin JL, Bettega G, et al. Mandibular advancement devices: rate of contraindications in 100 consecutive obstructive sleep apnea patients. Am J Respir Crit Care Med 2002; 166: 274–278.
10. Chan AS, Cistulli PA. Oral appliance treatment of obstructive sleep apnea: an update. Curr Opin Pulm Med 2009; 15: 591–596.
11. Gagnadoux F, Fleury B, Vielle B, et al. Titrated mandibular advancement versus positive airway pressure for sleep apnoea. Eur Respir J 2009; 34: 914–920.
12. Phillips CL, Grunstein RR, Darendeliler MA, et al. Health outcomes of continuous positive airway pressure versus oral appliance treatment for obstructive sleep apnea: a randomized controlled trial. Am J Respir Crit Care Med 2103; 187: 879–887.
13. Mayer G, Meier-Ewert K. Cephalometric predictors for orthopaedic mandibular advancement in obstructive sleep apnoea. Eur J Orthod 1995; 17: 35–43.
14. Ng AT, Qian J, Cistulli PA. Oropharyngeal collapse predicts treatment response with oral appliance therapy in obstructive sleep apnoea. Sleep 2006; 29: 666–671.
15. Zhao M, Barber T, Cistulli PA, et al. Computational fluid dynamics for the assessment of upper airway response to oral appliance treatment in obstructive sleep apnoea. J Biomech 2013; 46: 142–150.
16. Vroegop AV, Vanderveken OM, Dieltjens M, et al. Sleep endoscopy with simulation bite for prediction of oral appliance treatment outcome. J Sleep Res 2013; 22: 348–355.
17. Kato J, Isono S, Tanaka A, et al. Dose-dependent effects of mandibular advancement on pharyngeal mechanics and nocturnal oxygenation in patients with sleep-disordered breathing. Chest 2000; 117: 1065–1072.
18. Dieltjens M, Vanderveken OM, Heyning PH, et al. Current opinions and clinical practice in the titration of oral appliances in the treatment of sleep-disordered breathing. Sleep Med Rev 2012; 16: 177–185.
19. Petelle B, Vincent G, Gagnadoux F, et al. One-night mandibular advancement titration for obstructive sleep apnea syndrome: a pilot study. Am J Respir Crit Care Med 2002; 165: 1150–1153.
20. Tsai WH, Vazquez JC, Oshima T, et al. Remotely controlled mandibular positioner predicts efficacy of oral appliances in sleep apnea. Am J Respir Crit Care Med 2004; 170: 366–370.
21. Dort LC, Hadjuk E, Remmers JE. Mandibular advancement and obstructive sleep apnoea: a method for determining effective mandibular protrusion. Eur Respir J 2006; 27: 1003–1009.
22. Remmers J, Charkhandeh S, Grosse J, et al. Remotely controlled mandibular protrusion during sleep predicts therapeutic success with oral appliances in patients with obstructive sleep apnea. Sleep 2013; 36: 1517–1525.

23. Fleury B, Rakotonanahary D, Petelle B, *et al.* Mandibular advancement titration for obstructive sleep apnea: optimization of the procedure by combining clinical and oximetric parameters. *Chest* 2004; 125: 1761–1767.
24. Gindre L, Gagnadoux F, Meslier N, *et al.* Mandibular advancement for obstructive sleep apnea: dose effect on apnea, long-term use and tolerance. *Respiration* 2008; 76: 386–392.
25. Hoffstein V. Review of oral appliances for treatment of sleep-disordered breathing. *Sleep Breath* 2007; 11: 1–22.
26. Campbell AJ, Reynolds G, Trengrove H, *et al.* Mandibular advancement splint titration in obstructive sleep apnoea. *Sleep Breath* 2009; 13: 157–162.
27. Almeida FR, Parker JA, Hodges JS, *et al.* Effect of a titration polysomnogram on treatment success with a mandibular repositioning appliance. *J Clin Sleep Med* 2009; 5: 198–204.
28. Krishnan V, Collop NA, Scherr SC. An evaluation of a titration strategy for prescription of oral appliances for obstructive sleep apnea. *Chest* 2008; 133: 1135–1141.
29. Hans MG, Nelson S, Luks VG, *et al.* Comparison of two dental devices for treatment of obstructive sleep apnea syndrome (OSAS). *Am J Orthod Dentofacial Orthop* 1997; 111: 562–570.
30. Naismith SL, Winter VR, Hickie IB, *et al.* Effect of oral appliance therapy on neurobehavioral functioning in obstructive sleep apnea: a randomized controlled trial. *J Clin Sleep Med* 2005; 1: 374–380.
31. Blanco J, Zamarron C, Abeleira Pazos MT, *et al.* Prospective evaluation of an oral appliance in the treatment of obstructive sleep apnea syndrome. *Sleep Breath* 2005; 9: 20–25.
32. Petri N, Svanholt P, Solow B, *et al.* Mandibular advancement appliance for obstructive sleep apnoea: results of a randomised placebo controlled trial using parallel group design. *J Sleep Res* 2008; 17: 221–229.
33. Aarab G, Lobbezoo F, Hamburger HL, *et al.* Oral appliance therapy *versus* nasal continuous positive airway pressure in obstructive sleep apnea: a randomized, placebo-controlled trial. *Respiration* 2011; 81: 411–419.
34. Andren A, Hedberg P, Walker-Engstrom ML, *et al.* Effects of treatment with oral appliance on 24-h blood pressure in patients with obstructive sleep apnea and hypertension: a randomized clinical trial. *Sleep Breath* 2013; 17: 705–712.
35. Ferguson KA, Ono T, Lowe AA, *et al.* A short-term controlled trial of an adjustable oral appliance for the treatment of mild to moderate obstructive sleep apnoea. *Thorax* 1997; 52: 362–368.
36. Engleman HM, McDonald JP, Graham D, *et al.* Randomized crossover trial of two treatments for sleep apnea/hypopnea syndrome: continuous positive airway pressure and mandibular repositioning splint. *Am J Respir Crit Care Med* 2002; 166: 855–859.
37. Randerath WJ, Heise M, Hinz R, *et al.* An individually adjustable oral appliance *vs* continuous positive airway pressure in mild-to-moderate obstructive sleep apnea syndrome. *Chest* 2002; 122: 569–575.
38. Tan YK, L'Estrange PR, Luo YM, *et al.* Mandibular advancement splints and continuous positive airway pressure in patients with obstructive sleep apnoea: a randomized cross-over trial. *Eur J Orthod* 2002; 24: 239–249.
39. Barnes M, McEvoy RD, Banks S, *et al.* Efficacy of positive airway pressure and oral appliance in mild to moderate obstructive sleep apnea. *Am J Respir Crit Care Med* 2004; 170: 656–664.
40. Lam B, Sam K, Mok WY, *et al.* Randomised study of three non-surgical treatments in mild to moderate obstructive sleep apnoea. *Thorax* 2007; 62: 354–359.
41. Hoekema A, Stegenga B, Wijkstra PJ, *et al.* Obstructive sleep apnea therapy. *J Dent Res* 2008; 87: 882–887.
42. Li W, Xiao L, Hu J. The comparison of CPAP and oral appliances in treatment of patients with OSA: a systematic review and meta-analysis. *Respir Care* 2013; 58: 1184–1195.
43. Hoekema A, Stegenga B, Bakker M, *et al.* Simulated driving in obstructive sleep apnoea-hypopnoea; effects of oral appliances and continuous positive airway pressure. *Sleep Breath* 2007; 11: 129–138.
44. Bixler EO, Vgontzas AN, Lin HM, *et al.* Association of hypertension and sleep-disordered breathing. *Arch Intern Med* 2000; 160: 2289–2295.
45. Nieto FJ, Young TB, Lind BK, *et al.* Association of sleep-disordered breathing, sleep apnea, and hypertension in a large community-based study. Sleep Heart Health Study. *JAMA* 2000; 283: 1829–1836.
46. Peppard PE, Young T, Palta M, *et al.* Prospective study of the association between sleep-disordered breathing and hypertension. *N Engl J Med* 2000; 342: 1378–1384.
47. Lavie P, Herer P, Hoffstein V. Obstructive sleep apnoea syndrome as a risk factor for hypertension: population study. *BMJ* 2000; 320: 479–482.
48. Marin JM, Agusti A, Villar I, *et al.* Association between treated and untreated obstructive sleep apnea and risk of hypertension. *JAMA* 2012; 307: 2169–2176.
49. Montesi SB, Edwards BA, Malhotra A, *et al.* The effect of continuous positive airway pressure treatment on blood pressure: a systematic review and meta-analysis of randomized controlled trials. *J Clin Sleep Med* 2012; 8: 587–596.
50. Iftikhar IH, Hays ER, Iverson MA, *et al.* Effect of oral appliances on blood pressure in obstructive sleep apnea: a systematic review and meta-analysis. *J Clin Sleep Med* 2013; 9: 165–174.
51. Bradley TD, Floras JS. Obstructive sleep apnoea and its cardiovascular consequences. *Lancet* 2009; 373: 82–93.
52. Redline S, Yenokyan G, Gottlieb DJ, *et al.* Obstructive sleep apnea-hypopnea and incident stroke: the sleep heart health study. *Am J Respir Crit Care Med* 2010; 182: 269–277.
53. Gottlieb DJ, Yenokyan G, Newman AB, *et al.* Prospective study of obstructive sleep apnea and incident coronary heart disease and heart failure: the sleep heart health study. *Circulation* 2010; 122: 352–360.

54. Marin JM, Carrizo SJ, Vicente E, et al. Long-term cardiovascular outcomes in men with obstructive sleep apnoea-hypopnoea with or without treatment with continuous positive airway pressure: an observational study. Lancet 2005; 365: 1046–1053.

55. Barbe F, Duran-Cantolla J, Sanchez-de-la-Torre M, et al. Effect of continuous positive airway pressure on the incidence of hypertension and cardiovascular events in nonsleepy patients with obstructive sleep apnea: a randomized controlled trial. JAMA 2012; 307: 2161–2168.

56. Anandam A, Patil M, Akinnusi M, et al. Cardiovascular mortality in obstructive sleep apnoea treated with continuous positive airway pressure or oral appliance: an observational study. Respirology 2013; 18: 1184–1190.

57. Ross R. Atherosclerosis – an inflammatory disease. N Engl J Med 1999; 340: 115–126.

58. Perticone F, Ceravolo R, Pujia A, et al. Prognostic significance of endothelial dysfunction in hypertensive patients. Circulation 2001; 104: 191–196.

59. Trzepizur W, Gagnadoux F, Abraham P, et al. Microvascular endothelial function in obstructive sleep apnea: Impact of continuous positive airway pressure and mandibular advancement. Sleep Med 2009; 10: 746–752.

60. McGown AD, Makker HK, Battagel JM, et al. Long-term use of mandibular advancement splints for snoring and obstructive sleep apnoea: a questionnaire survey. Eur Respir J 2001; 17: 462–466.

61. Dort LC, Hussein J. Snoring and obstructive sleep apnea: compliance with oral appliance therapy. J Otolaryngol 2004; 33: 172–176.

62. Vanderveken OM, Devolder A, Marklund M, et al. Comparison of a custom-made and a thermoplastic oral appliance for the treatment of mild sleep apnea. Am J Respir Crit Care Med 2008; 178: 197–202.

63. Deane SA, Cistulli PA, Ng AT, et al. Comparison of mandibular advancement splint and tongue stabilizing device in obstructive sleep apnea: a randomized controlled trial. Sleep 2009; 32: 648–653.

64. Quinnell TG, Bennett M, Jordan J, et al. A crossover randomised controlled trial of oral mandibular advancement devices for obstructive sleep apnoea-hypopnoea (TOMADO). Thorax 2014; 69: 938–945.

65. de Almeida FR, Lowe AA, Tsuiki S, et al. Long-term compliance and side effects of oral appliances used for the treatment of snoring and obstructive sleep apnea syndrome. J Clin Sleep Med 2005; 1: 143–152.

66. Marklund M, Stenlund H, Franklin KA. Mandibular advancement devices in 630 men and women with obstructive sleep apnea and snoring: tolerability and predictors of treatment success. Chest 2004; 125: 1270–1278.

67. Clark GT, Sohn JW, Hong CN. Treating obstructive sleep apnea and snoring: assessment of an anterior mandibular positioning device. J Am Dent Assoc 2000; 131: 765–771.

68. Yoshida K. Effects of a mandibular advancement device for the treatment of sleep apnea syndrome and snoring on respiratory function and sleep quality. Cranio 2000; 18: 98–105.

69. Vanderveken OM, Dieltjens M, Wouters K, et al. Objective measurement of compliance during oral appliance therapy for sleep-disordered breathing. Thorax 2013; 68: 91–96.

70. Dieltjens M, Braem MJ, Vroegop AV, et al. Objectively measured vs self-reported compliance during oral appliance therapy for sleep-disordered breathing. Chest 2013; 144: 1495–1502.

71. Vanderveken OM, Braem MJ, Dieltjens M, et al. Objective measurement of the therapeutic effectiveness of continuous positive airway pressure versus oral appliance therapy for the treatment of obstructive sleep apnea. Am J Respir Crit Care Med 188: 1162.

72. Ferguson KA, Cartwright R, Rogers R, et al. Oral appliances for snoring and obstructive sleep apnea: a review. Sleep 2006; 29: 244–262.

73. de Almeida FR, Bittencourt LR, de Almeida CI, et al. Effects of mandibular posture on obstructive sleep apnea severity and the temporomandibular joint in patients fitted with an oral appliance. Sleep 2002; 25: 507–513.

74. Doff MH, Veldhuis SK, Hoekema A, et al. Long-term oral appliance therapy in obstructive sleep apnea syndrome: a controlled study on temporomandibular side effects. Clin Oral Investig 2012; 16: 689–697.

75. Almeida FR, Lowe AA, Otsuka R, et al. Long-term sequellae of oral appliance therapy in obstructive sleep apnea patients: Part 2. Study-model analysis. Am J Orthod Dentofacial Orthop 2006; 129: 205–213.

76. Almeida FR, Lowe AA, Sung JO, et al. Long-term sequellae of oral appliance therapy in obstructive sleep apnea patients: Part 1. Cephalometric analysis. Am J Orthod Dentofacial Orthop 2006; 129: 195–204.

77. Battagel JM, Kotecha B. Dental side-effects of mandibular advancement splint wear in patients who snore. Clin Otolaryngol 2005; 30: 149–156.

78. Hammond RJ, Gotsopoulos H, Shen G, et al. A follow-up study of dental and skeletal changes associated with mandibular advancement splint use in obstructive sleep apnea. Am J Orthod Dentofacial Orthop 2007; 132: 806–814.

79. Marklund M. Predictors of long-term orthodontic side effects from mandibular advancement devices in patients with snoring and obstructive sleep apnea. Am J Orthod Dentofacial Orthop 2006; 129: 214–221.

80. Pliska BT, Nam H, Chen H, et al. Obstructive sleep apnea and mandibular advancement splints: occlusal effects and progression of changes associated with a decade of treatment. J Clin Sleep Med 2014; 10: 1285–1291.

81. Doff MH, Finnema KJ, Hoekema A, et al. Long-term oral appliance therapy in obstructive sleep apnea syndrome: a controlled study on dental side effects. Clin Oral Investig 2013; 17: 475–482.

82. Marklund M, Franklin KA, Persson M. Orthodontic side-effects of mandibular advancement devices during treatment of snoring and sleep apnoea. *Eur J Orthod* 2001; 23: 135–144.

83. Martinez-Gomis J, Willaert E, Nogues L, *et al.* Five years of sleep apnea treatment with a mandibular advancement device. Side effects and technical complications. *Angle Orthod* 2010; 80: 30–36.

Disclosures: P. Cistulli is a chief investigator on sponsored clinical trials in obstructive sleep apnoea for ResMed Inc. and Exploramed Inc. His department receives equipment support for oral appliance research from SomnoMed Ltd, and he has a pecuniary interest in the company from previous involvement in product development. He is a medical advisor to Exploramed Inc. (a US medical device incubator) and Zephyr Sleep Technologies. He has received speaker fees/travel support from ResMed Inc., Fisher & Paykel Healthcare and SomnoMed Ltd. He receives book royalties from Quintessence Publishing. B. Fleury reports personal fees from Bluesom, outside the submitted work. In addition, B. Fleury has a patent on a thermoplastic oral appliance.

Chapter 19

New ventilator support in complex phenotypes: coexisting CSA and OSA

Winfried J. Randerath

Sleep-related breathing disorders can present with several phenotypes of OSA and CSA, and also hypoventilation. These include disorders with increased (*e.g.* high altitude or periodic breathing in CVDs) or reduced respiratory drive (*e.g.* opioid-induced sleep apnoea), and reduced minute ventilation in neuromuscular, skeletal or chronic pulmonary diseases. A subgroup of patients present with combinations of various phenotypes, which can be called a coexisting or complicated breathing pattern. The term "complex sleep apnoea" should be reserved for patients with newly emerging and persisting CSA under application of PAP. Optimal treatment requires precise determination of the underlying pathophysiology in order to select the best available therapy. New devices and algorithms combine fixed or automatically adapted expiratory pressure to overcome UA obstruction, variable pressure support to address increased or decreased ventilatory drive, and mandatory breaths to counterbalance CSA. The spectrum of PAP algorithms allows for individualised treatment and should be carefully adapted under polysomnographic control by experienced sleep specialists.

The complexity and heterogeneity of sleep-related breathing disorders (SRBDs) is currently being recognised and discussed intensively. This development was stimulated by the increasing awareness of SRBDs in several medical disciplines, caring for patients with cardiovascular, renal or chronic pain diseases. These patients often suffer not only from the classical phenotypes of OSA, CSA or hypoventilation syndromes, but also from various combinations of these phenotypes [1]. Moreover, sleep physicians are faced with periodic breathing, ataxic respiration and changing breathing patterns that evolve under therapy. Large and representative studies on the prevalence of these complicated breathing patterns are lacking. In addition, the terminology in the field of SRBDs is confusing, which impedes specific and individualised therapy. However, a clear diagnosis and discrimination of the phenotypes is urgently required in order to avoid inadequate or unnecessary treatments. New devices and algorithms have been developed to address the underlying pathophysiology of specific clinical situations [2, 3].

Institute of Pneumology at the University Witten/Herdecke, Clinic for Pneumology and Allergology, Centre of Sleep Medicine and Respiratory Care, Bethanien Hospital, Solingen, Germany

Correspondence: Winfried J. Randerath, Institute of Pneumology at the University Witten/Herdecke, Clinic for Pneumology and Allergology, Centre of Sleep Medicine and Respiratory Care, Bethanien Hospital, Aufderhöherstraße 169–175, 42699 Solingen, Germany. E-mail: randerath@klinik-bethanien.de

Copyright ©ERS 2015. Print ISBN: 978-1-84984-059-0. Online ISBN: 978-1-84984-060-6. Print ISSN: 2312-508X. Online ISSN: 2312-5098.

Phenotypes of non-obstructive breathing disturbances during sleep

CSA and periodic breathing

As a first approach, CSA may be differentiated into hypercapnic and non-hypercapnic CSA. Hypercapnic CSA and hypoventilation disorders are characterised by a reduction in the minute volume due to insufficient respiratory drive, impaired translation of breathing impulses to the muscles, or abnormalities of musculoskeletal function or morphology.

By contrast, respiratory drive or the sensitivity of the chemoreceptors to metabolic changes is increased and often leads to chronic hyperventilation in non-hypercapnic CSA. The function of the respiratory system has been described as a loop gain [4–8]. The feedback gain (central and peripheral chemoreceptors) measures any changes in the arterial carbon dioxide tension (PaCO_2) (and, less relevantly, the arterial oxygen tension) in the blood. Increases in the PaCO_2 induce elevations of the ventilatory impulses generated by the controller gain (the brain stem). The plant gain (lung and thoraco-skeletal system) executes these impulses by varying the minute ventilation. The level of the loop gain describes the relative change of the system to any breathing disturbance. Patients with non-hypercapnic CSA present with an elevated loop gain leading to over- and undershooting of minute ventilation, while loop gain is dampened in hypercapnic CSA. Periodic breathing at high altitude or Cheyne–Stokes respiration are clinical examples of a high loop gain.

Periodic breathing describes the polysomnographic phenotype of waxing and waning of respiratory flow and effort, *i.e.* a continuous shift between hyperventilation and hypoventilation up to central apnoea. The term Cheyne–Stokes respiration (or Hunter–Cheyne–Stokes respiration) should be reserved for the clinical syndrome composed of the polysomnographic pattern of periodic breathing on the one hand and typical underlying CVDs (especially HF) on the other [9–12].

Opioid-induced sleep apnoea

Patients who chronically use opioids often present with a variety of SRBDs, including obstructive disturbances, sustained hypoxia and hypoventilation or, most typically, ataxic breathing. The latter is characterised by a chaotic pattern of changing breathing frequency and amplitudes of the flow. PATTINSON [13] described shallow and irregular respiration leading to hypercapnia and hypoxia. The pathophysiology of opioid-induced sleep apnoea differs substantially from non-hypercapnic CSA. Opioids inhibit respiratory rhythms by suppressing brain stem activity, leading to reduced breathing frequency. Peripheral and central chemosensitivity play a major role, leading to a diminished hypoxic and hypercapnic ventilatory response. Moreover, opioids impede the activity of the UA muscles which predisposes to obstructive disturbances. In essence, opioid-induced sleep apnoea represents a hypercapnic phenotype of sleep apnoea [14].

CPAP-emerging CSA, complex sleep apnoea and coexisting breathing patterns

MORGENTHALER et al. [15] described the term complex sleep apnoea (CompSAS) in patients who were treated with CPAP for OSA. They found that the titration of CPAP eliminated obstructive disturbances, but that a central apnoea index of $\geqslant5$ events·h^{-1} remained or a Cheyne–Stokes pattern became prominent and sleep disruptive. JAVAHERI et al. [16]

differentiated CSA under CPAP into CPAP-emergent CSA, CPAP-resistant CSA and CPAP-persistent CSA. Patients with CPAP-emergent CSA present with OSA, but only rare CSA in the baseline PSG. However, CPAP titration evokes central disturbances, which disappear with continued CPAP use. Thus, CPAP-emergent CSA is acute and transient. By contrast, the central disturbances remain under continuous use in CPAP-persistent CSA. Conversely, CSA exists prior to treatment in CPAP-resistant CSA and is not induced by CPAP. CVDs or chronic opioid use are common risk factors for CPAP-resistant CSA (fig. 1). The transient character of a subgroup of CPAP-emergent CSA is confirmed by a prospective follow-up study in 675 OSA patients [17]. Interestingly, the majority of patients with CPAP-emergent CSA at baseline lost the phenomenon at follow-up, while others had newly developed CompSAS after 3 months. CompSAS was associated with impaired sleep quality and, thus, might be induced by arousals [17]. The pathophysiological background and the prevalence of CompSAS are under discussion. The substantial differences in prevalence may be due to different definitions and patient populations [18, 19].

In order to prevent misdiagnosis of CompSAS it is crucially important to identify and treat any underlying diseases. Their optimal treatment may reduce or eliminate breathing disturbances in pre-existing CSA (CPAP-resistant CSA). In a retrospective study, KUŹNIAR et al. [20] identified that 46.7% of 150 patients presented with one or more risk factors, such as arterial hypertension, coronary artery disease, congestive HF, atrial fibrillation or stroke (10–54%), diabetes and depression (28 and 30% respectively), or chronic opioid use (18.7%). Sleep insufficiency, insomnia and arousals can contribute to the emergence of CSA under PAP treatment [18, 19].

In addition, avoidable influences have to be recognised which do not fulfil the diagnosis of CompSAS. These include excessive titration, post-hyperventilation apnoea, post-arousal apnoea and misclassification of central hypopnoeas [21–24]. OSA and CSA may be heterogeneously distributed throughout the night [25]. If the diagnosis is build up on a split night PSG, the investigator may underestimate the relevance of central disturbances. However, PAP titration during the second part of the night will unmask these pre-existing central disturbances, which may be misdiagnosed as CompSAS (split night error). Finally, the resolution of UA obstruction allows for more effective elimination of CO_2. However, due to a higher CO_2 sensitivity in OSA, the prevailing CO_2 level may go under the individual apnoea threshold and induce central apnoea until the system adapts to a new set-point (ventilatory instability in OSA) [26–28].

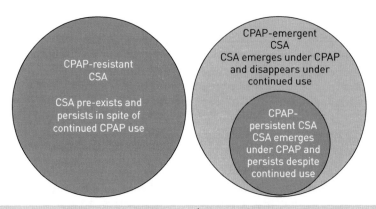

Figure 1. The phenotypes of CSA observed under CPAP (for a detailed explanation see the main text).

Putting these aspects together, the term CompSAS should be reserved for those patients with CSA newly developed under treatment and which persists under continuous use. By contrast, the combination of OSA on the one hand and CSA due to pre-existing comorbidities on the other describes the coexistence of two different diseases.

Other complicated breathing patterns, and the combination of OSA with any phenotype of central disturbances or hypoventilation should be described as "coexisting OSA and CSA (or Cheyne–Stokes respiration or hypoventilation)".

Hypoventilation disorders

Reduction of the minute volume is a common characteristic of hypoventilation disorders. They can generate from all levels of the respiratory system, including insufficient respiratory drive, impaired translation of the breathing impulses from the brain stem *via* the spinal cord and the peripheral nerves to the respiratory muscles, and functional or morphological abnormalities of the thorax and the muscles themselves.

Hypoventilation can be part of complicated breathing patterns and may be combined with other components as follows. 1) Neuromuscular diseases can be associated with passive closure of the UA. 2) The obesity hypoventilation syndrome is characterised by an impaired hypoxic and hypercapnic ventilatory response, leptin resistance, obstruction of the UA (in most cases OSA), an increased work of breathing and impaired ventilation–perfusion mismatch in the lungs. 3) The pathophysiology of COPD includes loss of vascular and parenchymal structures of the lungs, leading to impaired gas exchange, but also an imbalance of CO_2 production and minute ventilation. It is characterised by instability and obstruction of the small airways.

Therapeutic approach to complicated breathing patterns

The efficacy of oxygen, drugs, CPAP, BPAP and new ventilator support algorithms (including adaptive servo-ventilation (ASV)) differs substantially in patients with OSA, CSA and coexisting phenotypes.

The heterogeneous treatment response may be characterised by variable relative contributions of the loop gain [29–31], the respiratory drive and the airway obstruction to the evolution of the disease in an individual patient (fig. 2). ASV seems to be the best option to counterbalance the ventilatory instability in high loop gain (*e.g.* Cheyne–Stokes respiration or high altitude). BRADLEY *et al.* [32] have shown that CPAP reduces CSA by 50%, which may be due to an improvement in left ventricular function. However, CPAP fails to normalise CSA and the continuous application of PAP (CPAP, pressure support or controlled ventilation) may even propagate ventilatory instability by eliminating CO_2 [33, 34]. By contrast, these less variable, more controlled modes of ventilation may be indicated in patients with airway obstruction, reduced respiratory drive, reduced loop gain or other hypoventilatory disorders.

Thus, a practical approach to the patients with complicated breathing patterns can be based on the separation of the major pathophysiological components and on the individual adjustment of the device (fig. 3).

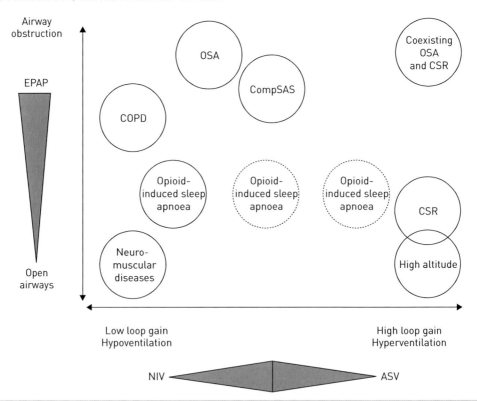

Figure 2. A description of the (hypothetical) relative contribution of level of the loop gain and the airway obstruction to the pathophysiology of various phenotypes of complicated breathing patterns. The higher the loop gain the higher the instability of the respiratory system. Periodic breathing at high altitude and Cheyne–Stokes respiration (CSR) represent high loop gain diseases. The loop gain may also be increased in complex sleep apnoea (CompSAS), although at a lower level. By contrast, hypoventilation disorders are characterised by reduced respiratory drive and low loop gain. The level of upper (OSA) and lower airway (COPD) obstruction is defined by the position on the y-axis. The diagram also illustrates that the individual components may vary and this defines their position in the diagram (as symbolised by the closed and dotted circles for opioid-induced sleep apnoea). In addition, the position of the components may lead the therapeutic approach. The higher the instability of the system is the more effective adaptive servo-ventilation (ASV) is. Whereas, the lower the respiratory drive and the instability the more ventilatory support is required. The level of obstruction defines the need for expiratory pressure to stabilise the upper and lower airways. NIV: noninvasive ventilation.

1) Obstruction of the upper or lower airways: airway obstruction can be addressed by increasing intraluminal pressure using CPAP or BPAP in the spontaneous mode (BPAP-S). These modes stabilise the UA, help avoid collapse of the small airways in COPD and improve the ventilation–perfusion mismatch. The reduction of the expiratory pressure in BPAP may ease respiration for the patient. Expiratory pressure relief algorithms apply different levels during early and end-expiration. These algorithms have not been shown to improve efficacy or adherence in general, but allow for an individualised approach.

2) Increased or decreased respiratory drive: reduced ventilatory drive can be addressed by the application of mandatory breaths. By contrast, the ventilatory over- and undershoot in high loop gain (Cheyne–Stokes respiration) may be counterbalanced by ASV.

3) Reduction of the minute ventilation: fixed or variable pressure support and mandatory breaths assure the necessary minute ventilation in hypoventilation disorders. While

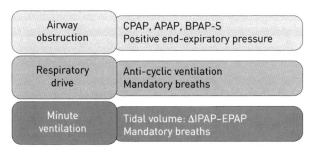

Figure 3. Pathophysiology-oriented therapeutic approach. For patients with complicated breathing patterns, the selection and setting of PAP devices can be based on analysis of the level of obstruction, the respiratory drive and the prevailing minute ventilation. The figure shows the therapeutic options for addressing the underlying pathophysiological component. BPAP-S: BPAP in the spontaneous mode; APAP: automatic PAP; ΔIPAP–EPAP: difference between IPAP and EPAP.

noninvasive ventilation (pressure or volume support, or controlled ventilation) is well established for patients with hypercapnic CSA, it may not be indicated or may even propagate the ventilatory overshoot.

New ventilator support algorithms

ASV, also called automatic servo-ventilation or anti-cyclic modulated ventilation (ACMV), primarily addresses breathing disturbances associated with high loop gain. ASV devices combine automatic CPAP, automatic pressure support and the application of mandatory breaths [2, 3]. The different ASV devices share several characteristics and features.

1) They measure the instantaneous airflow continuously in a moving time window and calculate an average of either peak inspiratory airflow or minute ventilation over the breaths during this window. The breaths contribute progressively less as new breaths are constantly added [3]. If a predefined range around the average is exceeded or missed, the algorithms modulate the pressure support anti-cyclically. The difference (ΔIPAP–EPAP) between the actual IPAP and the EPAP defines the pressure support [3].

2) The expiratory pressure serves to sustain UA patency. As in automatic CPAP, the EPAP level varies according to the prevailing obstruction in the most recent versions of ASV devices.

3) The variable pressure support in ASV differs substantially from the fixed ΔIPAP–EPAP in BPAP algorithms [35]. During periods of hyperventilation fixed pressure support increases CO_2 elimination and, therefore, propagates central disturbances and periodicity. By contrast, ASV reduces ΔIPAP–EPAP during hyperventilation and elevates it during hypoventilation so that the vicious circle can be interrupted.

4) Similar to BPAP (with backup frequency, *i.e.* BPAP in spontaneous-timed mode (BPAP-ST) or BPAP in timed mode), ASV applies mandatory breaths in central apnoeas.

The trilevel algorithm focuses on patients with coexisting OSA and CSA, and combinations of sleep apnoea phenotypes with sleep related hypoventilation. It combines variable pressure support and automatic adaptation of expiratory pressure (ASV) with the automatic adaptation of end-expiratory pressure (EEP). The relief of pressure during early expiration is based on endoscopic studies, which showed that the diameter of the UA is widest during early and narrowest during end-expiration. Therefore, the EEP is pivotal for the elimination of UA obstruction so that the pressure can be reduced during early expiration (EPAP). The difference between the pressure during inspiration and the early expiration pressure (equivalent to ΔIPAP−EPAP in ASV) defines tidal volume. Due to the lowering of the pressure during early expiration, the same tidal volume can be achieved with lower inspiratory pressures. Similar to automatic CPAP, the variation of the EEP overcomes UA obstruction, while pressure support eliminates CSA or counterbalances sustained hypoventilation. Recently, we compared the trilevel algorithm with CPAP in 35 patients in a cross-over study for 4 weeks [36]. The patients suffered from severe coexisting OSA and Cheyne–Stokes respiration. The study confirmed the equal efficacy of both algorithms in terms of OSA and superiority of the trilevel algorithm regarding central disturbances. Only the trilevel algorithm improved ejection fraction, while objective sleep quality and patient's adherence did not differ significantly [36]. However, further RCTs in different populations, including obesity hypoventilation are required.

Noninvasive ventilation generates the minute ventilation by a fixed difference between inspiratory and expiratory pressure (pressure support, pressure controlled ventilation) or tidal volume (volume support, volume controlled ventilation) together with a fixed breathing rate or back-up frequency. However, these rigid modes may be insufficient or unnecessary for clinical situations with varying requirements of the ventilation support, *e.g.* according to changes in the body position, sleep stage or patient's respiratory drive. To address these situations and complicated breathing patterns more closely, algorithms have been designed which allow for setting a fixed tidal volume but automatically adjust the tidal volume in order to ensure a predetermined target: pressure support ventilation with target volume (also known as average volume assured pressure support (AVAPS)) [37–39]. The most recent releases of the pressure support ventilation with target volume mode also include an automatic variation of the expiratory pressure to overcome UA obstruction.

Clinical efficacy of ASV

ASV in Cheyne–Stokes respiration

The efficacy of ASV in the treatment of Cheyne–Stokes respiration has been intensively studied over the short and long term, and compared with other PAP and non-PAP options [40–58]. TESCHLER *et al.* [56] compared ASV with oxygen, BPAP and CPAP in a randomised order for one night each in 14 stable HF patients under optimal medical treatment. CPAP reduced the AHI by half, while ASV improved SRBD by >80%. The effect of CPAP was similar to oxygen which confirmed previous findings [48, 56]. JAVAHERI *et al.* [44] compared CPAP and the two different modes of ASV, one with fixed and one with automatic adjustment of EPAP. CPAP reduced the total AHI and CSA by ~50%, while ASV was superior to CPAP in the suppression of hypopnoeas as well as central and mixed apnoeas. Interestingly, the advanced ASV device conferred an additional improvement in central disturbances compared with ASV with fixed EPAP [44, 54].

The superiority of ASV may be due to the fact that it interferes with the pathophysiology of Cheyne–Stokes respiration. Sufficient pressure support during hypoventilation normalises oxygen saturation and prevents a hypoxic ventilatory response. ASV reduces the sensitivity of the chemoreceptors to hypercapnia which dampens the overshoot of the system [49].

Moreover, several randomised and nonrandomised studies have shown improvements in left ventricular function [41, 43, 46, 52, 55]. In addition, a nonrandomised cohort study in patients with stable congestive HF and Cheyne–Stokes respiration found improvement of cardiac parameters and deaths or rehospitalisation [58], as well as glomerular filtration rate [47, 57]. ASV significantly reduced the stroke volume index in healthy controls, but not in chronic stable HF patients. The stroke volume index improved under ASV in a subgroup of HF patients with high pulmonary capillary wedge pressure and mitral regurgitation [58]. Therefore, the study is consistent with previous findings showing that PAP application improves cardiac function in HF by reducing preload, improving functional mitral regurgitation and the configuration of the heart [45, 51, 53].

Increased sympathetic activity is a marker of pour outcome. HARADA et al. [42] showed a modest positive correlation between muscle sympathetic nerve activity and respiratory instability in HF patients with periodic breathing in contrast to patients without periodic breathing. ASV reduced respiratory parameters and consequently muscle sympathetic nerve activity [42]. PEPPERELL et al. [50] performed a double-blind RCT comparing effective with subtherapeutic ASV over 1 month and found a significant improvement in EDS, brain natriuretic peptide (BNP) and metadrenaline excretion under therapeutic ASV.

PHILIPPE et al. [52] studied efficacy and compliance under ASV as compared with CPAP. While daily use decreased under CPAP, it improved under ASV at 6 months. There were no significant improvements in daytime sleepiness (ESS). However, the scores were low at baseline which is a typical finding in Cheyne–Stokes respiration. Therefore, there was only limited room for improvement. Nevertheless, the quality of life measured using the Minnesota questionnaire was significantly improved with ASV as compared with CPAP [52].

ASV in CompSAS, coexisting CSA and OSA, and other central disturbances

Most studies have primarily included patients with almost pure Cheyne–Stokes respiration or CSA. Based on the results of pilot studies [59], we conducted a randomised CPAP-controlled study for 12 months in 70 patients with coexisting OSA and CSA in mild-to-moderate HF [60]. ASV was equally effective in suppressing obstructive disturbances as CPAP, but was significantly superior with respect to central events and BNP as a marker of cardiac function [60]. The data on the efficacy of ASV for SRBD and BNP have been confirmed by ARZT et al. [61].

There are no prospective controlled trials on ASV in idiopathic CSA, high-altitude CSA or other forms of central disturbances. ASV has been compared with noninvasive positive pressure ventilation in CSA/Cheyne–Stokes respiration, CompSAS and mixed sleep apnoea. While both options sufficiently improved respiratory disturbances, ASV was more effective than noninvasive positive pressure ventilation [62]. Retrospective data from a heterogeneous population of CPAP non-responders demonstrated superiority of ASV as compared with the other PAP therapies [63].

ARZT et al. [64] described a subgroup of primary CPAP non-responders who improved over 3 months of ongoing CPAP therapy. Therefore, MORGENTHALER et al. [65] performed a multicentre RCT comparing optimised CPAP with ASV over 90 days. The patients suffered from a variety of underlying diseases or comorbidities, including cardiovascular disorders, insomnia and restless legs syndrome, or chronic opioid use. ASV was superior in terms of respiratory disturbances, both at the initial titration and after 90 days. The efficacy of CPAP improved substantially over time. Although the difference between ASV and CPAP was statistically significant, the clinical relevance was questionable. However, some questions remain: the initial CPAP titration did not show any difference as compared with the diagnostic study. This is surprising, as most previous studies showed a 50% reduction under CPAP. The remarkable reduction was shown on the second titration night after randomisation and needs further explanation. Moreover, the results are limited by the high number of non-evaluable data (30 out of 66 patients).

DELLWEG et al. [66] conducted a trial comparing ASV and BPAP-ST for noninvasive ventilation. They included patients with a predominantly obstructive AHI $\geqslant$15 events·h^{-1} at baseline who had a predominantly central AHI $\geqslant$15 events·h^{-1} after 6 weeks of CPAP therapy. Similar to other studies, CPAP reduced the mean±SD AHI from 42.2±14.9 events·h^{-1} to 28.1±8.1 events·h^{-1}, mainly due to a reduction in obstructive disturbances. Both BPAP-ST and ASV reduced the AHI significantly and substantially during the first night of treatment. However, after 6 weeks of treatment, the effect of BPAP-ST was minimised, while it was stable under ASV (BPAP-ST AHI: 16.5±8 events·h^{-1}; ASV AHI: 7.4±4.2 events·h^{-1}). Based on these findings, it is reasonable to make an early shift to ASV after a one night CPAP trial [66]. However, it has to be stated that sound evidence for the treatment of CompSAS is lacking at the moment.

ASV in opioid-induced sleep apnoea

Due to the complex pathophysiology, the optimal therapy for opioid-induced sleep apnoea is still debated [67, 68]. Recently, JAVAHERI et al. [69] discussed clinical findings from 20 patients who chronically used at least one opioid. The majority of the patients took additional psychotropic agents. At baseline, the patients suffered from severe sleep apnoea with overwhelming central disturbances. Prior to treatment with ASV, 16 out of 20 patients had undergone a CPAP trial showing a 50% reduction in the breathing disturbances. However, ASV reduced the final AHI to 12±14 events·h^{-1}, eliminated central apnoeas and improved parameters of oxygen saturation and arousals [69].

RAMAR et al. [70] recently retrospectively investigated CPAP non-responders with central breathing disturbances due to chronic HF or opioid use. They found that ASV enabled sufficient therapy in the majority of patients in both groups. Although this was not a RCT, the authors analysed the largest sample, to date, in a real-life situation [70]. A recent systematic review identified five studies involving 127 patients who used opioids for at least 6 months and were treated with different positive pressure algorithms. CPAP was proven mostly ineffective while BPAP and ASV achieved elimination of central apnoeas in 62% and 58%, respectively [71]. Future studies should address the question of why 30–40% of patients with HF and opioid-induced sleep apnoea could not be treated optimally.

Comparison of the ASV devices

To our knowledge, there are no clinical studies comparing the three available devices. ZHU et al. [72] performed a benchmarking test using a computer-controlled artificial lung and compared the reactions of the devices to central or obstructive breathing disturbances including Cheyne–Stokes respiration. While the devices sufficiently eliminated central apnoeas and obstructive events, central hypopnoeas still remained. There was a discrepancy between the number of manually scored and the stored events in the devices. In conclusion, the algorithms reacted as expected in accordance with the clinical experiences. However, the effects should be evaluated based on PSG as the internal evaluation underestimates hypopnoeas [72].

Titration and setting of ASV

The setting of maximum inspiratory pressure under ASV depends on suspected cardiovascular side-effects. High maximum pressure levels have been experimentally shown to reduce cardiac preload and output in healthy persons. This was clinically irrelevant in normals; however, it raised concerns that PAP may substantially impair cardiac function in patients with HF. The hypothesised negative effects have not been proven in chronic, stable HF [36, 41, 44, 46, 60]. However, the question is still open for acute, unstable HF. Nevertheless, the application of positive EEP is a basic option in lung oedema. In this situation the pressure level is elevated step by step in order to increase oxygen saturation until high pressure levels reduce BP, which limits further pressure increases. Accordingly, it is advisable to apply the maximum inspiratory pressure during wakefulness and control the arterial BP in severe or unstable HF. By contrast, to our knowledge and experience, negative effects on the cardiac output have not been reported in stable patients.

The minimal pressure support for home treatment can be set based on the findings of an in-hospital ASV trial using the largest possible inspiratory range. If the IPAP actually applied during this trial is on the lowest level for large time periods the minimal IPAP can be on the EPAP level. Otherwise, if the patient continuously needs higher pressure support during the trial it might be advantageous to predefine an additional support to stabilise breathing [35]. The former situations are typical for Cheyne–Stokes respiration/CSA in HF, while the latter may characterise combinations of sleep apnoea phenotypes with hypoventilation (*e.g.* obesity hypoventilation or COPD).

The most recent algorithms determine the expiratory pressure automatically. However, it can also be defined based on manual titration. Hence, a CPAP trial prior to ASV is reasonable for two reasons: 1) it allows the definition of the expiratory pressure level needed to overcome obstructive events; and 2) if CPAP efficiently normalises respiration, ASV can be avoided.

Clinical use of pressure support ventilation with target volume

MURPHY *et al.* [37] compared AVAPS and fixed pressure support ventilation in 50 patients with obesity hypoventilation syndrome. The authors showed equivalent impairments of $PaCO_2$, daytime performance and quality of life with both modes [37]. STORRE *et al.* [38] applied BPAP-ST and AVAPS in a cross-over design RCT to 10 patients with obesity hypoventilation syndrome who did not respond sufficiently to CPAP. While BPAP-ST improved parameters of quality of life and sleep quality and oxygenation, AVAPS additionally reduced transcutaneous CO_2 [38]. Most recently, BRIONES CLAUDETT *et al.* [39] compared AVAPS or BPAP-ST in 22 patients with acute exacerbation of COPD and hypercapnia with matched controls. They found more sufficient improvement in $PaCO_2$ and a higher maximum IPAP with AVAPS as compared with BPAP-ST. Although these studies did not prove benefits when compared with pressure support ventilation in general, the new algorithm allows more precise adaptation of treatment to individual patients.

Conclusions and open questions

ASV has been consistently proven to be highly effective for improving complicated breathing disturbances. It reduces distinct breathing disturbances more effectively than other PAP options, based on a limited number of high quality studies. However, additional

RCTs are required to address the long-term effects on cardiovascular parameters, comorbidities and outcome. As sufficient therapy has been shown to improve several parameters of heart function, it is still unclear if the treatment indication should be based on daytime symptoms in cardiac patients with breathing disturbances. The remaining questions about survival and severe cardiac events over the long-term are being addressed in two large international, multicentre RCTs (SERVE-HF and ADVENT-HF) [73].

Treatment failure in some patients should be interpreted on the basis of the underlying pathophysiology. It might also be associated with mask leakages [74], or active or passive closure of the UA [75]. The complexity of the breathing disturbances and the comorbidities underlines the relevance of close supervision and optimal management of the mask interface [35, 44].

Despite the lack of RCTs, our approach to patients with complicated breathing patterns includes the following steps. 1) Performing a PSG to clearly define obstructive and central apnoeas, hypopnoeas and hypoventilation. 2) Optimising treatment of any underlying disease, *e.g.* cardiovascular disorders, renal failure or chronic opioid intake. 3) Excluding avoidable causes of CSA, such as excessive titration, post-arousal CSA or post-hyperventilation apnoea. 4) Applying CPAP: to overcome UA obstruction and define EPAP; and/or to evaluate the individual response of CSA and Cheyne–Stokes respiration (expected 50%). 5) Applying new devices or algorithms, including ASV, trilevel or AVAPS on an individualised basis (personalised medicine) in CPAP failure.

References

1. Randerath W. Management of sleep disordered breathing in heart failure. *Minerva Pneumologica* 2013; 52: 111–122.
2. Javaheri S, Brown LK, Randerath WJ. Clinical applications of adaptive servoventilation devices: part 2. *Chest* 2014; 146: 858–868.
3. Javaheri S, Brown LK, Randerath WJ. Positive airway pressure therapy with adaptive servoventilation: part 1: operational algorithms. *Chest* 2014; 146: 514–523.
4. Wellman A, Malhotra A, Fogel RB, *et al.* Respiratory system loop gain in normal men and women measured with proportional-assist ventilation. *J Appl Physiol* 2003; 94: 205–212.
5. Pinna GD, Maestri R, Mortara A, *et al.* Periodic breathing in heart failure patients: testing the hypothesis of instability of the chemoreflex loop. *J Appl Physiol (1985)* 2000; 89: 2147–2157.
6. Hall MJ, Xie A, Rutherford R, *et al.* Cycle length of periodic breathing in patients with and without heart failure. *Am J Respir Crit Care Med* 1996; 154: 376–381.
7. Javaheri S. A mechanism of central sleep apnea in patients with heart failure. *N Engl J Med* 1999; 341: 949–954.
8. Naughton M, Benard D, Tam A, *et al.* Role of hyperventilation in the pathogenesis of central sleep apneas in patients with congestive heart failure. *Am Rev Respir Dis* 1993; 148: 330–338.
9. Javaheri S, Parker TJ, Liming JD, *et al.* Sleep apnea in 81 ambulatory male patients with stable heart failure. Types and their prevalences, consequences, and presentations. *Circulation* 1998; 97: 2154–2159.
10. Sin DD, Fitzgerald F, Parker JD, *et al.* Risk factors for central and obstructive sleep apnea in 450 men and women with congestive heart failure. *Am J Respir Crit Care Med* 1999; 160: 1101–1106.
11. Lanfranchi PA, Somers VK, Braghiroli A, *et al.* Central sleep apnea in left ventricular dysfunction: prevalence and implications for arrhythmic risk. *Circulation* 2003; 107: 727–732.
12. Javaheri S. Heart failure. *In*: Kryger M, Roth T, Dement W, eds. Principles and Practices of Sleep Medicine. 5th Edn. Philadelphia, WB Saunders, 2011; pp. 1400–1415.
13. Pattinson KT. Opioids and the control of respiration. *Br J Anaesth* 2008; 100: 747–758.
14. Wang D, Teichtahl H, Drummer O, *et al.* Central sleep apnea in stable methadone maintenance treatment patients. *Chest* 2005; 128: 1348–1356.
15. Morgenthaler TI, Kagramanov V, Hanak V, *et al.* Complex sleep apnea syndrome: is it a unique clinical syndrome? *Sleep* 2006; 29: 1203–1209.

16. Javaheri S, Smith J, Chung E. The prevalence and natural history of complex sleep apnea. *J Clin Sleep Med* 2009; 5: 205–211.

17. Cassel W, Canisius S, Becker HF, *et al.* A prospective polysomnographic study on the evolution of complex sleep apnoea. *Eur Respir J* 2011; 38: 329–337.

18. Dernaika T, Tawk M, Nazir S, *et al.* The significance and outcome of continuous positive airway pressure-related central sleep apnea during split-night sleep studies. *Chest* 2007; 132: 81–87.

19. Lehman S, Antic NA, Thompson C, *et al.* Central sleep apnea on commencement of continuous positive airway pressure in patients with a primary diagnosis of obstructive sleep apnea–hypopnea. *J Clin Sleep Med* 2007; 3: 462–466.

20. Kuźniar TJ, Kasibowska-Kuźniar K, Ray DW, *et al.* Clinical heterogeneity of patients with complex sleep apnea syndrome. *Sleep Breath* 2013; 17: 1209–1214.

21. Randerath WJ, Treml M, Priegnitz C, *et al.* Evaluation of a noninvasive algorithm for differentiation of obstructive and central hypopneas. *Sleep* 2013; 36: 363–368.

22. Eckert DJ, Jordan AS, Merchia P, *et al.* Central sleep apnea: pathophysiology and treatment. *Chest* 2007; 131: 595–607.

23. Lorenzi-Filho G, Rankin F, Bies I, *et al.* Effects of inhaled carbon dioxide and oxygen on Cheyne-Stokes respiration in patients with heart failure. *Am J Respir Crit Care Med* 1999; 159: 1490–1498.

24. Yumino D, Bradley TD. Central sleep apnea and Cheyne-Stokes respiration. *Proc Am Thorac Soc* 2008; 5: 226–236.

25. Tkacova R, Niroumand M, Lorenzi-Filho G, *et al.* Overnight shift from obstructive to central apneas in patients with heart failure: role of PCO$_2$ and circulatory delay. *Circulation* 2001; 103: 238–243.

26. Kuźniar TJ. The complexities of complex sleep apnea. *J Clin Sleep Med* 2013; 9: 1193–1194.

27. Skatrud JB, Dempsey JA, Badr S, *et al.* Effect of airway impedance on CO$_2$ retention and respiratory muscle activity during NREM sleep. *J Appl Physiol (1985)* 1988; 65: 1676–1685.

28. Salloum A, Rowley JA, Mateika JH, *et al.* Increased propensity for central apnea in patients with obstructive sleep apnea: effect of nasal continuous positive airway pressure. *Am J Respir Crit Care Med* 2010; 181: 189–193.

29. Orr J, Javaheri S, Malhotra A. Comparative effectiveness research in complex sleep apnea. *Sleep* 2014; 37: 833–834.

30. Sands SA, Edwards BA, Kee K, *et al.* Loop gain as a means to predict a positive airway pressure suppression of Cheyne-Stokes respiration in patients with heart failure. *Am J Respir Crit Care Med* 2011; 184: 1067–1075.

31. Javaheri S, Sands SA, Edwards BA. Acetazolamide attenuates Hunter-Cheyne-Stokes breathing but augments the hypercapnic ventilatory response in patients with heart failure. *Ann Am Thorac Soc* 2014; 11: 80–86.

32. Bradley TD, Logan AG, Kimoff RJ, *et al.* Continuous positive airway pressure for central sleep apnea and heart failure. *N Engl J Med* 2005; 353: 2025–2033.

33. Johnson KG, Johnson DC. Bilevel positive airway pressure worsens central apneas during sleep. *Chest* 2005; 128: 2141–2150.

34. Meza S, Mendez M, Ostrowski M, *et al.* Susceptibility to periodic breathing with assisted ventilation during sleep in normal subjects. *J Appl Physiol (1985)* 1998; 85: 1929–1940.

35. Randerath WJ. Therapeutical options for the treatment of Cheyne-Stokes respiration. *Swiss Med Wkly* 2009; 139: 135–139.

36. Galetke W, Ghassemi BM, Priegnitz C, *et al.* Anticyclic modulated ventilation *versus* continuous positive airway pressure in patients with coexisting obstructive sleep apnea and Cheyne-Stokes respiration: a randomized crossover trial. *Sleep Med* 2014; 15: 874–879.

37. Murphy PB, Davidson C, Hind MD, *et al.* Volume targeted *versus* pressure support non-invasive ventilation in patients with super obesity and chronic respiratory failure: a randomised controlled trial. *Thorax* 2012; 67: 727–734.

38. Storre JH, Seuthe B, Fiechter R, *et al.* Average volume-assured pressure support in obesity hypoventilation: a randomized crossover trial. *Chest* 2006; 130: 815–821.

39. Briones Claudett KH, Briones Claudett M, Chung Sang Wong M, *et al.* Noninvasive mechanical ventilation with average volume assured pressure support (AVAPS) in patients with chronic obstructive pulmonary disease and hypercapnic encephalopathy. *BMC Pulm Med* 2013; 13: 12.

40. Arzt M, Wensel R, Montalvan S, *et al.* Effects of dynamic bilevel positive airway pressure support on central sleep apnea in men with heart failure. *Chest* 2008; 134: 61–66.

41. Aurora RN, Chowdhuri S, Ramar K, *et al.* The treatment of central sleep apnea syndromes in adults: practice parameters with an evidence-based literature review and meta-analyses. *Sleep* 2012; 35: 17–40.

42. Harada D, Joho S, Oda Y, *et al.* Short term effect of adaptive servo-ventilation on muscle sympathetic nerve activity in patients with heart failure. *Auton Neurosci* 2011; 161: 95–102.

43. Hastings PC, Vazir A, Meadows GE, *et al.* Adaptive servo-ventilation in heart failure patients with sleep apnea: a real world study. *Int J Cardiol* 2010; 139: 17–24.

44. Javaheri S, Goetting MG, Khayat R, *et al.* The performance of two automatic servo-ventilation devices in the treatment of central sleep apnea. *Sleep* 2011; 34: 1693–1698.

45. Johnston WE, Vinten-Johansen J, Santamore WP, *et al.* Mechanism of reduced cardiac output during positive end-expiratory pressure in the dog. *Am Rev Respir Dis* 1989; 140: 1257–1264.

46. Kasai T, Usui Y, Yoshioka T, *et al.* Effect of flow-triggered adaptive servo-ventilation compared with continuous positive airway pressure in patients with chronic heart failure with coexisting obstructive sleep apnea and Cheyne-Stokes respiration. *Circ Heart Fail* 2010; 3: 140–148.

47. Koyama T, Watanabe H, Terada S, *et al.* Adaptive servo-ventilation improves renal function in patients with heart failure. *Respir Med* 2011; 105: 1946–1953.

48. Krachman SL, D'Alonzo GE, Berger TJ, *et al.* Comparison of oxygen therapy with nasal continuous positive airway pressure on Cheyne-Stokes respiration during sleep in congestive heart failure. *Chest* 1999; 116: 1550–1557.

49. Oldenburg O, Bitter T, Lehmann R, *et al.* Adaptive servoventilation improves cardiac function and respiratory stability. *Clin Res Cardiol* 2011; 100: 107–115.

50. Pepperell JC, Maskell NA, Jones DR, *et al.* A randomized controlled trial of adaptive ventilation for Cheyne-Stokes breathing in heart failure. *Am J Respir Crit Care Med* 2003; 168: 1109–1114.

51. Philip-Joët FF, Paganelli FF, Dutau HL, *et al.* Hemodynamic effects of bilevel nasal positive airway pressure ventilation in patients with heart failure. *Respiration* 1999; 66: 136–143.

52. Philippe C, Stoïca-Herman M, Drouot X, *et al.* Compliance with and effectiveness of adaptive servoventilation *versus* continuous positive airway pressure in the treatment of Cheyne-Stokes respiration in heart failure over a six month period. *Heart* 2006; 92: 337–342.

53. Pinsky MR, Matuschak GM, Klain M. Determinants of cardiac augmentation by elevations in intrathoracic pressure. *J Appl Physiol* 1985; 58: 1189–1198.

54. Randerath WJ. Every cloud has a silver lining–treatment of complicated breathing patterns during sleep. *Sleep* 2011; 34: 1625–1626.

55. Sharma BK, Bakker JP, McSharry DG, *et al.* Adaptive servoventilation for treatment of sleep-disordered breathing in heart failure: a systematic review and meta-analysis. *Chest* 2012; 142: 1211–1221.

56. Teschler H, Döhring J, Wang YM, *et al.* Adaptive pressure support servo-ventilation: a novel treatment for Cheyne-Stokes respiration in heart failure. *Am J Respir Crit Care Med* 2001; 164: 614–619.

57. Yamada S, Sakakibara M, Yokota T, *et al.* Acute hemodynamic effects of adaptive servo-ventilation in patients with heart failure. *Circ J* 2013; 77: 1214–1220.

58. Yoshihisa A, Shimizu T, Owada T, *et al.* Adaptive servo ventilation improves cardiac dysfunction and prognosis in chronic heart failure patients with Cheyne-Stokes respiration. *Int Heart J* 2011; 52: 218–223.

59. Galetke W, Anduleit N, Kenter M, *et al.* Evaluation of a new algorithm for patients with Cheyne-Stokes breathing and obstructive sleep apnea. *Am J Respir Crit Care Med* 2008; 177: A480.

60. Randerath WJ, Nothofer G, Priegnitz C, *et al.* Long-term auto-servoventilation or constant positive pressure in heart failure and coexisting central with obstructive sleep apnea. *Chest* 2012; 142: 440–447.

61. Arzt M, Schroll S, Series F, *et al.* Auto-servoventilation in heart failure with sleep apnoea: a randomised controlled trial. *Eur Respir J* 2013; 42: 1244–1254.

62. Morgenthaler TI, Gay PC, Gordon N, *et al.* Adaptive servoventilation *versus* noninvasive positive pressure ventilation for central, mixed, and complex sleep apnea syndromes. *Sleep* 2007; 30: 468–475.

63. Allam JS, Olson EJ, Gay PC, *et al.* Efficacy of adaptive servoventilation in treatment of complex and central sleep apnea syndromes. *Chest* 2007; 132: 1839–1846.

64. Arzt M, Schulz M, Schroll S, *et al.* Time course of continuous positive airway pressure effects on central sleep apnoea in patients with chronic heart failure. *J Sleep Res* 2009; 18: 20–25.

65. Morgenthaler TI, Kuzniar TJ, Wolfe LF, *et al.* The complex sleep apnea resolution study: a prospective randomized controlled trial of continuous positive airway pressure *versus* adaptive servoventilation therapy. *Sleep* 2014; 37: 927–934.

66. Dellweg D, Kerl J, Hoehn E, *et al.* Randomized controlled trial of noninvasive positive pressure ventilation (NPPV) *versus* servoventilation in patients with CPAP-induced central sleep apnea (complex sleep apnea). *Sleep* 2013; 36: 1163–1171.

67. Farney RJ, Walker JM, Boyle KM, *et al.* Adaptive servoventilation (ASV) in patients with sleep disordered breathing associated with chronic opioid medications for non-malignant pain. *J Clin Sleep Med* 2008; 4: 311–319.

68. Javaheri S, Malik A, Smith J, *et al.* Adaptive pressure support servoventilation: a novel treatment for sleep apnea associated with use of opioids. *J Clin Sleep Med* 2008; 4: 305–310.

69. Javaheri S, Harris N, Howard J, *et al.* Adaptive servoventilation for treatment of opioid-associated central sleep apnea. *J Clin Sleep Med* 2014; 10: 637–643.

70. Ramar K, Ramar P, Morgenthaler TI. Adaptive servoventilation in patients with central or complex sleep apnea related to chronic opioid use and congestive heart failure. *J Clin Sleep Med* 2012; 8: 569–576.

71. Reddy R, Adamo D, Kufel T, *et al.* Treatment of opioid-related central sleep apnea with positive airway pressure: a systematic review. *J Opioid Manag* 2014; 10: 57–62.

72. Zhu K, Kharboutly H, Ma J, *et al.* Bench test evaluation of adaptive servoventilation devices for sleep apnea treatment. *J Clin Sleep Med* 2013; 9: 861–871.

73. Cowie MR, Woehrle H, Wegscheider K, *et al.* Rationale and design of the SERVE-HF study: treatment of sleep-disordered breathing with predominant central sleep apnoea with adaptive servo-ventilation in patients with chronic heart failure. *Eur J Heart Fail* 2013; 15: 937–943.

74. Pusalavidyasagar SS, Olson EJ, Gay PC, *et al.* Treatment of complex sleep apnea syndrome: a retrospective comparative review. *Sleep Med* 2006; 7: 474–479.

75. Badr MS, Toiber F, Skatrud JB, *et al.* Pharyngeal narrowing/occlusion during central sleep apnea. *J Appl Physiol* 1995; 78: 1806–1815.

Disclosures: W.J. Randerath reports accommodation, travel grants and speaking fees from Weinmann, Respironics, Inspire and Resmed, outside the submitted work.

Chapter 20

Supporting patients receiving CPAP treatment: the role of training and telemedicine

Valentina Isetta[1,2], Mireia Ruiz[1], Ramon Farré[1,2] and Josep M. Montserrat[2,3,4]

Adequate adherence to treatment with CPAP is important, particularly during the first weeks of therapy. Therefore, different educational and training approaches have been suggested as potential tools to improve adherence, based on integrative and multidisciplinary networking. However, due to the current social and economic situation, overloaded sleep centres frequently have difficulties providing these services. Strategic changes towards alternative and more cost-effective methods of diagnosis and treatment are urgently needed. The use of telemedicine, defined as the use of information and communication technology to deliver healthcare at a distance, has significant potential for the management of patients with OSA. Together with its potential impact on healthcare utilisation and subsequent cost reductions, telemedicine promotes equity of access to healthcare. Moreover, its delivery is efficacious, facilitating the decentralisation of services and improvement of networking among different healthcare professionals. Nevertheless, further definitive long-term studies with cost-effectiveness analyses are needed.

OSA is considered to increase the risk of mild- and long-term morbidity, and is even associated with cardiovascular, metabolic and neurological mortality [1, 2]. OSA must be considered a chronic condition to ensure adequate management [3], with lifestyle recommendations and CPAP considered the optimal treatment. However, many patients do not tolerate CPAP and fail to adhere to the treatment, with adherence rates of approximately 50% or less depending on the country or health organisation involved [4–9]. Reasons for non-adherence include discomfort, skin irritation, noise and claustrophobia.

The definition of what constitutes adequate CPAP adherence to ensure optimal health outcomes is a crucial issue, but remains controversial [11–14]. Even with the widely accepted minimal use of 4 h per night, some studies have demonstrated greater improvement with longer use, while others have reported improvements with just 2–3 h of CPAP use. Furthermore, each organ or system may need different lengths of time to be fully

[1]Unitat de Biofísica i Bioenginyeria, Facultat de Medecina, Universitat de Barcelona - IDIBAPS, Barcelona, Spain. [2]CIBER de Enfermedades Respiratorias, Madrid, Spain. [3]Institut d'Investigacions Biomèdiques August Pi i Sunyer (IDIBAPS), Barcelona, Spain. [4]Pneumology Dept, Hospital Clinic, Barcelona, Spain.

Correspondence: Valentina Isetta, Unit of Biophysics and Bioengineering, Faculty of Medicine, University of Barcelona, Casanova 143, Barcelona, 08036, Spain. E-mail: valentina.isetta@ub.edu

Copyright ©ERS 2015. Print ISBN: 978-1-84984-059-0. Online ISBN: 978-1-84984-060-6. Print ISSN: 2312-508X. Online ISSN: 2312-5098.

restored. Nevertheless, many authors have demonstrated greater improvement with longer CPAP use [13, 14], or greater reductions in hypertension when used for at least 5 h per night [10, 11]. Based on these data, it seems reasonable to conclude that longer CPAP use is associated with greater improvement. Therefore, 4 h per night should be considered the minimum requirement, with use for more than 5.5 h considered optimal, representing the goal of CPAP use as Masa and Corral-Peñafiel [15] suggested in a recent editorial.

Given that improved adherence is key to the management of OSA patients receiving CPAP treatment, great inroads have been made in this direction. To increase adherence, two measures have been implemented: 1) technological optimisation of the CPAP devices themselves; and 2) special efforts in patient education, training, and clinical support during follow-up. Technological advances, including automatic [16], bilevel [17] or Bi-Flex [18] CPAP systems, have shown positive effects on improving patient adherence in a limited number of cases, for example patients requiring high therapeutic pressures [19]. The development of new CPAP masks that are designed to enhance patient comfort may also have a marked impact on CPAP adherence in the future [20, 21]. At the same time, different educational approaches have been suggested and successfully implemented that are based on integrative multidisciplinary training and support [4–9, 12–14]. These interventions include close management and follow-up focused on the quick resolution of treatment-related problems early in treatment, when long-term adherence patterns are usually determined [4–9, 12–14].

Educational support for CPAP treatment

Table 1 shows a suggested basic approach for the management of CPAP in patients with OSA. It comprises pre-titration, titration and post-titration support, with the latter specifically focused on the first days or weeks of treatment.Pre-titration support It is important to identify the predictors of treatment adherence early, so that the first weeks and months of follow-up can be personalised. In a 2014 Cochrane review, Wozniak et al. [22] reported that certain psychological and cognitive variables, including risk perception and expected treatment outcomes, and spousal involvement were modifiable predictors of CPAP adherence, which is consistent with the findings of other authors [23, 24]. Kohler et al. [25] found that the severity of sleep disordered breathing, rather than sleepiness, determines long-term adherence to CPAP therapy. Smith et al. [26] have suggested using the sentence "get in the habit of CPAP every day", and designed a programme that included different interventions such as music, a diary for recording nightly use and writing about CPAP benefits or problems, and softly spoken instructions for placing the CPAP mask comfortably among others. The intervention had a strong effect for improving adherence to CPAP at 1 month [26]. Other related factors have also been related to CPAP treatment adherence. For example, Law et al. [27] found that patients with depression had worse adherence rates. Other authors analysed the predictors of CPAP use during the first weeks of treatment, and identified that the main variables associated with reduced CPAP use were ethnicity and intimacy with partners [28]. Expert nurses are probably best placed to train most patients in the different aspects of CPAP management, including education, information, and the use of CPAP devices and masks in and out of hospitals [29, 30], with expertise being key. The most current technology for education or training should be used, or at least tested, to see if they can optimise sessions and improve cost-effectiveness [29, 31].

In summary, despite successful educational approaches, there are no common guidelines on training protocols for patient support during CPAP treatment. This is mainly due to the wide variety of variables implicated, including personal, social and disease-related characteristics.

Table 1. Recommended interventional scheme to guarantee adequate CPAP compliance

Pre-CPAP titration support
Consideration of the patient's personal and social characteristics
Adequate indication of treatment and symptoms
Assessment of physiological aspects (AHI, CT90%, etc.)
Careful initial educational CPAP and mask training session
Effort to reach patient's awareness of the need of treatment
Adequate mask choice

Support during CPAP titration (titration is an art)
Sometimes a slow increase of pressure is needed, depending of the patient
Assistance and guidance through the night (awake periods, perception of pressure, mask leaks or asynchronies)
A number of times not all the events can be corrected
A pleasant night is probably the most important point
Discussion of the procedure and problems in the morning

Post-CPAP titration follow-up
The intervals of the visits depend of the side-effects, compliance, characteristics of the patient and associated diseases
Early detection and treatment of side-effects is one of the most important points to control during the first weeks
Continuous educational and psychological support
First visit (1–2 weeks): individual face-to-face, group support or teleconsultation
Second visit (4–6 weeks): individual face-to-face, group support or teleconsultation
The next visits will depend on the patient's characteristics, comorbidities, side-effects, residual symptoms/events detected and compliance
All the procedures can be performed individually, in a group setting or by videoconference

The most important points are shown in bold font. CT90%: cumulative percentage of time spent at saturations below 90%.

Support during the titration process

As mentioned, poor CPAP adherence is usually associated with diagnostic variables, side-effects, health beliefs and disease severity, while the titration process itself is rarely considered. This phase typically represents the second exposure to CPAP, but can also be the first exposure if an initial training session was not performed. Few researchers have considered the sleep parameters assessed during CPAP titration as being predictors of adherence. DRAKE et al. [32] studied CPAP adherence in OSA patients after a mean follow-up of 47 days, and identified the best predictor of adherence to be improved sleep efficiency after the diagnostic/titration night, indicating that patients who slept better after the first titration night had the highest levels of subsequent adherence (more than 2 h). In addition, some authors report that patients who attended a PSG-assisted CPAP titration had significantly longer use during follow-up than those who were not assisted during titration [33]. However, MASA et al. [34] analysed the adherence of 360 OSA patients randomly allocated to three groups (standard, auto-adjusted and predicted formula titration with domiciliary adjustment), and after 3 months of CPAP treatment, similar improvement was seen in subjective and objective symptoms as well as adherence. FIETZE et al. [35] found similar results between CPAP titration performed in a sleep lab and portable sleep monitoring at home. In selected cases, the use of sedatives could be useful during CPAP titration [36]. The training approach and mask choice before titration could explain these discrepancies. These findings suggest that key aspects for CPAP adherence include what happens during the first night of titration, the perceived improvement when waking in the morning, and the resolution of any doubts in the morning.

Post-CPAP titration support

Although the schedule could change depending on patient characteristics, symptom evolution and the health system of the country in question, Spanish guidelines for optimal CPAP follow-up recommend monitoring at 1–2 weeks, 1 month and 3 months after CPAP titration. In the 2014 Cochrane review that analysed CPAP use, different interventions were found to be useful for increasing CPAP adherence [22]. Ongoing supportive interventions were more successful than usual care, increasing CPAP usage by 50 min per night. In addition, educational interventions resulted in modest improvements of 35 min per night, whereas behavioural therapy increased machine use by 1.5 h per night. However, some inconsistencies were noted between the results of individual studies, and it was occasionally unclear whether the interventions led to meaningful improvements in daytime symptoms or quality of life [22]. In a 12-month follow-up of OSA patients receiving CPAP therapy, the role of positive initial CPAP experiences (*i.e.*, adherence and side-effects at 1 month) was emphasised, suggesting that intensive early interventions could improve follow-up of OSA patients receiving CPAP treatment [37]. Age and initial adherence (as soon as 12 days after initiation) were identified as predictors of long-term adherence [37]. JANSON *et al.* [38] found side-effects such as nasal or pharyngeal problems, lack of perceived improvement, ageing and previous uvulopalatopharyngoplasty to be the main factors related to poor CPAP adherence. Similarly, in a 5-year follow-up of OSA patients receiving CPAP treatment, age and initial adherence (as soon as 12 days after initiation) were identified as predictors of long-term adherence [39]. Finally, LETTIERI *et al.* [40] compared the impact of a group educational programme *versus* individual education on CPAP adherence in a large number of patients. The main conclusion of the authors was that CPAP adherence was significantly greater in those participating in a group programme than in those receiving individual education [40]. Another noteworthy aspect is that the group approach enabled CPAP therapy to be initiated in 15–20 patients compared with just six patients over the same time period for individual counselling. Thus, good preparation before titration is important to convince the patient of the risks and benefits of good adherence to CPAP during the first days or weeks after CPAP initiation, trying to avoid and minimise side-effects.

The role of telemedicine in healthcare

As mentioned, different educational and training approaches based on integrative and multidisciplinary networking have been suggested to be the best tools to improve adherence [6], which raises several issues. First, the prevalence of OSA is likely to increase due to its strong correlation with the obesity epidemic and higher incidence among older adults and children. Together with a growing awareness about sleep disorders in the general population, this is likely to generate a large increase in demand for health visits and sleep studies. Second, to guarantee adequate treatment, side-effects that affect adherence, such as pressure intolerance, a claustrophobic reaction to the mask, and machine noise, need to be monitored very closely during the first days and weeks of therapy. Third, overloaded sleep centres in many countries have difficulties in providing their service because of recent healthcare cost reductions. Fourth, patients with impaired mobility from rural areas cannot always attend the hospital to which they are referred, and may not receive optimal healthcare. Therefore, providing adequate support to patients with sleep disorders is not always possible, and strategic changes toward alternative and more cost-effective methods of diagnosis and management are urgently needed.

The use of telemedicine, defined as the use of information and communication technology (ICT) to deliver healthcare at a distance [41], could resolve several of these issues in the management of patients with OSA. Together with its potential impact on healthcare utilisation and cost reduction [42], telemedicine promotes equity of access to healthcare. Moreover, its delivery is efficacious, improving networking among the different healthcare levels and facilitating the decentralisation of services [43]. In addition, it can enhance patient motivation and self-management skills through self-empowerment, and can strengthen the professional–patient relationship. However, different strategies must be developed to implement this approach. Figure 1 provides a representation of how the diagnostic and management processes could be performed in most patients at home using a telemedicine-based strategy, including teleconferencing, home study and clinical data transmission procedures.

Over recent decades, telemedicine has been considered increasingly relevant in closing the gap between the demand for and availability of home healthcare services [44–46]. Indeed, telemedicine services not only enable close follow-up of the patient at home but also provide home healthcare to prevent acute events that may lead to hospitalisation. Telemedicine now seems to offer credible solutions, tested in real medical settings, to major healthcare challenges facing our society, from the need to deal with an ageing population and spiralling health costs to the management of chronic disease. Publications have described the use of telemedicine for home monitoring of patients with respiratory diseases,

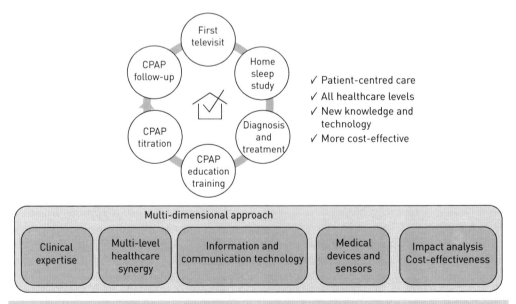

Figure 1. Fully integrated home-based management of sleep apnoea.

congestive HF, and in psychiatric and other chronic illnesses, as well as among geriatric patients with increased risk of falls. Together with portable electronic monitoring equipment, telemedicine can support home monitoring of blood glucose, pulmonary function and cardiac function [41–51].

Despite the evident potential of telemedicine-based interventions, the precise benefits, risks, and costs of this method to deliver healthcare remain unclear [42, 52, 53]. In a recent systematic review of the impact of telehealthcare on the quality and safety of different telemedicine-based models, limited differences were found in the outcomes between telemedicine and usual care [53]. Consequently, the authors suggested that policymakers and planners needed to be aware that investment in telemedicine would not inevitably yield clinical or economic benefits, and that long-term studies were needed to determine whether the benefits are sustained [53]. In an analysis of the clinical effects of home telemonitoring for diabetes, asthma, HF and hypertension, Paré and co-workers [41, 47] concluded that, although it appeared to be a promising approach, future study designers should consider ways to make the technology more effective while controlling possible mediating variables. Besides its clinical impact, another aspect of telemedicine-based strategies that requires further investigation is the economic impact and cost-effectiveness [52]. In a systematic review, telemedicine and telecare interventions were found to be no more cost-effective than conventional healthcare strategies [52]. However, another recent study considering the cost of a new Internet-based monitoring tool for neonatal care after discharge resulted in much lower costs than conventional hospital-based follow-up. It was found that the greater cost-effectiveness was especially due to the reduction in emergency department visits [54].

In "Another sobering result for home telehealth—and where we might go next" [53], Scott R. Wilson and Peter Cram considered the data for a recent randomised study in which older adults with multiple disease actually had worse mortality in the telemonitoring group [55]. They stressed the importance of care when choosing appropriate outcomes and patient populations for telemedicine-based strategies. It seems clear that, despite the many encouraging results, the widespread implementation of telemedicine should wait for these critical questions to be answered. Rigorous and large-scale trials continue to be needed to provide reliable data for assessing the actual clinical and economic impact of telemedicine.

Telemedicine interventions to support the management of sleep disorders

Several publications have described the use of telemedicine for respiratory diseases, congestive HF and other chronic illnesses [43–45, 47, 48]. Surprisingly, few telemedicine applications have been designed and implemented to support the diagnosis and management of OSA, for which novel social, healthcare and economic strategies are needed. Here, we explore the most recent applications of telemedicine in OSA and analyse their impact in patients, as identified in a PubMed search (using MeSH terminology). Table 2 summarises the key studies.

Telemedicine-based support of CPAP treatment

There are few long-term RCTs, and where they do exist, the results are often conflicting (table 2). In one, 75 CPAP naïve patients were divided into a group receiving standard treatment and another connected to a telemedicine monitoring system. CPAP adherence at

TABLE 2 Studies related to CPAP compliance using a telemedicine approach

First author [ref.]	Subjects n	Study title	ESS	AHI events·h⁻¹	Study length	Summary
Fox [56]	75	The impact of a telemedicine monitoring system on PAP adherence in patients with OSA: a RCT	9, 7	41	3 months	CPAP adherence can be improved with the use of a web-based telemedicine system; however, compliance was low in both groups#
Leseux [57]	101	Education of patients with OSA: feasibility of a phone coaching procedure. Phone-coaching and OSA			6 months	CPAP compliance increased in the intervention group but the difference was not statistically significant¶
Parikh [58]	90	Sleep telemedicine: patient satisfaction and treatment adherence			2 weeks	Similar compliance and satisfaction in both groups¶
Sparrow [59]	250	A telemedicine intervention to improve adherence to CPAP: a RCT	10, 5	38	12 months	Intervention group [weekly automatic voice responses and calls] improved CPAP compliance#
Stepnowsky [60]	45	Pilot randomised trial of the effect of wireless telemonitoring on compliance and treatment efficacy in OSA.	12, 6	39	2 months	Similar compliance in both groups. Intervention group significantly more likelihood of continuing to use CPAP¶
Smith [61]	19 (non-adherent)	Telehealth services to improve non-adherence: a placebo-controlled study			3 months	Telehealth intervention improves compliance and could be potentially cost-effective#
Taylor [62]	114	The role of telemedicine in CPAP compliance for patients with OSA syndrome	14		1 month	Telemedicine support improved compliance but no differences were found¶
DeMolles [63]	30	A pilot trial of a telecommunications system in sleep apnoea management		40	2 months	The use of an automated telephone monitoring system increased CPAP use¶
Chervin [64]	33	Compliance with nasal CPAP can be improved by simple interventions	10, 9	49	1 month	Intervention groups [literature and phone calls] had increased CPAP compliance#

#: adherence statistically significant; ¶: adherence not statistically significant.

3 months was significantly higher in the telemedicine arm (191 min·day^{-1}) *versus* the standard arm (105 min·day^{-1}), but there was no significant difference in the percentage of nights of use. The authors commented on the presence of important limitations in this study, such as the generally low adherence rates [56]. In another RCT based on telephone counselling, 101 patients with OSA using CPAP received usual follow-up or five sessions of support phone calls by appropriately trained staff [57]. Higher adherence to CPAP was observed at 6 months in the intervention group (94% *versus* 81%; p<0.05), with CPAP adherence at 3 months being 54 min higher in the intervention group than in the control group (4 h 39 min±2 h 17 min and 3 h 45 min±2 h 45 min, respectively; not statistically significant). The authors concluded that educational intervention dispensed by phone was applicable and affected CPAP adherence, but that its efficacy on long-term adherence must be confirmed in a larger group using a randomised procedure [57]. The possibility of a telephone-linked communication (TLC) system to improve CPAP adherence has also been studied in an RCT of 250 patients being started on CPAP therapy for OSA [59]. The control group received general health education *via* a TLC system, while the experimental group (TLC-CPAP) reported CPAP-related behaviour and symptoms, and received feedback and counselling to improve motivation. Adherence in the TLC-CPAP group was 1 h per night and 2 h per night higher after 6 and 12 months, respectively [59]. In addition, CPAP adherence was significantly associated with greater improvements in sleep apnoea symptoms, depressive symptoms and functional status. The use of a wireless device for the telemonitoring of CPAP adherence was studied by STEPNOWSKY *et al.* [60]. They analysed the efficacy CPAP use and other treatment in 45 patients recently diagnosed with OSA. After 2 months of follow-up, the telemonitored patients used CPAP for 4.1±1.8 h per night on 78±22% of the possible nights and rated that they had a high likelihood of continuing the treatment. By contrast, patients following the usual clinical care used CPAP for 2.8 ±2.2 h on 60±32% of the nights, but without significant differences in CPAP efficacy from the telemonitored group. The authors stressed the need for longer studies to confirm their promising results [60].

Patient satisfaction with telemedicine has also been analysed. TAYLOR *et al.* [62] compared functional status and client satisfaction during 30 days of CPAP use in patients with OSA randomised to a telemedicine group or to traditional care. The telemedicine group was assisted by a "Health Buddy" computer for information, support and feedback about CPAP treatment. Although no significant differences were found between groups in the usage patterns (hours of use per night and proportion of nights used), the authors reported good acceptance for this monitoring approach [62]. In another study, 90 patients with OSA completed a satisfaction questionnaire; although all were initially seen by a nurse practitioner and a sleep specialist, 56 were seen by a physician at the sleep centre and 34 by videoconference. Satisfaction did not differ between the groups [58]. DEMOLLES *et al.* [63] studied a group of 30 subjects who were randomly assigned to use a computer telephone system designed to improve CPAP adherence (TLC-CPAP) in addition to usual care (n=15) or to usual care alone (n=15) for a period of 2 months. The average nightly CPAP use in the TLC-CPAP group was 4.4 h compared with 2.9 h (p=0.076) in the usual care group [63]. Finally, CHERVIN *et al.* [64] performed a RCT among 33 subjects of two interventions to improve compliance. One group of subjects received weekly phone calls to uncover any problems and encourage use, a second group received written information about sleep apnoea and the importance of regular CPAP use, and a third group served as control subjects. The authors found that intervention improved CPAP compliance and that the effect was particularly strong when intervention occurred during the first month of CPAP treatment.

ISETTA et al. [29] have performed two important studies. In the first, 50 consecutive OSA patients received a teleconsultation with a physician and were asked to answer an anonymous questionnaire about the teleconsultation. Most patients were satisfied with the teleconsultation method, and 66% agreed that the teleconsultation could replace more than half of their CPAP follow-up visits. In the second study, they conducted an RCT in which 40 patients with OSA were divided into two groups for CPAP training; 20 received standard face-to-face training and 20 received the training *via* videoconference. After the session, they were blindly evaluated on what they had learned about OSA and mask placement. Patients who had received CPAP training *via* videoconference demonstrated comparable knowledge about OSA and CPAP therapy to those in the face-to-face group. Performance of practical skills (mask and headgear placement, and leak avoidance) was also similar between the two groups [29].

Telemedicine to support OSA diagnosis

Home-based procedures with simplified devices are often used to diagnose OSA, especially when there is a high pretest possibility of having OSA [65]. A few studies have explored the potential of telemedicine in OSA diagnosis. MASA et al. [66] compared both the diagnostic efficacy and cost of home respiratory polygraphy with in-hospital PSG in a large sample (n=348). Importantly, home respiratory polygraphy was a significantly lower cost alternative for the diagnosis of patients with OSA. Comparisons were also made between device transportation and telematic transmission of data, with comparable results. Having devices moved by a transportation company or sent telematically as raw data proved equally beneficial and cost-effective, and raise the possibility of application among patients with limited mobility or those who live a long way from the hospital [66]. In another study, 40 patients with OSA were analysed by respiratory polygraphy transmitted in real time [67]. Again, they were divided into a conventional face-to-face consultation group and a teleconsultation group, with 35 patients diagnosed with OSA based on an AHI $\geqslant$10 events·h^{-1}, and CPAP treatment started in 16 patients. The level of CPAP adherence was 85% at 6 months in patients attending the sleep centre and 75% in the teleconsultation arm. However, this study was not randomised, with small sample sizes and there was a bias toward including patients with suspected OSA in the study population. Nevertheless, the results indicate that new ICTs can help to establish diagnostic and therapeutic strategies for OSA while avoiding the need to travel.

Recently, BRUYNEEL and NINANE [68] analysed six prospective randomised crossover studies comparing home-based PSG and in-laboratory PSG. These studies convincingly showed that home-based PSG allowed complete sleep evaluation, with low failure rates despite the absence of supervision. In conclusion, home-based PSG can be used to diagnose or exclude OSA in patients, even in the presence of comorbidities [68]. At present, a considerable number of sensors and devices are available for OSA diagnosis, including mattress or contactless sensors, but most need further validation or testing in a larger number of patients [69–79]. Finally, large randomised studies are still lacking for home telemonitoring of mechanical ventilation, but it is a promising area in need of urgent exploration [80–85].

Technological support of CPAP treatment

CPAP is considered the treatment of choice for OSA, and many studies have shown a correlation between adherence and treatment outcomes. Consequently, new CPAP machines have been developed that can track adherence (*i.e.* hours of use), mask leak and residual AHI. The American Thoracic Society recently reviewed this topic [5] and assessed the reliability of the data (adherence, leak, efficacy and flow signals) obtained from CPAP adherence-tracking systems and the use of CPAP tracking systems in clinical practice. Their report was based on clinical experience and empirical evidence identified by a comprehensive literature review. They concluded that CPAP use could be reliably determined from CPAP tracking systems, but that residual events (apnoea/hypopnea) and leak data were not as easy to interpret, and that the definitions of these parameters differed among CPAP manufacturers. Nonetheless, the clinical extremes (*i.e.* very high or low values for residual events or mask leak) appear to have practical significance. Therefore, CPAP tracking systems can reliably monitor CPAP adherence providing practitioners can interpret the data of a given CPAP adherence-tracking system. In addition, it is clear that the nomenclature used in CPAP adherence-tracking system reports needs to be standardised between manufacturers, including the use of AHI/flow to describe residual events. Finally, studies should be performed examining the usefulness and effectiveness of CPAP tracking systems on OSA outcomes.

Conclusion

The use of telemedicine is useful for different aspects of the diagnosis and treatment of sleep disordered breathing, promoting equity and efficacy in access to healthcare and its delivery. However, there is an undoubted need for more definitive long-term studies with cost-effectiveness analysis. In addition, further research is needed to customise and optimise the target population, devices and situations in which telemedicine can be used with greatest benefit.

References

1. Eckert DJ, Malhotra A. Pathophysiology of adult obstructive sleep apnea. *Proc Am Thorac Soc* 2008; 5: 144–153.
2. Dempsey JA, Veasey SC, Morgan BJ, *et al.* Pathophysiology of sleep apnea. *Physiol Rev* 2010; 90: 47–112.
3. Heatley EM, Harris M, Battersby M, *et al.* Obstructive sleep apnoea in adults: a common chronic condition in need of a comprehensive chronic condition management approach. *Sleep Med Rev* 2013; 17: 349–355.
4. Sawyer AM, Gooneratne NS, Marcus CL, *et al.* A systematic review of CPAP adherence across age groups: clinical and empiric insights for developing CPAP adherence interventions. *Sleep Med Rev* 2011; 15: 343–356.
5. Schwab RJ, Badr SM, Epstein LJ, *et al.* An official American Thoracic Society statement: continuous positive airway pressure adherence tracking systems. The optimal monitoring strategies and outcome measures in adults. *Am J Respir Crit Care Med* 2013; 188: 613–620.
6. Crawford MR, Espie CA, Bartlett DJ, *et al.* Integrating psychology and medicine in CPAP adherence – new concepts? *Sleep Med Rev* 2014; 18: 123–139.
7. Shapiro GK, Shapiro CM. Factors that influence CPAP adherence: an overview. *Sleep Breath* 2010; 14: 323–335.
8. Weaver TE, Grunstein RR. Adherence to continuous positive airway pressure therapy: the challenge to effective treatment. *Proc Am Thorac Soc* 2008; 5: 173–178.
9. Engleman HM, Wild MR. Improving CPAP use by patients with the sleep apnoea/hypopnoea syndrome (SAHS). *Sleep Med Rev* 2003; 7: 81–99.
10. Barbé F, Durán-Cantolla J, Capote F, *et al.* Long-term effect of continuous positive airway pressure in hypertensive patients with sleep apnea. *Am J Respir Crit Care Med* 2010; 181: 718–726.
11. Martínez-García MA, Capote F, Campos-Rodríguez F, *et al.* Effect of CPAP on blood pressure in patients with obstructive sleep apnea and resistant hypertension: the HIPARCO randomized clinical trial. *JAMA* 2013; 310: 2407–2415.
12. Weaver TE. Don't start celebrating – CPAP adherence remains a problem. *J Clin Sleep Med* 2013; 9: 551–552.
13. Weaver TE, Sawyer AM. Adherence to continuous positive airway pressure treatment for obstructive sleep apnoea: implications for future interventions. *Ind J Med Res* 2010; 131: 245–258.
14. Weaver TE, Maislin G, Dinges DF, *et al.* Relationship between hours of CPAP use and achieving normal levels of sleepiness and daily functioning. *Sleep* 2007; 30: 711–719.

15. Masa JF, Corral-Peñafiel J. Should use of 4 hours continuous positive airway pressure per night be considered acceptable compliance? *Eur Respir J* 2014; 44: 1119–1120.

16. Ip S, D'Ambrosio C, Patel K, *et al.* Auto-titrating *versus* fixed continuous positive airway pressure for the treatment of obstructive sleep apnea: a systematic review with meta-analyses. *Syst Rev* 2012; 1: 20.

17. Gay PC, Herold DL, Olson EJ. A randomized, double-blind clinical trial comparing continuous positive airway pressure with a novel bilevel pressure system for treatment of obstructive sleep apnea syndrome. *Sleep* 2003; 26: 864–869.

18. Pépin JL, Muir JF, Gentina T, *et al.* Pressure reduction during exhalation in sleep apnea patients treated by continuous positive airway pressure. *Chest* 2009; 136: 490–497.

19. Massie CA, McArdle N, Hart RW, *et al.* Comparison between automatic and fixed positive airway pressure therapy in the home. *Am J Respir Crit Care Med* 2003; 167: 20–23.

20. Borel JC, Tamisier R, Dias-Domingos S, *et al.* Type of mask may impact on continuous positive airway pressure adherence in apneic patients. *PLoS One* 2013; 8: e64382.

21. Parthasarathy S. Mask interface and CPAP adherence. *J Clin Sleep Med* 2008; 4: 511–512.

22. Wozniak DR, Lasserson TJ, Smith I. Educational, supportive and behavioural interventions to improve usage of continuous positive airway pressure machines in adults with obstructive sleep apnoea. *Cochrane Database Syst Rev* 2014; 1: CD007736.

23. Wild MR, Engleman HM, Douglas NJ, *et al.* Can psychological factors help us to determine adherence to CPAP? A prospective study. *Eur Respir J* 2004; 24: 461–465.

24. Baron KG, Smith TW, Berg CA, *et al.* Spousal involvement in CPAP adherence among patients with obstructive sleep. *Sleep Breath* 2011; 15: 525–534.

25. Kohler M, Smith D, Tippett V, *et al.* Predictors of long-term compliance with continuous positive airway pressure. *Thorax* 2010; 65: 829–832.

26. Smith CE, Dauz E, Clements F, *et al.* Patient education combined in a music and habit-forming intervention for adherence to continuous positive airway (CPAP) prescribed for sleep apnea. *Patient Educ Couns* 2009; 74: 184–190.

27. Law M, Naughton M, Ho S, *et al.* Depression may reduce adherence during CPAP titration trial. *J Clin Sleep Med* 2014; 10: 163–169.

28. Ye L, Pack AI, Maislin G, *et al.* Predictors of continuous positive airway pressure use during the first week of treatment. *J Sleep Res* 2012; 21: 419–426.

29. Isetta V, León C, Torres M, *et al.* Telemedicine-based approach for obstructive sleep apnea management: building evidence. *Interact J Med Res* 2014; 3: e6.

30. Antic NA, Buchan C, Esterman A, *et al.* A randomized controlled trial of nurse-led care for symptomatic moderate-severe obstructive sleep apnea. *Am J Respir Crit Care Med* 2009; 179: 501–508.

31. Jean Wiese H, Boethel C, Phillips B, *et al.* CPAP compliance: video education may help! *Sleep Med* 2005; 6: 171–174.

32. Drake C, Day R, Hudgel D, *et al.* Sleep during titration predicts continuous positive airway pressure compliance. *Sleep* 2003; 26: 308–311.

33. Means MK, Edinger JD, Husain AM. CPAP compliance in sleep apnea patients with and without laboratory CPAP titration. *Sleep Breath* 2004; 8: 7–14.

34. Masa JF, Jiménez A, Durán J, *et al.* Alternative methods of titrating continuous positive airway pressure: a large multicenter study. *Am J Respir Crit Care Med* 2004; 170: 1218–1224.

35. Fietze I, Glos M, Moebus I, *et al.* Automatic pressure titration with APAP is as effective as manual titration with CPAP in patients with obstructive sleep apnea. *Respiration* 2007; 74: 279–286.

36. Collen J, Lettieri C, Kelly W, *et al.* Clinical and polysomnographic predictors of short-term continuous positive airway pressure compliance. *Chest* 2009; 135: 704–709.

37. Chai-Coetzer CL, Luo YM, Antic NA, *et al.* Predictors of long-term adherence to continuous positive airway pressure therapy in patients with obstructive sleep apnea and cardiovascular disease in the SAVE study. *Sleep* 2013; 36: 1929–1937.

38. Janson C, Nöges E, Svedberg-Randt S, *et al.* What characterizes patients who are unable to tolerate continuous positive airway pressure (CPAP) treatment? *Respir Med* 2000; 94: 145–149.

39. Van Zeller M, Severo M, Santos AC, *et al.* 5-years APAP adherence in OSA patients – do first impressions matter? *Respir Med* 2013; 107: 2046–2052.

40. Lettieri CJ, Walter RJ. Impact of group education on continuous positive airway pressure adherence. *J Clin Sleep Med* 2013; 9: 537–541.

41. Paré G, Jaana M, Sicotte C. Systematic review of home telemonitoring for chronic diseases: the evidence base. *J Am Med Inform Assoc* 2007; 14: 269–277.

42. Jennett PA, Affleck Hall L, Hailey D, *et al.* The socio-economic impact of telehealth: a systematic review. *J Telemed Telecare* 2003; 9: 311–320.

43. Craig J, Patterson V. Introduction to the practice of telemedicine. *J Telemed Telecare* 2005; 11: 3–9.

44. Bediang G, Perrin C, Ruiz de Castañeda R, *et al.* The RAFT telemedicine network: lessons learnt and perspectives from a decade of educational and clinical services in low- and middle-incomes countries. *Front Public Health* 2014; 2: 180.

45. Jenkins RL, White P. Telehealth advancing nursing practice. *Nurs Outlook* 2001; 49: 100–105.

46. McLean S, Sheikh A, Cresswell K, *et al.* The impact of telehealthcare on the quality and safety of care: a systematic overview. *PLoS One* 2013; 8: e71238.

47. Paré G, Moqadem K, Pineau G, *et al.* Clinical effects of home telemonitoring in the context of diabetes, asthma, heart failure and hypertension: a systematic review. *J Med Internet Res* 2010; 12: e21.

48. Free C, Phillips G, Galli L, *et al.* The effectiveness of mobile-health technology-based health behaviour change or disease management interventions for health care consumers: a systematic review. *PLoS Med* 2013; 10: e1001362.

49. Patterson V. Telemedicine for epilepsy support in resource-poor settings. *Front Public Health* 2014; 2: 120.

50. Zvornicanin E, Zvornicanin J, Hadziefendic B. The use of smart phones in ophthalmology. *Acta Inform Med* 2014; 22: 206–209.

51. Pietrzak E, Cotea C, Pullman S. Primary and secondary prevention of cardiovascular disease: is there a place for internet-based interventions? *J Cardiopulm Rehabil Prev* 2014; 34: 303–317.

52. Mistry H. Systematic review of studies of the cost-effectiveness of telemedicine and telecare. Changes in the economic evidence over twenty years. *J Telemed Telecare* 2012; 18: 1–6.

53. Wilson SR, Cram P. Another sobering result for home telehealth—and where we might go next. *Arch Intern Med* 2012; 172: 779–780.

54. Isetta V, Lopez-Agustina C, Lopez-Bernal E, *et al.* Cost-effectiveness of a new internet-based monitoring tool for neonatal post-discharge home care. *J Med Internet Res* 2013; 15: e38.

55. Takahashi PY, Pecina JL, Upatising B, *et al.* A randomized controlled trial of telemonitoring in older adults with multiple health issues to prevent hospitalizations and emergency department visits. *Arch Intern Med* 2012; 172: 773–779.

56. Fox N, Hirsch-Allen AJ, Goodfellow E, *et al.* The impact of a telemedicine monitoring system on positive airway pressure adherence in patients with obstructive sleep apnea: a randomized controlled trial. *Sleep* 2012; 35: 477–481.

57. Leseux L, Rossin N, Sedkaoui K, *et al.* Faisabilité du "coaching" téléphonique dans l'appareillage du syndrome d'apnée du sommeil. Coaching téléphonique et SAS. [Education of patients with sleep apnea syndrome: feasibility of a phone coaching procedure. Phone-coaching and SAS]. *Rev Mal Respir* 2012; 29: 40–46.

58. Parikh R, Touvelle MN, Wang H, *et al.* Sleep telemedicine: patient satisfaction and treatment adherence. *Telemed J E Health* 2011; 17: 609–614.

59. Sparrow D, Aloia M, Demolles DA, *et al.* A telemedicine intervention to improve adherence to continuous positive airway pressure: a randomised controlled trial. *Thorax* 2010; 65: 1061–1066.

60. Stepnowsky CJ, Palau JJ, Marler MR, *et al.* Pilot randomized trial of the effect of wireless telemonitoring on compliance and treatment efficacy in obstructive sleep apnea. *J Med Internet Res* 2007; 9: e14.

61. Smith CE, Dauz ER, Clements F, *et al.* Telehealth services to improve nonadherence: a placebo-controlled study. *Telemed J E Health* 2006; 12: 289–296.

62. Taylor Y, Eliasson A, Andrada T, *et al.* The role of telemedicine in CPAP compliance for patients with obstructive sleep apnea syndrome. *Sleep Breath* 2006; 10: 132–138.

63. DeMolles DA, Sparrow D, Gottlieb DJ, *et al.* A pilot trial of a telecommunications system in sleep apnea management. *Med Care* 2004; 42: 764–769.

64. Chervin RD, Theut S, Bassetti C, *et al.* Compliance with nasal CPAP can be improved by simple interventions. *Sleep* 1997; 20: 284–289.

65. Collop NA, Anderson WM, Boehlecke B, *et al.* Clinical guidelines for the use of unattended portable monitors in the diagnosis of obstructive sleep apnea in adult patients. *J Clin Sleep Med* 2007; 3: 737–747.

66. Masa JF, Corral J, Pereira R, *et al.* Effectiveness of home respiratory polygraphy for the diagnosis of sleep apnoea and hypopnoea syndrome. *Thorax* 2011; 66: 567–573.

67. Coma-Del-Corral MJ, Alonso-Álvarez ML, Allende M, *et al.* Reliability of telemedicine in the diagnosis and treatment of sleep apnea syndrome. *Telemed J E Health* 2013; 19: 7–12.

68. Bruyneel M, Ninane V. Unattended home-based polysomnography for sleep disordered breathing: current concepts and perspectives. *Sleep Med Rev* 2014; 18: 341–347.

69. Morillo DS, Gross N. Probabilistic neural network approach for the detection of SAHS from overnight pulse oximetry. *Med Biol Eng Comput* 2013; 51: 305–315.

70. Cao Z, Zhu R, Que RY. A wireless portable system with microsensors for monitoring respiratory diseases. *IEEE Trans Biomed Eng* 2012; 59: 3110–3116.

71. Morillo D, Rojas Ojeda JL, Crespo Foix LF, *et al.* An accelerometer-based device for sleep apnea screening. *IEEE Trans Inf Technol Biomed* 2010; 14: 491–499.

72. Arlotto P, Grimaldi M, Naeck R, *et al.* An ultrasonic contactless sensor for breathing monitoring. *Sensors (Basel)* 2014; 14: 15371–15386.

73. Hwang SH, Lee HJ, Yoon HN, *et al.* Unconstrained sleep apnea monitoring using polyvinylidene fluoride film-based sensor. *IEEE Trans Biomed Eng* 2014; 61: 2125–2134.

74. Sannino G, De Falco I, De Pietro G. Monitoring obstructive sleep apnea by means of a real-time mobile system based on the automatic extraction of sets of rules through differential evolution. *J Biomed Inform* 2014; 49: 84–100.

75. Defaye P, de la Cruz I, Martí-Almor J, *et al.* A pacemaker transthoracic impedance sensor with an advanced algorithm to identify severe sleep apnea: the DREAM European study. *Heart Rhythm* 2014; 11: 842–848.

76. Pallin M, O'Hare E, Zaffaroni A, *et al.* Comparison of a novel non-contact biomotion sensor with wrist actigraphy in estimating sleep quality in patients with obstructive sleep apnoea. *J Sleep Res* 2014; 23: 475–484.

77. Guerrero-Mora G, Palacios E, Bianchi AM, *et al.* Sleep-wake detection based on respiratory signal acquired through a pressure bed sensor. *Conf Proc IEEE Eng Med Biol Soc* 2012; 2012: 3452–3455.

78. Peltokangas M, Verho J, Vehkaoja A. Night-time EKG and HRV monitoring with bed sheet integrated textile electrodes. *IEEE Trans Inf Technol Biomed* 2012; 16: 935–942.

79. Hers V, Corbugy D, Joslet I, *et al.* New concept using Passive Infrared (PIR) technology for a contactless detection of breathing movement: a pilot study involving a cohort of 169 adult patients. *J Clin Monit Comput* 2013; 27: 521–529.

80. de Almeida JP, Pinto AC, Pereira J, *et al.* Implementation of a wireless device for real-time telemedical assistance of home-ventilated amyotrophic lateral sclerosis patients: a feasibility study. *Telemed J E Health* 2010; 16: 883–888.

81. Pinto A, Almeida JP, Pinto S, *et al.* Home telemonitoring of non-invasive ventilation decreases healthcare utilisation in a prospective controlled trial of patients with amyotrophic lateral sclerosis. *J Neurol Neurosurg Psychiatry* 2010; 81: 1238–1242.

82. Vitacca M, Guerra A, Assoni G, *et al.* Weaning from mechanical ventilation followed at home with the aid of a telemedicine program. *Telemed J E Health* 2007; 13: 445–449.

83. Vitacca M, Assoni G, Pizzocaro P, *et al.* A pilot study of nurse-led, home monitoring for patients with chronic respiratory failure and with mechanical ventilation assistance. *J Telemed Telecare* 2006; 12: 337–342.

84. Seifert GJ, Hedin DS, Dahlstrom RJ, *et al.* Telemedicine enabled remote critical care ventilator. *Conf Proc IEEE Eng Med Biol Soc* 2010; 2010: 1150–1153.

85. Swash M. Internet facilitated management improves home ventilation in amyotrophic lateral sclerosis. *J Neurol Neurosurg Psychiatry* 2010; 81: 1180.

Support statement: This work was supported in part by the Spanish Respiratory Society (SEPAR) and FIS PI11/01892.

Disclosures: None declared.

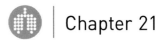

Chapter 21

Integrated care

Ching Li Chai-Coetzer[1,2], Nick Antic[1,2] and R. Doug McEvoy[1,2]

OSA is a highly prevalent, chronic condition that is frequently associated with modifiable risk factors and multiple medical comorbidities. Effective management of OSA requires a comprehensive, multidisciplinary, patient-centred approach that addresses not only the sleep disordered breathing events but also includes evaluation for and treatment of related medical comorbidities and strategies to optimise treatment adherence. Integrated care for OSA involves collaboration between health professionals from a variety of disciplines. There is significant potential for specialist nurses, as well as primary care physicians, to take greater responsibility for the diagnosis and management of OSA. Strategies aimed at promoting patient self-management and improving communication between patients and healthcare providers, including structured chronic disease self-management programmes and use of e-health interventions and related technologies, may be of benefit for patients with OSA.

A number of modifiable lifestyle factors are believed to be important contributors to the development of OSA, including obesity and excessive alcohol use. Furthermore, OSA patients often present with multiple chronic medical comorbidities, including depression, diabetes mellitus, hypertension and CVD. Therefore, effective management of OSA not only requires treatment to prevent the occurrence of sleep disordered breathing events, but must also address modifiable lifestyle factors as well as associated chronic medical conditions. OSA would ideally be suited to a comprehensive, integrated chronic disease management approach.

Chronic disease management

The concept of an integrated, patient-centred approach to chronic disease management using a chronic care model was originally described by WAGNER et al. [1] in the mid-1990s. It was proposed that, in order to deliver effective chronic disease management, there needed to be shift away from usual ambulatory care processes. These tended to focus on reactive treatment of acute symptoms, short appointments, brief and didactic patient education and patient-initiated follow-up. This lead to a system of regular, planned reviews involving patients and their caregivers, systematic assessment of disease, development and use of evidence-based guidelines, involvement of non-physician health providers, promotion of patient self-management aimed at prevention of disease exacerbations and/or complications and use of information systems to facilitate the initiation of disease registries

[1]Adelaide Institute for Sleep Health, Repatriation General Hospital, Daw Park, Australia. [2]School of Medicine, Faculty of Medicine, Nursing and Health Sciences, Flinders University, Bedford Park, Australia.

Correspondence: Doug McEvoy, Adelaide Institute for Sleep Health, Repatriation General Hospital, Daws Road, Daw Park, SA, Australia, 5041. E-mail: doug.mcevoy@health.sa.gov.au

Copyright ©ERS 2015. Print ISBN: 978-1-84984-059-0. Online ISBN: 978-1-84984-060-6. Print ISSN: 2312-508X. Online ISSN: 2312-5098.

and reminder systems to enable practise-initiated patient follow-up. The following six elements were identified as being essential aspects of the chronic care model [2]: 1) community resources and policies; 2) healthcare organisation; 3) self-management support; 4) delivery system design; 5) decision support; and 6) clinical information systems.

Integrated care models have increasingly been adopted for a wide range of chronic medical conditions, including COPD [3], diabetes mellitus [4], asthma [5], congestive cardiac failure [6], chronic kidney disease [7], depression [8] and arthritis [9]. For example, a multidimensional, patient-centred approach to the management of asthma and overlapping COPD in older adults that addresses medical comorbidities, risk factor modification and self-management skills, in addition to the treatment of airways disease, has been described previously [5]. A recent Cochrane review examined the effect of integrated disease management interventions of at least 3 months duration for patients with COPD [3]. The review, which included a total of 2997 participants from 26 trials, found statistically significant improvements in disease-specific quality of life and exercise capacity, as well as a reduction in hospital admissions and length of hospital stay compared to controls (*i.e.* standard care, no treatment, or single or mono-disciplinary interventions). Integrated care aimed at aggressive risk factor reduction for patients with atrial fibrillation improves long-term success of ablation therapy [10, 11]. A systematic review of interventions for diabetes mellitus in primary care has revealed that the most successful strategies to improve glycated haemoglobin (HbA1c) and cardiovascular risk factors are those that enable audit and feedback on performance, utilise clinical decision support systems, involve multidisciplinary teams and include patient education [4].

OSA fulfils the criteria for a chronic disease, which is defined as an illness that is prolonged in duration, often does not resolve spontaneously, and is rarely cured completely [12]. Although the 2009 American Academy for Sleep Medicine Clinical Guideline for the Evaluation, Management and Long Term Care of Obstructive Sleep Apnea in Adults recommends that the condition "should be approached as a chronic disease requiring long-term, multidisciplinary management" [13], available literature focussing on chronic disease management programmes for OSA remains scarce. Whilst previous studies have examined a role for health professionals other than sleep physicians, such as specialist nurses or primary care physicians, as principal providers of care for patients with OSA [14, 15], there have been no published studies specifically evaluating the effectiveness of comprehensive, integrated models of care for OSA.

Comorbidities associated with OSA

OSA and obesity

Patients with OSA often present with multiple chronic medical conditions, including hypertension, CVD, diabetes mellitus, depression and insomnia. A commonly shared risk factor is obesity, which is found in ~70% of patients with OSA and is associated with increasing OSA severity [16]. A 10% weight gain is associated with a 32% increase in AHI, whilst a 10% weight loss is associated with a 26% reduction in AHI [16]. Therefore, weight loss should be recommended for all overweight and obese patients with OSA. The recently published 2013 American Heart Association/American College of Cardiology/Obesity Society guidelines for the management of overweight and obesity in adults provides a treatment algorithm, "Chronic Disease Management Model for Primary Care of Patients with Overweight and Obesity" [17]. The algorithm includes recommendations for a comprehensive lifestyle intervention to achieve weight loss involving a multidisciplinary team of medical, nutritional and behavioural experts, with the use of additional strategies such as pharmacotherapy and bariatric surgery if required, as well as assessment and treatment of risk factors for CVD and other obesity-related comorbidities.

OSA and CVD risk

Observational cohort studies have reported an increase in hypertension [18], coronary artery disease [19, 20], cerebrovascular disease [21], congestive heart failure [22], cardiac arrhythmias [23] and cardiovascular mortality [24] in patients with OSA. Whilst most OSA patients with CVD will have one or more traditional risk factor, such as obesity, smoking, hypertension and hyperlipidaemia, mounting clinical and experimental data also point to a true independent association between OSA and CVD [25]. Hypertension is highly prevalent, affecting 35–80% of people with OSA, with higher rates seen in those with greater sleep apnoea severity [26]. Conversely, OSA has been found in ~40% of patients with hypertension, and in as many as 80% in those with resistant hypertension [27]. Type 2 diabetes mellitus, another important chronic illness and major risk factor for the development of CVD, has been found to be present in 30% of males with OSA in a sleep clinic population [28]. Prevalence of moderate-to-severe OSA (*i.e.* AHI $\geqslant$15 events·h^{-1}) has been found to be 36% (49% in men and 21% in women) in a group of consecutively recruited diabetic clinic patients [29]. A comprehensive chronic disease management approach to OSA involving multidisciplinary collaboration of healthcare providers at both primary care and specialty levels is, therefore, crucial to ensure that not only is OSA appropriately treated but that medical comorbidities are addressed and the risk for development of CVD is minimised. Identification and treatment of modifiable lifestyle factors, such as excessive alcohol intake and smoking, which may increase the risk of OSA and contribute to the development of CVD, would also be best undertaken using an integrative care approach. Referral for investigation of snoring and possible OSA provides an ideal opportunity to review and address traditional cardiovascular risk factors. Patients who are subsequently found not to have OSA, or are found to have OSA that is asymptomatic or minimally symptomatic and in whom OSA treatment is not accepted or considered suitable, should nevertheless have cardiovascular risk factors addressed [30]. When OSA treatment is initiated clinicians should be aware that it alone may not be sufficient to reverse or adequately treat the specific cardiovascular risk factor (s) involved [31].

OSA and depression

High rates of depression have been found in patients with OSA in both community and clinical settings, ranging from 17% to 41% [32]. OSA and depression share a number of overlapping symptoms, including complaints of daytime sleepiness or fatigue, poor concentration, low motivation and insomnia. Although excessive sleepiness is frequently reported to be an important symptom of OSA, a population study by BIXLER *et al.* [33] reported that depression was the strongest predictor of daytime sleepiness as defined by the ESS, followed by obesity, age, sleep duration, diabetes and smoking, ahead of OSA. Furthermore, residual sleepiness, as evidenced by a persistently abnormal ESS score, has been found to be present in over one-third of patients with moderate-to-severe OSA who have received treatment with 3 months of CPAP therapy at an optimal level of adherence (*i.e.* >6 h per night) [34]. Inadequately treated depression may be an important cause of ongoing daytime sleepiness in a significant number of these patients. Careful evaluation for mental health conditions and consideration of their potential impact on sleep health is important when assessing patients for sleep disorders, particularly those who report EDS. Mental health providers, such as psychologists and psychiatrists, should be incorporated into integrative sleep medicine teams.

OSA and insomnia

Sleep apnoea frequently coexists with other sleep disorders. A high prevalence of insomnia, ranging from 39% to 55%, has been reported in patients with OSA and 29– 67% of patients with insomnia have been found to have an AHI $\geqslant$5 events·h^{-1}[35]. Insomnia and OSA share common adverse health consequences, including a reduced quality of life, mood disturbances, an increased risk of motor vehicle or work-related accidents, and possibly increased cardiovascular risk. Treatment of OSA with CPAP could potentially worsen insomnia, and patients with insomnia may have difficulty accepting or adhering to CPAP in the long term due to increased feelings of anxiety and claustrophobia [36]. Use of benzodiazepines, which are commonly prescribed in primary care for patients who complain of insomnia, not only pose the problems of dependence, rebound and withdrawal effects, but may also increase the frequency and duration of sleep disordered breathing events in patients with OSA [37]. Effective therapy for comorbid insomnia and OSA will probably require investigation for and management of psychiatric conditions, and concurrent treatment of both insomnia and OSA using, for example, a combination of cognitive behaviour therapy for insomnia and CPAP.

Integrated sleep medicine service

Effective management of OSA requires a multidimensional approach that is tailored to the individual and addresses not only the problem of sleep disordered breathing, but also includes assessment for and treatment of related comorbidities and modifiable risk factors, and promotion of patient self-management skills.

Multidisciplinary sleep medicine team

A comprehensive, integrative sleep medicine service should have a patient-centred focus with involvement of health professionals from a broad range of disciplines that extend beyond the sleep specialist (fig. 1). Given that obesity is one of the leading causes, and a potentially modifiable risk factor for OSA, strategies aimed at successfully achieving and maintaining weight loss are crucial in the management of OSA. Therefore, the ability to access the services of health professionals, such as dieticians, exercise physiologists, psychologists, and surgeons specialising in bariatric surgery techniques, with capacity for intermittent multidisciplinary meetings to discuss complex patient cases would be important. Providing overweight and obese patients with information on available community resources to assist in and provide support for their weight loss efforts and to promote effective self-management behaviours is also critical.

As previously mentioned, mental health disorders such as depression and anxiety may be a consequence of, or commonly coexist with, OSA and other sleep disorders. Sleep physicians need to be aware of the potential overlap in those who present with sleep-related

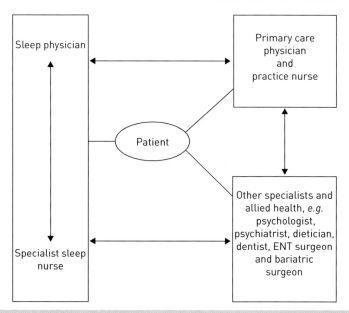

Figure 1. Integrated care for OSA. ENT: ear, nose and throat.

complaints, and ensure that patients are appropriately screened for mood disturbances with referral to mental health professionals, such as psychologists and psychiatrists, who should be part of the integrative sleep medicine team. Furthermore, psychologists (and other appropriately trained mental healthcare providers) can provide advice to patients on lifestyle changes to combat modifiable risk factors for OSA such as obesity, excessive alcohol intake and cigarette smoking, provide cognitive behaviour therapy for insomnia and help deliver effective CPAP adherence interventions (*e.g.* motivational interviewing or cognitive behaviour therapy).

There is a need for regular multidisciplinary clinical meetings between different healthcare providers to discuss complex patients, share ideas and learn from each other. Up-to-date teleconferencing software could be used to enable healthcare providers to link into these meetings from different locations, *e.g.* primary healthcare providers from their practise location, although it is important that face-to-face meetings also occur from time to time.

Optimising CPAP adherence

Although CPAP is a highly efficacious therapy for OSA, non-adherence to treatment can be problematic, with ~50% of patients either failing to commence CPAP therapy or using it for <4 h per night [38]. Although adherence has frequently been described as use of CPAP for at least 4 h·night^{-1} on 70% of nights, the precise amount of CPAP use that equates to optimal patient outcomes remains poorly defined and appears to be dependent on the outcome measure examined. Several studies have demonstrated a CPAP dose–response effect with greater improvements in both subjective and objective measures of sleepiness, as well as neurocognitive performance, seen in patients with longer average nightly CPAP use [34, 39, 40]. WEAVER *et al.* [39] demonstrated that after 3 months of treatment, subjective sleepiness was normalised (*i.e.* ESS ⩽10) in the greatest proportion of OSA patients with CPAP use of 4 h·night^{-1}. Objective sleepiness was normalised (*i.e.* multiple sleep latency test $\geqslant$7.5 min) in the largest proportion of patients with 6 h·night^{-1} of CPAP use, whilst normal functional outcomes, as measured by the Functional Outcomes of Sleep Questionnaire, was achieved in the greatest proportion of patients with CPAP use of 7.5 h·night^{-1}.

No individual factor has been consistently shown to predict CPAP adherence. The factors influencing CPAP adherence are multifactorial and highly variable between individuals, including patient and disease characteristics, technological factors, initial CPAP experience and psychosocial factors [41]. Although disease severity, as determined by the AHI, ODI and daytime sleepiness, has been demonstrated to be associated with CPAP use in some studies [42, 43], this has not been a consistent finding. Several studies have identified an association between early CPAP use and long-term adherence [44–46], thus efforts to optimise patients' early experiences with CPAP may be important in achieving long-term treatment success.

An abundance of published papers have emerged in recent years evaluating a multitude of strategies aimed at promoting CPAP adherence. These include educational [47], technological [48, 49], cognitive behavioural and psychosocial [50, 51], pharmacological, social [52] and multidimensional approaches, which have met with varying degrees of success. A multidisciplinary approach that is tailored to the individual appears to be necessary in order to optimise CPAP adherence in sleep clinic populations. For those who are unable to tolerate CPAP therapy, alternative treatment options will need to be provided. Therefore, an integrative sleep medicine service should also include dentists, who can evaluate patients for a mandibular advancement splint, and ear, nose and throat specialists, who can provide assessments to determine patient suitability for UA surgery.

Expanded role for specialist sleep nurses

With greater demand for improved and more efficient models of care for chronic disease, there has been increasing interest in specialist nurse roles for a wide range of medical conditions in both the primary care and specialist settings. A review of RCTs examining the effectiveness of specialised nurses with an autonomous role in chronic disease management in primary healthcare settings *versus* physicians for conditions such as diabetes, coronary artery disease and HF revealed comparable outcomes in health resource use, disease-specific measures, quality of life and patient satisfaction [53]. The studies included in this review were conducted in the USA, UK and the Netherlands. In trials of nurses working in collaboration with primary care physicians (PCPs) *versus* physicians working alone, disease-specific improvements and improved patient satisfaction were found and hospitalisation rates decreased for patients with coronary artery disease [53]. Another recent systematic review of RCTs of nurse-managed protocols for patients with diabetes, hyperlipidaemia and hypertension conducted in the USA and Western Europe reported positive findings with respect to HbA1c levels and BP control and a trend to improved serum lipids [54]. A previous randomised controlled study conducted in the Netherlands assessing a nurse-led clinic for the management of atrial fibrillation, which provided integrated care with use of clinical guidelines, software support and cardiologist supervision, *versus* usual care, revealed a superior outcome for nurse-led management, with a significant reduction in the composite outcome of cardiovascular hospitalisations and mortality after a mean follow-up of 22 months (14.3% *versus* 20.8%, HR 0.65 (95% CI 0.45–0.93); p=0.017) [55]. In the USA, the Department of Veterans Affairs is currently giving nurses and nurse practitioners a major role as care managers in the Patient Aligned Care Teams initiative, which is being developed to more effectively tackle the burden of chronic disease in the Veterans Affairs population [56].

We have previously evaluated a specialist nurse-led model of care for the management of OSA in three Australian tertiary care-based sleep centres [14]. In this study, 195 patients found to have moderate-to-severe OSA (*i.e.* >2% ODI >27 events·h^{-1} by home oximetry, ESS $\geqslant$8 and history of snoring) were randomised into either a simplified, nurse-led model of care consisting of home auto-adjusting PAP treatment to determine a fixed CPAP pressure, or to traditional, physician-led management including laboratory-based PSG and CPAP titration. After 3 months follow-up, specialist nurse-led management was not inferior to physician-led care in terms of the mean change in ESS score (4.02 *versus* 4.15, difference −0.13 (95% CI −1.52–1.25); non-inferiority margin −2.0). There were also no significant differences in objective sleepiness (maintenance of wakefulness test), quality of life (Functional Outcomes of Sleep Questionnaire and Short Form-36), executive neurocognitive function or CPAP adherence. Whilst overall patient satisfaction was no different, results for four out of nine items within the Visit-specific Satisfaction Questionnaire (relating to time waited, explanation, information provided and time spent with the healthcare professional) were in favour of the nurse-led model. Thus, selected patients with OSA can be managed by appropriately trained specialist nurses without compromising patient outcomes. Specialist, sleep-trained nurses also have the potential to take on an expanded role in the management of OSA, and might be ideally suited, for example, to assist in patient counselling to address issues such as obesity, excessive alcohol use, smoking cessation and CVD risk reduction, and delivering cognitive behavioural therapy and/or other psychosocial interventions to optimise CPAP adherence or as part of the management of depression and insomnia.

Primary care management of OSA

Collaboration with primary care-based physicians and allied health professionals is an integral part of chronic disease management for OSA. PCPs are ideally positioned to identify, monitor and coordinate care for patients with multiple chronic medical comorbidities. There is a potential role for either the incorporation of PCPs into sleep medicine teams, or development of hub-and-spoke models of care whereby OSA is managed predominantly in the primary care setting by physicians and practise nurses, with support from a tertiary care-based specialist sleep centre.

In our own research, we have demonstrated comparable clinical outcomes for patients managed using the latter approach. In a RCT [15], PCPs identified a total of 155 patients with moderate-to-severe OSA using a validated, two-step diagnostic strategy [57] of OSA50 screening questionnaire and home oximetry ($\geqslant$3% ODI $\geqslant$16 events·h^{-1}) plus daytime sleepiness (ESS $\geqslant$8) who were assigned to either ambulatory management by their PCP and a community-based nurse, or to usual laboratory-based care by a sleep specialist. (OSA50 is a questionnaire developed to screen primary care patients for high risk of OSA according to the presence or absence of obesity (by waist circumference measurement), troublesome snoring witnessed by sleep apnoeas, and age > or <50 years [57].) Prior to their involvement in the study, PCPs and community-based nurses were provided with training on OSA and its management in the form of a 6-h education module, and nursing staff undertook an additional week of intensive, in-service training at a specialist sleep centre. After a total of

6 months of follow-up, primary care management was not inferior to specialist management in terms of the mean change in ESS score, which was 5.8 for the primary care arm *versus* 5.4 for the specialist arm (adjusted difference −0.13 (lower bound one-sided 95% CI −1.5), p=0.43; non-inferiority margin −2.0). Also, no significant differences were found between groups for secondary outcome measures, including disease-specific and general quality of life, OSA symptoms, CPAP adherence and overall patient satisfaction. Furthermore, comparison of within-trial costs revealed that primary care management was less costly at an average of AUD$1606 per patient *versus* $2576 for specialist care.

Investigators in Spain have recently conducted a randomised controlled study, evaluating primary care follow-up of patients who were diagnosed with OSA (*i.e.* AHI $\geqslant$30 events·h^{-1}, ESS$\geqslant$10 and/or high CVD risk) and commenced on CPAP therapy, compared to standard care in a specialist sleep centre (F. Barbe, Respiratory Dept, Hospital Univ Arnau de Vilanova, Lleida, Spain; personal communication). At 6 months follow-up, the primary care-managed group were not inferior to the specialist group in terms of CPAP compliance. However, there appeared to be greater improvements in ESS scores and patient satisfaction in the specialist arm. Assessment of within-trial costs revealed cost-savings for the primary care group.

Although the results from these efficacy studies conducted in primary care appear promising, there are some important considerations. First, PCPs that were involved in these studies received training in OSA management and agreed to participate in a randomised controlled study; therefore, it is possible that they may have a higher level of motivation and interest in OSA compared to other PCPs. Also, patients involved in this study were a selected group of individuals, with symptomatic, moderate-to-severe disease and those with significant respiratory, cardiovascular and/or psychiatric comorbidities were excluded from participation. Furthermore, research trial participants may be more highly motivated or engaged in their care and may not be truly representative of the broader primary care population. Thus, these results will need to be confirmed and extended by larger "real-world" effectiveness RCTs and large-scale data registry studies.

Patient self-management

A crucial component of the chronic care model is the provision of appropriate resources and support to ensure that patients and their families have the skills and confidence to play an active role in the management of their chronic condition(s). Structured self-management support interventions, such as the Flinders Chronic Condition Management Programme (Flinders Programme) [58] and the Stanford Chronic Disease Self-Management Programme [59], have been developed to provide individuals with the tools and knowledge to promote effective self-management for a variety of chronic diseases. The Flinders Programme is a generic, health professional-led, self-management intervention derived from cognitive behaviour therapy and motivational interviewing approaches, which is designed to assess an individual's self-management behaviours, explore barriers to self-management, identify key problems and set goals that will result in sustained behaviour change [58]. Studies evaluating the Flinders Programme have demonstrated improved health outcomes for a variety of chronic medical conditions [60–63]. Therefore, a structured self-management support intervention such as the Flinders Programme could potentially be of benefit to patients with OSA.

With modern advances in technology, there has been growing interest in the use of computers and mobile devices to improve communication between patients and health professionals, and to deliver patient self-management programmes. A systematic review of e-health interventions for chronic diseases, (including monitoring, provision of treatment instructions, self-management training and provision of general information *via* interactive websites), either in addition to or instead of usual face-to-face care, revealed small-to-moderate improvements in several clinical health outcomes [64]. Technology is currently available which enables information from patients' CPAP devices, such as applied pressures, leaks, residual AHI and duration of machine usage, to be transmitted *via* a modem to healthcare providers, allowing for early identification of problems and appropriate intervention and could be adapted to provide relevant information directly to patients as part of self-management. A randomised study comparing the use of a telemedicine monitoring system in patients who commenced CPAP for moderate-to-severe OSA showed significant improvements in CPAP adherence compared to standard care alone [65]. Web-based and mobile technologies hold significant promise as a means for promoting patient self-management and facilitating communication between patients and healthcare providers; however, further research into their effectiveness in patients with OSA is needed.

Conclusion

OSA is a common chronic disease associated with a number of modifiable risk factors and multiple medical comorbidities which requires a comprehensive, integrated management approach. Treatment should be tailored around the needs of the patient, who should take an active role in their own treatment, and should involve collaboration amongst healthcare providers from multiple disciplines that extend beyond the sleep physician. There is growing evidence in support of an expanded role for nurses in the management of OSA both in the specialist and primary care settings. Structured self-management support interventions may be of potential benefit for patients with OSA, and future research should focus on assessing the effectiveness and cost-effectiveness of comprehensive, integrated management programmes for OSA.

References

1. Wagner EH, Austin BT, Von Korff M. Organizing care for patients with chronic illness. *Milbank Q* 1996; 74: 511–544.
2. Bodenheimer T, Wagner EH, Grumbach K. Improving primary care for patients with chronic illness. *JAMA* 2002; 288: 1775–1779.
3. Kruis AL, Smidt N, Assendelft WJ, *et al.* Integrated disease management interventions for patients with chronic obstructive pulmonary disease. *Cochrane Database Syst Rev* 2013; 10: CD009437.
4. Seitz P, Rosemann T, Gensichen J, *et al.* Interventions in primary care to improve cardiovascular risk factors and glycated haemoglobin (HbA1c) levels in patients with diabetes: a systematic review. *Diabetes Obes Metab* 2011; 13: 479–489.
5. Gibson PG, McDonald VM, Marks GB. Asthma in older adults. *Lancet* 2010; 376: 803–813.
6. Comin-Colet J, Verdu-Rotellar JM, Vela E, *et al.* Efficacy of an integrated hospital-primary care program for heart failure: a population-based analysis of 56,742 patients. *Rev Esp Cardiol (Engl Ed)* 2014; 67: 283–293.
7. Chen PM, Lai TS, Chen PY, *et al.* Multidisciplinary care program for advanced chronic kidney disease: reduces renal replacement and medical costs. *Am J Med* 2015; 128: 68–76.
8. Gellis ZD, Kenaley BL, Ten Have T. Integrated telehealth care for chronic illness and depression in geriatric home care patients: the Integrated Telehealth Education and Activation of Mood (I-TEAM) study. *J Am Geriatr Soc* 2014; 62: 889–895.
9. van Vilsteren M, Boot CR, Steenbeek R, *et al.* An intervention program with the aim to improve and maintain work productivity for workers with rheumatoid arthritis: design of a randomized controlled trial and cost-effectiveness study. *BMC Public Health* 2012; 12: 496.

10. Pathak R, Middeldorp M, Lau D, et al. Aggressive Risk factor Reduction Study for Atrial Fibrilliation (ARREST-AF Cohort Study): implications for the outcome of ablation. *J Am Coll Cardiol*; 2014; 64: 2222–2231.

11. Abed HS, Wittert GA, Leong DP, et al. Effect of weight reduction and cardiometabolic risk factor management on symptom burden and severity in patients with atrial fibrillation: a randomized clinical trial. *JAMA* 2013; 310: 2050–2060.

12. Dowrick C, Dixon-Woods M, Holman H, et al. What is chronic illness? *Chronic Illn* 2005; 1: 1–6.

13. Epstein LJ, Kristo D, Strollo PJ Jr, et al. Clinical guideline for the evaluation, management and long-term care of obstructive sleep apnea in adults. *J Clin Sleep Med* 2009; 5: 263–276.

14. Antic NA, Buchan C, Esterman A, et al. A randomized controlled trial of nurse-led care for symptomatic moderate-severe obstructive sleep apnea. *Am J Respir Crit Care Med* 2009; 179: 501–508.

15. Chai-Coetzer CL, Antic NA, Rowland LS, et al. Primary care *vs* specialist sleep center management of obstructive sleep apnea and daytime sleepiness and quality of life: a randomized trial. *JAMA* 2013; 309: 997–1004.

16. Peppard PE, Young T, Palta M, et al. Longitudinal study of moderate weight change and sleep-disordered breathing. *JAMA* 2000; 284: 3015–3021.

17. Jensen MD, Ryan DH, Apovian CM, et al. 2013 AHA/ACC/TOS guideline for the management of overweight and obesity in adults: a report of the American College of Cardiology/American Heart Association Task Force on Practice Guidelines and The Obesity Society. *J Am Coll Cardiol* 2014; 63: 2985–3023.

18. Peppard PE, Young T, Palta M, et al. Prospective study of the association between sleep-disordered breathing and hypertension. *N Eng J Med* 2000; 342: 1378–1384.

19. Marin JM, Carrizo SJ, Vicente E, et al. Long-term cardiovascular outcomes in men with obstructive sleep apnoea-hypopnoea with or without treatment with continuous positive airway pressure: an observational study. *Lancet* 2005; 365: 1046–1053

20. Shahar E, Whitney CW, Redline S, et al. Sleep-disordered breathing and cardiovascular disease. Cross-sectional results of the sleep heart health study. *Am J Respir Crit Care Med* 2001; 163: 19–25.

21. Redline S, Yenokyan G, Gottlieb DJ, et al. Obstructive sleep apnea-hypopnea and incident stroke: the Sleep Heart Health Study. *Am J Respir Crit Care Med* 2010; 182: 269–277.

22. Gottlieb DJ, Yenokyan G, Newman AB, et al. Prospective study of obstructive sleep apnea and incident coronary heart disease and heart failure: the sleep heart health study. *Circulation* 2010; 122: 352–360.

23. Mehra R, Benjamin EJ, Shahar E, et al. Association of nocturnal arrhythmias with sleep-disordered breathing: the Sleep Heart Health Study. *Am J Respir Crit Care Med* 2006; 173: 910–916.

24. Punjabi NM, Caffo BS, Goodwin JL, et al. Sleep-disordered breathing and mortality: a prospective cohort study. *PLoS Med* 2009; 6: e1000132.

25. Lévy P, Ryan S, Oldenburg O, et al. Sleep apnoea and the heart. *Eur Respir Rev* 2013; 22: 333–352.

26. Parati G, Lombardi C, Hedner J, et al. Recommendations for the management of patients with obstructive sleep apnoea and hypertension. *Eur Respir J* 2013; 41: 523–538.

27. Logan AG, Perlikowski SM, Mente A, et al. High prevalence of unrecognized sleep apnoea in drug-resistant hypertension. *J Hypertens* 2001; 19: 2271–2277.

28. Meslier N, Gagnadoux F, Giraud P, et al. Impaired glucose-insulin metabolism in males with obstructive sleep apnoea syndrome. *Eur Respir J* 2003; 22: 156–160.

29. Einhorn D, Stewart DA, Erman MK, et al. Prevalence of sleep apnea in a population of adults with type 2 diabetes mellitus. *Endocr Pract* 2007; 13: 355–362.

30. Grunstein RR, Phillips CL. Obstructive sleep apnoea – getting to the heart of the matter? *Med J Aust* 2008; 188: 324–325.

31. Pepin JL, Tamisier R, Barone-Rochette G, et al. Comparison of continuous positive airway pressure and valsartan in hypertensive patients with sleep apnea. *Am J Respir Crit Care Med* 2010; 182: 954–960.

32. Harris M, Glozier N, Ratnavadivel R, et al. Obstructive sleep apnea and depression. *Sleep Med Rev* 2009; 13: 437–444.

33. Bixler EO, Vgontzas AN, Lin HM, et al. Excessive daytime sleepiness in a general population sample: the role of sleep apnea, age, obesity, diabetes, and depression. *J Clin Endocrinol Metab* 2005; 90: 4510–4515.

34. Antic NA, Catcheside P, Buchan C, et al. The effect of CPAP in normalizing daytime sleepiness, quality of life, and neurocognitive function in patients with moderate to severe OSA. *Sleep* 2011; 34: 111–119.

35. Luyster FS, Buysse DJ, Strollo PJ Jr. Comorbid insomnia and obstructive sleep apnea: challenges for clinical practice and research. *J Clin Sleep Med* 2010; 6: 196–204.

36. Bjornsdottir E, Janson C, Sigurdsson JF, et al. Symptoms of insomnia among patients with obstructive sleep apnea before and after two years of positive airway pressure treatment. *Sleep* 2013; 36: 1901–1909.

37. Dolly FR, Block AJ. Effect of flurazepam on sleep-disordered breathing and nocturnal oxygen desaturation in asymptomatic subjects. *Am J Med* 1982; 73: 239–243.

38. Weaver TE, Grunstein RR. Adherence to continuous positive airway pressure therapy: the challenge to effective treatment. *Proc Am Thorac Soc* 2008; 5: 173–178.

39. Weaver TE, Maislin G, Dinges DF, *et al.* Relationship between hours of CPAP use and achieving normal levels of sleepiness and daily functioning. *Sleep* 2007; 30: 711–719.

40. Zimmerman ME, Arnedt JT, Stanchina M, *et al.* Normalization of memory performance and positive airway pressure adherence in memory-impaired patients with obstructive sleep apnea. *Chest* 2006; 130: 1772–1778.

41. Sawyer AM, Gooneratne NS, Marcus CL, *et al.* A systematic review of CPAP adherence across age groups: clinical and empiric insights for developing CPAP adherence interventions. *Sleep Med Rev* 2011; 15: 343–356.

42. McArdle N, Devereux G, Heidarnejad H, *et al.* Long-term use of CPAP therapy for sleep apnea/hypopnea syndrome. *Am J Respir Crit Care Med* 1999; 159: 1108–1114.

43. Kohler M, Smith D, Tippett V, *et al.* Predictors of long-term compliance with continuous positive airway pressure. *Thorax* 2010; 65: 829–832.

44. Weaver TE, Kribbs NB, Pack AI, *et al.* Night-to-night variability in CPAP use over the first three months of treatment. *Sleep* 1997; 20: 278–283.

45. Budhiraja R, Parthasarathy S, Drake CL, *et al.* Early CPAP use identifies subsequent adherence to CPAP therapy. *Sleep* 2007; 30: 320–324.

46. Chai-Coetzer CL, Luo YM, Antic NA, *et al.* Predictors of long-term adherence to continuous positive airway pressure therapy in patients with obstructive sleep apnea and cardiovascular disease in the SAVE study. *Sleep* 2013; 36: 1929–1937.

47. Lettieri CJ, Walter RJ. Impact of group education on continuous positive airway pressure adherence. *J Clin Sleep Med* 2013; 9: 537–541.

48. Chihara Y, Tsuboi T, Hitomi T, *et al.* Flexible positive airway pressure improves treatment adherence compared with auto-adjusting PAP. *Sleep* 2013; 36: 229–236.

49. Bakker JP, Marshall NS. Flexible pressure delivery modification of continuous positive airway pressure for obstructive sleep apnea does not improve compliance with therapy: systematic review and meta-analysis. *Chest* 2011; 139: 1322–1330.

50. Bartlett D, Wong K, Richards D, *et al.* Increasing adherence to obstructive sleep apnea treatment with a group social cognitive therapy treatment intervention: a randomized trial. *Sleep* 2013; 36: 1647–1654.

51. Aloia MS, Arnedt JT, Strand M, *et al.* Motivational enhancement to improve adherence to positive airway pressure in patients with obstructive sleep apnea: a randomized controlled trial. *Sleep* 2013; 36: 1655–1662.

52. Baron KG, Smith TW, Berg CA, *et al.* Spousal involvement in CPAP adherence among patients with obstructive sleep apnea. *Sleep Breath* 2011; 15: 525–534.

53. Health Quality Ontario. Specialized nursing practice for chronic disease management in the primary care setting: an evidence-based analysis. *Ont Health Technol Assess Ser* 2013; 13: 1–66.

54. Shaw RJ, McDuffie JR, Hendrix CC, *et al.* Effects of nurse-managed protocols in the outpatient management of adults with chronic conditions: a systematic review and meta-analysis. *Ann Intern Med* 2014; 161: 113–121.

55. Hendriks JM, de Wit R, Crijns HJ, *et al.* Nurse-led care *vs.* usual care for patients with atrial fibrillation: results of a randomized trial of integrated chronic care *vs.* routine clinical care in ambulatory patients with atrial fibrillation. *Eur Heart J* 2012; 33: 2692–2699.

56. Shaw RJ, McDuffie JR, Hendrix CC, *et al.* Effects of Nurse-Managed Protocols in the Outpatient Management of Adults with Chronic Conditions. Washington, Deptartment of Veterans Affairs, 2013.

57. Chai-Coetzer CL, Antic NA, Rowland LS, *et al.* A simplified model of screening questionnaire and home monitoring for obstructive sleep apnoea in primary care. *Thorax* 2011; 66: 213–219.

58. Reed RL, Battersby M, Osborne RH, *et al.* Protocol for a randomised controlled trial of chronic disease self-management support for older Australians with multiple chronic diseases. *Contemp Clin Trials* 2011; 32: 946–952.

59. Lorig KR, Sobel DS, Ritter PL, *et al.* Effect of a self-management program on patients with chronic disease. *Eff Clin Pract* 2001; 4: 256–262.

60. Crotty M, Prendergast J, Battersby MW, *et al.* Self-management and peer support among people with arthritis on a hospital joint replacement waiting list: a randomised controlled trial. *Osteoarthritis Cartilage* 2009; 17: 1428–1433.

61. Lawn S, Battersby MW, Pols RG, *et al.* The mental health expert patient: findings from a pilot study of a generic chronic condition self-management programme for people with mental illness. *Int J Soc Psychiatry* 2007; 53: 63–74.

62. Battersby M, Hoffmann S, Cadilhac D, *et al.* "Getting your life back on track after stroke": a Phase II multi-centered, single-blind, randomized, controlled trial of the Stroke Self-Management Program *vs.* the Stanford Chronic Condition Self-Management Program or standard care in stroke survivors. *Int J Stroke* 2009; 4: 137–144.

63. Harvey PW, Petkov JN, Misan G, *et al.* Self-management support and training for patients with chronic and complex conditions improves health-related behaviour and health outcomes. *Aust Health Rev* 2008; 32: 330–338.

64. Eland-de Kok P, van Os-Medendorp H, Vergouwe-Meijer A, *et al.* A systematic review of the effects of e-health on chronically ill patients. *J Clin Nurs* 2011; 20: 2997–3010.
65. Fox N, Hirsch-Allen AJ, Goodfellow E, *et al.* The impact of a telemedicine monitoring system on positive airway pressure adherence in patients with obstructive sleep apnea: a randomized controlled trial. *Sleep* 2012; 35: 477–481.

Disclosures: C.L. Chai-Coetzer has received grants from the National Health and Medical Research Council of Australia and other funding from ResMed, Philips Respironics and SomnoMed, outside the submitted work. N. Antic has received a grant from Philips-Respironics for a large RCT of CPAP therapy for OSA with additional equipment donations from Philips-Respironics, ResMed, Fisher and Paykel, and Compumedics (all sleep device companies) for this project. Equipment donations have also been received from Philips-Respironics, ResMed and Somnomed for a RCT of simplified management of OSA in specialist and primary care settings. N. Antic has received honoraria for educational presentations from Resmed and GSK. R.D. McEvoy is in receipt of a National Health and Medical Research Council Practitioner Fellowship, and several of the studies included in this chapter were funded by National Health and Medical Research Council project grants. He has received grants from Philips Respironics and Fisher and Paykel for the SAVE study. He has also received non-financial support from ResMed for equipment for the SAVE study and from Airliquide for equipment and in-kind support for two AISH-led clinical trials. R.D. McEvoy has received grants from the National Health and Medical Research Council during the conduct of the study. He has also received grants from Philips Respironics and Fisher and Paykel, and non-financial support from ResMed and Airliquide, outside the submitted work.

Chapter 22

Overall treatment strategies

Patrick Lévy[1,2,3], Jean-Louis Pépin[1,2,3], Renaud Tamisier[1,2,3] and Sandrine Launois-Rollinat[1,2,3]

Treatment of OSA has been extensively studied in the past 15 years. There has been a large number of controlled studies evaluating CPAP effects on sleepiness and daytime functioning, BP, cardiovascular outcomes, and metabolic parameters. These studies may help to determine to what extent CPAP is able to reverse the chronic consequences of OSA. Although there is a clinically significant impact of CPAP on EDS and daytime functioning as well as a reduction in BP, EDS may persist in a significant proportion of patients and BP may fall only modestly under CPAP, *i.e.* 1 to 3 mmHg. In addition, other cardiovascular morbidities seem to be moderately improved by CPAP. Other treatments, such as weight loss, positional treatment, oral appliances (MADs), UA stimulation and UA surgery, should be considered, although the degree of evidence is much less strong than that regarding CPAP. Using these data, in this chapter, we describe treatment strategies according to OSA severity. Lastly, we suggest that comparison and combination of treatment modalities, *e.g.* CPAP for OSA alleviation and specific cardiovascular or metabolic treatments, may be critical as regards full reversion of the chronic consequences of sleep apnoea.

Since 1981, nasal CPAP has been the first-line therapy for OSA [1]. However, there are limitations to CPAP use owing to side-effects and intolerability in some patients [2–4]. Thus, although there is no doubt that CPAP is nearly the only therapeutic possibility in severe OSA, alternatives are highly desirable in moderate OSA. Mild OSA is also part of the spectrum of the disease where CPAP is not the only desirable treatment, as there is no superiority of CPAP over MADs and MADs may be better tolerated [5–7].

The treatment of OSA during sleep should achieve three goals: 1) to alleviate symptoms and to improve quality of life [8]; 2) to reduce morbidity; and 3) to decrease mortality. Consequently, the choice of a particular treatment for a given patient should induce the lowest possible level of side-effects while addressing these outcomes.

Definitions

OSA has been redefined in the last 15 years [9–11]. To qualify as OSA, there should be EDS that is not better explained by other factors, or two or more "minor" symptoms (choking or

[1]Grenoble Alpes University, HP2 laboratory, Grenoble France. [2]Inserm U1042, Grenoble, France. [3]Clinique Universitaire de Physiologie et Sommeil, Pôle THORAX et VAISSEAUX, Hôpital A. Michallon, Grenoble, France.

Correspondence: Patrick Lévy, EFCR, Pôle Thorax et Vaisseaux, CHU de Grenoble, BP 217 X, 38043, Grenoble, France.
E-mail: patrick.levy@ujf-grenoble.fr

gasping during sleep, recurrent awakenings from sleep, unrefreshing sleep, daytime fatigue, or impaired concentration), plus an overnight monitoring demonstrating five or more obstructed breathing events per hour of sleep (*i.e.* apnoeas or hypopnoeas). The diagnosis may also be considered when the AHI is more than 15 even in the absence of symptoms.

The use of an event frequency of 5 per hour as a minimal threshold value was based on epidemiological data suggesting minimal health effects such as hypertension, sleepiness and motor vehicle accidents may be observed at an AHI threshold of 5 [12–15]. Additionally, data from interventional studies suggest a treatment-associated improvement in daytime function in mild-to-moderate sleep apnoea patients [16–18].

Defining the severity of OSA hypopnoea syndrome (OSAHS) is essential when establishing a strategy of treatment. It is usually suggested that the severity level should be based on two components: severity of daytime sleepiness and AHI based on overnight monitoring, the rating of severity being based on the most severe component. Sleepiness should be defined as mild, moderate or severe. The severity of sleep-related obstructive breathing events has been rated as follow. Mild: 5 to 15 events·h^{-1}; moderate: 15 to 30 events·h^{-1}; severe: greater than 30 events·h^{-1}.

There are currently no adequate prospective studies that have validated severity criteria for sleepiness. The data to justify a severity index based on event frequency are derived from various studies evidencing excess in morbidity at a given AHI [19]. It should be noted that SDB scoring definitions may significantly alter the outcomes [20], *e.g.* hypopnoea or oxygen desaturation quantification. Thus, comparison between studies is still difficult as AHI may vary significantly according to the scoring rules.

It is obvious from the literature that the severity of oxygen desaturation is a major predictive factor for OSA morbidity, especially cardiovascular consequences [21–23]. The most commonly used indices are the number of arterial oxygen saturation (SaO_2) drops (ODI), mean nocturnal SaO_2, minimal nocturnal SaO_2 and the cumulative time spent below a given value of SaO_2 (*e.g.* 90% or 85%). It is still unclear which SaO_2 parameter should be used. There had been debate regarding using 3% *versus* 4% desaturation when scoring hypopneas. In revising the 2007 American Academy of Sleep Medicine scoring manual, a task force reviewed the data supporting using a given level of desaturation [10]. For example, PUNJABI *et al.* [20] found respiratory events based on a desaturation of at least 4% were associated with an increased risk of cardiovascular consequences. Further analysis of Wisconsin Cohort data and Sleep Heart Health Study data suggests that the use of a ⩾3% desaturation criterion yields an AHI that is as predictive of adverse outcomes as an AHI based on a ⩾4% oxygen desaturation criterion [9, 24]. MEHRA *et al.* [25] used a definition of hypopnea based on ⩾3% desaturation, and found significant associations between AHI and the risk of atrial fibrillation or complex ventricular ectopy in older men without HF. Another study using a hypopnea definition requiring ⩾3% oxygen desaturation found an association between incident stroke and OSA [26]. Recognising the apparent equivalence of hypopnea definitions requiring ⩾3% or ⩾4% desaturation, this task force recommended adoption of the ⩾3% criterion. However, they pointed out that using ⩾3% instead of a ⩾4% desaturation requirement for defining hypopnea does increase the AHI substantially, with median AHI in a general community sample being almost twice as great using a ⩾3% as a ⩾4% criterion [10]. To our knowledge, there are limited data as regards other indices of oxygen desaturation, which makes difficult to propose specific thresholds.

Severe OSA

Since 1981, CPAP has progressively become the reference treatment in OSA hypopnoea (OSAH) [1]. Only very few alternatives should be discussed. UA surgery can be considered even in severe OSA but in selected populations. Bariatric surgery is becoming more popular and also marks the progression of obesity worldwide. There is some improvement in OSA after bariatric surgery. There are recent data suggesting that the stimulation of the hypoglossal nerve may be an option. Lastly, oral appliances are usually considered as less effective than CPAP in severe OSA.

CPAP: compliance, duration of treatment and relevant outcome measures

As mentioned earlier, CPAP remains the first-line therapy in OSA. However, compliance is a key point. Several studies, coming mainly from the USA [27–30], have demonstrated low compliance and irregular use of CPAP. However, many other studies have found a high rate of compliance (ranging from 65% to 80%) [31–33] and acceptance (about 15% of patients refusing this treatment after a single night's use in the laboratory) [31]. More recent reports confirmed these initial studies with persistent conflicting data [34]. The differences observed in compliance may merely reflect the respective efficacy of technical and medical follow-up in the different countries. However, there are significant side-effects affecting a majority of patients using CPAP [2, 31]. The reason for a high compliance despite side-effects (daily use between 5 and 6 h) [2] is obviously the clinical benefit obtained: only 1% of the patients had no subjective benefit induced by their therapy [2].

Another major issue is the optimal duration for CPAP use. Although there are few data to establish a clear threshold, there is growing evidence that a minimum duration of use of 4–5 h is required. EDS and daytime functioning including cognitive functioning improvements are highly dependent upon CPAP duration [35]. In this particular study, thresholds above which further improvements were less likely relative to nightly duration of CPAP were identified for ESS score (4 h), Multiple Sleep Latency Test (MSLT) (6 h) and Functional Outcomes of Sleep Questionnaire (FOSQ) (7.5 h). A linear dose–response relationship between increased use and achieving normal levels was shown for objective and subjective daytime sleepiness [35]. This also appears to be the case for BP and cardiovascular morbidity. It has been suggested from meta-analyses that the reduction in BP obtained with CPAP is more or less related to increasing use [36]. In addition, CPAP treatment for 1 year is associated with a small decrease in BP in nonsleepy OSA patients only in patients who use CPAP for more than 5.6 h per night [37]. Lastly, CPAP effects on cardiovascular events (occurrence of hypertension or nonfatal myocardial infarction, nonfatal stroke, transient ischaemic attack, hospitalisation for unstable angina or arrhythmia, HF, or cardiovascular death) when assessed in a large multicentre cohort (n=725) were nonsignificant in per-protocol analysis but became significant in the subgroup of OSA patients using CPAP for more than 4 h a day (table 1 and fig. 1) [38].

Lastly, an unanswered question is whether chronic consequences of OSA can be managed by CPAP alone. This is an issue for patients with persistent EDS despite adequate CPAP therapy [39, 40]. This should also be considered for hypertension, as antihypertensive drugs are far more effective than CPAP for controlling BP, although there is a beneficial effect when combining both treatments (fig. 2) [41]. In addition, CPAP has been found to

Table 1. Risk for new hypertension or cardiovascular event in intention-to-treat analysis, according to CPAP duration

	Intention-to-treat analysis		Analysis by adherence to CPAP use	
	Control	CPAP	CPAP <4 h per night	CPAP ⩾4 h per night
Persons	366	357	127	230
Events	110	96	37	59
Person-years	997.837	1043.436	296.4271	747.0089
Events per 100 person-years (95% CI)	11.02 (8.96–13.08)	9.20 (7.36–11.04)	12.48 (8.46–16.50)	7.90 (5.88–9.91)
IDR (95% CI)	1 (ref.)	0.83 (0.63–1.10)	1.13 (0.78–1.64)	0.72 (0.52–0.98)
p-value[#]		0.20	0.51	0.04

Data are presented as n, unless otherwise stated. There is a significant difference only when CPAP is used more than 4 h per night. IDR: incidence density ratio. [#]: Wald test. Reproduced and modified from [38] with permission from the publisher.

be effective in controlling BP in specific populations such as resistant hypertension [42]. Interestingly, in this last study, a greater reduction in BP was obtained when CPAP was used for more than 5.8 h per night. Another important question is whether CPAP is able to improve OSA associated metabolic changes [43]. This remains a conflicting issue [44]. Several RCTs have shown no significant improvement in metabolic anomalies including insulin sensitivity in obese OSA patients, whether diabetic or not [45–49], while others found the opposite [50]. EDS may play a role [51], but this is also much discussed [43].

UA surgery

Snoring and OSA are associated with recurrent sleep-induced narrowing or collapse of the pharyngeal airway at the level of the oropharynx and/or hypopharynx. The patency of this "floppy" segment is critically dependent upon UA anatomy and function.

Anatomical factors that predispose to UA narrowing during sleep are craniofacial skeletal abnormalities and/or increased tongue size and/or redundant pharyngeal soft tissues. The more frequent modifications in cranial structure are nasal abnormalities such as a deviated nasal septum, retroposition of the mandible associated with posterior displacement of the tongue and inferior position of hyoid bone. The tongue and pharyngeal soft tissues (soft palate, tonsils, adenoids, etc.) are usually larger than in normal subjects, and these abnormalities are worsened by fat deposition and oedema induced by vibration injury and/ or repeated UA collapse. Finally, UA size is also dependent upon lung volume and, therefore, smaller lung volume may also contribute to reduce UA size in obese subjects. However, UA anatomical abnormalities explain the major part of the variance in AHI only in young and lean subjects [52]. In obese and older patients, other factors such as changes in UA collapsibility, ventilatory instability, fragmented sleep, abnormalities in UA muscle function are predominant. As UA anatomical abnormalities seem to play an important

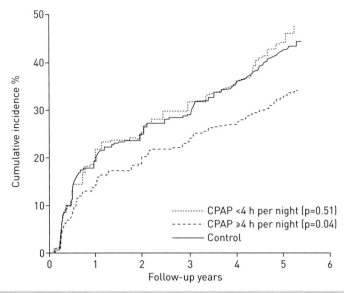

Figure 1. CPAP group stratified according to adherence (<4 *versus* ⩾4 h per night) and the p-values for their incidence density ratios in reference to the control group. Reproduced and modified from [38] with permission from the publisher.

pathophysiological role in young and lean patients, they may potentially be the best candidates for surgical therapy.

Uvulopalatopharyngoplasty (UPPP) aims to enlarge the oropharyngeal airway and reduce the collapsibility of this particular segment of the UA. The rate of success is approximately 40% [53, 54]. When using liberal success criteria (*e.g.* AHI less than 20 per hour and reduction of 50% or more from baseline), the rate of success is higher [55]. Nonresponders usually have a higher baseline AHI. Retropalatal collapse or narrowing is a factor of poor prognosis. Thus, when an imaging or endoscopic technique has undoubtedly shown an awake retrolingual narrowing or, more so, a retrolingual collapse during apnoeas, UPPP should be rejected. In summary, in OSA syndrome (OSAS) patients, palatal surgery has not evidenced a significant impact on short-term outcomes and long-term evolution remains uncertain [56]. Thus, UPPP indications, if any, should be restricted to patients with moderate disease and a presupposed retropalatal narrowing. It should also be remembered that, by increasing mouth leaks, UPPP may compromise CPAP therapy and reduce the maximal level of pressure that can be tolerated [57].

Maxillofacial surgery is presumably the only surgical procedure that reached high rates of success. Overall, maxillomandibular osteotomy is highly effective, with a success rate between 75% and 95% [58–61], as confirmed by a recent meta-analysis (average success of 86%) [60]. For a vast majority of the 627 OSA patients in that meta-analysis, however, the average follow-up was below 6 months, ranging between 3 and 7.7 months [60]. Only 56 patients were included in three long-term follow-up studies [59, 60]. At a mean follow-up of 43.7 ±29.5 months, 89% of patients were considered a surgical success with a significant reduction in the AHI (66.2±26.0 *versus* 7.9±6.4 events·h^{-1}; p<0.001), and there was no difference between the short- and long-term results [60]. Predictors of surgical success included younger age, lower pre-operative AHI, greater degree of maxillary advancement and lower preoperative BMI (individual-level data in multivariate analysis). The degree of mandibular

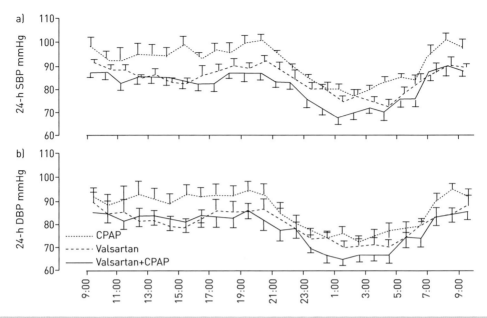

Figure 2. Open continuing study comparing valsartan and CPAP in OSA patients: ambulatory BP profile of patients receiving valsartan, CPAP or a combination of both. Reproduced and modified from [41] with permission from the publisher.

advancement was not predictive of surgical success with univariate or multivariate analysis [60]. In addition, an elegant study compared surgery and CPAP in a randomised controlled fashion in 50 moderately obese, severe OSA patients [62]. The authors did not find any difference in AHI or sleepiness improvement at 1-year follow-up [62]. It should also be remembered that this surgery is safe in expert hands but not without side-effects, *i.e.* facial paraesthesia that usually resolves but may persist in 15% cases at 1 year [60]. It represents overall a heavy procedure requiring well-informed and well-motivated subjects.

Weight loss

Approximately 60% to 70% of OSA patients are obese (BMI of more than 28 $kg·m^{-2}$ or a body weight in excess by more than 20% of the ideal weight) [63]. The relationship between obesity and OSA is still unclear; however, it is one of the most commonly recognised risk factors [63]. Obesity appears to be largely determined by genetic factors that influence metabolic rate, fat storage and eating behaviour, and are associated with autonomic, endocrine and hypothalamic function abnormalities. This is particularly true for regional fat distribution, which may be of particular relevance to the pathogenesis of OSA in which upper-body and visceral fat may be greater risk factors than whole-body fat [43, 64]. Weight loss or gain has significant impacts on the severity of sleep disordered breathing (SDB) [63, 65]. There is also a strong influence of weight reduction on snoring frequency and intensity. Both may result from the decrease in pharyngeal collapsibility obtained with weight loss. Weight loss is not only associated with a reduction in AHI and collapsibility but also with a nearly complete elimination of apnoea when the critical pressure reflecting collapsibility is lowered below −4 cmH_2O [66]. There are recent data looking at weight loss in various ways. A recent systematic review and meta-analysis showed that the published evidence suggests that weight loss through lifestyle and dietary interventions results in improvements in OSA parameters but is insufficient to normalise them. The changes in OSA parameters could, however, be clinically relevant in some patients by reducing OSA severity [67]. The effect of weight loss induced by a very low energy diet has been evaluated in a randomised fashion [68]. In the intervention group, mean body weight was 20 kg lower than in the control group, while mean AHI was 23 events·h^{-1} lower. In the intervention group, five (17%) of the 30 patients were disease free after the energy restricted diet (AHI <5 events·h^{-1}), with 15 (50%) out of 30 having mild disease (AHI 5–14.9 events·h^{-1}), whereas the AHI of all patients in the control group except one remained 15 events·h^{-1} or higher. In a subgroup analysis of the intervention group, baseline AHI significantly modified the effectiveness of treatment, with a greater improvement in AHI in patients with severe OSA (AHI >30 events·h^{-1}) at baseline compared with those with moderate (AHI 15–30 events·h^{-1}) sleep apnoea (AHI −38 *versus* −12 events·h^{-1}; p<0.001), despite similar weight loss (−19.2 *versus* −18.2 kg; p=0.55). Thus, it seems that severe OSA patients could be the best candidates for such caloric restriction [68].

In a very recent study, weight loss was compared to CPAP [69]. The authors randomly assigned 181 patients with obesity, moderate-to-severe OSA and serum levels of C-reactive protein (CRP) greater than 1.0 mg·L^{-1} to receive treatment with CPAP, a weight-loss intervention or CPAP plus a weight-loss intervention for 24 weeks. Weight loss significantly reduced CRP levels, insulin resistance, dyslipidaemia and BP. In contrast, CPAP therapy did not have a significant effect on CRP level, insulin sensitivity or dyslipidaemia, even among participants who adhered to the therapy [69]. However, in this CPAP-compliant population, there was a larger BP reduction in the combined intervention group than in either the weight-loss group or the CPAP group [69].

There have been several controlled trials looking at bariatric surgery. There have been positive results not only on sleep apnoea syndrome but also on metabolic consequences and comorbidities [70]. However, despite the usual massive weight loss obtained with bariatric surgery, cure of sleep apnoea is not systematically obtained. In a recent meta-analysis, bariatric surgery reduced mean BMI by 17.9 kg·m^{-2} (95% CI 16.5–19.3 kg·m^{-2}) from 55.3 kg·m^{-2} (95% CI 53.5–57.1 kg·m^{-2}) to 37.7 kg·m^{-2} (95% CI 36.6–38.9 kg·m^{-2}). Baseline AHI of 55 events·h^{-1} (95% CI 49.0–60.3 events·h^{-1}) was reduced by 38 events·h^{-1} (95% CI 31.9–44.4 events·h^{-1}) to a final value of 16 events·h^{-1} (95% CI 12.6–19.0 events·h^{-1}). The authors noted that a significant proportion of OSA patients will have to continue CPAP despite this major improvement [71]. In addition, more recently, obese OSA patients were randomised to a conventional weight-loss programme that included regular consultations with a dietician and physician, and the use of very low calorie diets as necessary (n=30), or to bariatric surgery (laparoscopic adjustable gastric banding; n=30). The use of bariatric surgery did not result in a statistically greater reduction in AHI compared with conventional weight-loss therapy, despite major differences in weight loss [72]. Lastly, it should be mentioned that OSA, along with deep vein thrombosis and impaired functional status, is associated with a risk of major adverse event in the peri- and post-operative period of bariatric surgery [73]. This strongly suggests the need to diagnose and treat OSA with CPAP at least for some time before and after such procedure.

Hypoglossal nerve stimulation

Oral appliances are usually recommended more for moderate sleep apnoea (see later in this chapter), and pharmacological treatment in OSA, although still very limited or in development, may also apply to moderate OSA (see later in this chapter). However, electrical stimulation of muscles and nerves has been tried in SDB. Several approaches have been tested: surface electrodes, muscular electrodes (on surface of muscles and intramuscular) and nerve electrodes placed directly on the XIIth cranial nerve in order to prevent UA collapse during sleep [74]. When electrodes were placed on the skin with the goal of stimulating the geniohyoid and genioglossus muscles, the results were disappointing. Although positive results were initially reported with this procedure in OSAH, further studies indicated that UA dilators needed a high stimulus intensity that consistently led to sleep fragmentation, even when applied chronically [75]. Direct stimulation of the XIIth nerve was then considered. With XIIth nerve stimulation, coordination with the thoracic muscles is needed and this problem has been handled by measurement of intrathoracic pressure changes. From preliminary reports, it appeared that several technical problems were still unsolved and that the rate of response is variable when using a unilateral stimulation [74, 76]. However, in the past 5 years, there is accumulated evidence suggesting that it might represent a valid therapeutic option [77–80] (fig. 3). After 12 months, 46 consecutive participants who had a response to therapy in a RCT were randomly assigned, in a 1:1 ratio, to the therapy-maintenance group or the therapy-withdrawal group. The therapy-withdrawal group had the device turned off for at least 5 days during this phase, and it remained off until PSG was performed. The therapy maintenance group continued nightly use of the device. There was a significant difference between the therapy-withdrawal group and the therapy-maintenance group with respect to the change in AHI from the assessment at 12 months of the cohort study to the assessment at the end of the therapy-withdrawal study (difference in changes in mean scores, 16.4 events·h^{-1}; p<0.001) [77]. There are currently on-going studies to evaluate the feasibility, safety and efficacy of this technique. One issue is the identification of responders to this treatment, which may be crucial in order to select the best candidates.

Mild-to-moderate OSA

Defining mild-to-moderate sleep apnoea is complex as the magnitude of overnight oxygen desaturation and the duration of the disease are difficult to assess, which affects the validity of intraindividual comparisons. Another factor is night-to-night variability, which is more pronounced in mild apnoeics, especially in the elderly. It raises also the question whether symptoms should be moderate, including sleepiness (*i.e.* ESS between 9 and 12). Defining outcomes in moderate sleep apnoea syndrome should be considered in two dimensions: 1) EDS and daytime functioning; and 2) cardiovascular outcomes.

There is compelling evidence that mild-to-moderate sleep apnoea syndromes are associated with less EDS and daytime impairment. This is true despite the absence of a linear relationship between AHI and symptoms. Sleep fragmentation, AHI, respiratory efforts or ODIs usually account for less than 10–15% each of the variance of either subjective or objective EDS [14, 81–86]. However, all these parameters are linked to OSA severity in a more or less similar manner, which makes it likely that there will be far fewer daytime symptoms in mild-to-moderate OSA. This is also true for cognitive deficits [87–90]. However, the outcome measures may be different than in severe OSA. Specifically, attentional deficits may exist and significantly alter daytime functioning without perceived subjective sleepiness [91, 92]. This may be a relevant outcome for OSA patients' driving ability [93].

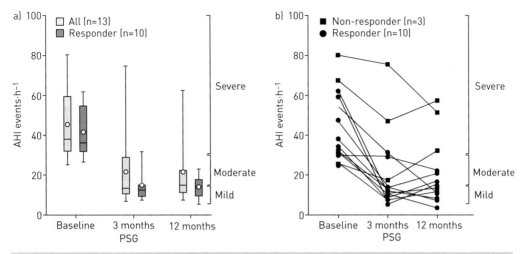

Figure 3. Effects of hypoglossal nerve stimulation in OSA. a and b) AHI scores at baseline, and at 3 and 12 months post-PSG for all patients. a) Boxplots of all subjects and responder groups showing the median (interquartile range). The open circle indicates the median values. Whiskers represent the maximum value (top) and the minimum value (bottom) of the dataset. b) Line graphs showing individual data of all 13 patients. Reproduced and modified from [78] with permission from the publisher.

Overall, cardiovascular consequences are also related to OSA severity, including AHI and oxygen desaturation severity indices. This is true, both in general and clinical populations, for hypertension [12, 94–96], coronary heart disease [97], nocturnal arrhythmias [98] and stroke [99, 100]. This was also found for vascular subclinical markers such as carotid intima-media thickness and pulse wave velocity [101–103]. However, cardiovascular changes are not restricted to severe OSA [21, 26, 104, 105].

Thus, from a clinical point of view, in moderate OSA, elimination of apnoeas and hypopnoeas should be obtained together with the suppression of snoring and EDS. However, additional outcomes could be suggested, such as attentional deficits and early cardiovascular changes. Regarding this last point, it would seem appropriate to use subclinical cardiovascular markers since they have been demonstrated to be predictive of future cardiovascular morbidity, *i.e.* myocardial infarction and stroke [104, 106].

CPAP treatment

CPAP in mild-to-moderate apnoeics raise two concerns: 1) is CPAP compliance acceptable; and 2) how does it compare to alternative treatments in terms of efficacy on symptoms and outcome measures, as defined earlier?

Long-term acceptance and mean rate of use was studied by KRIEGER *et al.* [107] in nonapnoeic snorers and mild apnoeics (RDI less than 15). The acceptance was greater than 60% at 3 years with a mean rate of daily use of CPAP at 5.6±1.4 h per day. However, although it actually resulted in significant improvements when compared with placebo, the compliance in mild apnoeics was significantly lower in the study by ENGLEMAN *et al.* [16] (*e.g.* less than 3 h). In further studies, compliance remained either close to 5 h per night [17, 108–110] or less [111, 112]. As a result, a meta-analysis found a mean compliance of 3.6 h [18], which is clearly less than in more severe OSA subjects [33].

Is CPAP effective on symptoms in mild-to-moderate OSA? Meta-analyses indicate that CPAP significantly reduces subjective daytime sleepiness (ESS) by 1.2 points (95% CI 0.5–1.9; p=0.001), improves objective daytime wakefulness (Maintenance of Wakefulness Test (MWT)) by 2.1 min (95% CI 0.5–3.7 min; p=0.011), and does not affect objective daytime sleepiness [18]. The two significant effects are small (effect size <0.30). The author concluded that CPAP elicits small improvements in subjective sleepiness and objective wakefulness in people with mild-to-moderate OSAS but that the effects on sleepiness are of limited clinical significance [18].

A more controversial issue is whether CPAP may alter cardiovascular outcomes in mild-to-moderate OSA. There is evidence of this for subclinical cardiovascular markers (*e.g.* pulse wave velocity and endothelial function). Critically, this may depend on the sample size [113] but there are usually significant changes that can be observed in RCTs [104]. For harder outcomes, *i.e.* cardiovascular morbidity and mortality, there is no evidence of improvement [114]. It has even been further estimated that future trials of CPAP *versus* no treatment would need to randomise approximately 2540 patients not to miss a real reduction in vascular events, and over 6000 for mortality [115].

How does CPAP compare to alternative treatments?

Several comparisons between CPAP and alternative treatments have been made in the past years in RCTs [108, 109, 112]. The evidence was recently reviewed [116], although not specifically in mild-to-moderate OSA. However, the analysis was stratified by symptom and disease severity at baseline. CPAP significantly reduced ESS score compared with placebo (mean difference (MD) −2.7, 95% CI −3.45–−1.96). The benefit was greatest in patients whose symptoms were severe at baseline: severely symptomatic population (MD −5.0, 95% CI −6.5–−3.5); moderate (MD −2.3, 95% CI −3.0–−1.6); mild (MD −1.1, 95% CI −1.8–−0.3). CPAP significantly improved MWT score compared to control (MD 3.3, 95% CI 1.3–5.3) but not on the MSLT. There was no statistically significant difference between CPAP and dental devices on the ESS, MWT or MSLT, in a population with moderate symptoms. The authors concluded that CPAP is an effective treatment for OSAHS in moderate-to-severe symptomatic patients and there may be benefits for mild symptoms. Dental devices may be a treatment option for mild-to-moderate symptoms. In a more recent comparison between CPAP and an oral appliance in moderate-to-severe OSA (126 patients with AHI 25.6±12.3) [6], sleepiness, driving simulator performance and disease-specific quality of life improved on both treatments by similar amounts, although MADs were superior to CPAP for improving four general quality-of-life domains (FOSQ and SF-36) [6].

In the cardiovascular field, there are several studies showing a significant benefit on BP [112, 117] and endothelial function [118, 119]. There is little, if any, difference between CPAP and oral appliance effects on BP [6, 112, 120].

Pharmacological treatment

A huge number of drugs have been tested in OSA with very little success and the feasibility of an effective drug for preventing UA collapse has been questioned [121, 122]. Drug research into OSA has been hampered by the lack of useful experimental systems and animal models for drug screening. In addition, the phenotypic characterisation of OSA seems to be incomplete, thus limiting the possibility of using stringent criteria for patient selection in drug studies. Finally, the criteria for defining the severity of OSA and disease impact seem to be insufficient for adequate definition of efficacy end-points in clinical trials [122].

Most of the studies have been small and many trials had methodological limitations [123]. Six drugs had some impact on OSA severity and two altered daytime symptoms. One study reported that AHI was lower following treatment with intranasal fluticasone compared with placebo (23.3 versus 30.3) in 24 participants with sleep apnoea and rhinitis [124]. Daytime alertness also improved. Physostigmine reduced AHI to 41 events·h^{-1} compared with 54 events·h^{-1} on placebo [125] and in a similar study, mirtazapine 15 mg produced a 50% improvement in AHI [126]. However, this was not confirmed by a more recent and larger RCT [127]. Paroxetine was also shown to reduce apnoeas by 35%, exclusively in non-REM sleep and, amazingly, with no effects on hypopnoeas. In that study, there was no improvement in daytime symptoms [128]. Protriptyline is probably the drug that has been the most commonly used for treating OSA. Several studies report protriptyline to be effective in 50% to 70% of cases of OSA [129–131] but its usefulness is limited by anticholinergic side-effects.

Until now, pharmacological treatment has demonstrated little effect on apnoea and hypopnoea. There are, however, important potential targets that remain insufficiently explored. The brainstem neurons represent a potentially important pharmacological target [121, 122, 132]. The ultimate goal of pharmacological approaches for snoring and OSA is the prevention of sleep-related reduction in pharyngeal muscle activity and the subsequent alleviation of sleep-related airway narrowing and closure. Although it is difficult to selectively target the proper neuronal structures, both increase in UA muscle activity and induced changes in sleep structure might be of interest. Recently, a proof-of-principle study demonstrated that targeting blockade of certain potassium channels at the hypoglossal motor pool is an effective strategy for reversing UA hypotonia and causing sustained reactivation of genioglossus throughout non-REM and REM sleep [133]. We are still lacking an appropriate drug to stimulate the UA during sleep, although several potential candidates have been tested in early phase II studies in the last 10 years. Such a strategy has been proposed in animal models using a specific potassium channel blocker administered topically to the UA that dose-dependently inhibited UA collapsibility [134]. For instance, 10 mg of this specific compound (AVE0118) prevented UA collapse against negative pressures of −150 mbar (p<0.01) for >4 h in pigs [135] (fig. 4). Although there have been early-phase studies in normal volunteers and OSA patients using this type of compound, further research in this direction is needed.

As regards sleep structure, arousal threshold could be possibly manipulated in order to promote ventilatory stability [135, 136]. However, until now, this has not proven to be feasible or effective in reducing SDB.

Further developments are expected in the field of combined treatment targeting OSA consequences or comorbidities, e.g. CPAP or oral appliance plus pharmacotherapy, which applies both to severe and mild-to-moderate SDB. As already mentioned, there may be a need to use antihypertensive drugs in combination with CPAP to control BP [41]. In addition, residual EDS is relatively prevalent in OSA despite adequate CPAP treatment [39, 40], which may require, after excluding any specific cause and improving CPAP duration if feasible [35], the use of wakefulness stimulants [137]. Finally, exercise [138], and antioxidant and anti-inflammatory drugs [139] are currently being evaluated in comparison or in addition to CPAP.

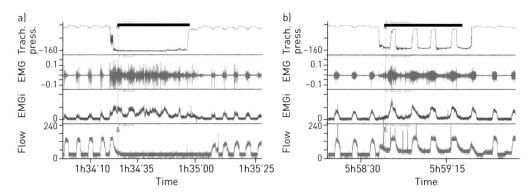

Figure 4. Sensitisation of UA mechanoreceptors as a new pharmacological principle to treat OSA. AVE0118 is potassium channel blocker administered topically to the UA in doses of 1, 3 and 10 mg per nostril, which sensitised the negative pressure reflex, shifting the mechanoreceptor response threshold for the genioglossus muscle to more positive pressures. Traces illustrating a collapsibility test in an anaesthetised pig a) before and b) after nasal administration of AVE0118, 10 mg per nostril. a) UA collapse is indicated by an interruption of flow (lowest trace) and a sublaryngeal pressure close to the negative device pressure (upper trace) during both the inspiratory and expiratory phase. Second and third traces: genioglossus raw electromyogram (EMG) and integrated EMG (EMGi), respectively. b) After AVE0118, the UA is open during the inspiratory phase, as indicated by flow to the negative pressure device and sublaryngeal pressure approaching atmospheric pressure. Time of application of negative pressure is labelled by a black line. Airflow during this period is directed to the negative pressure device. EMG activity is given in arbitrary units, tracheal pressure (Trach. press.) in mbar and airflow in $mL \cdot s^{-1}$. Reproduced and modified from [134] with permission from the publisher.

Weight loss

Bariatric surgery is not an option in mild-to-moderate OSA. Massive obesity is usually associated with severe OSA. OSA, when moderate, is not a major target for treatment with bariatric surgery. Thus, in mild-to-moderate OSA, weight loss has rather been performed using caloric restriction programmes and, more recently, anorexigens or other drugs used in weight control.

There are few RCTs comparing weight control to other modalities. In a relatively small group of moderate OSA patients (AHI 21 events·h⁻¹), LAM et al. [120] compared CPAP, oral appliance and conservative measures including sleep hygiene and a weight-loss programme. The patients were randomised in parallel groups for 10 weeks. CPAP produced the best improvement in terms of physiological, symptomatic and quality-of-life measures, while oral appliances were slightly less effective. Weight loss, if achieved, resulted in an improvement in sleep parameters, but weight control alone was not uniformly effective.

Sibutramine has been evaluated both on weight changes and OSA control [140, 141], with positive results for both as well as metabolic improvement [142]. However, sibutramine has been removed from the European market because data from SCOUT (Sibutramine Cardiovascular Outcome Trial) [143] showed an increased risk of serious, nonfatal cardiovascular events, such as stroke or heart attack, with sibutramine compared with placebo [144].

Sleep posture

It has been long recognised that snoring patients do so most loudly in the supine position. Similarly, it has been well proven that a large proportion of unselected patients with a diagnosis of OSAS demonstrate a different rate of apnoeic events in the lateral than in the supine position [145]. Positional sleep apnoea syndrome has been defined as an AHI during the time in supine sleep that is two or more times the AHI during sleep in the lateral position [146]. In a group of nearly 600 patients, OKSENBERG et al. [147] found, among positional sleep apnoea patients, a slightly reduced BMI and age, a better sleep efficiency, increased slow-wave sleep, less wake after sleep onset and fewer microarousals, smaller AHI and fewer oxygen desaturations, as well as longer sleep latencies on MSLT, compared with patients with nonpositional OSA. All these characteristics correspond to a moderate sleep apnoea syndrome. In logistic regression analysis, both RDI (upper limit at 40 events·h^{-1}) and BMI were negatively correlated with the occurrence of positional sleep apnoea [147]. In terms of prevalence, this was confirmed, as 49.5% of positional sleep apnoea was found in mild OSA (AHI between 5 and 15 events·h^{-1}), 19.4% in moderate OSA (AHI between 15 and 30 events·h^{-1}) and only 6% in severe OSA (AHI >30 events·h^{-1}) [148]. Is positional treatment effective and feasible? It has been tested since the 1980s [149], compared with other treatment modalities [150, 151], further evaluated at 6 months [152] and, lastly, included in clinical practice guidelines [153, 154]. In patients trained to sleep on their side, using a sound alarm to prevent supine position, about 50% are able to avoid supine position on a long-term basis. There is, however, a lack of standardisation and innovation designed to provide patients with an adequate system for long-term positional treatment in OSA. The tennis ball technique, where a tennis ball is placed into a pocket of a wide cloth band or belt attached around the abdomen so that the ball lies in the centre of the back, is the first technique that was used. When the patient rolls onto their back, they feel the pressure of the ball and instinctively roll back onto their side again. Several other methods have been used [146]. Some may use a T-shirt with a long vertical pocket holding three or four tennis balls along the back. This is perhaps less likely to slip out of place during sleep. Others have found that a large device consisting of a polyvinylchloride pipe wrapped in foam (about the size of an American football) is more effective than the tennis ball [146]. A comparison between all these devices on effectiveness, acceptance and compliance would be beneficial. When using the tennis ball technique, compliance appears to be around 40%, with 24% being still able to avoid supine sleep position after treatment cessation [152]. Regarding effectiveness, there is a randomised cross-over study comparing CPAP and positional treatment for 2 weeks in moderate positional OSA (AHI 17±8 events·h^{-1}) [151]. There was a significant difference regarding AHI (MD 6 events·h^{-1}) and oxygen saturation (MD of 4% for nocturnal minimal $S_{a}O_2$) in favour of CPAP, but no difference regarding symptoms, sleep structure, objective vigilance, cognitive tests and quality of life [151]. In clinical guidelines, favouring factors for positional sleep apnoea are mentioned (i.e. low AHI, low-to-moderate BMI and younger subjects) and only two studies are considered sufficiently evidence-based [150, 151]. It is also underlined that normalisation of AHI should be checked owing to incomplete or variable responses to treatment [153].

Oral appliances

There is accumulated evidence that oral appliances are effective in mild OSA [155]. Oral appliances improve subjective sleepiness and SDB compared with control. CPAP appears to be more effective in improving SDB than oral appliances. However, the difference in symptomatic response between these two treatments is not significant. Thus, OA may be recommended to patients with mild symptomatic OSA and those patients who are unwilling or unable to tolerate CPAP therapy [155].

There are several possible primary contraindications to oral appliances, *i.e.* insufficient teeth to support the device, periodontal problems inducing tooth mobility or active temporomandibular joint (TMJ) disorder [156]. We found primary contraindication in 34% of 100 consecutive patients, mainly owing to dental problems. Moreover, another subgroup of patients (16%) required close supervision and follow-up to avoid impairment of pre-existing TMJ and dental problems [156]. Side-effects, tolerance and compliance have been studied [157–160]. Side-effects are common: mucosal dryness (86% of patients), tooth discomfort (59%), hypersalivation (55%) [157] and increased in TMJ symptoms [159]. However, this does not seem to affect oral appliance use [157, 159]. Compliance is declarative, which makes more difficult to compare with CPAP. However, during long-term use, there are more than 60% of patients who declare using their device almost every night [159, 160]. Oral appliances appear to be an effective therapy in moderately sleepy and overweight OSA patients. Although eventually less effective than CPAP, successfully titrated oral appliances are very effective at reducing AHI and were associated with a higher reported compliance, with >70% of patients preferring this treatment [7].

In summary, oral appliances are indicated for use in patients with mild-to-moderate OSA, possibly in addition to behavioural measures such as weight loss or positional treatment. Patients with moderate-to-severe OSA could have an initial trial of nasal CPAP, although greater effectiveness has not been shown systematically with this intervention compared with oral appliances.

Strategies of treatment

In cases of severe OSA, there is no doubt that CPAP remains the first-line treatment. Only maxillofacial surgery should be considered as a potential alternative in a limited number of young, non-obese and well-motivated subjects. We may also suggest that specific maxillofacial anomalies should be present. Whether hypoglossal nerve stimulation may be a significant option should be further studied. In the case of CPAP intolerance, if UA surgery is not possible, oral appliances should be evaluated, being possibly effective even in some severe OSA.

In mild-to-moderate OSA, the following strategy may be suggested. 1) A CPAP trial may be recommended, at least to establish whether CPAP, in normalising sleep and respiration, leads to the relief of the symptoms attributed to SDB. It should be remembered, however, that a significant placebo effect has been demonstrated when initiating CPAP treatment [161]. 2) Oral appliances may, however, be indicated if feasible, particularly from a dental point of view. oral appliances should also be tried either initially or in cases of primary or secondary failure of CPAP (patients refusing CPAP or becoming noncompliant). 3) Surgical indications are limited regarding OSA.

Conclusion

Sleep apnoea syndrome outcomes have been extensively studied in the past decade, as well-controlled studies have been published since 1999. Sleepiness, attentional deficits, BP and metabolic changes have been assessed in RCTs. There are on-going studies currently being performed in Spain [37, 162] and in Australia and China (www.savetrial.org). This will provide additional information to the longitudinal cohort studies [163] and short-term intervention studies [161, 164]. Although there is growing evidence that CPAP is effective for sleepiness, daytime functioning and BP, it is also obvious that most chronic consequences of OSA may not be fully reversed by CPAP alone. Residual sleepiness may persist despite CPAP treatment [35, 39], although longer CPAP use may be required. BP may not be fully controlled with CPAP [41]. However, symptoms (*i.e.* sleepiness) do not necessarily need to be present to obtain a significant change in BP with CPAP [37]. CPAP-induced metabolic changes are much more discussed, at least in obese subjects [43]. Combined therapy with CPAP and drugs targeting oxidative stress or inflammation should be further validated. Oral appliances have been extensively studied and used in clinical practice in the past decade. Their effectiveness on symptoms in mild-to-moderate OSA seems comparable to CPAP [7, 155]. Oral appliance effects on cardiovascular and metabolic outcomes remain to be further studied. However, in mild OSA, oral appliances have become the first-line treatment when feasible. Other treatments remain to be developed (*e.g.* drugs targeting UA muscle activity and hypoglossal nerve stimulation). In the context of epidemic obesity, weight loss, either using a very low energy diet or bariatric surgery, should be considered in obese subjects [68, 71].

References

1. Sullivan CE, Issa FG, Berthon-Jones M, *et al.* Reversal of obstructive sleep apnoea by continuous positive airway pressure applied through the nares. *Lancet* 1981; 1: 862–865.
2. Pepin JL, Leger P, Veale D, *et al.* Side effects of nasal continuous positive airway pressure in sleep apnea syndrome. Study of 193 patients in two French sleep centers. *Chest* 1995; 107: 375–381.
3. Giles TL, Lasserson TJ, Smith BJ, *et al.* Continuous positive airways pressure for obstructive sleep apnoea in adults. *Cochrane Database Syst Rev* 2006; CD001106.
4. McDaid C, Griffin S, Weatherly H, *et al.* Continuous positive airway pressure devices for the treatment of obstructive sleep apnoea-hypopnoea syndrome: a systematic review and economic analysis. *Health Technol Assess* 2009; 13: 143–274.
5. Levy P, Pepin JL, Mayer P, *et al.* Management of simple snoring, upper airway resistance syndrome, and moderate sleep apnea syndrome. *Sleep* 1996; 19: Suppl. 9, S101–S110.
6. Phillips CL, Grunstein RR, Darendeliler MA, *et al.* Health outcomes of continuous positive airway pressure *versus* oral appliance treatment for obstructive sleep apnea: a randomized controlled trial. *Am J Respir Crit Care Med* 2013; 187: 879–887.
7. Gagnadoux F, Fleury B, Vielle B, *et al.* Titrated mandibular advancement *versus* positive airway pressure for sleep apnoea. *Eur Respir J* 2009; 34: 914–920.
8. Veale D, Poussin G, Benes F, *et al.* Identification of quality of life concerns of patients with obstructive sleep apnoea at the time of initiation of continuous positive airway pressure: a discourse analysis. *Qual Life Res* 2002; 11: 389–399.
9. Sleep-related breathing disorders in adults: recommendations for syndrome definition and measurement techniques in clinical research. The Report of an American Academy of Sleep Medicine Task Force. *Sleep* 1999; 22: 667–689.
10. Berry RB, Budhiraja R, Gottlieb DJ, *et al.* Rules for scoring respiratory events in sleep: update of the 2007 AASM Manual for the Scoring of Sleep and Associated Events. Deliberations of the Sleep Apnea Definitions Task Force of the American Academy of Sleep Medicine. *J Clin Sleep Med* 2012; 8: 597–619.
11. Qaseem A, Dallas P, Owens DK, *et al.* Diagnosis of obstructive sleep apnea in adults: a clinical practice guideline from the American college of physicians diagnosis of obstructive sleep apnea in adults. *Ann Intern Med* 2014; 161: 210–220.
12. Peppard PE, Young T, Palta M, *et al.* Prospective study of the association between sleep-disordered breathing and hypertension. *N Engl J Med* 2000; 342: 1378–1384.
13. Kim HC, Young T, Matthews CG, *et al.* Sleep-disordered breathing and neuropsychological deficits. A population-based study. *Am J Respir Crit Care Med* 1997; 156: 1813–1819.
14. Gottlieb DJ, Whitney CW, Bonekat WH, *et al.* Relation of sleepiness to respiratory disturbance index: the Sleep Heart Health Study. *Am J Respir Crit Care Med* 1999; 159: 502–507.
15. Kapur VK, Baldwin CM, Resnick HE, *et al.* Sleepiness in patients with moderate to severe sleep-disordered breathing. *Sleep* 2005; 28: 472–477.
16. Engleman H, Kingshott R, Wraith P, *et al.* Randomized placebo-controlled crossover trial of continuous positive airway pressure for mild sleep apnea/hypopnea syndrome. *Am J Respir Crit Care Med* 1999; 159: 461–467.

17. Monasterio C, Vidal S, Duran J, et al. Effectiveness of continuous positive airway pressure in mild sleep apnea-hypopnea syndrome. Am J Respir Crit Care Med 2001; 164: 939–943.

18. Marshall NS, Barnes M, Travier N, et al. Continuous positive airway pressure reduces daytime sleepiness in mild to moderate obstructive sleep apnoea: a meta-analysis. Thorax 2006; 61: 430–434.

19. Punjabi NM. The epidemiology of adult obstructive sleep apnea. Proc Am Thorac Soc 2008; 5: 136–143.

20. Punjabi NM, Newman AB, Young TB, et al.. Sleep-disordered breathing and cardiovascular disease: an outcome-based definition of hypopneas. Am J Respir Crit Care Med 2008; 177: 1150–1155.

21. Levy P, Pepin JL, Arnaud C, et al. Obstructive sleep apnea and atherosclerosis. Prog Cardiovasc Dis 2009; 51: 400–410.

22. McNicholas WT, Bonsignore MR, Management Committee of EU COST ACTION B26. Sleep apnoea as an independent risk factor for cardiovascular disease: current evidence, basic mechanisms and research priorities. Eur Respir J 2007; 29: 156–178.

23. Levy P, Pepin JL, Arnaud C, et al. Intermittent hypoxia and sleep-disordered breathing: current concepts and perspectives. Eur Respir J 2008; 32: 1082–1095.

24. Redline S, Budhiraja R, Kapur V, et al. The scoring of respiratory events in sleep: reliability and validity. J Clin Sleep Med 2007; 3: 169–200.

25. Mehra R, Stone KL, Varosy PD, et al. Nocturnal arrhythmias across a spectrum of obstructive and central sleep-disordered breathing in older men: outcomes of sleep disorders in older men (MrOS sleep) study. Arch Intern Med 2009; 169: 1147–1155.

26. Redline S, Yenokyan G, Gottlieb DJ, et al. Obstructive sleep apnea-hypopnea and incident stroke: the sleep heart health study. Am J Respir Crit Care Med 2010; 182: 269–277.

27. Kribbs NB, Pack AI, Kline LR, et al. Objective measurement of patterns of nasal CPAP use by patients with obstructive sleep apnea. Am Rev Respir Dis 1993; 147: 887–895.

28. Reeves-Hoche MK, Meck R, Zwillich CW. Nasal CPAP: an objective evaluation of patient compliance. Am J Respir Crit Care Med 1994; 149: 149–154.

29. Engleman HM, Martin SE, Deary IJ, et al. Effect of continuous positive airway pressure treatment on daytime function in sleep apnoea/hypopnoea syndrome. Lancet 1994; 343: 572–575.

30. Gay P, Weaver T, Loube D, et al. Evaluation of positive airway pressure treatment for sleep related breathing disorders in adults. Sleep 2006; 29: 381–401.

31. Krieger J. Long-term compliance with nasal continuous positive airway pressure (CPAP) in obstructive sleep apnea patients and nonapneic snorers. Sleep 1992; 15: Suppl. 6, S42–S46.

32. Fleury B, Rakotonanahary D, Hausser-Hauw C, et al. Objective patient compliance in long-term use of nCPAP. Eur Respir J 1996; 9: 2356–2359.

33. Pepin JL, Krieger J, Rodenstein D, et al. Effective compliance during the first 3 months of continuous positive airway pressure. A European prospective study of 121 patients. Am J Respir Crit Care Med 1999; 160: 1124–1129.

34. Weaver TE, Grunstein RR. Adherence to continuous positive airway pressure therapy: the challenge to effective treatment. Proc Am Thorac Soc 2008; 5: 173–178.

35. Weaver TE, Maislin G, Dinges DF, et al. Relationship between hours of CPAP use and achieving normal levels of sleepiness and daily functioning. Sleep 2007; 30: 711–719.

36. Haentjens P, Van Meerhaeghe A, Moscariello A, et al. The impact of continuous positive airway pressure on blood pressure in patients with obstructive sleep apnea syndrome: evidence from a meta-analysis of placebo-controlled randomized trials. Arch Intern Med 2007; 167: 757–764.

37. Barbe F, Duran-Cantolla J, Capote F, et al. Long-term effect of continuous positive airway pressure in hypertensive patients with sleep apnea. Am J Respir Crit Care Med 2010; 181: 718–726.

38. Barbe F, Duran-Cantolla J, Sanchez-de-la-Torre M, et al. Effect of continuous positive airway pressure on the incidence of hypertension and cardiovascular events in nonsleepy patients with obstructive sleep apnea: a randomized controlled trial. JAMA 2012; 307: 2161–2168.

39. Pepin JL, Viot-Blanc V, Escourrou P, et al. Prevalence of residual excessive sleepiness in CPAP-treated sleep apnoea patients: the French multicentre study. Eur Respir J 2009; 33: 1062–1067.

40. Gasa M, Tamisier R, Launois SH, et al. Residual sleepiness in sleep apnea patients treated by continuous positive airway pressure. J Sleep Res 2013; 22: 389–397.

41. Pepin J-L, Tamisier R, Barone-Rochette G, et al. Comparison of continuous positive airway pressure and valsartan in hypertensive patients with sleep apnea. Am J Respir Crit Care Med 2010; 182: 954–960.

42. Lozano L, Tovar JL, Sampol G, et al. Continuous positive airway pressure treatment in sleep apnea patients with resistant hypertension: a randomized, controlled trial. J Hypertens 2010; 28: 2161–2168.

43. Levy P, Bonsignore MR, Eckel J. Sleep, sleep-disordered breathing and metabolic consequences. Eur Respir J 2009; 34: 243–260.

44. Pepin JL, Tamisier R, Levy P. Obstructive sleep apnoea and metabolic syndrome: put CPAP efficacy in a more realistic perspective. Thorax 2012; 67: 1025–1027.

45. Coughlin SR, Mawdsley L, Mugarza JA, et al. Cardiovascular and metabolic effects of CPAP in obese males with OSA. Eur Respir J 2007; 29: 720–727.

46. West SD, Nicoll DJ, Wallace TM, et al. The effect of CPAP on insulin resistance and HbA1c in men with obstructive sleep apnoea and type 2 diabetes. Thorax 2007; 62: 969–974.

47. Weinstock TG, Wang X, Rueschman M, et al. A controlled trial of CPAP therapy on metabolic control in individuals with impaired glucose tolerance and sleep apnea. Sleep 2012; 35: 617B–625B.

48. Sivam S, Phillips CL, Trenell MI, et al. Effects of 8 weeks of continuous positive airway pressure on abdominal adiposity in obstructive sleep apnoea. Eur Respir J 2012; 40: 913–918.

49. Hoyos CM, Killick R, Yee BJ, et al. Cardiometabolic changes after continuous positive airway pressure for obstructive sleep apnoea: a randomised sham-controlled study. Thorax 2012; 67: 1081–1089.

50. Lam JC, Lam B, Yao TJ, et al. A randomised controlled trial of nasal continuous positive airway pressure on insulin sensitivity in obstructive sleep apnoea. Eur Respir J 2010; 35: 138–145.

51. Barcelo A, Barbe F, de la Pena M, et al. Insulin resistance and daytime sleepiness in patients with sleep apnoea. Thorax 2008; 63: 946–950.

52. Mayer P, Pepin JL, Bettega G, et al. Relationship between body mass index, age and upper airway measurements in snorers and sleep apnoea patients. Eur Respir J 1996; 9: 1801–1809.

53. Pepin JL, Veale D, Mayer P, et al. Critical analysis of the results of surgery in the treatment of snoring, upper airway resistance syndrome (UARS), and obstructive sleep apnea (OSA). Sleep 1996; 19: Suppl. 9, S90–S100.

54. Sher AE, Schechtman KB, Piccirillo JF. The efficacy of surgical modifications of the upper airway in adults with obstructive sleep apnea syndrome. Sleep 1996; 19: 156–177.

55. Xiong YP, Yi HL, Yin SK, et al. Predictors of surgical outcomes of uvulopalatopharyngoplasty for obstructive sleep apnea hypopnea syndrome. Otolaryngol Head Neck Surg 2011; 145: 1049–1054.

56. Sundaram S, Bridgman SA, Lim J, et al. Surgery for obstructive sleep apnoea. Cochrane Database Syst Rev 2005; CD001004.

57. Mortimore IL, Bradley PA, Murray JA, et al. Uvulopalatopharyngoplasty may compromise nasal CPAP therapy in sleep apnea syndrome. Am J Respir Crit Care Med 1996; 154: 1759–1762.

58. Riley RW, Powell NB, Guilleminault C. Obstructive sleep apnea syndrome: a review of 306 consecutively treated surgical patients. Otolaryngol Head Neck Surg 1993; 108: 117–125.

59. Conradt R, Hochban W, Brandenburg U, et al. Long-term follow-up after surgical treatment of obstructive sleep apnoea by maxillomandibular advancement. Eur Respir J 1997; 10: 123–128.

60. Holty JE, Guilleminault C. Maxillomandibular advancement for the treatment of obstructive sleep apnea: A systematic review and meta-analysis. Sleep Med Rev 2010; 14: 287–297.

61. Bettega G, Pepin JL, Veale D, et al. Obstructive sleep apnea syndrome. fifty-one consecutive patients treated by maxillofacial surgery. Am J Respir Crit Care Med 2000; 162: 641–649.

62. Vicini C, Dallan I, Campanini A, et al. Surgery vs ventilation in adult severe obstructive sleep apnea syndrome. Am J Otolaryngol 2010; 31: 14–20.

63. Young T, Peppard PE, Taheri S. Excess weight and sleep-disordered breathing. J Appl Physiol 2005; 99: 1592–1599.

64. Fantuzzi G, Mazzone T. Adipose tissue and atherosclerosis: exploring the connection. Arterioscler Thromb Vasc Biol 2007; 27: 996–1003.

65. Newman AB, Foster G, Givelber R, et al. Progression and regression of sleep-disordered breathing with changes in weight: the sleep heart health study. Arch Intern Med 2005; 165: 2408–2413.

66. Schwartz AR, Gold AR, Schubert N, et al. Effect of weight loss on upper airway collapsibility in obstructive sleep apnea. Am Rev Respir Dis 1991; 144: 494–498.

67. Araghi MH, Chen YF, Jagielski A, et al. Effectiveness of lifestyle interventions on obstructive sleep apnea (OSA): systematic review and meta-analysis. Sleep 2013; 36: 1553–1562.

68. Johansson K, Neovius M, Lagerros YT, et al. Effect of a very low energy diet on moderate and severe obstructive sleep apnoea in obese men: a randomised controlled trial. BMJ 2009; 339: b4609.

69. Chirinos JA, Gurubhagavatula I, Teff K, et al. CPAP, weight loss, or both for obstructive sleep apnea. N Engl J Med 2014; 370: 2265–2275.

70. Grunstein RR, Stenlof K, Hedner JA, et al. Two year reduction in sleep apnea symptoms and associated diabetes incidence after weight loss in severe obesity. Sleep 2007; 30: 703–710.

71. Greenburg DL, Lettieri CJ, Eliasson AH. Effects of surgical weight loss on measures of obstructive sleep apnea: a meta-analysis. Am J Med 2009; 122: 535–542.

72. Dixon JB, Schachter LM, O'Brien PE, et al. Surgical vs conventional therapy for weight loss treatment of obstructive sleep apnea: a randomized controlled trial. JAMA 2012; 308: 1142–1149.

73. Flum DR, Belle SH, King WC, et al. Perioperative safety in the longitudinal assessment of bariatric surgery. N Engl J Med 2009; 361: 445–454.

74. Kezirian EJ, Boudewyns A, Eisele DW, et al. Electrical stimulation of the hypoglossal nerve in the treatment of obstructive sleep apnea. Sleep Med Rev 2010; 14: 299–305.

75.   Guilleminault C, Powell N, Bowman B, et al. The effect of electrical stimulation on obstructive sleep apnea syndrome. Chest 1995; 107: 67–73.

76.   Eisele DW, Smith PL, Alam DS, et al. Direct hypoglossal nerve stimulation in obstructive sleep apnea. Arch Otolaryngol Head Neck Surg 1997; 123: 57–61.

77.   Strollo PJ Jr, Soose RJ, Maurer JT, et al. Upper-airway stimulation for obstructive sleep apnea. N Engl J Med 2014; 370: 139–149.

78.   Mwenge GB, Rombaux P, Dury M, et al. Targeted hypoglossal neurostimulation for obstructive sleep apnoea: a 1-year pilot study. Eur Respir J 2013; 41: 360–367.

79.   Rodenstein D, Rombaux P, Lengele B, et al. Residual effect of THN hypoglossal stimulation in obstructive sleep apnea: a disease-modifying therapy. Am J Respir Crit Care Med 2013; 187: 1276–1278.

80.   Schwartz AR, Barnes M, Hillman D, et al. Acute upper airway responses to hypoglossal nerve stimulation during sleep in obstructive sleep apnea. Am J Respir Crit Care Med 2012; 185: 420–426.

81.   Chervin RD, Aldrich MS. Characteristics of apneas and hypopneas during sleep and relation to excessive daytime sleepiness. Sleep 1998; 21: 799–806.

82.   Kingshott RN, Engleman HM, Deary IJ, et al. Does arousal frequency predict daytime function? Eur Respir J 1998; 12: 1264–1270.

83.   Bennett Lesley S, Barbour C, Langford B, et al. Health status in obstructive sleep apnea. Relationship with sleep fragmentation and daytime sleepiness, and effects of continuous positive airway pressure treatment. Am J Respir Crit Care Med 1999; 159: 1884–1890.

84.   Punjabi NM, O'Hearn DJ, Neubauer DN, et al. Modeling hypersomnolence in sleep-disordered breathing. A novel approach using survival analysis. Am J Respir Crit Care Med 1999; 159: 1703–1709.

85.   Adams N, Strauss M, Schluchter M, et al. Relation of measures of sleep-disordered breathing to neuropsychological functioning. Am J Respir Crit Care Med 2001; 163: 1626–1631.

86.   Cheshire K, Engleman H, Deary I, et al. Factors impairing daytime performance in patients with sleep apnea/hypopnea syndrome. Arch Intern Med 1992; 152: 538–541.

87.   Naegele B, Thouvard V, Pepin JL, et al. Deficits of cognitive executive functions in patients with sleep apnea syndrome. Sleep 1995; 18: 43–52.

88.   Naegele B, Launois SH, Mazza S, et al. Which memory processes are affected in patients with obstructive sleep apnea? An evaluation of 3 types of memory. Sleep 2006; 29: 533–544.

89.   Bedard MA, Montplaisir J, Richer F, et al. Obstructive sleep apnea syndrome: pathogenesis of neuropsychological deficits. J Clin Exp Neuropsychol 1991; 13: 950–964.

90.   Engleman HM, Kingshott RN, Martin SE, et al. Cognitive function in the sleep apnea/hypopnea syndrome (SAHS). Sleep 2000; 23: Suppl. 4, S102–S108.

91.   Mazza S, Pepin JL, Naegele B, et al. Most obstructive sleep apnoea patients exhibit vigilance and attention deficits on an extended battery of tests. Eur Respir J 2005; 25: 75–80.

92.   Mazza S, Pepin JL, Deschaux C, et al. Analysis of error profiles occurring during the OSLER test: a sensitive mean of detecting fluctuations in vigilance in patients with obstructive sleep apnea syndrome. Am J Respir Crit Care Med 2002; 166: 474–478.

93.   Mazza S, Pepin JL, Naegele B, et al. Driving ability in sleep apnoea patients before and after CPAP treatment: evaluation on a road safety platform. Eur Respir J 2006; 28: 1020–1028.

94.   Hla KM, Young TB, Bidwell T, et al. Sleep apnea and hypertension. A population-based study. Ann Intern Med 1994; 120: 382–388.

95.   Young T, Peppard P, Palta M, et al. Population-based study of sleep-disordered breathing as a risk factor for hypertension. Arch Intern Med 1997; 157: 1746–1752.

96.   Nieto FJ, Young TB, Lind BK, et al. Association of sleep-disordered breathing, sleep apnea, and hypertension in a large community-based study. Sleep Heart Health Study. JAMA 2000; 283: 1829–1836.

97.   Peker Y, Kraiczi H, Hedner J, et al. An independent association between obstructive sleep apnoea and coronary artery disease. Eur Respir J 1999; 14: 179–184.

98.   Mehra R, Benjamin EJ, Shahar E, et al. Association of nocturnal arrhythmias with sleep-disordered breathing: The Sleep Heart Health Study. Am J Respir Crit Care Med 2006; 173: 910–916.

99.   Yaggi HK, Concato J, Kernan WN, et al. Obstructive sleep apnea as a risk factor for stroke and death. N Engl J Med 2005; 353: 2034–2041.

100.   Arzt M, Young T, Finn L, et al. Association of sleep-disordered breathing and the occurrence of stroke. Am J Respir Crit Care Med 2005; 172: 1447–1451.

101.   Baguet JP, Hammer L, Levy P, et al. The severity of oxygen desaturation is predictive of carotid wall thickening and plaque occurrence. Chest 2005; 128: 3407–3412.

102.   Drager LF, Bortolotto LA, Lorenzi MC, et al. Early signs of atherosclerosis in obstructive sleep apnea. Am J Respir Crit Care Med 2005; 172: 613–618.

103. Monneret D, Pepin J-L, Godin-Ribuot D, et al. Association of urinary 15-F2t-isoprostane level with oxygen desaturation and carotid intima-media thickness in nonobese sleep apnea patients. Free Radic Biol Med 2010; 48: 619–625.

104. Kohler M, Craig S, Nicoll D, et al. Endothelial function and arterial stiffness in minimally symptomatic obstructive sleep apnea. Am J Respir Crit Care Med 2008; 178: 984–988.

105. Saletu M, Nosiska D, Kapfhammer G, et al. Structural and serum surrogate markers of cerebrovascular disease in obstructive sleep apnea (OSA): association of mild OSA with early atherosclerosis. J Neurol 2006; 253: 746–752.

106. Lorenz MW, Markus HS, Bots ML, et al. Prediction of clinical cardiovascular events with carotid intima-media thickness: a systematic review and meta-analysis. Circulation 2007; 115: 459–467.

107. Krieger J, Kurtz D, Petiau C, et al. Long-term compliance with CPAP therapy in obstructive sleep apnea patients and in snorers. Sleep 1996; 19: Suppl. 9, S136–S143.

108. Engleman HM, McDonald JP, Graham D, et al. Randomized crossover trial of two treatments for sleep apnea/ hypopnea syndrome: continuous positive airway pressure and mandibular repositioning splint. Am J Respir Crit Care Med 2002; 166: 855–859.

109. Randerath WJ, Heise M, Hinz R, et al. An individually adjustable oral appliance vs continuous positive airway pressure in mild-to-moderate obstructive sleep apnea syndrome. Chest 2002; 122: 569–575.

110. Marshall NS, Neill AM, Campbell AJ, et al. Randomised controlled crossover trial of humidified continuous positive airway pressure in mild obstructive sleep apnoea. Thorax 2005; 60: 427–432.

111. Barnes M, Houston D, Worsnop C, et al. A randomized controlled trial of continuous positive airway pressure in mild obstructive sleep apnea. Am J Respir Crit Care Med 2002; 165: 773–780.

112. Barnes M, McEvoy RD, Banks S, et al. Efficacy of positive airway pressure and oral appliance in mild to moderate obstructive sleep apnea. Am J Respir Crit Care Med 2004; 170: 656–664.

113. Comondore VR, Cheema R, Fox J, et al. The impact of CPAP on cardiovascular biomarkers in minimally symptomatic patients with obstructive sleep apnea: a pilot feasibility randomized crossover trial. Lung 2009; 187: 17–22.

114. Craig SE, Kohler M, Nicoll D, et al. Continuous positive airway pressure improves sleepiness but not calculated vascular risk in patients with minimally symptomatic obstructive sleep apnoea: the MOSAIC randomised controlled trial. Thorax 2012; 67: 1090–1096.

115. Turnbull CD, Craig SE, Kohler M, et al. Cardiovascular event rates in the MOSAIC trial: 2-year follow-up data. Thorax 2014; 69: 950.

116. McDaid C, Duree KH, Griffin SC, et al. A systematic review of continuous positive airway pressure for obstructive sleep apnoea-hypopnoea syndrome. Sleep Med Rev 2009; 13: 427–436.

117. Gotsopoulos H, Kelly JJ, Cistulli PA. Oral appliance therapy reduces blood pressure in obstructive sleep apnea: a randomized, controlled trial. Sleep 2004; 27: 934–941.

118. Itzhaki S, Dorchin H, Clark G, et al. The effects of 1-year treatment with a herbst mandibular advancement splint on obstructive sleep apnea, oxidative stress, and endothelial function. Chest 2007; 131: 740–749.

119. Trzepizur W, Gagnadoux F, Abraham P, et al. Microvascular endothelial function in obstructive sleep apnea: Impact of continuous positive airway pressure and mandibular advancement. Sleep Med 2009; 10: 746–752.

120. Lam B, Sam K, Mok WY, et al. Randomised study of three non-surgical treatments in mild to moderate obstructive sleep apnoea. Thorax 2007; 62: 354–359.

121. Veasey SC. Will we ever have an effective pharmacotherapy for obstructive sleep apnoea? Sleep 2005; 28: 18–19.

122. Hedner J, Grote L, Zou D. Pharmacological treatment of sleep apnea: current situation and future strategies. Sleep Med Rev 2008; 12: 33–47.

123. Smith I, Lasserson TJ, Wright J. Drug therapy for obstructive sleep apnoea in adults. Cochrane Database Syst Rev 2006; CD003002.

124. Kiely JL, Nolan P, McNicholas WT. Intranasal corticosteroid therapy for obstructive sleep apnoea in patients with co-existing rhinitis. Thorax 2004; 59: 50–55.

125. Hedner J, Kraiczi H, Peker Y, et al. Reduction of sleep-disordered breathing after physostigmine. Am J Respir Crit Care Med 2003; 168: 1246–1251.

126. Carley DW, Olopade C, Ruigt GS, et al. Efficacy of mirtazapine in obstructive sleep apnea syndrome. Sleep 2007; 30: 35–41.

127. Marshall NS, Yee BJ, Desai AV, et al. Two randomized placebo-controlled trials to evaluate the efficacy and tolerability of mirtazapine for the treatment of obstructive sleep apnea. Sleep 2008; 31: 824–831.

128. Kraiczi H, Hedner J, Dahlof P, et al. Effect of serotonin uptake inhibition on breathing during sleep and daytime symptoms in obstructive sleep apnea. Sleep 1999; 22: 61–67.

129. Brownell LG, West P, Sweatman P, et al. Protriptyline in obstructive sleep apnea: a double-blind trial. N Engl J Med 1982; 307: 1037–1042.

130. Smith PL, Haponik EF, Allen RP, et al. The effects of protriptyline in sleep-disordered breathing. Am Rev Respir Dis 1983; 127: 8–13.

131. Whyte KF, Gould GA, Airlie MA, *et al.* Role of protriptyline and acetazolamide in the sleep apnea/hypopnea syndrome. *Sleep* 1988; 11: 463–472.

132. Horner RL. Impact of brainstem sleep mechanisms on pharyngeal motor control. *Respir Physiol* 2000; 119: 113–121.

133. Grace KP, Hughes SW, Horner RL. Identification of a pharmacological target for genioglossus reactivation throughout sleep. *Sleep* 2014; 37: 41–50.

134. Wirth KJ, Steinmeyer K, Ruetten H. Sensitization of upper airway mechanoreceptors as a new pharmacologic principle to treat obstructive sleep apnea: investigations with AVE0118 in anesthetized pigs. *Sleep* 2013; 36: 699–708.

135. Wang D, Eckert DJ, Grunstein RR. Drug effects on ventilatory control and upper airway physiology related to sleep apnea. *Respir Physiol Neurobiol* 2013; 188: 257–266.

136. Eckert DJ, White DP, Jordan AS, *et al.* Defining phenotypic causes of obstructive sleep apnea. Identification of novel therapeutic targets. *Am J Respir Crit Care Med* 2013; 188: 996–1004.

137. Santamaria J, Iranzo A, Ma Montserrat J, *et al.* Persistent sleepiness in CPAP treated obstructive sleep apnea patients: evaluation and treatment. *Sleep Med Rev* 2007; 11: 195–207.

138. Mendelson M, Tamisier R, Laplaud D, *et al.* Low physical activity is a determinant for elevated blood pressure in high cardiovascular risk obstructive sleep apnea. *Respir Care* 2014; 59: 1218–1227.

139. Joyeux-Faure M, Tamisier R, Baguet JP, *et al.* Response to statin therapy in obstructive sleep apnea syndrome: a multicenter randomized controlled trial. *Mediators Inflamm* 2014; 2014: 423120.

140. Yee BJ, Phillips CL, Banerjee D, *et al.* The effect of sibutramine-assisted weight loss in men with obstructive sleep apnoea. *Int J Obes (Lond)* 2007; 31: 161–168.

141. Ferland A, Poirier P, Series F. Sibutramine *versus* continuous positive airway pressure in obese obstructive sleep apnoea patients. *Eur Respir J* 2009; 34: 694–701.

142. Phillips CL, Yee BJ, Trenell MI, *et al.* Changes in regional adiposity and cardio-metabolic function following a weight loss program with sibutramine in obese men with obstructive sleep apnea. *J Clin Sleep Med* 2009; 5: 416–421.

143. Torp-Pedersen C, Caterson I, Coutinho W, *et al.* Cardiovascular responses to weight management and sibutramine in high-risk subjects: an analysis from the SCOUT trial. *Eur Heart J* 2007; 28: 2915–2923.

144. European Medicines Agency. Sibutramine. www.ema.europa.eu/ema/index.jsp?curl=pages/medicines/human/referrals/Sibutramine/human_referral_000219.jsp&mid=WC0b01ac05805c516f

145. Cartwright RD. Effect of sleep position on sleep apnea severity. *Sleep* 1984; 7: 110–114.

146. Oksenberg A, Silverberg DS. The effect of body posture on sleep-related breathing disorders: facts and therapeutic implications. *Sleep Med Rev* 1998; 2: 139–162.

147. Oksenberg A, Silverberg DS, Arons E, *et al.* Positional *vs* nonpositional obstructive sleep apnea patients: anthropomorphic, nocturnal polysomnographic, and multiple sleep latency test data. *Chest* 1997; 112: 629–639.

148. Mador MJ, Kufel TJ, Magalang UJ, *et al.* Prevalence of positional sleep apnea in patients undergoing polysomnography. *Chest* 2005; 128: 2130–2137.

149. Cartwright RD, Lloyd S, Lilie J, *et al.* Sleep position training as treatment for sleep apnea syndrome: a preliminary study. *Sleep* 1985; 8: 87–94.

150. Cartwright R, Ristanovic R, Diaz F, *et al.* A comparative study of treatments for positional sleep apnea. *Sleep* 1991; 14: 546–552.

151. Jokic R, Klimaszewski A, Crossley M, *et al.* Positional treatment vs continuous positive airway pressure in patients with positional obstructive sleep apnea syndrome. *Chest* 1999; 115: 771–781.

152. Oksenberg A, Silverberg D, Offenbach D, *et al.* Positional therapy for obstructive sleep apnea patients: a 6-month follow-up study. *Laryngoscope* 2006; 116: 1995–2000.

153. Morgenthaler TI, Kapen S, Lee-Chiong T, *et al.* Practice parameters for the medical therapy of obstructive sleep apnea. *Sleep* 2006; 29: 1031–1035.

154. Veasey SC, Guilleminault C, Strohl KP, *et al.* Medical therapy for obstructive sleep apnea: a review by the Medical Therapy for Obstructive Sleep Apnea Task Force of the Standards of Practice Committee of the American Academy of Sleep Medicine. *Sleep* 2006; 29: 1036–1044.

155. Lim J, Lasserson TJ, Fleetham J, *et al.* Oral appliances for obstructive sleep apnoea. *Cochrane Database Syst Rev* 2006; CD004435.

156. Petit FX, Pepin JL, Bettega G, *et al.* Mandibular advancement devices: rate of contraindications in 100 consecutive obstructive sleep apnea patients. *Am J Respir Crit Care Med* 2002; 166: 274–278.

157. Fritsch KM, Iseli A, Russi EW, *et al.* Side effects of mandibular advancement devices for sleep apnea treatment. *Am J Respir Crit Care Med* 2001; 164: 813–818.

158. Rose EC, Staats R, Virchow C Jr, *et al.* Occlusal and skeletal effects of an oral appliance in the treatment of obstructive sleep apnea. *Chest* 2002; 122: 871–877.

159. de Almeida FR, Lowe AA, Tsuiki S, *et al.* Long-term compliance and side effects of oral appliances used for the treatment of snoring and obstructive sleep apnea syndrome. *J Clin Sleep Med* 2005; 1: 143–152.

160. Gindre L, Gagnadoux F, Meslier N, *et al.* Mandibular advancement for obstructive sleep apnea: dose effect on apnea, long-term use and tolerance. *Respiration* 2008; 76: 386–392.

161. Jenkinson C, Davies RJ, Mullins R, *et al.* Comparison of therapeutic and subtherapeutic nasal continuous positive airway pressure for obstructive sleep apnoea: a randomised prospective parallel trial. *Lancet* 1999; 353: 2100–2105.

162. Phillips B. Your tax dollars at work! or the APPLES trial bears fruit. *J Clin Sleep Med* 2008; 4: 419–420.

163. Marin JM, Carrizo SJ, Vicente E, *et al.* Long-term cardiovascular outcomes in men with obstructive sleep apnoea-hypopnoea with or without treatment with continuous positive airway pressure: an observational study. *Lancet* 2005; 365: 1046–1053.

164. Pepperell JC, Ramdassingh-Dow S, Crosthwaite N, *et al.* Ambulatory blood pressure after therapeutic and subtherapeutic nasal continuous positive airway pressure for obstructive sleep apnoea: a randomised parallel trial. *Lancet* 2002; 359: 204–210.

Disclosures: None declared.

Other titles in the series

ORDER INFORMATION

Monographs are individually priced.
Visit the European Respiratory Society bookshop
www.ersbookshop.com
For bulk purchases contact the Publications Office directly.
European Respiratory Society Publications Office,
442 Glossop Road, Sheffield, S10 2PX, UK.
Tel: 44 (0)114 267 2860; Fax: 44 (0)114 266 5064; E-mail: sales@ersj.org.uk